Sensory Cue Integration

COMPUTATIONAL NEUROSCIENCE

SERIES EDITORS
Michael Stryker
Terrence J. Sejnowski

*Biophysics of Computation*
Christof Koch

*23 Problems in Systems Neuroscience*
Edited by J. Leo van Hemmen and Terrence J. Sejnowski

*Sensory Cue Integration*
Edited by Julia Trommershäuser, Konrad P. Körding, and Michael S. Landy

# Sensory Cue Integration

*Edited by*

Julia Trommershäuser

Konrad P. Körding

Michael S. Landy

OXFORD
UNIVERSITY PRESS

OXFORD
UNIVERSITY PRESS

Oxford University Press, Inc., publishes works that further
Oxford University's objective of excellence
in research, scholarship, and education.

Oxford New York
Auckland Cape Town Dar es Salaam Hong Kong Karachi
Kuala Lumpur Madrid Melbourne Mexico City Nairobi
New Delhi Shanghai Taipei Toronto

With offices in
Argentina Austria Brazil Chile Czech Republic France Greece
Guatemala Hungary Italy Japan Poland Portugal Singapore
South Korea Switzerland Thailand Turkey Ukraine Vietnam



Published by Oxford University Press, Inc.
198 Madison Avenue, New York, New York 10016
www.oup.com



Library of Congress Cataloging-in-Publication Data
Sensory cue integration / edited by Julia Trommershäuser, Konrad Körding, and
Michael S. Landy.
p. cm. – (Computational neuroscience)
Includes bibliographical references and index.
ISBN 978-0-19-538724-7 (hardback : alk. paper)
1. Computational neuroscience. 2. Cognitive neuroscience. 3. Senses and sensation.
I. Trommershäuser, Julia. II. Körding, Konrad. III. Landy, Michael S.
QP357.5.S46 2011
612.8′2–dc22 2010049048

1 3 5 7 9 8 6 4 2

Printed in China
on acid-free paper

# PREFACE

Aristotle distinguished five senses—sight, hearing, touch, smell, and taste—that provide cues about the outside world to the nervous system. The modern perceptual literature has found a host of additional senses and has also found that many senses provide more than one cue. For example, if we want to estimate how heavy an object is, then vision will provide us both with size cues (larger objects tend to be heavier) as well as surface textural cues (objects with visible metal texture tend to be denser). Cues can be thought of as largely independent pieces of sensory information that are used by the nervous system.

In most situations we make use of a multitude of cues. Thus, one of the central objectives of the nervous system is the combination of all cues into useful estimates of the properties of the world, a notion often attributed to Helmholtz (1856/1962), but already present in the work of Alhazen (1021/1989) in the 11th century. Based on this information we can then successfully interact with the world. The study of cue combination asks under which circumstances and how cues are combined toward this purpose.

There are several reasons why the nervous system needs to combine cues (see Chapter 1). Cues tend to be noisy. For example, the auditory system cannot estimate the location of the source of a sound perfectly. Moreover, cues can be ambiguous. For example, vision alone cannot always discriminate metal from plastic that has been painted to look like metal. If we combine vision with touch, however, we can more readily distinguish between different materials. Cue combination allows the nervous system to reduce noise and ambiguity.

This book focuses on the emerging probabilistic way of thinking about cue combination in terms of uncertainty. These probabilistic approaches derive from the realization that all our sensors are noisy and, moreover, are often affected by ambiguity. For example, our mechanoreceptors are noisy and they cannot distinguish whether a perceived force is caused by the weight of an object or by the force we are producing ourselves. The probabilistic approaches elaborated in this book aim at formalizing the uncertainty of cues. They describe cue combination as the nervous system's attempt to minimize uncertainty in its estimates and to choose successful actions. Some computational approaches described in the chapters of this book are concerned with the application of such statistical ideas to real-world cue-combination problems. Others ask how uncertainty may be represented in the nervous system and used for cue combination. Notably, across behavioral, electrophysiological, and theoretical approaches, Bayesian statistics is emerging as a common language in which cue-combination problems can be expressed.

The broadening scope of probabilistic approaches to cue combination is highlighted in the breadth of topics covered in this book. The different chapters summarize and discuss computational approaches and behavioral evidence aimed at understanding the combination of visual, auditory, proprioceptive, and haptic cues. Some chapters address the combination of cues within a single modality, whereas others address the combination across modalities. Neural implementation, behavior, and theory are considered. The unifying aspect of this book is the focus on the uncertainty intrinsic to sensory cues and the underlying question of how the nervous system deals with this uncertainty.

Following David Marr's taxonomy of three different levels of modeling of the nervous system (Dayan & Abbott, 2001; Marr, 1982), we can divide models of the nervous system into those that describe the implementation of computation (level 3), the algorithm used (level 2), and the objective of computation (level 1). This book derives from considerations about the computational objective (level 1) of cue combination (primarily dealing with uncertainty). The first section of the book gives an overview of the fundamental concepts and mathematics. Chapters in the subsequent two sections are concerned with the specific algorithms used by the brain and how they are implemented.

This book is divided into three sections. The first section, "Theory and Fundamentals," introduces the mathematical ideas needed to formalize cues and uncertainty. The second section, "Behavioral Studies," asks how human subjects behave, comparing human behavior with the behavior of an optimal cue-integration scheme. The chapters in the final section, "Neural Implementation," ask how the nervous system is able to produce behavior that is impressively close to the predictions that arise from optimal algorithms.

This book is the result of a workshop that was held in the autumn of 2008 at the beautiful German castle Rauischholzhausen, and we gratefully acknowledge the support we received from the German Science Foundation (DFG) for organizing this workshop. Scientists from many parts of the cue-combination community participated. The discussions we had at that workshop highlighted that scientists who study a wide range of distinct cue-combination phenomena are converging onto a common set of open questions and are starting to use a common language to frame and analyze experimentally observable phenomena. During the workshop it became clear that this unified quantitative language for talking about cue combination enables researchers from a broad spectrum of backgrounds and research areas to communicate effectively about their research progress and current theoretical issues. While earlier research had already started to move in that direction (Knill & Richards, 1996), recent research has broadened the scope of phenomena that can now be described in a coherent and consistent framework.

## REFERENCES

Alhazen (1021/1989). *The optics of Ibn al-Haytham. Volume I. Translation* (Translated by A. I. Sabra), London: Warburg Institute, University of London.

Dayan, P., & Abbott, L. F. (2001). *Theoretical neuroscience: Computational, mathematical modeling of neural systems.* Cambridge, MA: MIT Press.

Helmholtz, H. L. F. (1856/1962). *Treatise on physiological optics.* Translated from the third German edition by J. P. C. Southall. New York: Dover.

Knill, D., & Richards, W. (1996). *Perception as Bayesian inference.* New York: Cambridge University Press.

Marr, D. (1982). *Vision.* San Francisco, CA: W. H. Freeman.

# CONTENTS

# CONTRIBUTORS

**Dora E. Angelaki**
Washington University School of Medicine
Anatomy and Neurobiology
St. Louis, MO

**Gregory Apker**
School of Biological and Health Systems Engineering
Arizona State University
Tempe, AZ

**Benjamin T. Backus**
Graduate Program in Vision Science
SUNY College of Optometry
New York, NY

**Martin S. Banks**
School of Optometry
University of California, Berkeley
Berkeley, CA

**Peter W. Battaglia**
Brain & Cognitive Sciences
Computer Science & Artificial Intelligence Laboratory
Massachusetts Institute of Technology
Cambridge, MA

**Jeff Beck**
Gatsby Computational Neuroscience Unit
University College London
London, England

**Ulrik Beierholm**
Gatsby Computational Neuroscience Unit
University College London
London, England

**Paola Binda**
Institute of Neuroscience
CNR
Pisa, Italy

**Anne-Marie Brouwer**
TNO Human Factors
Soesterberg, The Netherlands

**Christopher A. Buneo**
School of Biological and Health Systems Engineering
Arizona State University
Tempe, AZ

**Johannes Burge**
Center for Perceptual Systems
Department of Psychology
The University of Texas
Austin, TX

**David Burr**
Department of Psychology
Università degli Studi di Firenze
Florence, Italy

**Corrado Caudek**
Department of Psychology
Università degli Studi di Firenze
Florence, Italy

**Gregory C. DeAngelis**
Department of Brain & Cognitive Sciences
University of Rochester
Rochester, NY

**Sophie Denève**
Group for Neural Theory, DEC
Ecole Normale Supérieure
Paris, France

**Massimiliano Di Luca**
MPI for Biological Cybernetics
Tübingen, Germany

**Fulvio Domini**
Cognitive and Linguistic Sciences
Brown University
Providence, RI

**Marc O. Ernst**
MPI for Biological Cybernetics
Tübingen, Germany

**Christopher R. Fetsch**
Washington University School of Medicine
Anatomy and Neurobiology
St. Louis, MO

**Monica Gori**
Robotics, Brain and Technical Science Department
Italian Institute of Technology
University of Genoa
Genoa, Italy

**Yong Gu**
Washington University School of Medicine
Anatomy and Neurobiology
St. Louis, MO

**Adrian Haith**
Department of Biomedical Engineering
Johns Hopkins University
Baltimore, MD

**Robert T. Held**
Joint Graduate Group in Bioengineering
University of California, San Francisco and
University of California, Berkeley
Berkeley, CA

**Yun-Xian Ho**
Department of Biomedical Informatics
Vanderbilt University Medical Center
Nashville, TN

**Timothy Hospedales**
Department of Computer Science
Queen Mary University of London
London, England

**Robert A. Jacobs**
Center for Visual Science
Department of Brain & Cognitive Sciences
University of Rochester
Rochester, NY

**Daniel Kersten**
Department of Psychology
University of Minnesota
Minneapolis, MN

**David C. Knill**
Center for Visual Science
University of Rochester
Rochester, NY

**Konrad P. Körding**
Department of Physiology, Physical Medicine and Rehabilitation
Rehabilitation Institute of Chicago
Northwestern University
Chicago, IL

**Michael S. Landy**
Department of Psychology and Center for Neural Science
New York University
New York, NY

**Timm Lochmann**
Group for Neural Theory, DEC
Ecole Normale Supérieure
Paris, France

**Wei Ji Ma**
Department of Neuroscience
Baylor College of Medicine
Houston, TX

**Laurence T. Maloney**
Department of Psychology and Center for Neural Science
New York University
New York, NY

**Melchi M. Michel**
Center for Perceptual Systems
Department of Psychology
The University of Texas
Austin, TX

**Rama Natarajan**
Center for Neural Science
New York University
New York, NY

**Alexandre Pouget**
Center for Visual Sciences
Brain and Cognitive Science Department
University of Rochester
Rochester, NY

**Pedro Rosas**
Institute of Biomedical Sciences
Faculty of Medicine
Universidad de Chile
Santiago, Chile

**Benjamin A. Rowland**
Department of Neurobiology & Anatomy
Wake Forest University School of Medicine
Winston-Salem, NC

**Maneesh Sahani**
Gatsby Computational Neuroscience Unit
University College London
London, England

**Paul Schrater**
Department of Psychology & Computer Science
University of Minnesota
Minneapolis, MN

**Sascha Serwe**
FernUniversität in Hagen
Institute for Psychology
Hagen, Germany

**Anna Seydell**
Laboratory of Integrative Neuroscience and Cognition
Department of Physiology & Biophysics
Georgetown University Medical Center
Washington, D.C.

**Ladan Shams**
Department of Psychology
University of California, Los Angeles
Los Angeles, CA

**Ying Shi**
School of Biological and Health Systems Engineering
Arizona State University
Tempe, AZ

**Terrence R. Stanford**
Department of Neurobiology & Anatomy
Wake Forest University School of Medicine
Winston-Salem, NC

**Barry E. Stein**
Department of Neurobiology & Anatomy
Wake Forest University School of Medicine
Winston-Salem, NC

**Julia Trommershäuser**
Center for Neural Science
New York University
New York, NY

**Sethu Vijayakumar**
1.28 Informatics Forum
School of Informatics
University of Edinburgh
Edinburgh, Scotland

**Kunlin Wei**
Department of Physiology, Physical Medicine and Rehabilitation
Rehabilitation Institute of Chicago
Northwestern University
Chicago, IL

**Andrew E. Welchman**
School of Psychology
University of Birmingham
Birmingham, England

**Louise Whiteley**
National Core for Neuroethics
University of British Columbia
Vancouver, Canada

**Felix A. Wichmann**
Cognitive Process Modeling
Technical University of Berlin and
Bernstein Center for Computational Neuroscience
Berlin, Germany

**Richard S. Zemel**
Department of Computer Science
University of Toronto
Toronto, Canada

# WORKSHOP ATTENDEES

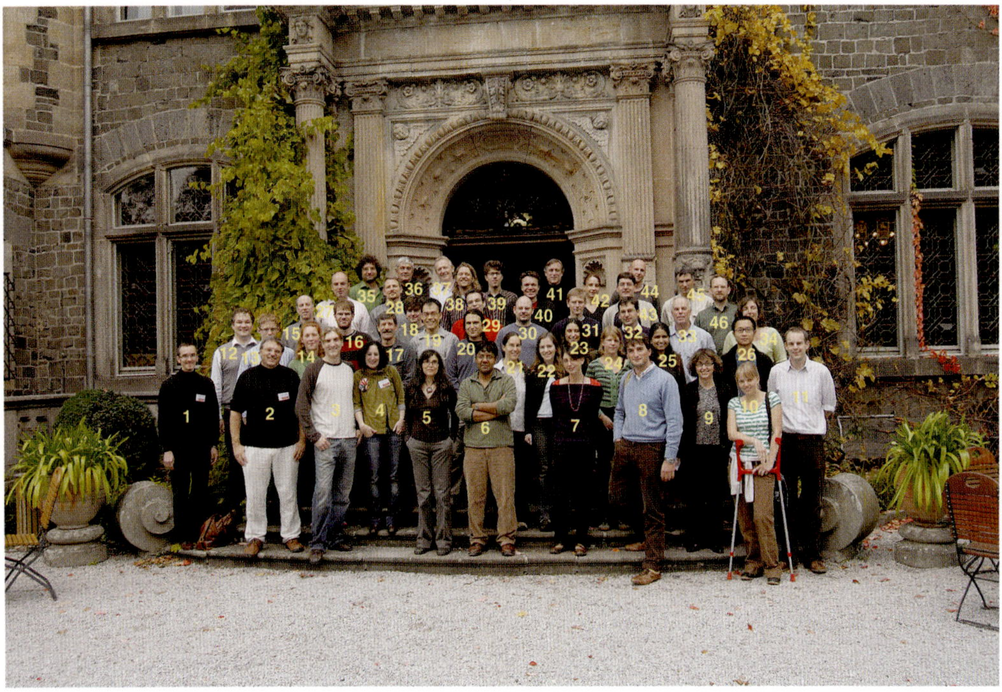

1) Alexander Schütz, 2) Laurence Harris, 3) David Wozny, 4) Jess Hartcher, 5) Ladan Shams, 6) Sethu Vijayakumar, 7) Monica Gori, 8) Claudio Simoncini, 9) Dora E. Angelaki, 10) Stephanie Westendorff, 11) Andrew E. Welchman, 12) Jan Drewes, 13) Stephen M. Fleming, 14) Christa M. van Mierlo, 15) Robert A. Jacobs, 16) Jonas Knöll, 17) Michael S. Landy, 18) Scott Love, 19) Wei Ji Ma, 20) Massimiliano Di Luca, 21) Anna Seydell, 22) Carmel Levitan, 23) Paola Binda, 24) Katinka van der Kooij, 25) Rama Natarajan, 26) Luo Jie, 27) Charles Spence, 28) Paul Schrater, 29) Wolfgang Einhäuser, 30) Sascha Serwe, 31) Mathias Reiser, 32) Pascal Mamassian, 33) Martin S. Banks, 34) Sophie Denève, 35) Marc O. Ernst, 36) David Burr, 37) Karl Gegenfurtner, 38) Ulrik Beierholm, 39) Konrad P. Körding, 40) Fulvio Domini, 41) Stuart Fuller, 42) Julia Trommershäuser, 43) Daniel Berger, 44) Heiko Maurer, 45) Hermann Müller, 46) Benjamin T. Backus

# Sensory Cue Integration

# SECTION I

# Introduction to Section I: Theory and Fundamentals

The chapters in Section I formalize the computational problems that need to be solved for successful cue combination. They focus on the issue of uncertainty and the Bayesian ways of solving such problems. Through the sequence of chapters in Section I, the reader will get a thorough overview and introduction into the current Bayesian formalization of sensory cue combination.

This section highlights the fundamental similarity between seemingly distinct problems of cue combination. The computational objectives and the algorithms that can be used to find the optimal solution do not depend on the modality or kind of cue that is considered. The solutions to progressively more complicated problems are largely derived using essentially the same statistical techniques.

The first five chapters of Section I are concerned with Bayesian theories of optimal cue combination. The book starts with an introductory chapter by Landy, Banks, and Knill that gives an overview of the basic philosophy and the mathematics that is used to calculate how an ideal observer would combine cues. These models form the backbone of much of the cue-combination research presented in this book. The following computational chapters provide more detailed insights into the basic techniques, computational tools, and behavioral evidence necessary to test the predictions arising from these models. Wei and Körding focus on ideal-observer models for cases where it is not a priori certain that the cues belong together. In this particular case, the nervous system needs to determine whether the cues belong together or, in other words, to determine their causal relationship. Battaglia, Kersten, and Schrater focus on object perception. They ask how the kinds of causal knowledge we have about the way objects are made can be used to constrain estimates of attributes such as shape and size. Vijayakumar, Hospedales, and Haith extend these ideas to model cue combination for sensorimotor integration. This is complicated because sensorimotor tasks depend on a set of variables that must be estimated simultaneously. Lastly, Sahani and Whiteley extend these concepts to cue integration in cluttered environments. They point out that complicated visual scenes are a special case of situations in which we are uncertain about the causal relationship between cues. These chapters use a coherent probabilistic language to develop methods appropriate for a wide range of problems.

The last three chapters of Section I highlight limitations of the standard ideas of probabilistic cue combination. They point out interesting ways in which human observers fall short of optimal predictions. Backus explains how novel cues can be recruited for perception. In the next chapter of the section, Domini and Caudek propose an alternative to the Bayesian ideal observer for combining cues to depth. The simple algorithm they present results in an affine estimate of depth (i.e., depth up to an unknown scale factor) and yet, perhaps surprisingly, is closely related to the Bayesian weighted-linear model discussed in Chapter 1. Finally, Rosas and Wichmann discuss limits of sensory cue integration, suggesting that simple ideas of optimality may be inappropriate in a complex world.

# CHAPTER 1

## Ideal-Observer Models of Cue Integration

*Michael S. Landy, Martin S. Banks, and David C. Knill*

When an organism estimates a property of the environment so as to make a decision ("Do I flee or do I fight?") or plan an action ("How do I grab that salt shaker without tipping my wine glass along the way?"), there are typically multiple sources of information (signals or "cues") that are useful. These may include different features of the input from one sense, such as vision, where a variety of cues—texture, motion, binocular disparity, and so forth—aid the estimation of the three-dimensional (3D) layout of the environment and shapes of objects within it. Information may also derive from multiple senses such as visual and haptic information about object size, or visual and auditory cues about the location of a sound. In most cases, the organism can make more accurate estimates of environmental properties or more beneficial decisions by integrating these multiple sources of information. In this chapter, we review models of cue integration and discuss benefits and possible pitfalls in applying these ideas to models of behavior.

Consider the problem of estimating the 3D orientation (i.e., slant and tilt) of a smooth surface (Hillis, Ernst, Banks, & Landy, 2002; Hillis, Watt, Landy, & Banks, 2004; Knill & Saunders, 2003; Rosas, Wagemans, Ernst, & Wichmann, 2005). An estimate of surface orientation is useful for guiding a variety of actions, ranging from reaching for and grasping an object (Knill, 2005) to judging whether one can safely walk or crawl down an incline (Adolph, 1997). Errors in the estimate may lead to failures of execution of the motor plan (and a fumbled grasp) or incorrect motor decisions (and a risky descent possibly leading to a fall). Thus, estimation accuracy can be very important, so the observer should use all sources of information effectively.

The sensory information available to an observer may come in the form of multiple visual cues (the pattern of binocular disparity, linear perspective and foreshortening, shading, etc.) as well as haptic cues (feeling the surface with the hand, testing the slope with a foot). If one of the cues always provided the observer with a perfect estimate, there would be no need to incorporate information from other cues. But cues are often imperfectly related to environmental properties because of variability in the mapping between the cue value and a given property and because of errors in the nervous system's measurement of the cue value. Thus, measured cue values will vary somewhat unpredictably across viewing conditions and scenes. For example, stereopsis provides more accurate estimates of surface orientation for near than for far surfaces. This is due to the geometry underlying binocular disparity: A small amount of measurement error translates into a larger depth error at long distances than at short ones. In addition, estimates may be based on assumptions about the scene and will be flawed if those assumptions are invalid. For example, the use of texture perspective cues is generally based on the assumption that texture is homogeneously distributed across the surface, so estimates based on this assumption will be incorrect if the texture itself varies across the surface. For example, viewing a frontoparallel photograph of a slanted, textured surface could yield the erroneous estimate that the photograph is slanted. Unlike stereopsis, the reliability of texture perspective as a cue to surface orientation does not diminish with viewing distance.

Because of this uncertain relationship between a cue measurement and the environmental property to be estimated, the observer can generally improve the reliability of an estimate of an environmental property by combining multiple cues in a rational fashion. The combination rule needs to take into account the uncertainties associated with the individual cues, and those depend on many factors.

Along with the benefit of improving the reliability of perceptual estimates, there is also a clear benefit of knowing how uncertain the final estimate is and how to make decisions given that uncertainty. Consider, for example, estimating the distance to a precipitous drop-off (Maloney, 2002). An observer can estimate that distance most reliably by using all available cues, but knowing the uncertainty of that estimate can be crucial for guiding future behavior. If the future task is to toss a ball as close as possible to the drop-off, one would use the most likely distance estimate to plan the toss; the plan would be unaffected by the uncertainty of the distance estimate. If, however, the future task is to walk blindfolded toward the drop-off, the decision of how far to meander toward the drop would most certainly be influenced by the uncertainty of the distance estimate.

Much of the research in this area has focused on the question of whether cue integration is optimal. This focus has been fruitful for a variety of reasons. First, to determine whether the nervous system is performing optimally requires a clear, quantitative specification of the task, the stimulus, and the relationship between the stimulus and the specified environmental property. As Gibson (1966) argued, it forces the researcher to investigate and define the information available for the task. As Marr (1982) put it, it forces one to construct a quantitative, predictive account of perceptual performance. Second, for tasks that have been important for survival, it seems quite plausible that the organism has evolved mechanisms that utilize the available information optimally. Therefore, the hypothesis that sensory information is used optimally in tasks that are important to the organism is a reasonable starting point. Indeed, given the efficacy of natural selection and developmental learning mechanisms, it seems unlikely to us that the nervous system would perform suboptimally in an important task with stimuli that are good exemplars of the natural environment (as opposed to impoverished or unusual stimuli that are only encountered in the laboratory). Third, using optimality as a starting point, the observation of suboptimal behavior can be particularly informative. It can indicate flaws in our characterization of the perceptual problem posed to or solved by the observer; for example, it could indicate that the perceptual system is optimized for tasks other than one we have studied or that the assumptions made in our formulation of an ideal-observer model fail to capture the problem posed to observers in naturalistic situations. Of course, there remains the possibility that we have characterized the sensory information and the task correctly, but the nervous system simply has not developed the mechanisms for performing optimally (e.g., Domini & Braunstein, 1998; Todd, 2004). We expect that such occurrences are rare, but emerging scientific investigations will ultimately determine this.

In this way, "ideal-observer" analysis is a critical step in the iterative scientific process of studying perceptual computations. At perhaps a deeper level, ideal-observer models help us to understand the computational structure of what are generally complex problems posed to observers. This can in turn lead to understanding complex behavior patterns by relating them to the features of the problems from which they arise (e.g., statistics of natural environments or noise characteristics of sensory systems). Ideal-observer models provide a framework for constructing quantitative, predictive accounts of perceptual performance at Marr's computational level for describing the brain (Marr, 1982).

Several studies have found that humans combine sensory signals in an optimal fashion, taking into account the variation of cue reliability with viewing conditions, and resulting in estimates with maximum reliability (e.g., Alais & Burr, 2004; Ernst & Banks, 2002; Hillis et al., 2004; Knill & Saunders, 2003; Landy & Kojima, 2001; Tassinari, Hudson, & Landy, 2006). These results suggest that human observers are optimal for a wide variety of perceptual and sensorimotor tasks.

This chapter is intended to provide a general introduction to the field of cue combination from the perspective of optimal cue integration. We work through a number of qualitatively different problems, and we hope thereby to illustrate how building ideal observers helps formulate the scientific questions that need to be answered before we can understand how the brain solves these problems. We begin with a simple example of integration leading to a linear model of cue integration. This is followed by a summary of a general approach to optimality: Bayesian estimation and decision theory. We then review situations in which realistic generative models of sensory data lead to nonlinear ideal-observer models. Subsequent sections review empirical studies of cue combination and issues they raise, as well as open questions in the field.

## LINEAR MODELS FOR MAXIMUM RELIABILITY

There is a wide variety of approaches to cue integration. The specific approach depends on the assumptions the modeler makes about the sources of uncertainty in sensory signals as well as what the observer is trying to optimize. Quantitative empirical evidence can then determine whether those assumptions are valid.

The simplest such models result in linear cue integration. For the case of Gaussian noise, linear cue integration is optimal for an observer who tries to maximize the precision (i.e., minimize the variance) of the estimate made based on the cues. Suppose you have samples $x_i$, $i = 1, \cdots, n$, of $n$ independent, Gaussian random variables $X_i$ that share a common mean $\mu$ and have variances $\sigma_i^2$. The minimum-variance unbiased estimator of $\mu$ is a weighted average

$$\hat{x} = \sum_{i=1}^{n} w_i x_i, \tag{1.1}$$

where the weight $w_i$ of cue $i$ is proportional to that cue's *reliability* $r_i$ (defined as its inverse variance, $r_i = 1/\sigma_i^2$):

$$w_i = \frac{r_i}{\sum_{j=1}^{n} r_j} \tag{1.2}$$

(Cochran, 1937). The reliability $r$ of this integrated estimate is

$$r = \sum_{i=1}^{n} r_i. \tag{1.3}$$

As a result, the variance of the integrated estimate is generally lower than the variance of the individual estimates and never worse than the least variable of them. Thus, if an observer has access to unbiased estimates of a particular world property from each cue, and the cues are Gaussian distributed and conditionally independent (meaning that for a given value of the world property being estimated, errors in the estimates derived from each cue are independent), the minimum-variance estimate is a weighted average of the individual estimates from each cue (Landy, Maloney, Johnston, & Young, 1995; Maloney & Landy, 1989).

To form this estimate, an observer needs to represent and compute with estimates of cue uncertainty. The estimates could be implicit in the neural population code derived from the sensory features associated with a cue or might be explicitly computed, for example, by measuring the stability of each cue's estimates over repeated views of the scene. They could also be assessed online by using ancillary information (viewing distance, amount of self-motion, etc.) that impacts cue reliability (Landy et al., 1995). Estimates of reliability need not be explicitly represented by the nervous system, but they might be implicit in the form of the neural population code (Ma, Beck, Latham, & Pouget, 2006).

If the variability in different cue estimates is correlated, the minimum-variance unbiased estimator will not necessarily be a weighted average. For some distributions, it is a nonlinear function of the individual estimates; for others, including the Gaussian, it is still a weighted average, but the weights take into account the covariance of the cues (Oruç, Maloney, & Landy, 2003).

## BAYESIAN ESTIMATION AND DECISION MAKING

The linear model has dominated cue-integration research and has provided important insights into human perceptual and sensorimotor processing. However, most perceptual and sensorimotor problems encountered by an observer in the natural world cannot be accurately characterized by the linear model. In many cases, the linear model provides a reasonable "local" approximation to the ideal observer. In those cases, the complexity of the problem is reduced in the laboratory setting and this reduction is assumed to be known by the observer. To characterize the complex problems presented to observers in the real world, a more general computational framework is needed. Bayesian decision theory provides such a framework.

### Priors, Likelihoods, and Posteriors

In the Bayesian framework, the information provided by sensory information to estimate a scene property or make a decision related to that property is represented by a "posterior" probability distribution

$$P(s|d) = \frac{P(d|s)P(s)}{P(d)}, \tag{1.4}$$

where $s$ represents the scene property or properties of interest (possibly multidimensional) and $d$ is a vector of sensory data. In this formulation, it is important to delineate what is known by the observer from what is unknown. The data, $d$, are given to and therefore known by the observer. The scene properties, $s$, are unknown. The probability distribution, $P(s|d)$, represents the probabilities of different values of $s$ being "true," given the observed data. If the distribution is narrowly concentrated around one value of $s$, it represents reliable data; if broad, it represents unreliable data. If it is narrow in one dimension and broad in others, it reflects a situation in which the information provided by $d$ reliably determines $s$ along the narrow dimension but does not along the other dimensions.

Bayes' rule (Eq. 1.4) shows how to compute the posterior distribution from prior knowledge about the statistics of $s$—represented by the prior distribution $P(s)$ (that is, which values of $s$ are more likely in the environment than others)—and knowledge about how likely scenes with different values of $s$ are to give rise to the observed data $d$, which is represented by the likelihood function $P(d|s)$. Because $d$ is given, the likelihood is a function of the conditioning variable and does not behave like a probability distribution (i.e., it need not integrate to one), and hence it is often notated as $L(s|d)$. The third term in the denominator, $P(d)$, is a constant, normalizing term (so that the full expression integrates to one), and it can generally be ignored in formulating an estimation procedure. From a computational point of view, if one has a good "generative" model for how the data are generated by different scenes (e.g., the geometry of disparity and the noise associated with measuring disparity) and a good model of the statistics of scenes, one can use Bayes' rule to compute the posterior distribution, $P(s|d)$, and hence derive a full representation of the information provided by some observed sensory data about scene properties of interest.

### Gain/Loss Functions, Estimation, and Decision Making

Having computed the posterior distribution, the Bayesian decision maker next chooses a course of action. For that action to be optimal, one must have a definition of optimality. That is, one must have a loss function that defines the consequences of the decision maker's action. Optimality is defined as making decisions that minimize expected loss. For Bayesian estimation, the observer's task is to choose an estimate, and often the loss is defined as a function of estimation error (the difference between the chosen estimate and the true value of the parameter in the world). In other situations, the observer makes a discrete decision (e.g., categorizing the stimulus as signal or noise) or forms a motor plan (e.g., a planned trajectory to grasp an observed object).

Bayesian decision theory prescribes the optimal choice of action based on several ingredients. First, one needs a model of the environment: that is, a set of possible states of the world or *scenes* and a prior distribution across them (random variable $S$ with prior distribution $P(s)$). This world leads to noisy sensory data $d$ conditioned on a particular state of the world (with distribution $P(d|s)$). The task of the observer is to choose an optimal action $a(d)$, which might be an estimate of a scene parameter, a button press in an experiment, or a plan for movement in a visuomotor task. For experimental tasks or estimation, the action is the final output of the decision-making task upon which gain or loss is based. In other situations, like visuomotor control, the outcome itself—the executed movement—may be stochastic. So we distinguish the outcome of the plan (e.g., the movement trajectory) $t$ as distinct from the selected action $a(d)$ (with distribution $P(t|a(d))$). The final ingredient is typically called the loss function, although we also use the negative of loss, or gain $g(t, s)$. Note that $g$ is a function only of the actual scene $s$ and actual outcome of the decision $t$. An optimal choice of action is one that maximizes expected gain

$$a_{\text{opt}} = \arg\max_a EG(a), \text{ where}$$

$$EG(a) = \iiint g(t, s)P(t|a(d))P(d|s) P(s)dt\, dd\, ds. \quad (1.5)$$

It is worth reviewing some special cases of this general method. For estimation, the final output is the estimate itself ($t \equiv a(d)$). If the prior distribution is uniform over the domain of interest ($P(s) = c$, a constant) and the gain function only rewards perfectly correct estimates (a delta function centered on the correct value of the parameter), then Eq. 1.5 results in maximum-likelihood estimation: that is, choosing the mode of $P(d|s)$ over possible scenes $s$. If the prior distribution is not uniform, the optimal method is maximum a posteriori (MAP) estimation, that is, choosing the mode of the posterior $P(s|d)$. If the gain function is not a delta function, but treats estimation errors symmetrically (i.e., is a function of $|\hat{s} - s|$, where $\hat{s}$ is the estimate and $s$ is the true value in the scene), the optimal estimation procedure corresponds to first convolving the gain function with the posterior distribution, and then choosing the estimate corresponding to the peak of that function. For example, the oft-used squared-error loss function leads the optimal observer to use a minimum-variance criterion and hence the mean of the posterior as the estimate.

## Bayesian Decision Theory and Cue Integration

The most straightforward application of Bayesian decision theory to cue integration involves the case in which the sensory data associated with each cue are conditionally independent. In that case, we can write the likelihood function for all of the data as the product of likelihood functions for the data associated with each cue,

$$P(d_1, \cdots, d_n|s) = \prod_{i=1}^{n} P(d_i|s), \quad (1.6)$$

where $d_i$ is a data vector representing the sensory data associated with cue $i$ (e.g., disparity for the stereo cue) and $s$ is the scene variable being estimated. Combining Eqs. 1.4 and 1.6, we have

$$P(s|d_1, \cdots, d_n) \propto P(s)\prod_{i=1}^{n} P(d_i|s), \quad (1.7)$$

where we have dropped the constant denominator term for simplicity.

If the individual likelihood functions and the prior distribution are Gaussian, with variances $\sigma_i^2$ and $\sigma_{\text{prior}}^2$, then the posterior distribution will be Gaussian with mean and variance identical to the minimum-variance estimate; that is, for Gaussian distributions, the MAP estimate and the mean of the posterior both yield a linear estimation procedure identical to that of the minimum-variance unbiased estimator expressed in Eqs. 1.1–1.3. If the prior distribution is flat or significantly broader than the likelihood function, the posterior is simply the product of individual cue likelihoods and the mode and mean correspond to the maximum-likelihood estimate of *s*. If the Gaussian assumption holds, but the data associated with the different cues are not conditionally independent, the MAP estimate will remain linear, but the cue weights have to take into account the covariance structure of the data, resulting in the same weighted linear combination as the minimum-variance, unbiased estimate (Oruç et al., 2003).

While a linear system can characterize the optimal estimator when the estimates are Gaussian distributed and conditionally independent, the Bayesian formulation offers an equally simple, but much more general formulation. In essence, it replaces the averaging of estimates with the combining of information as represented by multiplying likelihood functions and priors. It also replaces the notion of perceptual estimates as point representations (single, specific values) with a notion of perceptual estimates as probability distributions. This allows one to separate information (as represented by the posterior distribution) from the task, as represented by a gain function.

Figure 1.1 illustrates Bayesian integration in two simple cases: estimation of a scalar variable (size) from a pair of cues (visual and haptic) with Gaussian likelihood functions, and estimation of a two-dimensional variable (slant and tilt) from a pair of cues, one of which is decidedly non-Gaussian (skew symmetry). While the latter may appear more complex than the former, the ideal observer operates similarly by multiplying likelihood functions and priors.

## NONLINEAR MODELS: GENERATIVE MODELS AND HIDDEN VARIABLES

We now turn to conditions under which optimal cue integration is not linear. We will describe three qualitatively different features of cue-integration problems that make the linear model inappropriate. One such situation is when the information provided by two cues interacts because each cue disambiguates scene or viewing variables that the other cue requires to determine a scene property. Another problem is that the information provided by many cues, particularly visual depth cues, depends on what prior assumptions about the world hold true and cues can interact by jointly determining the appropriate world model. A special case of this is a situation in which an observer has to decide whether different sensory cues should or should not be combined into one estimate at all.

### Cue Disambiguation

The raw sensory data from different cues are often incommensurate in the sense that they specify a scene property in different coordinate frames of reference. For example, auditory cues provide information about the location of a sound source in head-centered coordinates, whereas visual cues provide information in retinal coordinates. To apply a linear scheme for combining these sources of information, one would first need to use an estimate of gaze direction relative to the head to convert visual position estimates to head-centered coordinates or auditory position estimates to retinal coordinates, so that the two location estimates are in the same coordinates. Similarly, visual depth estimates based on relative motion should theoretically be scaled by an estimate of the viewing distance to provide an estimate of metric depth (i.e., an estimate in centimeters). On the other hand, depth derived from disparity needs to be scaled approximately by the square of the viewing distance to put it in the same units. Landy et al. (1995) called this preliminary conversion into common units *promotion*.

A normative Bayesian model finesses the problem in a very elegant way. Figure 1.2 illustrates the structure of the computations as applied to disparity and velocity cues to relative depth. The key observation is that the generative model for the sensory data associated with both the disparity and velocity cues depends not only on the scene property being estimated (relative depth) but also on the viewing distance to the fixated point. We will refer to viewing

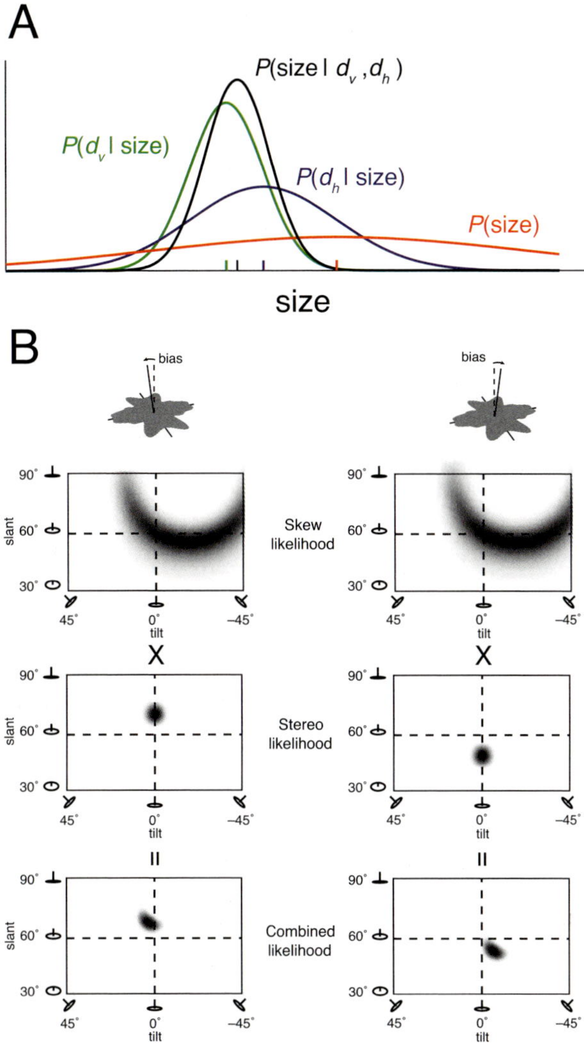


**Figure 1.1** Bayesian integration of sensory cues. (A) Two cues to object size, visual and haptic, each have Gaussian likelihoods (as in Ernst & Banks, 2002). The resulting joint likelihood is Gaussian with mean and variance as predicted by Eqs. 1.1–1.3. (B) Two visual cues to surface orientation are provided: skew symmetry (a figural cue) and stereo disparity (as in Saunders & Knill, 2001). Surface orientation is parameterized as slant and tilt angles. Skew-symmetric figures appear as figures slanted in depth because the brain assumes that the figures are projected from bilaterally symmetric figures in the world. The information provided by skew symmetry is given by the angle between the projected symmetry axes of a figure, shown here as solid lines superimposed on the figure. Assuming that visual measurements of the orientations of these angles in the image are corrupted by Gaussian noise, one can compute a likelihood function for three-dimensional (3D) surface orientation from skew. The result, as shown here, is highly non-Gaussian. The shape of the likelihood function is highly dependent on the spin of the figure around its 3D surface normal. Top row of graphs: skew likelihood for the figure shown at the top. Middle row: two stereo likelihoods centered on larger (left) and smaller (right) values of slant. Bottom row: When combined with stereoscopic information from binocular disparities, assuming the prior on surface orientation is flat. This leads to the prediction that perceptual biases will depend on the spin of the figure. It also leads to the somewhat counterintuitive prediction illustrated here that changing the slant suggested by stereo disparities should change the perceived tilt of symmetric figures. This is exactly the pattern of behavior shown by subjects.

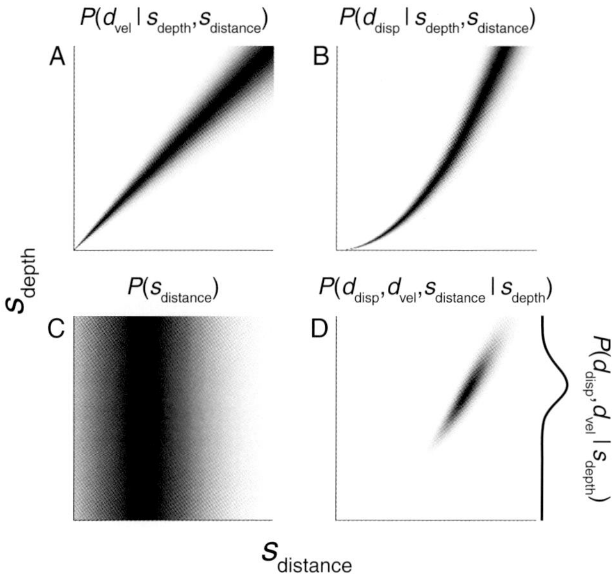


**Figure 1.2** Cue disambiguation. (A) Likelihood function for the motion cue as a function of depth and viewing distance $P(d_{\mathrm{vel}}|s_{\mathrm{depth}}, s_{\mathrm{distance}})$. The depth implied by a given retinal velocity is proportional to the viewing distance. (B) Likelihood function for the disparity cue $P(d_{\mathrm{disp}}|s_{\mathrm{depth}}, s_{\mathrm{distance}})$. The depth implied by a given retinal disparity is approximately proportional to the square of the viewing distance. (C) A Gaussian prior on viewing distance. (D) Combined likelihood function $P(d_{\mathrm{disp}}, d_{\mathrm{vel}}, s_{\mathrm{distance}}|s_{\mathrm{depth}})$. The right-hand side of the plot illustrates the likelihood for depth alone, $P(d_{\mathrm{disp}}, d_{\mathrm{vel}}|s_{\mathrm{depth}})$, integrating out the unknown distance.

distance as a hidden variable in the problem (statisticians refer to these kinds of variables as nuisance parameters; for more discussion of the role of hidden variables and marginalization in visual cue integration, see Knill, 2003). The generative model for both the relative-disparity and relative-velocity measurements requires that both relative depth and viewing distance be specified. This allows one to compute likelihood functions for both cues, $d_{\mathrm{vel}}$ and $d_{\mathrm{disp}}$, $P(d_{\mathrm{vel}}|s_{\mathrm{depth}}, s_{\mathrm{distance}})$ and $P(d_{\mathrm{disp}}|s_{\mathrm{depth}}, s_{\mathrm{distance}})$ (assuming one knows the noise characteristics of the disparity and motion sensors). Assuming that the noises in the two sensor systems are independent, we can write the likelihood function for the two cues as the product of the likelihood functions for the individual cues,

$$
\begin{aligned}
&P(d_{\mathrm{disp}} d_{\mathrm{vel}}|s_{\mathrm{depth}}, s_{\mathrm{distance}}) \\
&= P(d_{\mathrm{disp}}|s_{\mathrm{depth}}, s_{\mathrm{distance}}) \\
&\quad \times P(d_{\mathrm{vel}}|s_{\mathrm{depth}}, s_{\mathrm{distance}}). \qquad (1.8)
\end{aligned}
$$

This is not quite what we want, however. What we want is the likelihood function for depth alone, $P(d_{\mathrm{disp}}, d_{\mathrm{vel}}|s_{\mathrm{depth}})$. This is derived by integrating ("marginalizing") over the hidden variable, $s_{\mathrm{distance}}$:

$$
\begin{aligned}
&P(d_{\mathrm{disp}} d_{\mathrm{vel}}|s_{\mathrm{depth}}) \\
&= \int P(d_{\mathrm{disp}}, d_{\mathrm{vel}}, s_{\mathrm{distance}}|s_{\mathrm{depth}})\, ds_{\mathrm{distance}} \\
&= \int P(d_{\mathrm{disp}}, d_{\mathrm{vel}}|s_{\mathrm{distance}}, s_{\mathrm{depth}}) \\
&\quad \times P(s_{\mathrm{distance}})\, ds_{\mathrm{distance}} \\
&= \int P(d_{\mathrm{disp}}|s_{\mathrm{depth}}, s_{\mathrm{distance}}) \\
&\quad \times P(d_{\mathrm{vel}}|s_{\mathrm{depth}}, s_{\mathrm{distance}}) P(s_{\mathrm{distance}})\, ds_{\mathrm{distance}}. \qquad (1.9)
\end{aligned}
$$

(Note that the second step required that depth and distance be independent.) The important thing to note is that the joint likelihood for $s_{\mathrm{depth}}$ is not the product of the individual cue likelihoods, $P(d_{disp}|s_{depth})$ and $P(d_{vel}|s_{depth})$. Rather, we had to expand the representational space for the scene to include viewing distance, express both likelihood functions in that space, multiply the likelihoods in the expanded space and then integrate over the hidden variable to obtain a final likelihood. If we had a nonuniform prior on relative depth, we would then multiply the likelihood function by the prior and normalize to obtain the posterior distribution. As illustrated in Figure 1.2, both cues are consistent with a large range of relative depths (depending on the viewing distance assumed), but because the cues depend differently on viewing distance, when combined they can disambiguate both relative depth and viewing distance (Richards, 1985).

An alternative to this approach would be to estimate the viewing distance from ancillary information (e.g., vergence signals from the oculomotor system). With these parameters fixed, optimal cue integration will again be linear. However, this approach is almost certainly suboptimal because it ignores the noise in the ancillary signals. The optimal approach is to incorporate the information from ancillary signals in the same Bayesian formulation. In this case, extraretinal vergence signals specify a likelihood function in depth-distance space that is simply stretched out along the depth dimension (because those signals say nothing about relative depth) (much like the prior in the lower-left panel of Fig. 1.2). In this way, vergence signals disambiguate viewing distance only in so much as the noise in the signals allows. If that noise is high, the disambiguating effects of the nonlinear interaction between the relative disparity and relative motion signals will dominate the perceptual estimate.

### Robust Estimation and Mixture Priors

One might ask how a normative system should behave when cues suggest very different values for some scene property. Consider a case in which disparity indicates a frontoparallel surface, but the texture pattern in the image suggests a surface slanted away from frontoparallel by 60°. A linear system would choose some intermediate slant as its best estimate, but if the relative reliabilities of the two cues (i.e., the inverse of the variances of the associated likelihood functions) were similar, this estimate would be at a slant (say 30°) that is wildly inconsistent with both cues.

On the face of it, this appears like a standard problem in robust statistics. For example, the mean of a set of samples can be influenced strongly by a single outlier, and robust, nonlinear statistical methods, such as the trimmed mean, are intended to alleviate such problems (Hampel, 1974; Huber, 1981). The trimmed mean and related methods reduce the weight of a given data point as the value of that data point becomes increasingly discrepant from the bulk of the sample. The application of robust statistical methods to cue integration is difficult, however, because one is usually dealing with a small number of cues rather than a large sample, so it is often unclear which cue should be treated as the discrepant outlier.

A discrepant cue may result from a particularly noisy sample, but it may also indicate that the estimate from that cue was fallacious due to a mistaken assumption (Landy et al., 1995). The second problem is more common than the first. The observation that outliers may arise from fallacious assumptions suggests a reconceptualization of the outlier problem. Consider the case of depth perception. All pictorial depth cues rely on prior assumptions about objects in the world (texture relies on homogeneity, linear perspective on parallelism, relative motion on rigidity, etc.). A notable and very simple example is that provided by the compression cue (Fig. 1.3A). The visual system interprets figures that are very compressed in one direction as being slanted in 3D in that direction. For example, the visual system uses the aspect ratio of ellipses in the retinal image as a cue to the 3D slant of a figure, so much so that it gives nearly equal weight to that cue and disparity in a variety of viewing conditions (Hillis et al., 2004; Knill & Saunders, 2003). Of course, the aspect ratio of an ellipse on the retina is only useful if one can assume that the figure from which it projects is a circle. This is usually a reasonable assumption because most ellipses in an image are circular in the world. When disparities suggest a slant differing by only a small amount from that suggested by the compression cue, it makes sense to combine the two cues linearly. When disparities suggest a very different slant, however, the discrepancy provides evidence that one is viewing a noncircular ellipse. In this situation, an observer should down-weight the compression cue or even ignore it.

Figure 1.3 illustrates how these observations are incorporated into a Bayesian model (see Chapter 9 and Knill, 2007b, for details). The generative model for the aspect ratio of an ellipse in the image depends on both the 3D slant of a surface and the aspect ratio of the ellipse in the world. The aspect ratio of the ellipse in the world is a hidden variable and must be integrated out to derive the likelihood for slant. The prior distribution on ellipse aspect ratios plays a critical role here. The true prior is

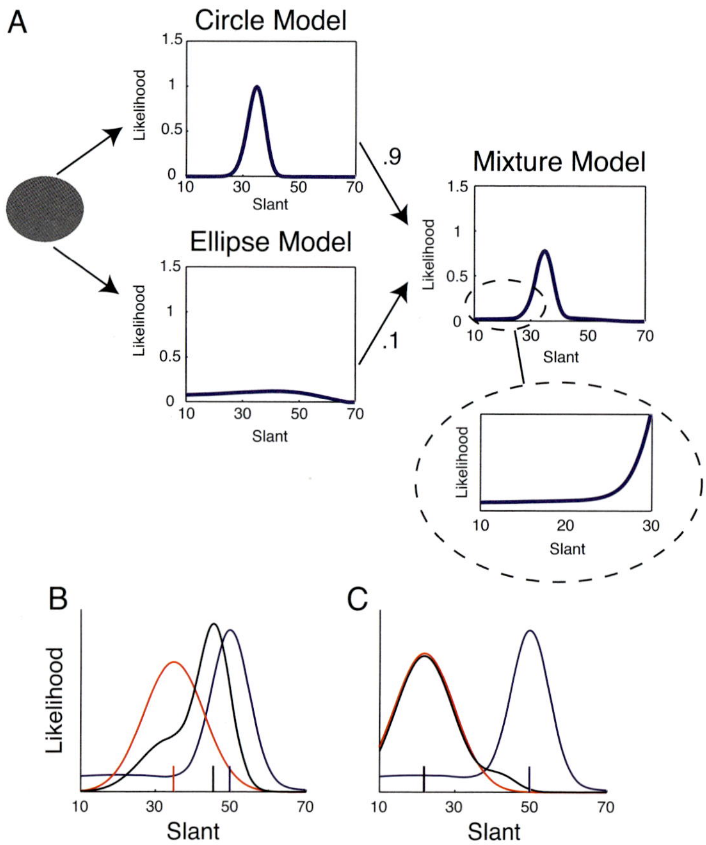


**Figure 1.3** Bayesian model of slant from texture (Knill, 2003). (A) Given the shape of an ellipse in the retinal image, the likelihood function for slant is a mixture of likelihood functions derived from different prior models on the aspect ratios of ellipses in the world. The illustrated likelihoods were derived by assuming that noise associated with sensory measurements of aspect ratio has a standard deviation of 0.03, that the prior distribution of aspect ratios of randomly shaped ellipses in the world has a standard deviation of 0.25, and that 90% of ellipses in the world are circles. The mixture of narrow and broad likelihood functions creates a likelihood function with long tails, as shown in the blow-up. (B) Combination of a long-tailed likelihood function from compression (blue) and a Gaussian likelihood function from disparity (red) yields a joint likelihood function that peaks between the two individual estimates when the individual estimates are similar, much as with the linear, Gaussian model of cue integration. (C) When the cue conflict is increased, the heavy tail of the compression likelihood results in a joint likelihood that peaks at the disparity estimate, effectively vetoing the compression cue.

a mixture of distributions, each corresponding to different categories of shapes in the world. A simple first-order model is that the prior distribution is a mixture of a delta function at one (i.e., all of the probability massed at one) representing circles and a broader distribution over other possible aspect ratios representing randomly shaped ellipses. In Figure 1.3, the width of the likelihood for the circle model is due to sensory noise in measurement of ellipse aspect ratio. The result is a likelihood function that is a mixture of two likelihood functions—one derived for circles, in which the uncertainty in slant is caused only by noise in sensory measurements of shape on the retina, and one derived for randomly shaped ellipses, in which the uncertainty in slant is a combination of sensory noise and the variance in aspect ratios of ellipses in the world. The result is a likelihood function for the compression cue that is peaked at the slant consistent with a circle interpretation of the measured aspect ratio but has broad tails (Fig. 1.3A).

The likelihood function for both the compression cue and the disparity cue results from multiplying the likelihood function for disparity (which presumably does not have broad tails; but see Girshick and Banks, 2009, for evidence that the disparity likelihood also has broad tails) with the likelihood function for the compression cue. The resulting likelihood function peaks at a point either between the peaks of the two cue likelihood functions when they are close to one another (small cue conflicts, Fig. 1.3B) or very near the peak of the disparity likelihood function when they are not close (large cue conflicts, Fig. 1.3C). The latter condition appears behaviorally as a down-weighting or vetoing of the compression cue. Thus, multiplying likelihood functions can result in a form of model selection, thereby determining which prior constraint is used to interpret a cue. Similar behavior can be predicted for many different depth cues because they also derive their informativeness from a mixture of prior constraints that hold for different categories of objects. This behavior of integrating with small cue conflicts and vetoing with large ones is a form of model switching and has been observed with disparity-perspective conflict stimuli (Girshick & Banks, 2009; Knill, 2007b) and with auditory-visual conflict stimuli (Wallace et al., 2004).

### Causal Inference

The development of the linear cue-combination model is based on the assumption that the individual cues are all estimating the same feature of the world (e.g., the depth or location of the same object). However, the observer may not know for sure that the cues derive from the same source in the world. The observer has to first infer whether the scene that gave rise to the sensory input consists of one or two sources (i.e., one or two objects) before determining whether the sources should be integrated. That is, the observer is faced with inferring the structure of the scene, not merely producing a single estimate.

Consider the problem of interpreting auditory and visual location cues. When presented with both a visual and auditory stimulus, an observer should take into account the possibility that the two signals come from different sources in the world. If they come from one source, it is sensible to integrate them. If they come from different sources, integration would be counterproductive. As we mentioned in the previous section, behavior consistent with model switching has been observed in auditory-visual integration experiments (Wallace et al., 2004). Specifically, when auditory and visual stimuli are presented in nearby locations, subjects' estimates of the auditory stimulus are pulled toward the visual stimulus (the ventriloquist effect). When they are presented far apart, the auditory and visual signals appear to be separate sources in the world and do not affect one another.

Recent work has approached this *causal-inference* problem using Bayesian inference of structural models (see Chapters 2, 3, 4, and 13). These models typically begin with a representation of the causal structure of the sensory input in the form of a Bayes net (Pearl, 1988). For example, Körding and colleagues (2007) used a structural model to analyze data on auditory-visual cue interactions in location judgments. The structural model (Fig. 1.4) is a probabilistic description of a generative model of the scene. According to this model, the generation of auditory and visual signals can be thought of as a two-step process. First, a weighted coin flip determines whether the scene consists of one cause (with probability $p_{\text{common}}$, left-hand branch) or separate causes for the auditory and visual stimuli (right-hand branch). If there is one cause, the location of that cause, $x$, is then determined (as a random sample from a prior distribution of locations), and the source at that location then gives rise independently to visual and auditory signals. If there are two causes, each has its own independently chosen location, giving rise to unrelated signals.

An observer has to invert the generative model and infer the locations of the visual and auditory sources (and whether they are one and the same). While there are numerous, mathematically equivalent ways to formulate the ideal observer, the formulation that is consistent with the others in this chapter is one in which an observer computes a posterior distribution on both the auditory and visual locations, $x_a$ and $x_v$. The prior in this case is a mixture of a delta function along the diagonal in $x_a - x_v$ space (corresponding to situations in which the auditory and visual signals derive from the same source) and a broad distribution over the entire space (corresponding to situations in which the locations are independent). In this formulation, the prior distribution has broad tails, but the result is similar. If the two signals indicate locations near one another, the posterior is peaked at a point on the diagonal corresponding to a position between the two. If they are far apart, it peaks at the same point as the likelihood function. The joint likelihood function for the location of the visual and auditory sources can be described by the same sort of mixture model used in the earlier slant example (for further discussion of causal and mixture models, see Chapters 2, 3, 4, 12, and 13).

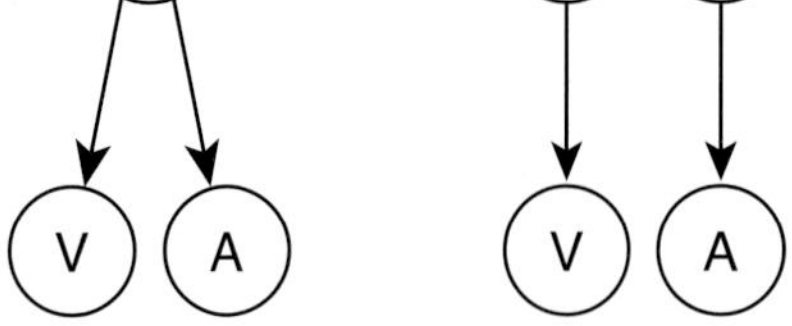


**Figure 1.4** A causal-inference model of the ventriloquist effect. The stimulus either comes from a common source or from two independent sources (governed by probability $p_{\text{common}}$). If there is a common source, the auditory and visual cues both depend on that common source's location. If not, each cue depends upon an independent location.

### Conclusions (Theory)

The previous theoretical discussion has a number of important take-home messages. First, Bayesian decision theory provides a completely general normative framework for cue integration. A linear approximation can characterize the average behavior of an optimal integrator in limited circumstances, but many realistic problems require the full machinery of Bayesian inference. This implies that the same framework can be used to build models of human performance, for example, by constructing and testing model priors that are incorporated into human perceptual mechanisms or by modeling the tasks human perceptual systems are designed to solve using appropriate gain functions. Second, the representational framework used to model specific problems depends critically on the structure of the information available and the observer's task. In the aforementioned examples, appropriate representational primitives include "average" cue estimates (in linear models), additive mixtures of likelihood functions, and graphical models. Finally, constructing normative models of cue integration serves to highlight the qualitative structure of specific problems. This implies that normative models can suggest the appropriate scientific questions that need to be answered to understand, at a computational level, how the brain solves specific problems. In some cases, this may mean that appropriate questions revolve around the weights that observers use to integrate cues. In others, they may revolve around the mixture components of the priors people use. In still others, they center on the causal structure assumed by observers in their models of the generative process that gives rise to sensory data.

## THEORY MEETS DATA

### Methodology

A variety of experimental techniques has been used to test theories of cue integration. Many researchers have used variants of the perturbation-analysis technique introduced by Young and colleagues (Landy et al., 1995; Maloney & Landy, 1989; Young, Landy, & Maloney, 1993) and later extended to intersensory cue combination (Ernst & Banks, 2002). Consider the combination of visual and haptic cues to size (Ernst & Banks, 2002). The visual stimuli are stereoscopic random-dot displays that depict a raised bar on a flat background (Fig. 1.5). The haptic stimuli are also a raised bar presented with force-feedback devices attached to the index finger and thumb. Four kinds of stimuli are used: visual-only (the stimulus is seen but not felt); haptic-only (felt but not seen); two-cue, consistent stimuli (seen and felt, and both cues depict the same size); and

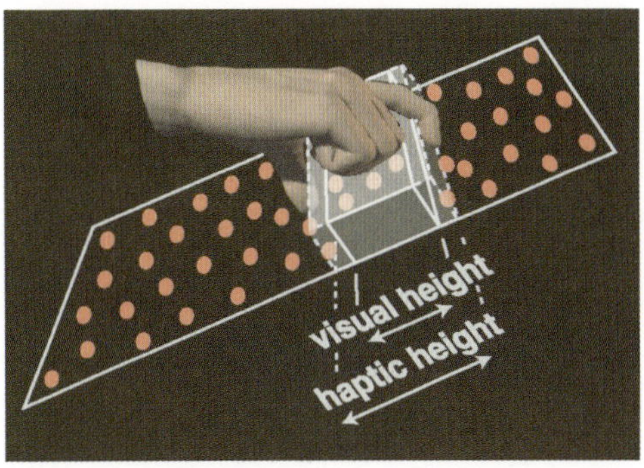


**Figure 1.5** Multisensory stimulus used by Ernst and Banks (2002). A raised bar was presented visually as a random-dot stimulus with binocular disparity displaying a bar height $x_v$ and, in inconsistent-cues stimuli, haptically with a height $x_h = x_v + \Delta x$.

two-cue, inconsistent stimuli (in which the visual stimulus depicts one size $x_v$ and the haptic stimulus indicates a different size $x_h$). Subjects are presented with two stimuli sequentially and indicate which was larger. For example, a subject is shown two visual-only stimuli that depict bars with heights $x_v$ and $x_v + \Delta x_v$. The threshold value of $\Delta x_v$ (the just-noticeable difference or JND) is used to estimate the underlying single-cue noise $\sigma_v$. An analogous single-cue experiment is used to estimate the haptic-cue noise $\sigma_h$. Interleaved with the visual-only and haptic-only trials, the two-cue stimuli are also presented. On such trials, subjects discriminate the perceived size of an inconsistent-cues stimulus in which the size depicted by haptics is perturbed from that depicted visually, $x_h = x_v + \Delta x$, as compared to a consistent-cues stimulus in which $x'_h = x'_v = x'$. The size $x'$ of the consistent-cues stimulus is varied to find the point of subjective equality (PSE), that is, the pair of stimuli $((x_h, x_v)$ and $(x'_h, x'_v))$ that are perceived as being equal in size. Linear, weighted cue integration implies that $x'$ is a linear function of $\Delta x$ with slope $w_h$ (the weight applied to the perturbed cue). The weight may be predicted independently from the estimates of the individual cue variances and Eq. 1.2.

There are a few issues with this method. First, one might argue that the artificial stimuli create cue conflicts that exceed those experienced under natural conditions and therefore that observers might use a different integration method than would be used in the natural environment. One can ask whether the results are similar across conflict sizes to determine whether this is a serious concern in a particular set of conditions.

Second, the method does not necessarily detect a situation in which the results have been affected by other unmodeled information such as another cue or a prior. Consider, for example, an experiment in which texture and motion cues to depth were manipulated, and the perturbation method was used to estimate the two cue weights (Young et al., 1993). The observers estimated depth by using texture and motion cues, but they may also have incorporated other cues such as blur and accommodation that specify flatness and/or a Bayesian prior favoring flatness (Watt, Akeley, Ernst, & Banks, 2005). As a result of using these other cues, observers should perceive all of the stimuli as flatter than specified by texture and motion, and therefore the texture and motion weights should sum to less than one ($w_t + w_m < 1$). This perceptual flattening would occur equally with both the consistent- and inconsistent-cues stimuli, and therefore would not affect points of subjective equality. In particular, the inconsistent-cues stimulus for which $\Delta x = 0$ is identical to the consistent-cues stimulus in which $x' = x_t = x_m$ and thus these two stimuli must be subjectively equivalent (except for measurement error). In this experimental design, the consistent-cues stimuli are used as a "yardstick" to measure the perceived depth of the inconsistent-cues stimulus. To uncover a bias in the percept, the yardstick must be qualitatively different from the inconsistent-cues stimulus. In the texture-motion case, for example, when the inconsistent-cues stimuli have reduced texture or motion reliability (by adding noise to texture shapes or velocities), but the consistent-cues stimuli do not have the added stimulus noise, the relative flattening of the noisy stimuli becomes apparent, and the separately measured weights sum to less than one (Young et al., 1993).

This experimental design is still useful if the observer incorporates a nonuniform prior into the computation of the environmental property of interest. For example, suppose the observer has a Gaussian prior on perceived depth centered on zero depth (i.e., a prior for flatness) and that the reliability $r_i$ of each experimenter-manipulated cue $i$ is unchanging across experimental conditions. The prior has the form of a probability distribution, but it is a fixed (nonstochastic) contributor to the computation. That is, as measured in stimulus units, the use of the prior will have no effect on the estimation of single-cue JNDs, nor on the estimation of relative cue weights. All percepts will be biased toward zero depth, but that will occur equally for the two discriminanda in each phase of the experiment and should not affect the results. Thus, the prior has no effect when the cue reliabilities $\{r_i\}$ are the same for the two stimuli being compared. The prior does have an effect when observers compare stimuli that differ in reliability: The stimulus with lower reliability displays a stronger bias toward the mean of the prior (Stocker & Simoncelli, 2006). This would occur in comparisons of single-cue to two-cue stimuli because cue integration typically increases reliability. Critically, it would also occur in conditions in which cue reliability depends on the resulting estimate so that reliability for each cue varies from trial to trial as, for example, occurs in the estimation of slant from texture (Knill, 1998).

### Overview of Results

Many studies have supported optimal linear cue integration as a model of human perception for stimuli involving relatively small cue conflicts. By and large, these studies have confirmed the two main predictions of the model: With small cue conflicts, cue weights are proportional to cue reliability, and the reliability for stimuli with multiple cues is equal to the sum of individual cue reliabilities. Such studies have been carried out for combinations of visual cues to depth, slant, shape (Hillis et al., 2002; Hillis et al., 2004; Johnston, Cumming, & Landy, 1994; Knill & Saunders, 2003; Young et al., 1993), and location (Landy & Kojima, 2001). Multisensory studies have also been consistent with the model, including combinations of visual and haptic cues to size (Ernst & Banks, 2002; Gepshtein & Banks, 2003; Hillis et al., 2002) and visual and auditory cues to location (Alais & Burr, 2004). Some studies have found suboptimal choices of cue weights (Battaglia, Jacobs, & Aslin, 2003; Rosas et al., 2005; Rosas, Wichmann, & Wagemans, 2007).

Cue promotion is an issue for many cue-integration problems. Consider, for example, the visual estimation of depth. Stereo stimuli are misperceived in a manner that suggests that near viewing distances are overestimated, and far viewing distances underestimated, for the purposes of scaling depth from retinal disparity (Gogel, 1990; Johnston, 1991; Rogers & Bradshaw, 1995; Watt et al., 2005). This misscaling could be ameliorated by combining disparity and relative-motion cues to shape. However, the evidence for this particular cue interaction has been equivocal (Brenner &

Landy, 1999; Johnston et al., 1994; Landy & Brenner, 2001). It is important to note that people are essentially veridical at taking distance into account—little if any overestimation of near distances and little if any underestimation of far distances—when all cues to flatness are eliminated (Watt et al., 2005). In other words, failures to observe depth constancy may be due to the influence of unmodeled flatness cues such as blur and accommodation.

There is some evidence for robustness in intrasensory cue combination; that is, evidence that individual cues are down-weighted as they become too discrepant from estimates based on other cues. Most laboratory studies involve only two experimenter-manipulated cues with small conflicts, but some have looked at cue integration with large discrepancies. Bayesian estimation using a mixture prior can lead to robust behavior. For example, Knill (2007b; also see Chapter 9) has described two models for estimation of slant from texture, a more constrained and accurate model that assumes the texture is isotropic and a second that does not make this assumption. By assuming a mixture prior over scenes (between isotropic and nonisotropic surface textures), one can predict a smooth switch from the predictions of one model to the other as the presented surface texture becomes increasingly nonisotropic. Human performance appears to be consistent with the predictions of this mixture-prior model (Knill, 2007b). Recently, Girshick and Banks (2009) confirmed Knill's result that observers' percepts are intermediate between cue values for disparity and texture when the discrepancy between the two cues is small, and that percepts migrate toward one cue when the discrepancy is large. Like Knill, they found that the cue dictating the large-conflict percept was consistently disparity in some conditions. But unlike Knill, they also found other conditions in which the large-conflict percept was consistently dictated by texture. Girshick and Banks showed that their data were well predicted by a Bayesian model in which both the texture and disparity likelihoods had broader tails than Gaussians.

Empirical studies suggest that integration is impeded when the display indicates the two cues do not come from the same source. For example, optimal cue integration is found in combinations of visual and haptic cues to object size (Ernst & Banks, 2002), but if the haptic object is in a different location from the visual object, observers no longer integrate the two estimates (Gepshtein, Burge, Ernst, & Banks, 2005). Bayesian structural models have been successful at modeling phenomena like this, for example, in the ventriloquist effect (Körding et al., 2007).

Humans also appear to be optimal or nearly so in movement tasks involving experimenter-imposed rewards and penalties for movement outcome (Trommershäuser, Maloney, & Landy, 2003a, 2003b, 2008). Yet when analogous tasks are carried out involving visual estimation and integration of visual cues, many observers use suboptimal strategies (Landy, Goutcher, Trommershäuser, & Mamassian, 2007). As we argued earlier, observers should be more likely to approach optimal behavior in tasks that are important for survival. It seems reasonable that accurate visuomotor planning in risky environments is such a task and that the visual analog of these movement-planning tasks is not such a task. There remain many open questions in determining the limits of optimal behavior by humans in perceptual and visuomotor decision-making tasks with experimenter-imposed loss functions (i.e., decision making under risk).

## ISSUES AND CONCERNS

### Realism and Unmodeled Cues

Perceptual systems evolved to perform useful tasks in the natural environment. Accordingly, these systems were designed to make accurate estimates of environmental properties in settings in which many cues are present and large cue conflicts are rare. The lack of realism and the dearth of sensory cues in the laboratory give the experimenter greater stimulus control, but they may place the perceiver in situations for which the nervous system is ill suited and therefore may perform suboptimally.

Bülthoff (1991) describes an experiment in which the perceived depth of a monocularly viewed display is gauged by comparison with a stereo display. Depth from texture alone, and depth from shading alone were both underestimated, but when the two pictorial cues were combined, depth was approximately veridical. The depth values appeared to sum rather than average in the two-cue display. Bülthoff and Yuille (1991) interpreted this as an example of "strong fusion" of cues (in contrast with the "weak fusion" of weighted averaging). However, these were impoverished displays and contained other visual cues (blur, accommodation, etc.) that indicated the display was flat. Bayesian cue integration predicts that the addition of cues to a display will have the effect of reducing the weight given to these cues to flatness (because increasing the amount of information about depth increases the reliability of that information), resulting in greater perceived depth than that with either of the experimenter-controlled cues alone.

There is now clear evidence that display cues to flatness can provide a substantial contribution to perceived depth. Buckley and Frisby (1993) observed a striking effect that illustrates the importance of considering unmodeled cues in general and specifically the role of cues from the computer display itself. Their observers viewed raised ridges presented as real objects or as computer-graphic images. In one experiment, the stimuli were stereograms viewed on a computer display. Disparity- and texture-specified depths were varied independently and observers indicated the amount of perceived depth. The data revealed clear effects of both cues. Disparity dominated when the texture-specified depth was large, and texture dominated when the texture depth was small. In the framework of the linear cue-combination model, the disparity and texture weights changed depending on the texture-specified depth.

Buckley and Frisby next asked whether the results would differ if the stimuli were real objects. They constructed 3D ridges consisting of a textured card wrapped onto a wooden form. Disparity-specified depth was varied by using forms of different shapes. Texture-specified depth was varied by distorting the texture pattern on the card so that the projected pattern created the desired texture depth once the card was bent onto the form. The results differed dramatically: Now the disparity-specified depth dominated the percept. Buckley and Frisby speculated that unmodeled focus cues—blur and accommodation—played an important role in the difference between the computer display and real results.

We can quantify their argument by translating it into the framework of the linear model. There are three depth cues in their experiments: disparity, texture, and focus cues; focus cues specify flatness on the computer-display images and the true shape on the real objects.

The real-ridge experiment is easier to interpret, so we start there. In the linear Gaussian model, perceived depth is based on the sum of all available depth cues, each weighted according to its reliability:

$$\begin{aligned} \hat{d} &= w_d d_d + w_t d_t + w_f d_f \\ w_d &+ w_t + w_f = 1, \end{aligned} \tag{1.10}$$

where the subscripts refer to the cues of disparity, texture, and focus. The depth specified by the focus cues was equal to the depth specified by disparity: $d_f = d_d$. Thus, Eq. 1.10 becomes:

$$\hat{d} = (w_d + w_f)d_d + w_t d_t. \tag{1.11}$$

The texture cue $d_t$ had a constant value $k$ for each curve in their data figure (their Fig. 3); therefore,

$$\hat{d} = (w_d + w_f)d_d + (1 - w_d - w_f)k. \tag{1.12}$$

For this reason, when perceived depth is plotted against disparity-specified depth ($d_d$), the slope corresponds to the sum of the weights given to the disparity and focus cues: $w_d + w_f$. The experimentally observed slope was ~0.95. Thus, the texture weight $w_t$ was small in the real-ridge experiment.

In the computer-display experiment, focus cues always signaled a flat surface ($D_f = 0$); therefore,

$$\hat{d} = w_d d_d + w_t d_t = w_d d_d + (1 - w_d - w_f)k. \tag{1.13}$$

Thus, the slope of the data in their figures was an estimate of the disparity weight $w_d$. The slope was always lower in the computer-display data than in the real data, and this probably reflects the influence of focus cues.

Frisby, Buckley, and Horsman (1995) further explored the cause of increased reliance on disparity cues with real as opposed to computer-displayed stimuli. Observers viewed the real-ridge and computer-display stimuli through pinholes, which greatly increased depth of focus, thereby rendering all distances roughly equally well focused. The computer-display data were unaffected by the pinholes, but the real-ridge data were significantly affected: Those data became similar to the computer-display data. This result makes good sense. Viewing through a pinhole renders the blur in the retinal image similar for a wide range of distances and causes the eye to adopt a fixed focal distance. This causes no change in the signals arising from stereograms on a flat display, so the computer-display results were unaffected. The increased depth of focus does cause a change in the signals arising from real 3D objects—focus cues now signal flatness as they did with computer-displayed images—so the real ridge results became similar to the computer-display results. The work of Frisby and colleagues, therefore, demonstrates a clear effect of focus cues. Tangentially, their work shows that using pinholes is not an adequate method for eliminating the influence of focus cues.

Computer-displayed images are far and away the most frequent means of presenting visual stimuli in depth-perception research. Very frequently, the potential influence of unmodeled cues is not considered and so, as we have seen in the earlier analysis, the interpretation of empirical observations can be suspect. One worries that many findings in the depth-perception literature have been misinterpreted and therefore that theories constructed to explain those findings are working toward the wrong goal.

Watt et al. (2005) and Hoffman, Girshick, Akeley, and Banks (2008) explicitly examined the role of focus cues in depth perception. They found that differences in the distance specified by disparity and the physical distance of the stimuli (which determines blur and the stimulus to accommodation) had a systematic effect on perceived distance and therefore had a consistent and predictable effect on the perception of the 3D shape of an object.

### Estimation of Uncertainty

The standard experimental procedure for testing optimality includes measurements of the reliability of individual cues ($\sigma \propto$ JND). For some cue-integration problems, such as the combination of auditory, haptic, and/or visual cues to spatial location, this is relatively straightforward. However, for intramodal cue integration, difficulties arise in isolating a cue. And as we argued earlier in the analysis of the Buckley and Frisby (1993) study, this can lead to errors in interpretation. Consider, for example, the estimation of surface slant from the visual cues of surface texture and disparity. It is easy to isolate the texture cue by viewing the stimulus monocularly. In contrast, it is impossible to produce disparity without surface markings from which disparities can be estimated.

The best one can do in these situations is to generate stimuli in which the information provided by one of the two cues is demonstrably so unreliable as to be useless for performing the psychophysical task. For the stereo-texture example, Hillis et al. (2004) and Knill and Saunders (2003) did this by using sparse random-dot textures when measuring slant-from-disparity thresholds. While a random-dot texture generates strong disparity cues to shape, the texture cue provided by perspective distortions (changes in dot density) is so unreliable that its contribution is likely to be small (Hillis et al., 2004; Knill & Saunders, 2003). Hillis and colleagues (2004) showed this by examining cases in the two-cue experiment in which the texture weight was nearly zero; in those cases, a texture signal was present, but the percepts were dictated by the disparity signal. They found that those two-cue JNDs were the same as the disparity-only JNDs. The close correspondence supports the assumption that the disparity-alone discrimination thresholds provided an estimate of the appropriate reliability for the two-cue experiment. Knill and Saunders (2003) took a different approach. In their study, the random-dot textures used in the stimuli to measure slant-from-stereo thresholds were projected from the same slant as indicated by disparities and thus contained perspective distortions that could in theory be used to judge slant. They showed, however, that when discriminating the slants of these stimuli viewed monocularly, subjects were at chance regardless of the pedestal slant or the difference in slant between two stimuli.

Single-cue discrimination experiments are typically used to estimate the uncertainty associated with individual cues. Suppose that, in addition to the uncertainty inherent in the individual cues (which we model as additive noise sources $N_1$ and $N_2$), there is uncertainty due to additional noise late in the process, which we term *decision noise* ($N_d$, Fig. 1.6). Suppose further that this noise corrupts the estimate after the cues are combined but prior to any decisions involving this estimate. If this is the case, the single-cue experiments will provide estimates of the sum of the cue uncertainty and the uncertainty created by the added late noise (e.g., $\sigma_1^2 + \sigma_d^2$). The optimal cue weights are still those defined by Eq. 1.2 (based on the individual cue reliabilities, e.g., $r_1 = 1/\sigma_1^2$). By using the results of the single-cue discrimination experiments, the experimenter will estimate the single-cue reliabilities as, for example, $r_1' = 1/(\sigma_1^2 + \sigma_d^2)$. The resulting predictions of optimal cue weights based on Eq. 1.2 will be biased toward equality

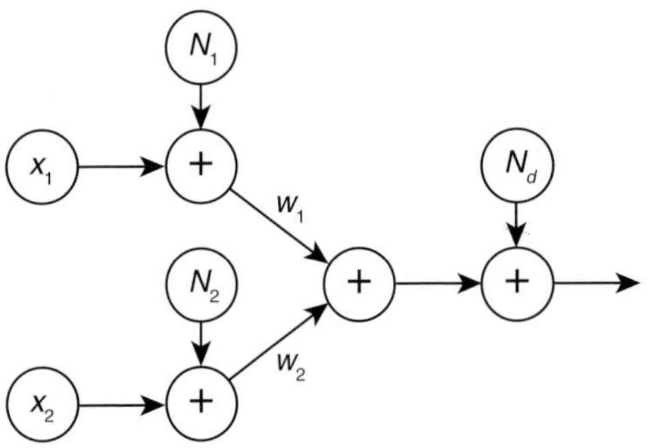


**Figure 1.6** Illustration of a model that incorporates both early, single-cue noise terms ($N_1$ and $N_2$) as well as a late, postcombination, decision-noise term ($N_d$).

(weights of 0.5 for each cue in the slant/disparity experiment). Fortunately, decision noise affects PSEs and JNDs in a predictable way, and so one can gauge the degree to which decision noise affected the measurements. Both Knill and Saunders (2003) and Hillis and colleagues (2004) concluded the effects of decision noise were negligible.

Another important assumption of these methods is that subjects use the same information in the stimulus to make the single-cue judgments as the multiple-cue judgments. This can be a particular concern when the single-cue stimuli do not generate a compelling percept of whatever one is studying. In the depth domain, one has to be concerned about interpreting thresholds derived from monocular displays with limited depth information, particularly when presented on computer displays. One way around this is to use subjects' ability to discriminate changes in the sensory features (e.g., texture compression) that are the source of information in a cue and use an ideal-observer model to map the measured sensory uncertainty onto the consequent uncertainty in perceptual judgments from that cue. Good examples of this outside the cue-integration literature are work on how motion acuity limits structure-from-motion judgments (Eagle & Blake, 1995) and heading judgments form optic flow (Crowell & Banks, 1996), and how disparity acuity limits judgments of surface orientation at different eccentricities and distances from the horopter (Greenwald & Knill, 2009). In a visuomotor context, Saunders and Knill (Saunders & Knill, 2004) used estimates of position and motion acuity to parameterize an optimal feedback-control model and showed that the resulting model did a good job at predicting how subjects integrate position and motion information about the moving hand to control pointing movements. Knill (2007b) used psychophysical measures of aspect-ratio discrimination thresholds to parameterize a Bayesian model for integrating figural compression and disparity cues to slant, but he did not test optimality with the model.

Finally, it is important to note that the implications of optimal integration differ for displays in which a cue is missing (e.g., the focus cue when viewing a display through a pinhole) and displays in which the cue is present but is fixed. When two cues are present rather than just one, both contribute to perceived depth, but both of their uncertainties contribute to the uncertainty of the result. For example, Eq. 1.3 implies that the JNDs for depth should satisfy

$$\frac{1}{\mathrm{JND}_c^2} = \frac{1}{\mathrm{JND}_1^2} + \frac{1}{\mathrm{JND}_2^2}, \tag{1.14}$$

where $\mathrm{JND}_c$ is the threshold for discriminating consistent-cues, two-cue stimuli, and $\mathrm{JND}_1$ and $\mathrm{JND}_2$ are the individual uncertainties of the two cues (proportional to the standard deviation of estimates based on each cue), typically measured by isolating each cue.

Suppose an experimenter fails to isolate each cue when measuring the single-cue thresholds and, instead, single-cue thresholds are measured with both cues present in the stimulus, with one cue held fixed while discrimination threshold is measured for the other, variable cue. For such an experiment, the relationship between thresholds measured for each cue is different. Subjects' JNDs should instead satisfy[1]

$$\frac{1}{\mathrm{JND}_c} = \frac{1}{\mathrm{JND}_1'} + \frac{1}{\mathrm{JND}_2'}, \tag{1.15}$$

where $\mathrm{JND}_1'$ and $\mathrm{JND}_2'$ are the JNDs measured for each cue in the presence of the other, fixed cue. In fact, this relationship applies regardless of the weights that subjects give to the cues, optimal or not. It only depends on the linearity assumption.

Bradshaw and Rogers (1996) ran such an experiment, measuring the JNDs of the two constituent cues in the presence of the other cue, but the depth indicated by the second cue was fixed at zero (flat). That is, both cues' noise sources were involved. Bradshaw and Rogers interpreted the resulting improvement in JND for two-cue displays as indicative of a nonlinear interaction of the cues. But, their data were, in fact, reasonably consistent with the predictions of Eq. 1.15, that is, with the predictions of linear cue combination (optimal or not).

### Estimator Bias

In introducing the cue-combination models in the theory section of this chapter, we made the common assumption that perceptual estimates derived from different cues are unbiased; that is, we assumed that for any given value of a physical stimulus variable (e.g., depth or slant), the average perceptual estimate of that variable is equal to the true value. This assumption is generally incorporated in descriptions of optimal models because it simplifies exposition: Disregarding bias allows one to focus only on minimizing variance as an optimality criterion. However, it seems to us that it is generally impossible to determine whether sensory estimates derived from different cues prior to integration are unbiased relative to ground truth, largely because we only have access to the outputs of systems that operate on perceptual estimates (decision or motor processes) that may themselves introduce unknown biases. It is possible, however, to determine whether they are internally consistent, that is, whether their estimates agree with one another on average.

If the estimators in the optimal combination model (Eq. 1.1) are not internally calibrated, problems may arise. Consider presenting a 3D stimulus with a slant of 0° to the eye and hand. Let us say that vision and touch are equally reliable, but that vision is biased by 20° because the person is wearing spectacles. The internal inconsistency introduces a serious problem: If the stimulus is seen but not felt, its perceived slant will be 20°. If it is felt but

[1] To see this, assume that JNDs are defined to be the standard deviation of the noise that must be matched by the change in perceived depth to reach threshold. Thus, in the normal perturbation experiment in which single-cue JNDs are measured in isolation, $\mathrm{JND}_1 = \sigma_1$, $\mathrm{JND}_2 = \sigma_2$, and by Eq. 1.3, $\mathrm{JND}_c = \sigma_c = 1/\left[(1/\sigma_1^2) + (1/\sigma_2^2)\right]^{1/2}$ from which Eq. 1.14 follows. In the Bradshaw and Rogers (1996) experiment, when only cue 1 is manipulated and cue 2 is fixed, the weighted combination of the cues must overcome the combined noise, so that $w_1\Delta_1 + w_2\Delta_2 = w_1\mathrm{JND}_1' + w_2(0) = \sigma_c$ and similarly for $\mathrm{JND}_2$, where $\Delta_i$ is the difference in cue value for cue $i$ between the two discriminanda at threshold. Because the weights are assumed to sum to 1, Eq. 1.15 follows.

not seen, the percept will be 0°. If it seen and felt, the percept will be 10° (assuming equal cue weights in Eq. 1.1). The internal inconsistency of the estimators has undermined one of the great achievements of perception: the ability to perceive a given environmental property as constant despite changes in the proximal stimuli used to estimate the property. Thus, it is clearly important for sensory estimators to maintain internal consistency with respect to one another (see Chapter 12).

There is a rich literature on how sensory estimators maintain internal consistency and external accuracy (Burian, 1943; Miles, 1948; Morrison, 1972; Ogle, 1950). The problem is referred to as sensory recalibration. Adams, Banks, and van Ee (2001) studied recalibration of estimates of slant from texture and slant from disparity by exposing people to a horizontally magnifying lens in front of one eye. The lens was worn continuously for 6 days. People were tested before, during, and after wearing the lens with three types of stimuli: slanted planes specified by texture and viewed monocularly, slanted planes specified by disparity and viewed binocularly, and two-cue, disparity-texture stimuli viewed binocularly. The introduction of the lens caused a change in the disparities measured at the two eyes such that a binocularly viewed plane that was previously perceived as frontoparallel was now perceived as slanted by ~ 10°. The apparent slant of monocularly viewed planes did not change. Thus, the introduction of the lens had created a conflict between the perceived slants for disparity- and texture-based stimuli even when they specified the same physical slant. Over the six days, observers adapted until frontoparallel planes, whether they were defined by texture alone, disparity alone, or both, were again perceived as frontoparallel. When the lens was removed, everyone experienced a negative after-effect: A disparity-defined frontoparallel plane appeared slanted in the opposite direction (and a texture-defined plane did not). The negative after-effect also went away in a few days as the observers adapted back to the original no-lens condition. These observations clearly show that the visual system maintains internal consistency between the perceived slants of disparity and texture stimuli even when the two cues are put into large conflict by optical manipulation. Because they maintain calibration with respect to one another, the visual system can achieve greater accuracy and precision by appropriate cue combination as described earlier in the chapter.

Girshick and Banks (2009) also obtained persuasive data that disparity and texture estimators maintain calibration relative to one another. They measured the slants of single-cue stimuli that matched the apparent slant of two-cue stimuli. Specifically, they measured the slant of a disparity-only stimulus that matched the perceived slant of a two-cue, disparity-texture conflict stimulus and they measured the slant of a texture-only stimulus that matched the perceived slant of the same disparity-texture conflict stimulus. The disparity-only stimulus was a sparse random-dot textured plane viewed binocularly and the texture-only stimulus was a Voronoi-textured plane viewed monocularly. On each trial, one interval contained a two-cue stimulus, and the other contained one of the two single-cue stimuli. Observers indicated the one containing the greater perceived slant. No feedback was provided. The slant of the single-cue stimulus was varied according to a staircase procedure to find the value that appeared the same as the two-cue stimulus. Figure 1.7 shows the results. Each data point represents the disparity- and texture-specified slants that yielded the same perceived slant as a particular two-cue, disparity-texture stimulus. Clearly, the disparity- and texture-specified slants were highly correlated and one was not biased relative to the other, showing that the disparity and texture estimators were calibrated relative to one another.

### Variable Cue Weights

This discussion brings up one last point: Cue weights need not be constant, independent of the value of the parameter being estimated. Effective cue reliability can vary with conditions, including with changes in the parameter itself. This phenomenon has been observed, for example, with estimation of surface slant.

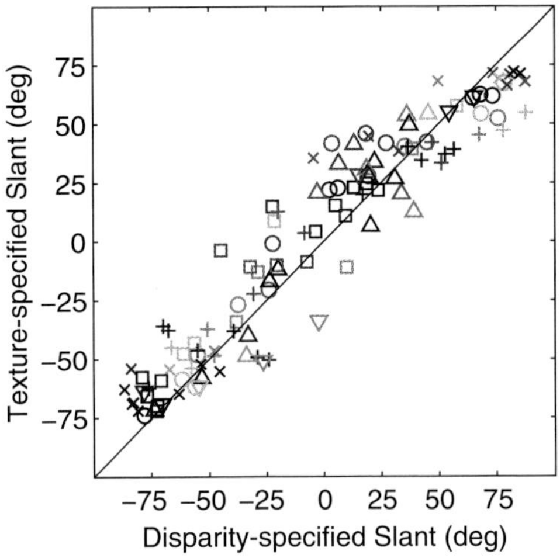


**Figure 1.7** The slants of single-cue stimuli that matched the apparent slant of two-cue stimuli. The data are from Experiment 2 of Girshick and Banks (2009). On each trial, two stimuli were presented in sequence. One was a single-cue stimulus: either texture only or disparity only. The other was a two-cue stimulus: texture plus disparity. The two-cue, texture-disparity stimulus had various amounts of conflict between the slants specified by the two cues; some conflicts were as large as 75°. After each trial, observers indicated which of the two stimuli had the greater perceived slant. Each data point represents the disparity- and texture-specified slants that yielded the same perceived slant as a particular two-cue, disparity-texture stimulus. Different symbols represent different conflicts between the texture- and disparity-specified slants and different observers. (Adapted from Girshick & Banks, 2009.)

The JND for discrimination of surface slant from texture varies substantially with base slant (Knill, 1998) and the JND for slant from disparity varies with base slant as well (Hillis et al., 2004). Of course, JNDs can also vary with other stimulus parameters. For example, the reliability of slant estimates based on disparity varies with viewing distance (Hillis et al., 2004). As a result, one predicts changes in the relative weights of texture and disparity with changes in base slant (Hillis et al., 2004; Knill & Saunders, 2003) and distance (Hillis et al., 2004). For a large, slanted surface, one predicts changes in cue weights for different locations along the surface itself (Hillis et al., 2004).

The interesting point is that the optimal cue weights can change rapidly, from moment to moment or from location to location, sensitive to local conditions. These optimal weight settings are in response to changes in estimated cue reliability. This raises the question of how human observers estimate and represent cue reliability. One suggestion is that a neural population code can simultaneously encode both the estimate and its associated uncertainty (see Chapter 21 and Beck, Ma, Latham, & Pouget, 2007; Ma et al., 2006).

### Simulation of the Observer

In the development of the linear model for a Bayesian observer, we pointed out that observers make measurements for each cue, then form the product of likelihood functions derived from these measurements and the prior distribution (Eq. 1.7). This results in the linear rule for Gaussian distributions. One can prove this by multiplying the likelihood functions corresponding to the expected cue measurements and the prior. But real observers do not have access to the expected cue measurement on any given trial. Rather, they have samples and must derive (and multiply) likelihood functions based on those samples. For symmetric likelihood functions like Gaussians, the predictions do not differ from those based on the expected measurements. However, for non-Gaussian likelihood functions or priors (e.g., mixture priors), one is forced to consider the variability of the cue estimates in formulating predictions.

In formulating Bayesian models incorporating both likelihoods and priors, one must confront the issue of where the prior comes from and how to estimate it. Three different approaches have been used in recent years. In one line of research, natural-image statistics are gathered and used to estimate a given prior distribution, and then human behavior is compared to the performance of a Bayesian ideal observer using that prior (see Chapter 11 and Elder & Goldberg, 2002; Fowlkes, Martin, & Malik, 2007; Geisler, Perry, Super, & Gallogly, 2001). An alternative approach is to ask what prior distribution is consistent with observers' behavior independent of whether it accurately reflects the statistics of the environment. The technique of Stocker and Simoncelli (2006) provides such an approach, by taking advantage of the differential effect of a prior on stimuli that differ in reliability. Others have fit parametric models of the prior distribution to psychophysical data (Knill, 2007b; Mamassian & Landy, 2001). Finally, Knill (2007a) has examined how the visual system adapts its internal prior to the current statistics of the environment.

## OPEN QUESTIONS

The research on cue integration has been wide ranging, and it has led to interesting data and many successful models. Nevertheless, there is plenty of room for further progress. Here is a short list of interesting open questions:

1. How is cue reliability estimated and represented in the nervous system? Observers seem to be able to estimate cue reliability in novel environments, so this is presumably not learned in specific environments and then applied when one of the learned environments is encountered again. Clearly, cue reliability depends on many factors, and thus estimation of reliability is itself a problem of cue integration.
2. Are there general methods the perceptual system uses to determine when cues should be integrated and when, instead, they should be kept separate and attributed to different environmental causes? This problem can be cast as a statistical problem of causal inference.
3. How optimal is cue integration with respect to the information that is available in the environment? Scientists tend to classify environmental properties into distinct categories. The classical list of depth cues is an example. There are surely many other sources of depth information that observers' brains know about, but scientists' brains do not. A rigorous analysis of the linkages between information in natural scenes and human perceptual behavior should reveal previously unappreciated cues.
4. When human cue integration is demonstrably suboptimal, what design considerations does the suboptimality reflect? Are there examples in which the task and required mechanisms have been characterized correctly and the task is undeniably important to the organism, yet perception is nonetheless suboptimal?
5. There are now many examples in which Bayesian priors are invoked to explain aspects of human perception: a prior for slowness, light from above, shape convexity, and many more. Do these priors actually correspond to the probability distributions encountered in the natural environment?

## REFERENCES


Adams, W. J., Banks, M. S., & van Ee, R. (2001). Adaptation to three-dimensional distortions in human vision. *Nature Neuroscience, 4,* 1063–1064.

Adolph, K. E. (1997). Learning in the development of infant locomotion. *Monographs of the Society for Research in Child Development, 62,* 1–158.

Alais, D., & Burr, D. (2004). The ventriloquist effect results from near-optimal bimodal integration. *Current Biology, 14,* 257–262.

Battaglia, P. W., Jacobs, R. A., & Aslin, R. N. (2003). Bayesian integration of visual and auditory signals for spatial localization. *Journal of the Optical Society of America A: Optics, Image Science, and Vision, 20,* 1391–1397.

Beck, J., Ma, W. J., Latham, P. E., & Pouget, A. (2007). Probabilistic population codes and the exponential family of distributions. *Progress in Brain Research, 165,* 509–519.

Bradshaw, M. F., & Rogers, B. J. (1996). The interaction of binocular disparity and motion parallax in the computation of depth. *Vision Research, 36,* 3457–3468.

Brenner, E., & Landy, M. S. (1999). Interaction between the perceived shape of two objects. *Vision Research, 39,* 3834–3848.

Buckley, D., & Frisby, J. P. (1993). Interaction of stereo, texture and outline cues in the shape perception of three-dimensional ridges. *Vision Research, 33,* 919–933.

Bülthoff, H. H. (1991). Shape from X: Psychophysics and computation. In M. S. Landy & J. A. Movshon (Eds.), *Computational models of visual processing* (pp. 305–330). Cambridge, MA: MIT Press.

Bülthoff, H. H., & Yuille, A. L. (1991). Shape-from-X: Psychophysics and computation. In P. S. Schencker (Ed.), *Sensor fusion III: 3-D perception and recognition, Proceedings of the SPIE* (Vol. 1383, pp. 235–246). Bellingham, WA: SPIE.

Burian, H. M. (1943). Influence of prolonged wearing of meridional size lenses on spatial localization. *Archives of Ophthalmology, 30,* 645–666.

Cochran, W. G. (1937). Problems arising in the analysis of a series of similar experiments. *Journal of the Royal Statistical Society, 4*(Suppl.), 102–118.

Crowell, J. A., & Banks, M. S. (1996). Ideal observer for heading judgments. *Vision Research, 36,* 471–490.

Domini, F., & Braunstein, M. L. (1998). Recovery of 3-D structure from motion is neither Euclidean nor affine. *Journal of Experimental Psychology: Human Perception and Performance, 24,* 1273–1295.

Eagle, R. A., & Blake, A. (1995). Two-dimensional constraints on three-dimensional structure from motion tasks. *Vision Research, 35,* 2927–2941.

Elder, J. H., & Goldberg, R. M. (2002). Ecological statistics of Gestalt laws for the perceptual organization of contours. *Journal of Vision, 2,* 324–353.

Ernst, M. O., & Banks, M. S. (2002). Humans integrate visual and haptic information in a statistically optimal fashion. *Nature, 415,* 429–433.

Fowlkes, C. C., Martin, D. R., & Malik, J. (2007). Local figure-ground cues are valid for natural images. *Journal of Vision, 7*(8):2, 1–9.

Frisby, J. P., Buckley, D., & Horsman, J. M. (1995). Integration of stereo, texture, and outline cues during pinhole viewing of real ridge-shaped objects and stereograms of ridges. *Perception, 24,* 181–198.

Geisler, W. S., Perry, J. S., Super, B. J., & Gallogly, D. P. (2001). Edge co-occurrence in natural images predicts contour grouping performance. *Vision Research, 41,* 711–724.

Gepshtein, S., & Banks, M. S. (2003). Viewing geometry determines how vision and haptics combine in size perception. *Current Biology, 13,* 483–488.

Gepshtein, S., Burge, J., Ernst, M. O., & Banks, M. S. (2005). The combination of vision and touch depends on spatial proximity. *Journal of Vision, 5,* 1013–1023.

Gibson, J. J. (1966). *The senses considered as perceptual systems.* Boston, MA: Houghton-Mifflin.

Girshick, A. R., & Banks, M. S. (2009). Probabilistic combination of slant information: Weighted averaging and robustness as optimal percepts. *Journal of Vision, 9*(9):8, 1–20.

Gogel, W. C. (1990). A theory of phenomenal geometry and its applications. *Perception and Psychophysics, 48,* 105–123.

Greenwald, H. S., & Knill, D. C. (2009). Cue integration outside central fixation: A study of grasping in depth. *Journal of Vision, 9*(2):11, 1–16.

Hampel, F. R. (1974). The influence curve and its role in robust estimation. *Journal of the American Statistical Association, 69,* 383–393.

Hillis, J. M., Ernst, M. O., Banks, M. S., & Landy, M. S. (2002). Combining sensory information: Mandatory fusion within, but not between, senses. *Science, 298,* 1627–1630.

Hillis, J. M., Watt, S. J., Landy, M. S., & Banks, M. S. (2004). Slant from texture and disparity cues: Optimal cue combination. *Journal of Vision, 4,* 967–992.

Hoffman, D. M., Girshick, A. R., Akeley, K., & Banks, M. S. (2008). Vergence-accommodation conflicts hinder visual performance and cause visual fatigue. *Journal of Vision, 8*(3):33, 1–30.

Huber, P. J. (1981). *Robust statistics.* New York, NY: Wiley.

Johnston, E. B. (1991). Systematic distortions of shape from stereopsis. *Vision Research, 31,* 1351–1360.

Johnston, E. B., Cumming, B. G., & Landy, M. S. (1994). Integration of stereopsis and motion shape cues. *Vision Research, 34,* 2259–2275.

Knill, D. C. (1998). Discrimination of planar surface slant from texture: Human and ideal observers compared. *Vision Research, 38,* 1683–1711.

Knill, D. C. (2003). Mixture models and the probabilistic structure of depth cues. *Vision Research, 43,* 831–854.

Knill, D. C. (2005). Reaching for visual cues to depth: The brain combines depth cues differently for motor control and perception. *Journal of Vision, 5,* 103–115.

Knill, D. C. (2007a). Learning Bayesian priors for depth perception. *Journal of Vision, 7*(8):13, 1–20.

Knill, D. C. (2007b). Robust cue integration: A Bayesian model and evidence from cue-conflict studies with stereoscopic and figure cues to slant. *Journal of Vision, 7*(7):5, 1–24.

Knill, D. C., & Saunders, J. A. (2003). Do humans optimally integrate stereo and texture information for judgments of surface slant? *Vision Research, 43*, 2539–2558.

Körding, K. P., Beierholm, U., Ma, W. J., Quartz, S., Tenenbaum, J. B., & Shams, L. (2007). Causal inference in multisensory perception. *PLoS ONE, 2*, e943.

Landy, M. S., & Brenner, E. (2001). Motion-disparity interaction and the scaling of stereoscopic disparity. In L. R. Harris & M. R. M. Jenkin (Eds.), *Vision and attention* (pp. 129–151). New York, NY: Springer-Verlag.

Landy, M. S., Goutcher, R., Trommershäuser, J., & Mamassian, P. (2007). Visual estimation under risk. *Journal of Vision, 7*(6):4, 1–15.

Landy, M. S., & Kojima, H. (2001). Ideal cue combination for localizing texture-defined edges. *Journal of the Optical Society of America A: Optics, Image Science, and Vision, 18*, 2307–2320.

Landy, M. S., Maloney, L. T., Johnston, E. B., & Young, M. (1995). Measurement and modeling of depth cue combination: In defense of weak fusion. *Vision Research, 35*, 389–412.

Ma, W. J., Beck, J. M., Latham, P. E., & Pouget, A. (2006). Bayesian inference with probabilistic population codes. *Nature Neuroscience, 9*, 1432–1438.

Maloney, L. T. (2002). Statistical decision theory and biological vision. In D. Heyer & R. Mausfeld (Eds.), *Perception and the physical world: Psychological and philosophical issues in perception* (pp. 145–189). New York, NY: Wiley.

Maloney, L. T., & Landy, M. S. (1989). A statistical framework for robust fusion of depth information. In W. A. Pearlman (Ed.), *Visual communications and image processing IV. Proceedings of the SPIE* (Vol. 1199, pp. 1154–1163). Bellingham, WA: SPIE.

Mamassian, P., & Landy, M. S. (2001). Interaction of visual prior constraints. *Vision Research, 41*, 2653–2668.

Marr, D. (1982). *Vision.* San Francisco, CA: W. H. Freeman.

Miles, P. W. (1948). A comparison of aniseikonic test instruments and prolonged induction of artificial aniseikonia. *American Journal of Ophthalmology, 31*, 687–696.

Morrison, L. (1972). Further studies on the adaptation to artificially-induced aniseikonia. *British Journal of Physiological Optics, 27*, 84–101.

Ogle, K. N. (1950). *Researches in binocular vision.* Philadelphia, PA: Saunders.

Oruç, I., Maloney, L. T., & Landy, M. S. (2003). Weighted linear cue combination with possibly correlated error. *Vision Research, 43*, 2451–2468.

Pearl, J. (1988). *Probabilistic reasoning in intelligent systems: Networks of plausible inference.* San Francisco, CA: Morgan Kaufmann.

Richards, W. (1985). Structure from stereo and motion. *Journal of the Optical Society of America A: Optics, Image Science, and Vision, 2*, 343–349.

Rogers, B. J., & Bradshaw, M. F. (1995). Disparity scaling and the perception of frontoparallel surfaces. *Perception, 24*, 155–179.

Rosas, P., Wagemans, J., Ernst, M. O., & Wichmann, F. A. (2005). Texture and haptic cues in slant discrimination: Reliability-based cue weighting without statistically optimal cue combination. *Journal of the Optical Society of America A: Optics, Image Science, and Vision, 22*, 801–809.

Rosas, P., Wichmann, F. A., & Wagemans, J. (2007). Texture and object motion in slant discrimination: Failure of reliability-based weighting of cues may be evidence for strong fusion. *Journal of Vision, 7*(6):3, 1–21.

Saunders, J. A., & Knill, D. C. (2001). Perception of 3D surface orientation from skew symmetry. *Vision Research, 41*, 3163–3183.

Saunders, J. A., & Knill, D. C. (2004). Visual feedback control of hand movements. *Journal of Neuroscience, 24*, 3223–3234.

Stocker, A. A., & Simoncelli, E. P. (2006). Noise characteristics and prior expectations in human visual speed perception. *Nature Neuroscience, 9*, 578–585.

Tassinari, H., Hudson, T. E., & Landy, M. S. (2006). Combining priors and noisy visual cues in a rapid pointing task. *Journal of Neuroscience, 26*, 10154–10163.

Todd, J. T. (2004). The visual perception of 3D shape. *Trends in Cognitive Sciences, 8*, 115–121.

Trommershäuser, J., Maloney, L. T., & Landy, M. S. (2003a). Statistical decision theory and the selection of rapid, goal-directed movements. *Journal of the Optical Society of America A: Optics, Image Science, and Vision, 20*, 1419–1433.

Trommershäuser, J., Maloney, L. T., & Landy, M. S. (2003b). Statistical decision theory and trade-offs in the control of motor response. *Spatial Vision, 16*, 255–275.

Trommershäuser, J., Maloney, L. T., & Landy, M. S. (2008). Decision making, movement planning and statistical decision theory. *Trends in Cognitive Sciences, 12*, 291–297.

Wallace, M. T., Roberson, G. E., Hairston, W. D., Stein, B. E., Vaughan, J. W., & Schirillo, J. A. (2004). Unifying multisensory signals across time and space. *Experimental Brain Research, 158*, 252–258.

Watt, S. J., Akeley, K., Ernst, M. O., & Banks, M. S. (2005). Focus cues affect perceived depth. *Journal of Vision, 5*, 834–862.

Young, M. J., Landy, M. S., & Maloney, L. T. (1993). A perturbation analysis of depth perception from combinations of texture and motion cues. *Vision Research, 33*, 2685–2696.

# CHAPTER 2

# Causal Inference in Sensorimotor Learning and Control

*Kunlin Wei and Konrad P. Körding*

## INTRODUCTION

### Cue Combination and Causal Inference

People are constantly surrounded by sights, sounds, odors, and tactile stimuli, and they combine these sensory cues into their percepts. We construct a coherent understanding of various properties of our bodies and the external world and use our percepts to choose actions. The nature of this process has been a long-standing question for philosophers, psychologists, and neuroscientists, and it continues to captivate our interest.

Von Helmholtz, in the late 19th century, when considering spatial perception, formalized perception as unconscious inference of the state of the world from elementary sensations (Hatfield, 1990). In Helmholtz's terms, sensations are only signs (cues) for the properties of the external world, and perception is their interpretation. Over the last decade, many scientists followed this idea. Realizing the probabilistic nature of cues, recent research has studied perception as a statistical inference problem.

Sensory cues may be affected by various external and internal factors, and they only provide inaccurate and noisy measurements of the estimated property of the world. For example, vision is limited under dim lights or extrafoveal conditions, hearing becomes unreliable for weak sounds, and proprioception drifts without calibration from vision (Brown, Rosenbaum, & Sainburg, 2003). However, by combining multiple cues, the effect of noise can be reduced and better estimates can be formed (see Chapter 1).

Another issue with sensory cues is that they are often ambiguous to the nervous system. For instance, the same moving image on the retina can be caused by a moving scene, self-motion, or a combination of both. To form a correct percept, the nervous system may need to infer the causes of the cues and their relative contributions. For the motion signal problem, this can be achieved by incorporating visual signals with proprioceptive and vestibular signals as well as efference copies of motor commands (e.g. Brandt, Dichgans, & Büchele, 1974; see also Chapter 16 for a discussion of self-motion).

This chapter focuses on the issue of causal inference in perception and action. We argue that ambiguous sensory cues only make sense when the brain understands their causes. Interestingly, this necessity of inferring the cause of a stimulus was also proposed by Helmholtz (Hatfield, 1990; McDonald, 2003) who stated that "we can never emerge from the world of our sensations to the representation of an external world, except through an inference from the changing sensations to external objects as the cause of this change . . . ."

Perception thus may be formalized as the process of inferring the causes of our sensory cues. When you listen to a friend's speech, you are watching the mouth movement of the speaker and hearing his words and combining the two. Combining these two signals allows us to use our visual perception to improve speech recognition (McGurk & MacDonald, 1976; Munhall, Gribble, Sacco, & Ward, 1996). In fact, this process can be tricked by ventriloquists who manage to speak without moving their mouths while moving the mouth of a puppet in synchrony with their speech. This produces a powerful illusion of a puppet that can actually talk. This illusion highlights the importance of causal inference in cue combination: The percept from cue combination is tightly related to the causal relationship between cues. We will discuss evidence from experiments that ask whether the nervous system estimates the causes that give rise to the perceived cues.

Our movement system also needs to combine cues for proper motor control and, as such, it also needs to solve the causal-inference problem. For example, if you participate in a pistol shooting game, the shooting error is an important cue for updating the aiming direction in the practice. This visual cue needs to be combined with other cues like proprioceptive cues about limb configuration and visual cues of the alignment between the pistol and the arm. If the shooting game is held outdoors on a windy day, the visually perceived error may be caused by an external perturbation and thus lose its informative role for movement control. In this case, the nervous system needs to react to the same errors differently than it should in sunny and calm weather when the causes of errors may be different. Thus, causal inference plays a central role in motor learning and motor control.

## Causal Inference in Psychology

Scientists have long recognized that causality is a pivotal organizing principle of the human perception of the physical world. If we see a billiard ball move toward a second ball and the latter starts to move in the same direction while the first ball stops rolling, we will perceive that the first ball *causes* the second ball to move (Michotte & Miles, 1963). We perceive this sort of causation effortlessly in a seemingly automatic way during our daily life. However, the nature of this percept of causality has long been an intriguing question for researchers. Philosophers in the 18th century inspired psychologists to pursue the question of causation. David Hume recognized that sensory information does not explicitly contain the cause–effect information and the nervous system must compute the causality through *covariation* between a potential cause and the effect (Hume, 1987/1739). Immanuel Kant proposed that we have a priori knowledge that all events are caused (Kant, 1965/1781). His view has been taken by later researchers to mean that causes can be inferred only when people have prior knowledge that a certain effect is *generated* by a cause (e.g., Bullock, Gelman, & Baillargeon, 1982; Michotte & Miles, 1963). Despite these divergent views about the basis of causal inference, scientists generally agree that humans perceive the external world in terms of causal relationships.

In the area of psychology, extensive studies have been conducted on cognitive processing related to causal inference (Sperber & Premack, 1995). Studies on the perception of causality, which focus on causal inference in perceptual processing, have generated a large body of interesting findings. Albert Michotte's seminal work on the perception of billiard ball collisions (Michotte & Miles, 1963) has sparked a wide range of research on causation in collisions (e.g., Scholl & Tremoulet, 2000). Several aspects of these findings are of particular relevance for causal inference in sensorimotor integration. First, the perception of causality exists even in early infancy (Leslie, 1982; Saxe & Carey, 2006), despite a heated debate as to what degree this ability is innate (Cohen & Oakes, 1993; Leslie, 1986; Scholl & Leslie, 1999). Second, the perception of causality is fairly fast, automatic, and more important, distinct from causal inference on the cognitive level (Michotte & Miles, 1963; Schlottmann & Shanks, 1992; Scholl & Tremoulet, 2000). Third, the perception of causality is affected by many factors such as the details of cues, perceptual grouping, attention, context, and so forth (Scholl & Tremoulet, 2000). A recent development in the area of psychology is that researchers have started to apply Bayesian theory in studying causal inference (Gopnik et al., 2004; Griffiths & Tenenbaum, 2005; Tenenbaum,

Griffiths, & Kemp, 2006). Causal inference allows humans to estimate the relationships between cues that are sensed about the environment. In this chapter, we focus on how causal inference can affect cue combination and sensorimotor integration in human behavior.

### Preview

The nervous system should not simply combine cues. If cues are indicative of the same cause, which is the property that the nervous system is really interested in, they should be combined. If cues are from independent causes and our nervous system knows that for sure, they should be processed independently. Here we discuss a model of how the nervous system may *estimate* the cause of individual cues and decide whether it should process cues separately or combine them into a joint estimate. As sensory cues are inherently noisy, Bayesian statistics is a proper, systematic way of predicting how the cues should be combined optimally to infer the underlying variables. We will introduce the Bayesian treatment of causal-inference problems in sensorimotor learning and control.

This chapter takes a normative view, which focuses on how the nervous system could optimally infer properties of the body or world for perception and sensorimotor control given assumptions about noise in the body and the environment. The normative approach aims to understand why the nervous system works the way it does and not the specific mechanisms that give rise to behavior. Specifically, we ask how the nervous system *should* estimate the causal relation of events (e.g., errors and movements) and then compare the predictions of these optimal inference models to the way humans actually behave.

## LINEAR MODELS

### Optimal Cue Combination with a Common Cause

Most studies on cue combination find that cues are combined linearly with weights proportional to the reliability of individual cues (see Chapter 1). This is the optimal strategy if the cues are conditionally independent and associated with Gaussian noise (see Chapter 1). These models implicitly contain the assumption that all cues originate from the same source. Thus, all the cues are relevant for estimating variables and should be integrated.

To illustrate the linear model using a cue-combination task with two modalities, consider the problem of locating an object in space when only visual cues $v$ and auditory cues $a$ are available. Assuming a common cause, the underlying variable (source) that generates these two cues is the position of the object $s$ (see the graphic model of this *Common*- or *c*-cause case in Fig. 2.1, left). The object's position can also be assumed to be drawn from some prior distribution; for simplicity, we assume a Gaussian distribution $p(s) = N(\mu, \sigma_S)$ with mean $\mu$ and standard deviation $\sigma_S$ here. Linear models usually assume the cues are noisy copies of the underlying variables and that the visual and auditory cues are drawn according to Gaussian distributions that depend on the real position $s : p(v|s) = N(s, \sigma_V)$ and $p(a|s) = N(s, \sigma_A)$, respectively. The two distributions are centered on the actual location of the object $s$. The standard deviation $\sigma_V$ and $\sigma_A$ characterize how precise the visual and the auditory sense are. To estimate the location $s$ optimally, Bayes' rule can be applied:

$$p(s|v, a) = \frac{p(v, a|s)p(s)}{p(v, a)} = \frac{p(v|s)p(a|s)p(s)}{p(v, a)}. \tag{2.1}$$

Here $p(v, a|s)$ is the conditional probability of both cues given a common cause, and $p(s)$ is the prior distribution of the underlying variable $s$. This derivation assumes conditional independence of the cues. If the nervous system applies maximum a posteriori (MAP) estimation, its optimal estimate $\hat{s}$ will be a weighted average of individual cues (see Chapter 1 for details),

$$\hat{s} = w_V v + w_A a + w_\mu \mu, \tag{2.2}$$

where $v$ and $a$ are visual and auditory cues on a specific trial, respectively. $\mu$ is the mean of the prior distribution of object location. The weights

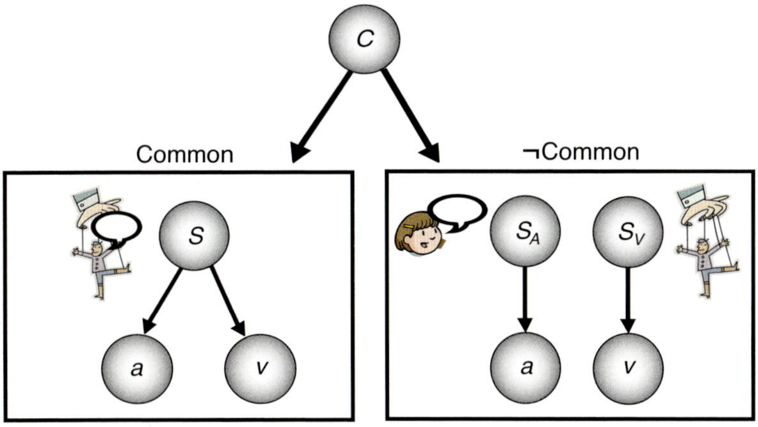


**Figure 2.1** Graphic representation of a causal-inference model. (Left) The visual and auditory cues can be from the same source $s$. This is the default scenario that the linear model of cue combination considers. (Right) Alternatively, the visual and auditory cues are from different sources. The mixture model of causal inference considers both scenarios and infers the probability of each case. The final estimate is a weighted average of the estimates from both cases with weights equal to their corresponding probabilities (Eq. 2.12).

$w_V$, $w_A$, and $w_\mu$ are proportional to the reliabilities, the inverse variances of visual percept, auditory percept, and the prior, respectively. It is important to note that the final estimates are more precise than the individual cues and are optimal in the Bayesian sense. A large array of studies on sensory integration have provided evidence that in many situations human behavior is similar to predictions of linear models of this sort (see Chapter 1 for details and bibliography).

### Violations of the Linearity of Cue Combination

Not all cues that arrive at the nervous system originate from a single object of interest. If the nervous system treats cues differently depending on their relevance to the task and their causal relationship, then, as we will see below, optimal cue combination will no longer be linear.

Many sensory-integration studies have found that spatiotemporal difference between cues is a key factor in determining how strongly and even if cues are integrated, which is in violation of the simple linear cue-combination model (see also Calvert & Thesen, 2004). It has long been known that auditory-visual integration is weakened for large spatial and temporal differences (Hairston et al., 2003; Jack & Thurlow, 1973; Munhall et al., 1996; Radeau, 1994; Slutsky & Recanzone, 2001). Thus, the integration is no longer linear. This breakdown also occurs between other modalities (see Chapters 12 and 13). This effect of reduced cue combination with increasing spatiotemporal difference is known intuitively to many of us. If we go to an outdoor movie or concert and the loudspeakers are far away from the stage, we often perceive the breakdown of the ventriloquist effect; that is, we actually hear the sound as coming out of the loudspeaker, not the speaker's mouth.

Another line of evidence relating to the breakdown of linear integration is from studies where incorrect causal attribution leads to illusions. Simultaneous but irrelevant auditory stimuli can bias visual perception (Frassinetti, Pavani, & Ladavas, 2002; Shams, Kamitani, & Shimojo, 2000; Shams, Ma, & Beierholm, 2005) or tactile perceptions (Hotting & Roder, 2004). For example, if human subjects hear three beeps while seeing two visual flashes, they will sometimes report the perception of three visual flashes (Shams et al., 2000). Analogously, if human subjects hear three beeps while their finger is touched twice, they sometimes report three touches (Bresciani et al., 2005). It has been argued that this kind of illusion may be consistent with the model of optimal linear sensory integration (Shams et al., 2005). These illusions, however, also appear to be reduced in strength with increasing spatiotemporal difference (Bresciani et al., 2005).

In many cue-combination tasks, subjects were asked to make a single decision, either a perceptual judgment or a behavioral response, with multiple conflicting cues presented. This single decision prompts for mandatory sensory integration. Recent studies on cross-modality cue combination strived to bypass this limitation by asking subjects to make a judgment for each modality (Beierholm, Körding, Shams, & Ma, 2008; Roach, Heron, & McGraw, 2006) or to explicitly indicate whether cues from multiple modalities came from the same source (Wallace et al., 2004). Again, these studies found that cues are only partially combined and, more important, cues that are closer together spatially and temporally are integrated more strongly.

In summary, numerous findings indicate that cues are not always combined linearly and that this incomplete integration is a function of spatiotemporal difference between cues.

### Early Studies of Causal Inference in Perception

Studies of how linear sensory integration breaks down give us an indication of the potential role of causal inference in cue combination. There is also direct evidence for causal inference from a range of studies. It has been found that if subjects are told that cues with disparities are from different sources, this significantly reduces cross-modal cue combination (Welch, 1972; Welch & Warren, 1986). However, even when subjects are fully aware of the fact that some cues are from a different object, they cannot ignore them completely (Helbig & Ernst, 2007). On the other hand, if subjects are instructed that cues came from the same source, they tend to integrate stimuli more, despite the lack of an actual common cause (Warren, Welch, & McCarthy, 1981). There is a positive correlation between verbal reports of a unified percept of visual and auditory stimuli and the measured interaction between these cues (Hairston et al., 2003). It seems that the more certain the nervous system is about a common cause of cues, the more it will integrate these cues (also see Fig. 2.2 for an illustration).

## MIXTURE MODELS FOR CAUSAL INFERENCE

### Optimal Cue Combination with Unknown Causal Structure

How does the nervous system *know* whether certain cues belong together and thus should be combined? To combine cues when they belong together and to process them independently otherwise, the nervous system needs to estimate the causal relations between cues. Models of optimal integration thus require the combination of causal inference ideas from cognitive science with ideas from classical cue combination (ideal observers). Here, we continue with the simple example of visuoauditory cue combination to illustrate optimal cue combination, assuming an unknown causal relationship between cues.

In our example of locating an object in space, the visual cue and the auditory cue may have different causes. For example, the ventriloquist can synchronize his or her voice with the mouth movement of the puppet to deliver an impression of a talking puppet although these two cues are from unrelated sources. This dissociation of cues is not uncommon in experimental studies. For example, most cross-modal cue-combination studies create discrepancies between cues. Visual cues are created by computer display, haptic cues by robotic linkage (e.g., Ernst & Banks, 2002), and auditory cues by speakers (e.g., Alais & Burr, 2004; Shams et al., 2005). If, in our example, the visual and the auditory cues do not share a common cause, we can only assume that they are drawn from two different Gaussian distributions $p(v) = N(s_V, \sigma_V)$ and $p(a) = N(s_A, \sigma_A)$ with different means. $s_V$ and $s_A$ are the actual positions of the sources of visual and auditory cues, respectively. $\sigma_V$ and $\sigma_A$ are the corresponding sensory standard deviations. Ultimately we want to come up with estimates of $s_V$ and $s_A$, and we will call these optimal estimates $\hat{s}_V$ and $\hat{s}_A$ (Table 2.1).

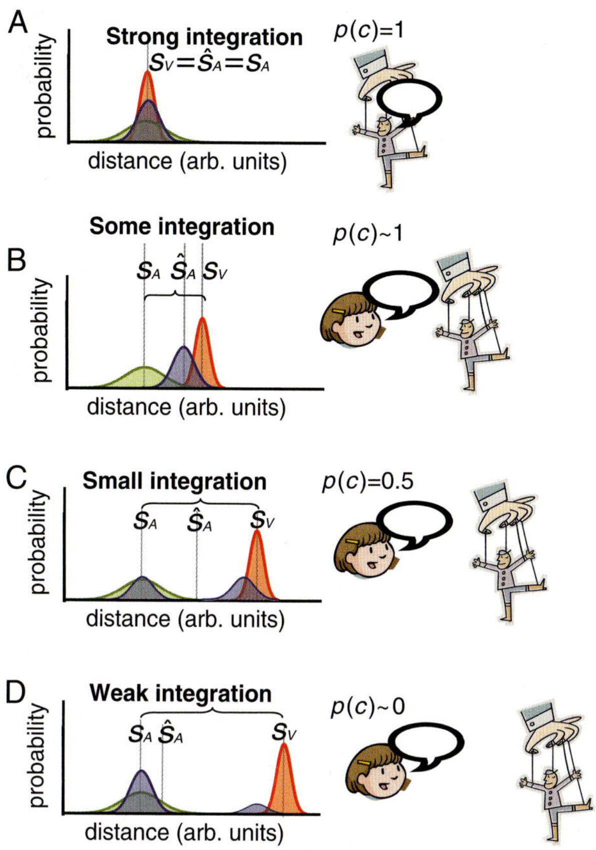


**Figure 2.2** Example of audiovisual cue combination. Subjects estimate the position of an auditory cue. The green distribution is the auditory likelihood. The red distribution is the visual likelihood. The blue distribution is the posterior distribution of the location of the auditory source. (A and B) When two cues are very similar to one another (in terms of spatial distance in this example), they will be combined in good approximation as though they have a common source as p(c) is close to 1. (C) If there is more spatial disparity between the two cues, p($c$) can be close to 0.5. Under these circumstances both peaks are important and the mean-squared error function results in an intermediate estimate. (D) As the disparity increases further, p($c$) approaches 0 and the cues are processed independently.

**Table 2.1 Mixture-Model Notation**

| | |
|---|---|
| $s_V$ and $s_A$ | Actual locations of visual and auditory stimuli |
| $v$ and $a$ | (Noisy) estimates obtained by the visual and auditory modalities separately |
| $\hat{s}_V$ and $\hat{s}_A$ | Optimal estimates of the positions of visual and auditory stimuli |

The nervous system only has access to noisy cues; thus, it has to *estimate* whether they share a common cause. We can express this in probabilistic terms as the probability of a common cause given the cues $p(c|v, a)$ and the probability of separate causes $p(\neg c|v, a) = 1 - p(c|v, a)$. Applying Bayes' rule, we can compute

$$p(c|v, a) = \frac{p(v, a|c)p(c)}{p(v, a)}. \tag{2.3}$$

In Eq. 2.3, $p(v, a|c)$ is the joint probability of both cues given a common cause. $p(c)$ is the prior probability that both of the visual and proprioceptive cues share a common cause. $p(v, a)$ is the joint probability of the two cues, which is given by marginalizing over both causal interpretations,

$$p(v, a) = p(c)p(v, a|c) + p(\neg c)p(v, a|\neg c). \tag{2.4}$$

Eq. 2.4 does not imply that the nervous system tries to choose between a $c$ model and a $\neg c$ model. Given the ambiguity of available perceptual cues, it instead estimates the probability of each case. Eq. 2.4 shows why this model is called a mixture model: The probability of $v$ and $a$ is obtained by mixing components for a common cause and the noncommon causes. Our particular example of causal inference is about inference of a causal *structure* instead of *parameters.*

For the mathematical derivation, we need to calculate the probability of possible stimulus locations *assuming* hypothetical knowledge of causality. For the $c$ case we can write,

$$\begin{aligned} p(v, a|c) &= \int p(v, a|s)p(s)ds \\ &= \int p(v|s)p(a|s)p(s)ds. \end{aligned} \tag{2.5}$$

Both cues are drawn relative to a single underlying cause $s$. This cause $s$ in turn is drawn from the prior $p(s)$ whose distribution is assumed to be $N(\mu, \sigma_S)$. We marginalize over this unobserved variable to calculate the joint distribution of $v$ and $a$ given the assumption of a cause.

For the $\neg c$ case in turn we can write:

$$\begin{aligned} p(v,a|\neg c) &= \iint p(v,a|s_V,s_A) \\ &\quad \times p(s_V,s_A)ds_V\,ds_A \\ &= \left(\int p(v|s_V)p(s_V)ds_V\right) \\ &\quad \times \left(\int p(a|s_A)p(s_A)ds_A\right). \end{aligned} \tag{2.6}$$

The two cues are independently drawn from their own distributions and we marginalize over those unobserved positions separately in Eq. 2.6. Since the terms in Eqs. 2.5 and 2.6 are Gaussian distributions, we can write analytic solutions for them:

$$\begin{aligned} p(v,a|c) &= \frac{1}{2\pi\sqrt{\sigma_V^2\sigma_A^2+\sigma_S^2\sigma_V^2+\sigma_S^2\sigma_A^2}} \\ &\quad \times exp\left[-\frac{1}{2}\left(\frac{(v-a)^2\sigma_S^2+(v-\mu)^2\sigma_A^2+(a-\mu)^2\sigma_V^2}{\sigma_V^2\sigma_A^2+\sigma_S^2\sigma_V^2+\sigma_S^2\sigma_A^2}\right)\right] \end{aligned} \tag{2.7}$$

$$\begin{aligned} p(v,a|\neg c) &= \frac{1}{2\pi\sqrt{(\sigma_V^2+\sigma_S^2)(\sigma_A^2+\sigma_S^2)}} \\ &\quad \times exp\left[-\frac{1}{2}\left(\frac{(v-\mu)^2}{\sigma_V^2+\sigma_S^2}+\frac{(a-\mu)^2}{\sigma_A^2+\sigma_S^2}\right)\right]. \end{aligned} \tag{2.8}$$

Note that by combining Eqs. 2.4, 2.7, and 2.8, we can derive analytic solutions of the probability of a common cause. Interestingly, it is a function of the difference between the cues as well as the difference between the cues and the prior, as shown in Eqs. 2.7 and 2.8. This makes intuitive sense as we know from the literature that the difference between cues appears to influence cue integration (Lewald, Ehrenstein, & Guski, 2001; Wallace et al., 2004).

For the $c$ case, the best estimate of the position will result from a complete integration of the cues with the prior (just as in the linear model of cue combination):

$$\hat{s}_C = \frac{\frac{v}{\sigma_V^2}+\frac{a}{\sigma_A^2}+\frac{\mu}{\sigma_S^2}}{\frac{1}{\sigma_V^2}+\frac{1}{\sigma_a^2}+\frac{1}{\sigma_S^2}}. \tag{2.9}$$

The estimated position is thus a weighted average of individual cues and the prior with weights proportional to the reliability. For the $\neg c$ case, the cues are not related to one another and thus should not be combined. An optimal integration strategy will thus ignore the irrelevant other cue and base the estimate only on the relevant cue and the prior.

$$\hat{s}_{V,\neg c} = \frac{\frac{v}{\sigma_V^2}+\frac{\mu}{\sigma_S^2}}{\frac{1}{\sigma_V^2}+\frac{1}{\sigma_S^2}} \quad \text{or} \quad \hat{s}_{A,\neg c} = \frac{\frac{a}{\sigma_A^2}+\frac{\mu}{\sigma_S^2}}{\frac{1}{\sigma_A^1}+\frac{1}{\sigma_S^2}}. \tag{2.10}$$

To estimate the probabilities of the visual and auditory positions, the nervous system needs to consider both possible causal structures, each according to its probability. We thus obtain

$$p(s_A|v, a) = p(c|v, a)p(s_A|v, a, c) + p(\neg c|v, a)p(s_A|v, a, \neg c). \quad (2.11)$$

Here, $p(s_A|v, a)$ is the probability distribution over the (unobserved) potential source of the auditory stimulus. An analogous equation can be written for the source of the visual cue. This inference thus results from a mixture of two probabilities, a so-called *mixture model.*

If the task of subjects is to report the location of a visual source or the location of an auditory source, the nervous system needs to combine the estimates from the two cases. Because the task does not differentiate the directions of errors, we choose to minimize the quadratic error. The best estimate that minimizes the expected quadratic error is the weighted average of estimated positions from both cases,

$$\hat{s}_V = p(c|v, a)\hat{s}_c + p(\neg c|v, a)\hat{s}_{\neg c,v} \quad \text{or}$$
$$\hat{s}_A = p(c|v, a)\hat{s}_c + p(\neg c|v, a)\hat{s}_{\neg c,a}. \quad (2.12)$$

This estimate is no longer a linear function of the various cues but exhibits interesting nonlinear properties. While both estimates ($\hat{s}_c$ and $\hat{s}_{\neg c,v}$ or $\hat{s}_{\neg c,a}$) are linearly dependent on cues, their combination is nonlinear (see also Stevenson & Körding, 2009).

### Causal Inference in Perception

Mixture models have recently been applied to a range of different problems in perception (also see Chapters 12 and 13). They have been applied to visuoauditory integration, in which subjects were not only required to locate visual and auditory stimuli but also to report whether these two stimuli share the same source (Körding et al., 2007). The model successfully predicts the effect of spatiotemporal difference on the degree of cue combination (data not shown) and the chance of reporting a common cause (Fig. 2.3A).

This mixture model also explains a counterintuitive biasing effect (Fig. 2.3B and C). When subjects reported that they perceived distinct causes for visual and auditory stimuli, they tended to judge the auditory stimulus to come from a location further away from the visual stimulus than where it really was. Standard linear models of cue combination

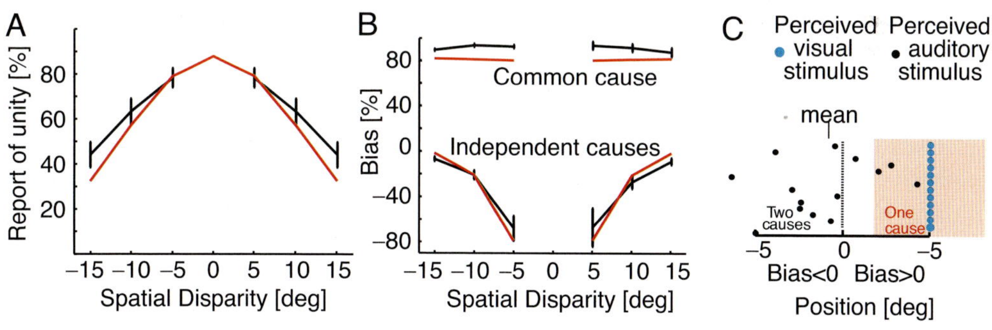


**Figure 2.3** Experimental data (Wallace et al., 2004) and corresponding predictions from the mixture model of causal inference (Körding et al., 2007). (A) The relative frequency of subjects reporting one cause (black) is shown with the predictions of the causal-inference model (red). The probability of reporting a common cause depends on the spatial difference between the visual and auditory stimuli. (B) The bias, that is, the linear influence of vision on the perceived auditory position is shown (black). A bias of zero implies that vision has no influence. A bias of one would imply that subjects only use vision when estimating the auditory position. The predictions of the model are shown in red. Data from trials in which subjects report a common cause and trials in which subjects report independent causes are plotted separately. (C) A schematic illustration explaining the finding of negative biases. Blue and black dots represent the perceived visual and auditory stimuli, respectively. In the pink area people report having perceived a common cause.

do not predict this result, and they normally predict that one cue will always be attracted by another cue.

In the mixture model, this effect is predicted naturally. The auditory stimuli that are close to the visual stimuli are likely to be interpreted as having the same cause. The auditory stimuli that are judged to be from independent causes were only trials where the auditory stimuli were randomly perceived to be perturbed away from the visual stimulus. Their distribution is thus truncated (Fig. 2.3C). The mean of this truncated distribution is then biased away from the visual stimulus, which results in a negative biasing effect. This effect is a so-called selection bias and arises because the same piece of information is used to both select the category and also to compute the estimate. This effect cannot be accounted for by the linear cue-combination model, which only predicts a positive biasing effect. The mixture model has also been found to fit the data better than the linear cue-combination model (Körding et al., 2007).

The causal-inference (mixture) model shares some assumptions with the typical linear model of cue combination such as cues being noisy copies of the underlying source(s), conditional independence of individual cues and Gaussian noise associated with individual cues as well as Gaussian prior distributions. However, the causal-inference model assumes that the nervous system needs to *infer* the cause of sensory cues. It is a mixture model because it contains two causal models: Cues are either caused by the underlying variable of interest or caused by some irrelevant factor. The model estimates the probability of each case or mixture component. In the visuoauditory integration example mentioned earlier, the probability of two cues coming from the same cause is determined by their spatial difference. In other contexts, factors that a causal-inference model needs to consider might include difference in time, task goal, attention, environmental context, and so on. We argue that models of cue combination need to incorporate elements of causal inference as soon as there is significant difference between the cues.

## Causal Inference in Motor Learning and Control

So far, causal inference has been discussed in the domain of perception and cognitive psychology. Given its success in explaining salient aspects of the way the nervous system processes sensory information, it should also be relevant for human sensorimotor control. Motor adaptation has been an extensively studied topic in sensorimotor control. It focuses on how people respond to changes in their motor apparatus and in the surrounding environment. Perceptual information is of particular importance for this type of behavior because the motor system needs to perceive changes and perturbations and make corrections accordingly.

During motor adaptation, the motor system changes its behavior in response to movement errors. Many models of motor adaptation and motor learning assume that the nervous system uses errors in a linear fashion (Baddeley, Ingram, & Miall, 2003; Kawato, Furukawa, & Suzuki, 1987; Scheidt, Dingwell, & Mussa-Ivaldi, 2001; Thoroughman & Shadmehr, 2000; Wolpert & Kawato, 1998). This means that if the nervous system detects an error, it will make a correction to future movements with a magnitude that is linearly proportional to the error size. However, this linear error-compensation strategy could be problematic in some situations. If we reach for a cup and our hand does not move far enough by a few millimeters, it makes sense to adapt and use larger motor commands in the future. If, on the other hand, we miss it by more than the length of our arm, it is very likely that this error was not caused by our body (for example, someone may have played a practical joke on us) and we should not adapt linearly in response to this error. Hence, the optimal strategy is not simply to scale linearly the corrective action to the error size but also to consider the cause of the error.

Whenever the nervous system detects an error, the nervous system needs to consider two scenarios. The error may be induced by extrinsic factors, unrelated to the motor plant such as the displaced cup in the earlier example. Alternatively, the error may be induced by intrinsic factors within the motor plant, such as

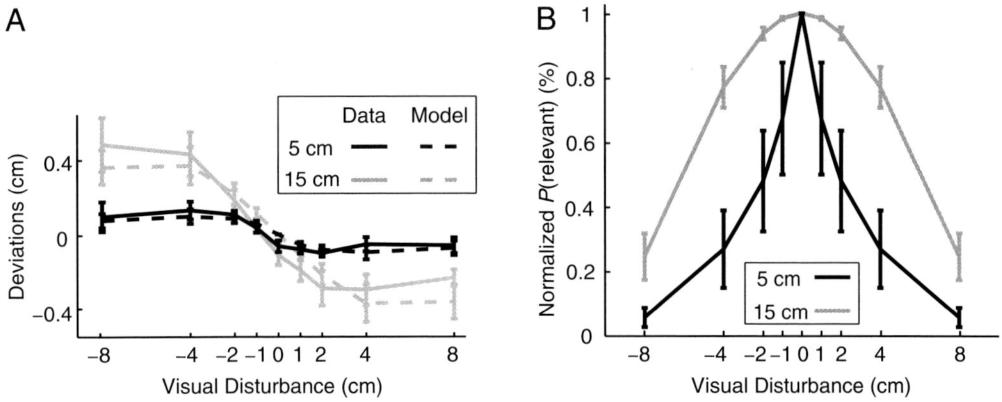


**Figure 2.4** Experimental data and predictions from the mixture model of causal inference (Wei & Körding, 2008). Error bars denote standard errors over subjects. (A) Deviations of hand (from trials following perturbations; an indicator of adaptation) and the corresponding model predictions are plotted as a function of the size of visual disturbance (displacement of cursor relative to hand) for all subjects. Results from 5 and 15 cm movements are plotted separately. The deviations take the opposite sign as the disturbance, indicating adaptation aiming to compensate for errors. The adaptation is a nonlinear function of applied visual disturbance. The same disturbances elicit less adaptation when the hand movement is smaller (5 cm vs. 15 cm). (B) The normalized probability of visual error being relevant as a function of the size of the visual disturbance. This probability is equivalent to the conditional probability of a common cause given the sensory cues in the mixture model described earlier. The probability is highest when there is no visual disturbance (equivalent to the case of no difference between cues); it drops with increasingly larger disturbances. In the experiment with smaller movement amplitude (5 cm vs. 15 cm), the inferred probability of a common cause is smaller and it drops faster.

muscle fatigue. The size of the perceived error could be used by the nervous system to calculate how likely each of the two scenarios is. In this particular example, the nervous system should strongly adapt to small errors (more likely to be caused by the body) and only weakly adapt to very large errors (less likely to be caused by the body).

These theoretical predictions have been tested in a reaching experiment where the size of errors was systematically varied (Wei & Körding, 2008). The experiment required subjects to make straight reaching movements to a target in a virtual-reality setting where the visual feedback of the hand was represented as a cursor. The actual hand was occluded as the hand moved underneath a projection screen. The cursor was only shown at the end of the reaching movement. For each trial, its position was perturbed from its actual position by a random amount. The visual disturbance specified the size of a one-dimensional visual error for each reach. To quantify the amount of adaptation in the very next trial following perturbation, the deviation of the actual hand position from the baseline level in unperturbed trials was measured. Proprioception and vision are two perceptual cues available for estimating the actual error; thus, the mixture model we introduced earlier for visuoauditory integration can be applied directly to this question by replacing the auditory cue with the proprioceptive cue.

Results demonstrate that subjects adapt to the visual error and move in the opposite direction of error following perturbations (Fig. 2.4A, gray lines). Positive disturbances (the cursor is shown above the actual hand location) lead to negative corrections and vice versa. More important, the adaptation is a nonlinear function of error size: When the error size is small, adaptation depends linearly on the size of visual errors but becomes sublinear when the visual error increases further. This nonlinear behavior is well predicted by the mixture model of causal inference. The model also predicts that large errors lead to very small probabilities of the cursor's position being caused by the hand position (Fig. 2.4B, gray line). Model comparison indicates that a linear model cannot fully account for this nonlinearity in motor adaptation (Wei & Körding, 2008). Hence, the linear model of cue combination also breaks down for motor adaptation.

The causal-inference model further predicts that it is easier for the nervous system to infer the cause of an error if there is less motor variance, allowing it to be more certain that the movement error is not self-produced but rather caused by irrelevant external factors. To test this hypothesis, a second experiment was conducted with the same subjects with a smaller movement amplitude of 5 cm. Motor variance is smaller for this experiment; other studies have shown that variability in the final position decreases when the movement amplitude becomes smaller (Harris & Wolpert, 1998). The adaptation is again a nonlinear function of error size (Fig. 2.4A, black line). By fitting the model with actual responses, it was found that subjects also inferred a smaller probability of a common cause for the same error as in the first experiment (Fig. 2.4B, black line).

Some recent experimental studies have found evidence of similar nonlinear relationships between the size or the rate of adaptation and the size of the error (Fine & Thoroughman, 2007; Harris & Wolpert, 1998; Wei, Bajaj, Scheidt, & Patton, 2005). These studies share a common experimental design; in all cases, perturbations were rather large compared to typical movement errors.

Fine and Thoroughman (2007) investigated how people adapted to a velocity-dependent force field that perturbed a straight reaching movement. The force field's gain, which determined the strength of the perturbing force, changed randomly from trial to trial. Results indicated that adaptation showed a nonlinear scaling relationship to the perturbation amplitude, a pattern similar to our results (Fig. 2.5A).

Wei and colleagues (2005) investigated adaptation in a reaching task in a virtual reality setup where the visual representation of the hand movement was rotated around the origin of the movement. The visual error feedback was amplified by a variable gain factor. It was found that the rate of adaptation increased for small gains but decreased when the gain increased further. This finding indicated that the effect of visual error on adaptation rate is a nonlinear function of error size (Fig. 2.5B).

Robinson, Noto, and Bevans (2003) studied saccadic adaptation in monkeys by systematically varying the size of visual errors introduced after the initiation of saccades. The visual error signal elicited adaptation in saccades in subsequent trials. Expressed as the percentage of initially intended saccade size, the visual error had a nonlinear relationship with the adaptation gain (Fig. 2.5C).

The implication from these studies is that though they used different experimental paradigms (arm movements and saccades) and different types of perturbations (visual and mechanical), the nonlinear relationship between adaptation and error size persisted. The mixture model of causal inference provides good fits to the nonlinear relationship between error size and adaptation (Fig. 2.5, black symbols). The model can explain 99.4% and 65% of the total variance of the Fine and Thoroughman (2007) and Robinson et al. (2003) data, respectively.

The dependence of motor adaptation on the size of error strongly suggests that the nervous system constantly infers the cause of movement errors. The same mixture model that successfully fits cue combination for perception can explain a wide range of findings in the literature of motor adaptation and generalization.

### Attribution of Errors to Multiple Sources

In the mixture models that we have discussed thus far, only relatively simple situations are considered: whether two sensory cues belong together, and whether motor errors are relevant. Real-life situations in sensorimotor control may be much more complicated. The same observed movement error may be caused by different factors. For example, our body changes in terms of location, configuration, muscle fatigue, and so on. Various properties of the environment such as properties of the objects we interact with (weight, friction, etc) also vary over time.

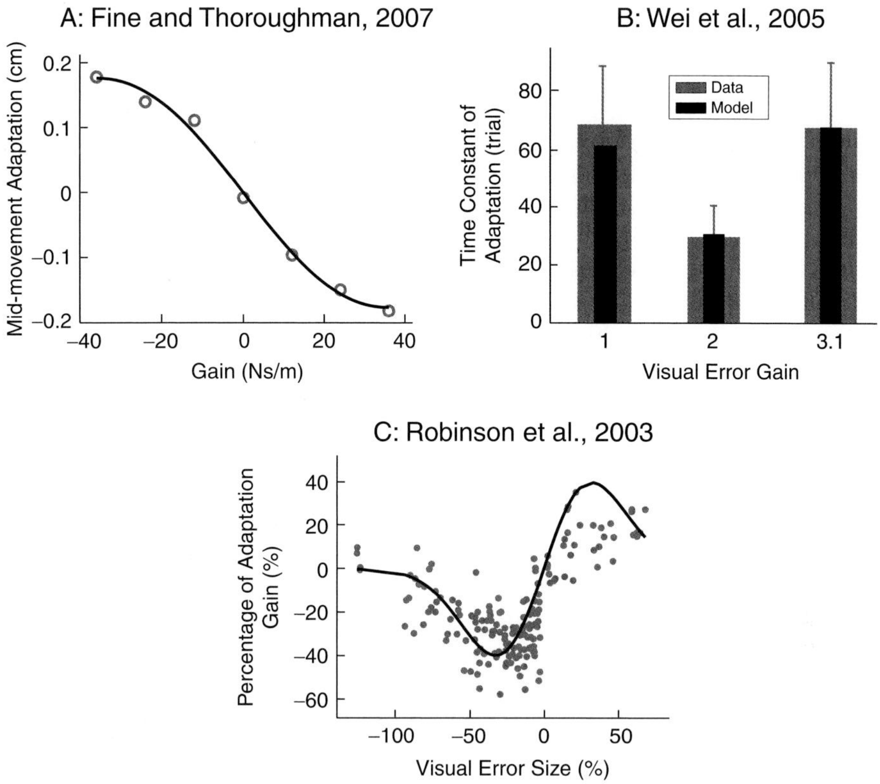


**Figure 2.5** Empirical data from three motor-adaptation studies and the corresponding predictions from the mixture model of causal inference (Wei & Körding, 2008). Gray symbols are for data, and black symbols are for model predictions. (A) Study by Fine and Thoroughman (2007): The amount of adaptation in reaching movements is plotted as a function of the gain of the viscous perturbation (B) Study by Wei et al. (2005): The inverse of the adaptation rate in a visuomotoradaptation task is plotted as a function of visual error gain. (C) Study by Robinson et al (2003): The adaptation gain of saccades is plotted as a function of the visual error size.

To process sensory information for movements correctly, the nervous system should infer the complicated causes in the body and the environment that give rise to the observed error.

Traditional models of motor learning do not assume that the nervous system learns from errors by estimating the sources of errors in terms of the body and the environment. Instead these models usually use a joint representation of the body and the environment. This makes the problem of how to generalize errors to new movements ill defined. If I know that I made an error because my arm is weaker than normal, I will generalize to any movement of that arm but not the other arm. If instead that same error was caused by a different weight of an object in my hand, I will generalize to any movement of the same object but not movements without that object. Without representing the explicit cause of motor errors, this kind of generalization would not be possible.

A recent model has phrased the problem of motor adaptation and generalization in terms of a complicated source-estimation model, in which the causes of errors are inferred (Berniker & Körding, 2008). This model was able to predict correctly experimental results about the way humans generalize from one part of space to another (Shadmehr & Mussa-Ivaldi, 1994). It also explains salient aspects of the way humans generalize from one arm to another (Criscimagna-Hemminger, Donchin,

Gazzaniga, & Shadmehr, 2003; Wang & Sainburg, 2004). Notably, the source-estimation model explains the asymmetry of generalization, where skills learned with the right hand generalize to the left hand but not vice versa. When we make an error with our right hand—whose properties we are very certain of—then we will be inclined to attribute the error to the environment. Alternatively, if we make an error with our left hand, we will be inclined to attribute it to a misestimation of our hand because we are more uncertain about it. It appears that the nervous system naturally interprets movement errors in terms of their underlying causes (Berniker & Körding, 2008).

The many studies on motor adaptation such as the ones listed earlier are typically formulated as questions about whether the nervous system represents the properties of the body (intrinsic) or the environment (extrinsic). A relatively large number of papers present evidence in favor of one or the other of these ideas. In a causal-inference framework, naturally both of these representations exist and any error is attributed to many possible sources depending on the evidence in the observed cues.

### Interaction-Prior Models as an Alternative to Mixture Models

An alternative model to mixture models that has been used to explain nonlinear cue combination is the use of a joint or interaction prior over the cues. Such an interaction prior may be Gaussian or a general lookup table for probabilities (Bresciani, Dammeier, & Ernst, 2006; Ernst & Bülthoff, 2004; Roach et al., 2006; Shams et al., 2005). This prior formalizes the interaction between cues (equivalent to the term $p(v, a)$ in the mixture models example). This model was also formulated in a Bayesian way and has been applied to perceptual tasks where subjects were asked to count the numbers of simultaneously presented visual and tactile stimuli (Bresciani et al., 2006) or of sequentially presented visual and auditory stimuli (Shams et al., 2005), or to perceive the rate of a sequence of visual and auditory stimuli (Roach et al., 2006). All these studies found that increasing temporal difference between cues made subjects more likely to infer distinct causes and induced less interaction between cues. The interaction-prior model produced good fits to these experimental findings.

This type of model is different from mixture models in two aspects. First, it is structurally different (for a detailed mathematical comparison, see Beierholm et al., 2008). The interaction-prior model does not assume two alternative causal relationships between sensory cues and their underlying variables. Instead it simply proposes a prior over the two variables that represent the measurements. In the mixture model, cues can have their own underlying variables, and they can also share the same cause. However, by integrating out the latent (unobserved) variable $C$, the causal-inference model reduces to an interaction prior. However, in this representation we can no longer resolve whether the two cues come from the same cause.

Second, the interaction-prior model either estimates the distribution of the interaction prior via subjects' responses (Shams et al., 2005), or makes assumptions about its specific form (Bresciani et al., 2006; Roach et al., 2006). The mixture model approach, on the other hand, views the prior as the result of causal structure that the nervous system tries to infer. Thus, it offers a normative explanation for the nonlinear effects in cue combination. It has also been found that causal inference explains a number of experimental datasets better than interaction-prior models (Beierholm et al., 2008). However, interaction priors with Gaussian form often result in predicted behavior that is very similar to that found in mixture models, and the nervous system may be using such priors as simple heuristics. Future research will need to discover to what extent humans solve the causal-inference problem or use approximations thereof.

## OPEN QUESTIONS

Causal inference was originally studied in the domain of cognitive science. Studies on perceptual causality revealed that inferring the causality of perceptual cues is an automatic process, and it is largely dissociated from high-level cognitive judgment. Because it is also influenced by high-level factors such as attention, it was postulated that causal inference in perception resides at the intersection of cognitive and perceptual processing (Scholl & Tremoulet, 2000). Evidence of causal inference in cue combination and sensorimotor control in human behavior raises the question of how various cognitive and sensorimotor processes interact.

Causal inference is tightly related to the within-modality binding problem, where the nervous system has to determine which set of stimuli correspond to the same object and should be bound together (Knill, 2003; Reynolds & Desimone, 1999; Treisman, 1996). The link between causal inference (small number of cues) and the binding problems (many cues) is an open question in cue combination.

Lastly, up to now, causal inference has mostly been applied to very simple problems. However, many domains, such as sensorimotor control, have complicated structures and the level to which the nervous system can model complicated causal relations is currently unknown. Many high-level causes exist: Agents have objectives, objects are affected by physics, and the world exhibits many kinds of structure. To what extent the nervous system efficiently accounts for these many levels of structure is an area of intense debate in the field of cognitive science (e.g., Tenenbaum et al., 2006), and it is, in our opinion, a central open question for future research in cue combination and sensorimotor control.

## REFERENCES


Alais, D., & Burr, D. (2004). The ventriloquist effect results from near-optimal bimodal integration. *Current Biology, 14*, 257–262.

Baddeley, R. J., Ingram, H. A., & Miall, R. C. (2003). System identification applied to a visuomotor task: Near-optimal human performance in a noisy changing task. *Journal of Neuroscience, 23*, 3066–3075.

Beierholm, U., Körding, K., Shams, L., & Ma, W. (2008). Comparing Bayesian models for multisensory cue combination without mandatory integration. *Advances in Neural Information Processing Systems, 20*, 81–88.

Berniker, M., & Körding, K. (2008). Estimating the sources of motor errors for adaptation and generalization. *Nature Neuroscience, 11*, 1454–1461.

Brandt, T., Dichgans, J., & Büchele, W. (1974). Motion habituation: Inverted self-motion perception and optokinetic after-nystagmus. *Experimental Brain Research, 21*, 337–352.

Bresciani, J. P., Dammeier, F., & Ernst, M. O. (2006). Vision and touch are automatically integrated for the perception of sequences of events. *Journal of Vision, 6*, 554–564.

Bresciani, J. P., Ernst, M. O., Drewing, K., Bouyer, G., Maury, V., & Kheddar, A. (2005). Feeling what you hear: Auditory signals can modulate tactile tap perception. *Experimental Brain Research, 162*, 172–180.

Brown, L. E., Rosenbaum, D. A., & Sainburg, R. L. (2003). Limb position drift: Implications for control of posture and movement. *Journal of Neurophysiology, 90*, 3105–3118.

Bullock, M., Gelman, R., & Baillargeon, R. (1982). The development of causal reasoning. In W. J. Friedman (Ed.), *The developmental psychology of time* (pp. 209–254). New York, NY: Academic Press.

Calvert, G., & Thesen, T. (2004). Multisensory integration: Methodological approaches and emerging principles in the human brain. *Journal of Physiology, 98*, 191–205.

Cohen, L. B., & Oakes, L. M. (1993). How infants perceive a simple causal event. *Developmental Psychology, 29*, 421–433.

Criscimagna-Hemminger, S. E., Donchin, O., Gazzaniga, M. S., & Shadmehr, R. (2003). Learned dynamics of reaching movements generalize from dominant to nondominant arm. *Journal of Neurophysiology, 89*, 168–176.

Ernst, M. O., & Banks, M. S. (2002). Humans integrate visual and haptic information in a statistically optimal fashion. *Nature, 415*, 429–433.

Ernst, M. O., & Bülthoff, H. H. (2004). Merging the senses into a robust percept. *Trends in Cognitive Sciences, 8*, 162–169.

Fine, M. S., & Thoroughman, K. A. (2007). Trial-by-trial transformation of error into sensorimotor adaptation changes with environmental dynamics. *Journal of Neurophysiology, 98*, 1392–1404.

Frassinetti, F., Pavani, F., & Ladavas, E. (2002). Acoustical vision of neglected stimuli: Interaction among spatially converging audiovisual inputs in neglect patients. *Journal of Cognitive Neuroscience, 14*, 62–69.

Gopnik, A., Glymour, C., Sobel, D. M., Schulz, L. E., Kushnir, T., & Danks, D. (2004). A theory of causal learning in children: Causal maps and Bayes nets. *Psychological Review, 111*, 3–32.

Griffiths, T. L., & Tenenbaum, J. B. (2005). Structure and strength in causal induction. *Cognitive Psychology, 51*, 334–384.

Hairston, W. D., Wallace, M. T., Vaughan, J. W., Stein, B. E., Norris, J. L., & Schirillo, J. A. (2003). Visual localization ability influences cross-modal bias. *Journal of Cognitive Neuroscience, 15*, 20–29.

Harris, C. M., & Wolpert, D. M. (1998). Signal-dependent noise determines motor planning. *Nature, 394*, 780–784.

Hatfield, G. C. (1990). *The natural and normative: Theories of spatial perception from Kant to Helmholtz.* Cambridge, MA: MIT Press.

Helbig, H. B., & Ernst, M. O. (2007). Knowledge about a common source can promote visual-haptic integration. *Perception, 36*, 1523–1533.

Hotting, K., & Roder, B. (2004). Hearing cheats touch, but less in congenitally blind than in sighted individuals. *Psychological Science, 15*, 60–64.

Hume, D. (1987/1739). *A treatise on human nature* (2nd ed.). Oxford, England: Clarendon Press.

Jack, C. E., & Thurlow, W. R. (1973). Effects of degree of visual association and angle of displacement on the "ventriloquism" effect. *Perceptual and Motor Skills, 37*, 967–979.

Kant, I. (1965/1781). *Critique of pure reason.* London, England: Macmillan.

Kawato, M., Furukawa, K., & Suzuki, R. (1987). A hierarchical neural-network model for control and learning of voluntary movement. *Biological Cybernetics, 57*, 169–185.

Knill, D. (2003). Mixture models and the probabilistic structure of depth cues. *Vision Research, 43*, 831–854.

Körding, K., Beierholm, U., Ma, W., Quartz, S., Tenenbaum, J., & Shams, L. (2007). Causal inference in multisensory perception. *PLoS One, 2*(9), e943.

Leslie, A. M. (1982). The perception of causality in infants. *Perception, 11*, 173–186.

Leslie, A. M. (1986). Getting development off the ground: Modularity and the infant perception of causality. In P. van Geert (Ed.), *Theory building in development* (pp. 405–437). New York, NY: North-Holland.

Lewald, J., Ehrenstein, W. H., & Guski, R. (2001). Spatio-temporal constraints for auditory-visual integration. *Behavioral Brain Research, 121*, 69–79.

McDonald, P. (2003). Demonstration by simulation: The philosophical significance of experiment in Helmholtz's theory of perception. *Perspectives on Science, 11*, 170–207.

McGurk, H., & MacDonald, J. (1976). Hearing lips and seeing voices. *Nature, 264*, 746–748.

Michotte, A., & Miles, T. (1963). *The perception of causality.* London, England: Methuen.

Munhall, K., Gribble, P., Sacco, L., & Ward, M. (1996). Temporal constraints on the McGurk effect. *Perception and Psychophysics, 58*, 351–362.

Radeau, M. (1994). Auditory-visual spatial interaction and modularity. *Current Psychology of Cognition, 13*, 3–51.

Reynolds, J. H., & Desimone, R. (1999). The role of neural mechanisms of attention in solving the binding problem. *Neuron, 24*, 19–29, 111–125.

Roach, N., Heron, J., & McGraw, P. (2006). Resolving multisensory conflict: A strategy for balancing the costs and benefits of audio-visual integration. *Proceedings of the Royal Society of London B: Biological Sciences, 273*, 2159–2168.

Robinson, F. R., Noto, C. T., & Bevans, S. E. (2003). Effect of visual error size on saccade adaptation in monkey. *Journal of Neurophysiology, 90*, 1235–1244.

Saxe, R., & Carey, S. (2006). The perception of causality in infancy. *Acta Psychologica, 123*, 144–165.

Scheidt, R. A., Dingwell, J. B., & Mussa-Ivaldi, F. A. (2001). Learning to move amid uncertainty. *Journal of Neurophysiology, 86*, 971–985.

Schlottmann, A., & Shanks, D. R. (1992). Evidence for a distinction between judged and perceived causality. *The Quarterly Journal of Experimental Psychology Section A, 44*, 321–342.

Scholl, B. J., & Leslie, A. M. (1999). Modularity, development and "theory of mind." *Mind and Language, 14*, 131–153.

Scholl, B. J., & Tremoulet, P. D. (2000). Perceptual causality and animacy. *Trends in Cognitive Sciences, 4*, 299–309.

Shadmehr, R., & Mussa-Ivaldi, F. A. (1994). Adaptive representation of dynamics during learning of a motor task. *Journal of Neuroscience, 14*, 3208–3224.

Shams, L., Kamitani, Y., & Shimojo, S. (2000). What you see is what you hear. *Nature, 408*, 788.

Shams, L., Ma, W. J., & Beierholm, U. (2005). Sound-induced flash illusion as an optimal percept. *Neuroreport, 16*, 1923–1927.

Slutsky, D. A., & Recanzone, G. H. (2001). Temporal and spatial dependency of the ventriloquism effect. *Neuroreport, 12*, 7–10.

Sperber, D., & Premack, D. (1995). *Causal cognition: A multidisciplinary debate.* Oxford, England: Oxford University Press.

Stevenson, I., & Körding, K. (2009). *Structural inference affects depth perception in the context of potential occlusion.* In Y. Bengio, D. Schuurmans, J. Lafferty, C. K. I. Williams, & A. Culotta (Eds.). *Advances in Neural Information Processing Systems 22*, 1777–1784.

Tenenbaum, J. B., Griffiths, T. L., & Kemp, C. (2006). Theory–based Bayesian models of inductive learning and reasoning. *Trends in Cognitive Sciences, 10*, 309–318.

Thoroughman, K. A., & Shadmehr, R. (2000). Learning of action through adaptive combination of motor primitives. *Nature, 407*, 742–747.

Treisman, A. (1996). The binding problem. *Current Opinion in Neurobiology, 6*, 171–178.

Wallace, M. T., Roberson, G. E., Hairston, W. D., Stein, B. E., Vaughan, J. W., & Schirillo, J. A. (2004). Unifying multisensory signals across time and space. *Experimental Brain Research, 158*, 252–258.

Wang, J., & Sainburg, R. L. (2004). Interlimb transfer of novel inertial dynamics is asymmetrical. *Journal of Neurophysiology, 92*, 349–360.

Warren, D. H., Welch, R. B., & McCarthy, T. J. (1981). The role of visual-auditory "compellingness" in the ventriloquism effect: Implications for transitivity among the spatial senses. *Perception and Psychophysics, 30*, 557–564.

Wei, K., & Körding, K. P. (2008). Relevance of error: What drives motor adaptation? *Journal of Neurophysiology, 101*, 655–664.

Wei, Y., Bajaj, P., Scheidt, R., & Patton, J. L. (2005). A real-time haptic/graphic demonstration of how error augmentation can enhance learning. *Proceedings of the 2005 IEEE Conference on Robotics and Automation* (pp. 4406–4411). New York, NY: IEEE.

Welch, R. B. (1972). The effect of experienced limb identity upon adaptation to simulated displacement of the visual field. *Perception and Psychophysics, 12*, 453–456.

Welch, R. B., & Warren, D. (1986). Intersensory interactions. In K. R. Boff, L. Kaufman, & J. P. Thomas (Eds.), *Handbook of perception and human performance* (Vol. 1, pp. 25–21). New York, NY: Wiley.

Wolpert, D., & Kawato, M. (1998). Multiple paired forward and inverse models for motor control. *Neural Networks, 11*, 1317–1329.

# CHAPTER 3

## The Role of Generative Knowledge in Object Perception

*Peter W. Battaglia, Daniel Kersten, and Paul Schrater*

## INTRODUCTION

Combining multiple sensory cues is an effective strategy for improving perceptual judgments in principle, but in practice it demands sophisticated processing to extract useful information. Sensory cues are signals from the environment available through sensory modalities; perceptions are internal estimates about the world's state derived from sensory cues and prior assumptions about the world. The influence that world properties have on sensory cues is inherently complicated, so recovering information about the world from sensations is a difficult problem. Imagine trying to analyze measurements from a scientific experiment without knowing the experimental protocol: It is impossible to draw conclusions without knowing the methods by which the raw data were produced. Likewise, converting raw neural sensory signals into perceptual judgments, like the distance to a nearby object or the material it is made of, requires the application of knowledge that is both structured and flexible. In this chapter, we discuss "generative knowledge" as a unifying framework regarding how biological brains overcome these difficulties to interpret sensory cues.

### Challenges for Perception

Perceptual processes translate raw sensory data into high-level interpretations. In doing so, perception solves several major computational challenges:

1) The mapping from sensory data to interpretations can be complex and ill posed. For example, extracting three-dimensional (3D) geometry from two-dimensional (2D) images is fundamentally ambiguous because a multitude of 3D structures can project to any single 2D pattern (Marroquin, Mitter, & Poggio, 1987). More generally, the relationship between each sensory cue and the environmental properties that caused it may be intricate and convoluted (the acoustic vibrations arriving at the eardrum or the pattern of light intensities on the retina have no simple, unambiguous relationship with the position of an object's sound source or its geometric shape).
2) Many sensory cues do not relate directly to the environmental properties of interest, but rather contain "auxiliary" information related to the quality and meaning of other cues. For instance, when judging the distance to a face, knowing its physical size is

irrelevant in isolation, but it can be used to disambiguate the visual image size (Yonas, Pettersen, & Granrud, 1982). Employing auxiliary information is important, but it requires understanding of how the multiple cues are related to each other.

3) Sensory cues vary in quality:
    i) Relative to each other. For instance, vision provides higher spatial resolution than audition, whereas audition provides higher temporal resolution than vision.
    ii) Depending on external factors. For instance, in fog visual cues may provide worse spatial information than auditory cues.
    iii) Depending on internal factors. For instance, cataracts and uncorrected myopia diminish visual acuity.
    iv) As a function of the world state. For instance, binocular stereo cues to slant decrease in reliability as surface slant increases, whereas texture compression cues to slant increase in reliability as the slant increases (Knill, 1998a, 1998b).

    Because of variability in the quality of cues, the brain must know when, and how much, to trust cues' information and when they are too unreliable to be informative (see Chapter 1; Ernst & Banks, 2002; Jacobs, 1999).

4) The arrangements of objects' spatial and material properties in the world follow highly predictable patterns. Though it's possible for objects to appear in an infinite variety of arrangements, we only ever encounter a very small subset of the possible configurations. For instance, water faucets almost exclusively appear in bathrooms and kitchens near waist level. In the absence of particularly strong sensory evidence to the contrary, such knowledge can be used to immediately exclude perceptual scene interpretations that involve a water faucet on the ceiling. Statistical distributions about object properties and context can be learned; these distributions are termed *priors*. Priors offer tremendous benefits for perception by helping overcome ambiguity and impoverished sensations, but because of the vastness and complexity of scene knowledge, knowing how to organize and use it is neither obvious nor trivial (Strat & Fischler, 1991).

### Overcoming Perception's Challenges Using Generative Knowledge

The challenges presented earlier are a consequence of the complex relationships among the set of immediate world properties and the sensory cues they generate. The brain draws percepts from sensations by taking advantage of knowledge about these complex relationships. To study how observers use their knowledge for perception, it is useful to precisely identify the potential sources of this knowledge.

We use the term *sensory generative process* to characterize how sensations are caused by the world. This includes the physical factors that lead to the stimulation of the sensory organs, and the relationships among world properties that make some situations more common than others. Some examples include the optical projection process by which light stimulates the retina, and the typical arrangements of objects in an office that favor large objects being placed on the floor and smaller objects being placed on desks and shelves. In general, the generative process refers to those events that happen before the sensations arrive at the brain and which constrain sensory input in a physically predictable manner.

The term *sensory generative knowledge* refers to built-in assumptions held by the brain about the sensory generative process—it links sensory cues back to the world properties that caused them. An observer who interprets sensory cues in the context of their generative process can make more accurate judgments about the world by combining sensory cues and prior information to constrain possible scene interpretations, which leads to more accurate and robust perceptions.

As an example, consider the relationship between retinal image size and object size. An object's image size on the retina is influenced by two factors, the object's physical size and distance. Image size alone does not allow an observer to unambiguously determine the size or distance: The object could be small and near, or large and far; either situation

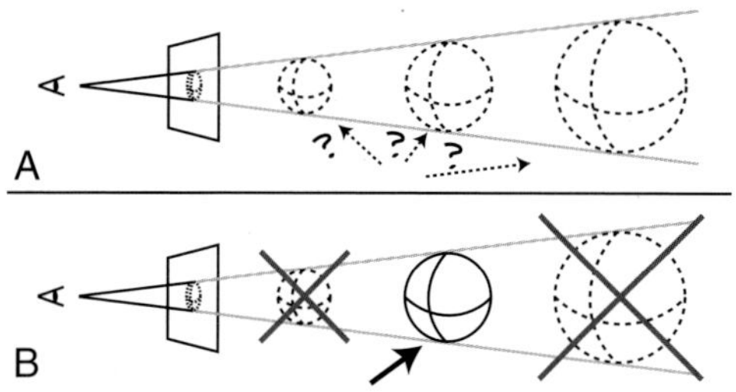

**Figure 3.1** (A) The size of an object's image does not uniquely specify its physical size and distance, only a set of size and distance combinations consistent with the image. (B) If one knows the distance, the size can be uniquely determined; likewise, if one knows the size, the distance can be uniquely determined.

may produce the same image size (Fig. 3.1A). Now, consider the sensory generative process. Because of perspective projection, two factors play a dominant role in determining monocular image size ($I$) (measured in visual angle): the object's physical size ($S$) and distance ($D$). The generative relationship between $S$, $D$, and $I$ can be summarized by the function

$$\frac{S}{D} = I. \tag{3.1}$$

For an observer that has this generative knowledge and can measure $I$, several facts about $S$ and $D$ are immediately apparent. First, it is possible to solve for the precise value of $S$ only if $D$ is known, and it is possible to solve for $D$ precisely only if $S$ is known: It is not possible to solve one equation for two unknowns. However, if an auxiliary cue to size or distance is available, estimating the other becomes possible (Fig. 3.1B). Second, if information about either $S$ or $D$ is available, but uncertain, this provides uncertain information about the other. For instance, if you are told that $S$ is between 1 and 2 meters in diameter, and $I$ is 1/10 radians, you can infer that $D$ is between 10 and 20 meters.

This simple illustration shows how generative knowledge can help overcome the ill-posed, ambiguous nature of perception through auxiliary cues (challenges 1 and 2 presented earlier). When judging an object's distance, cues to its physical size, although independent of distance, can nonetheless be used to disambiguate the causes of the extent of the image on the retina.

Sensory cues vary in quality (challenge 3), and an observer who knows the relative reliability of available sensory cues can differentially incorporate cues of varying quality to form more accurate perceptions. Consider an experiment in which an object is viewed binocularly and the observer also reaches out and touches it. Thus, at least two cues are available to the object distance: vergence angle and felt arm position while touching the object (haptic cue). If one cue were less reliable than the other, it should be allowed less influence on the perceptual judgment. For instance, if vergence angle is a more reliable cue to the distance, then in an experiment in which the two cues are set in conflict (meaning they indicate different distances), the observer's perceptual distance judgment would more closely reflect the vergence-indicated distance than the haptic-indicated distance.

Exploiting knowledge of how world properties relate to other world properties (challenge 4) can be useful for constraining possible perceptual interpretations. In the size/distance example, if the observer recognizes that the object whose size is being judged is a face, this provides a strong restriction on possible sizes because the variance among face sizes is very small. Alternatively, if the observer is trying to judge the distance to the object, the prior knowledge that face sizes fall in a tight range can be used to rule out size/distance combinations that are inconsistent with the size prior. More generally, almost every perceptual behavior is heavily influenced by contextual information (Biederman, 1972; Oliva & Torralba, 2007). For instance, a large, horizontally extended object on a street is likely a car, whereas a vertically extended object indoors is likely a person.

### Generating Perceptual Samples

Although some kinds of generative knowledge can be embodied in a purely feedforward inference process, mechanisms that use generative knowledge to hypothesize new instances that have never been experienced can provide considerably more flexible and robust visual inferences (Yuille & Kersten, 2006). Such generative models of the world provide a functional link between world properties and sensory cues that can take a hypothesized world property and compute its probable sensory consequences. Such generative knowledge is believed to form a critical part of the motor control system, called a *forward model* (Kawato, 1999), that predicts the afferent sensations that will result from motor commands. Much less is known about the existence of sophisticated generative models for perception; however, neural predictive-coding models posit that the brain has higher level perceptual processing sites that generate predictions of sensory input at lower levels (Mumford, 1992; Rao & Ballard, 1999). In addition, humans' dreams and visual imagery abilities suggest generating perceptual samples is possible. For example, imagine you are looking at a kitchen. Immediately items like refrigerators, stoves, sinks, and tables come to mind, and you can provide likely colors, sizes, and positions of such objects. The particular kitchen you conjure may be a kitchen you have seen in the past, but it is also possible to imagine a new kitchen you have never before seen. The ability to visualize and imaginatively construct unobserved scenes may reflect the operation of complex generative models of the visual world. Lastly, predicting causal chains of events, like a tennis ball's future position after a series of bounces, can be aided by an approximate generative model of elastic collisions and momentum.

In the next (second) section, we introduce the theoretical issues concerning generative knowledge in the context of Bayesian inference and the joint roles of sensory cues and prior knowledge for perceptual inference. In the third section, we present empirical results that support the brain's use of sensory generative knowledge. In the fourth section, we discuss inference of world properties when nuisance properties confound available cues.

## THE BAYESIAN OBSERVER MODEL

### Background

Bayesian inference is a model for perception that has achieved broad support for several reasons (Knill & Pouget, 2004; Körding & Wolpert, 2006). Methodologically, it is a principled, rigorous language for probabilistic models suitable for characterizing perceptual inference based on sensations and prior knowledge. As described earlier, perception solves the frequent problem of ambiguity due to the noninvertibility of sensations; formally, inference is a process of inversion under uncertainty in which a set of possibilities are obtained, rather than a unique solution. Bayesian models naturally describe the combination of prior knowledge and available sensory cues, as well as how observers learn from experience to make better-informed judgments in the future, both of which are common phenomena in biological perception. Through Bayesian models, numerous studies have reported optimal and near-optimal performance across a gamut of perception tasks (for a review, see Kersten, Mamassian, & Yuille, 2004). Of equal importance, failures of optimality provide an opportunity for identifying limitations in neural processing and deviations between human and model assumptions (see Chapter 8).

### Perception as Bayesian Inference

As presented in Chapter 1, Bayes' rule specifies how to optimally combine measurements and prior information to gain information about unobserved quantities, a computation termed *Bayesian inference.* In biological perception, the brain directly measures sensory cues but does not directly measure external world properties. By treating both cues and world properties as *random variables*, and quantifying their respective conditional and marginal probability distributions, Bayesian inference provides a probability distribution over possible world states that can be used to make optimal scene estimates. Bayesian models provide a powerful normative framework for describing and evaluating theories of perceptual behavior.

Let the relevant state of the world, or those properties the observer is interested in, be represented by $R$, and direct sensory measurements by $D$. Bayes' rule specifies:

$$P(R|D) = \frac{P(D|R)P(R)}{P(D)}, \quad (3.2)$$

where $P(D|R)$ is the *conditional likelihood* of D given $R$, $P(R)$ is the *prior probability* of $R$, $P(D)$ is the *marginal likelihood* of D, and $P(R|D)$ is the *posterior probability* of $R$ given $D$. The term $P(D|R)$ represents the generative relationship between world properties $R$ and sensory cues $D$.

We can use these variables to represent elements from the size- and distance-perception example in the previous section. Consider an observer who is trying to judge the distance to a ball; we represent distance as the relevant variable, $R$. Assume the observer reaches out and touches the ball, so that the felt arm position provides a direct distance cue, $D$. We represent the conditional relationship of the sensory cue given the relevant world property as $P(D|R)$ (Fig. 3.2, dashed curve). We represent prior knowledge about different ball distances as $P(R)$ (Fig. 3.2, dotted curve). For this example the prior specifies the ball's probable distance before

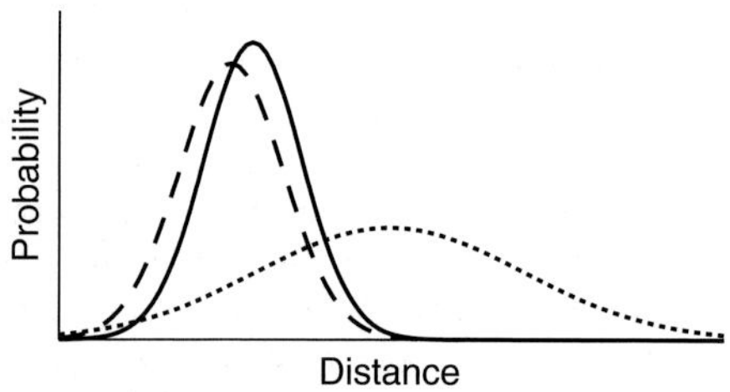


**Figure 3.2** The dashed curve represents the conditional likelihood of a sensory cue given different distances. The dotted curve represents the prior probability distribution over different distances. The solid curve represents the posterior probability distribution over different distances given the cue; note that its peak lies between the likelihood and prior peaks—closer to the peak specified by the more reliable, likelihood function.

considering specific sensory cues; in this case, it may reflect knowledge that the ball is between 1 and 2 meters from the observer. The term $P(D)$ characterizes the probability of receiving cue $D$. For any particular sensory cue, $P(D)$ is constant and because the right-hand side is a probability distribution (that integrates to one), $P(D)$ is fully determined by $P(D|R)P(R)$. Bayesian inference proceeds by merging the cue likelihood and distance prior to form a posterior probability distribution over the possible ball distances.

## Bayes' Nets

Pearl (1988) introduced Bayes' nets (see examples in Fig. 3.3) as directed, acyclic graphical models that express the conditional probability relationships among multiple random variables and their prior probability distributions. Bayes' nets are a useful tool for describing sensory generative processes and the requisite inference rules because they allow graphical expressions of properties that otherwise must be represented by dense symbolic notation. And perhaps more important, they allow similarities among seemingly unrelated sensation-perception behaviors to be recognized by the modeler. The circles, called *nodes* (Fig. 3.3), represent random variables. Nodes that have no parents, termed *roots,* have prior probability distributions over their possible values. The arrows connecting the nodes, called *edges,* represent conditional probability distributions among random variables. In sensory generation, conditional dependencies (edges) typically represent causal relationships. For instance, the node labeled $R$ in Figure 3.3A can represent the ball's distance and $D$ can represent the haptically sensed arm position cue from the size-distance example in the previous subsection. The arrow connecting them represents the conditional likelihood function of sensory cue given distance. In general, the direction of an edge is arbitrary (the edge in Fig. 3.3A represents $P(D|R)$, but if its direction were reversed would represent $P(R|D)$). Modelers choose directions that best suit the problem and system being modeled. For perceptual inference, the generative process relates to the forward direction from world to sensations; the inference process is the reverse

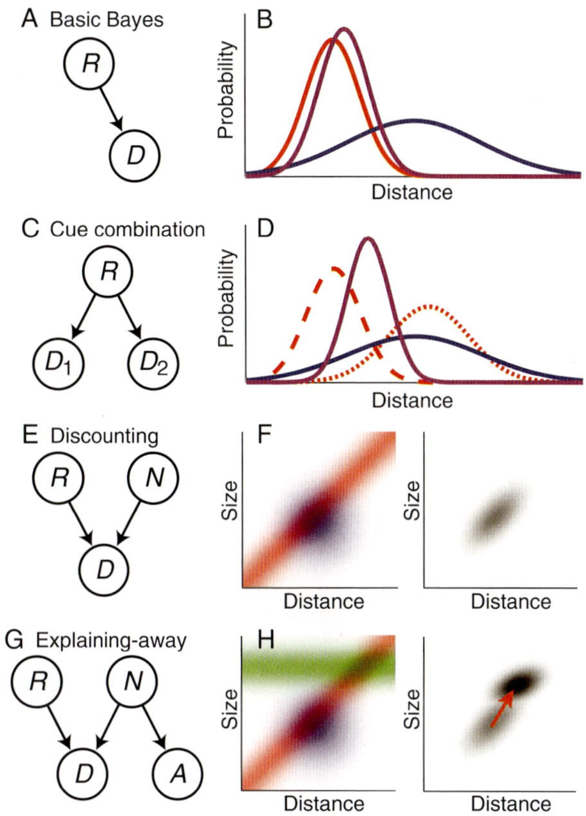


**Figure 3.3** (A) Basic Bayes: A relevant world property, *R*, causes a direct cue, *D*. (B) The optimal inference strategy is to combine cue likelihood (red curve) with the prior assumption about the relevant property (blue curve) to compute a posterior probability distribution (purple curve). Note that the prior probability distribution is over the root node, *R*. (C) Cue combination: A relevant world property, *R*, causes two likelihood (red dashed/dotted curves) with the prior assumption about the relevant property (flat, blue curve) to compute a posterior probability distribution (purple curve). Bayes' rule prescribes calculating their product. (E) Discounting: Two world properties cause a direct cue, *D*. The observer needs to perceive the relevant world property, *R*, and not the nuisance property, *N*, but *R* is ambiguous given only the sensory cue. (F) The optimal inference strategy is to combine the cue likelihood (red distribution, left) with the prior assumptions about the nuisance and relevant properties (blue distribution, left) to compute a posterior probability distribution (gray distribution, right). Bayes' rule prescribes calculating their product. The prior assumptions disambiguate the sensory measurement. (G) Explaining away: Two world properties, relevant, *R*, and nuisance, *N*, cause a direct cue, *D*, and auxiliary cue, *A*. The observer needs to perceive *R*, but not *N*, but *R* is ambiguous given only the cue. Though *A* is not directly related to *R*, it provides information about *N* that can disambiguate *R*. (H) The optimal inference strategy is to combine the direct (red distribution, left) and auxiliary cue likelihoods (green distribution, left) with the prior assumptions about the nuisance and relevant properties (blue distribution, left) to compute a posterior probability distribution (black distribution, right). The prior assumptions and auxiliary cues disambiguate the sensory measurement. The arrow shows how the discounting posterior distribution (panel F) shifts (as well as tightening to become more peaked) as a result of the auxiliary cue.

direction, from sensory cues to world properties. As a terminology note, we use the term *direct* to refer to cues that are connected to relevant states by an edge. In contrast, the term *auxiliary* is used to refer to cues that do not share an edge with any relevant states but are connected by a sequence of edges between intermediate nodes.

### Generative Knowledge in Bayesian Inference

Figure 3.3 illustrates four elementary sensory generative process models (Kersten et al., 2004). These are not unique or exclusive; there may be more than one way to characterize a sensory circumstance. Instead they can be thought of as choices made by the modeler to characterize particular sensation-perception events in an accurate yet succinct manner. As an extreme example, ambient air temperature affects the index of refraction between air and eye, and thus influences the visual generative process, but the impact is negligible so the modeler can choose to ignore it.

Figures 3.3A and 3.3B represent situations in which a single world property causes a single cue and follows a relatively straightforward generative process. Some examples include a moving object producing a moving image on an observer's retina, the distance to an object being measured by binocular vergence, and the position of a sound source being sensed through interaural auditory differences. Inference in this situation, termed *basic Bayes*, is performed by inverting the nondeterministic functional relationship between the cue and world property, and combining this information with prior knowledge about the world property like the example in the previous subsection.

Figures 3.3C and 3.3D represent situations in which a single world property causes multiple cues. Some examples include a surface producing binocular stereo and texture compression cues to its slant, the distance to an object being measured by binocular vergence and felt arm position, and the position of a sound source being sensed through interaural auditory differences and visual cues. Inference here, termed *cue combination*, is similar to the basic Bayes case. It is performed by inverting the direction of influence between each cue and world property, and combining these inverted relationships with prior knowledge about the world property.

Figures 3.3E and 3.3F represent situations in which multiple world properties influence one cue. Some examples include illuminant intensity and surface reflectance causing a sensed luminance cue, or an object's size and distance each influencing its monocular image size. When an observer infers one (relevant) world property among other, nuisance properties, termed *discounting*, the cue only can constrain the possible relevant property values to a set of relevant-/nuisance-value combinations. Prior knowledge about the nuisance property must be used to rule out unlikely relevant/nuisance combinations.

Figures 3.3G and 3.3H represent situations in which multiple world properties influence multiple cues; the cues can be divided into those that are *directly* influenced by the relevant world property, and auxiliary ones that are only *indirectly* related to the relevant world variable. Some examples include a surface's shape and reflectance each influencing a sensed luminance cue and the shape also influencing a visual geometry cue, an object's size and distance each influencing its sensed image size and the distance also influencing a binocular vergence cue, and two spatially separated sound sources each causing interaural auditory difference cues and one source also causing a visual cue to its position. When an observer infers one (relevant) world property among other, nuisance properties, termed *explaining away*, the direct, confounded cue only can constrain the possible relevant property values to a set of possible relevant/nuisance value combinations (as in discounting). However, auxiliary cues (those not directly related to the relevant world property) and prior knowledge about the nuisance property can be used to rule out unlikely relevant/nuisance combinations.

The conditional-likelihood and prior-probability terms implicitly dictate how strongly the sensory cues and prior knowledge should influence the final perceptual inference. When sensory information propagates backward through the generative structure in inference, the uncertainty in the conditional distribution determines the relative impact of the information: For conditional dependencies with low uncertainty the information is very influential; for high uncertainty the information plays a lesser role. The same is true for the uncertainty in prior probability distributions.

### Discounting and Explaining Away

Discounting and explaining-away inference processes critically depend on generative knowledge. It is easier to conceive noninferential, associative learning systems that conduct cue-combination-like inference, even using relative cue reliability, but it is difficult to contrive reasoning patterns like "explaining away" without generative knowledge and Bayesian inference. Thus, discounting and explaining-away phenomena form stronger tests of humans' use of generative knowledge for perceptual inference than cue combination. However, new analysis tools must be developed for testing discounting and explaining-away phenomena that entail more complex ideal-observer models. The fourth section presents a novel framework for analyzing more complex ideal-observer models.

The following section reviews qualitative reports of perceptual discounting and explaining away.

## EXPERIMENTAL EVIDENCE FOR THE USE OF GENERATIVE KNOWLEDGE: DISCOUNTING AND EXPLAINING AWAY

Observers frequently receive ambiguous sensory input, which makes interpreting the scene challenging because more than one possible interpretation could be correct. Perceptual discounting and explaining away are behaviors that overcome this problem using generative knowledge.

### Discounting

Studies of perceptual discounting have found evidence that shape-from-shading perception is influenced by prior assumptions about illuminant direction in accordance with the generative relationship between shape, illumination, and sensed luminance. Mamassian and Goutcher (2001) measured human observers' estimates of an object's shape from shading cues, which require an assumption about what direction the light arrives from, to be useful. This prior knowledge helps to disambiguate the otherwise ambiguous shading cue. Mamassian and Landy (2001) investigated how multiple priors' weights are decided by the brain, specifically lighting direction and surface slant priors, and concluded that the weights reflect their relative reliabilities. Adams, Graf, and Ernst (2004) modified observers' light direction priors by providing haptic feedback that suggested a different lighting direction than the default overhead assumption.

### Explaining Away

Some of the most striking examples of perceptual explaining away can be demonstrated with ambiguous, especially bistable, stimuli. Bistable stimuli are those that have more than one perceptual interpretation, and when viewing the stimuli the perceptual experience spontaneously "flips" between interpretations with a period of roughly 5–45 seconds, though sometimes much longer. Examples include the "Necker cube" and kinetic-depth-effect rotating cylinders (see Chapter 9 for a picture). Studies have shown (Blake, Sobel, & James, 2004; James & Blake, 2004) that by providing an auxiliary sensory cue, like binocular stereo or haptic input, the bistability can be reduced or removed altogether. This auxiliary cue serves to explain away particular stable interpretations that are inconsistent with the cue.

Knill and Kersten (1991) reported a clear instance of perceptual explaining away in which an object's surface shape affects observers' judgments of albedo, consistent with a generative model that explains away the effect of the shape on the luminance. Figure 3.4 illustrates Knill and Kersten's (1991) stimuli in which generative knowledge allows auxiliary shape cues to disambiguate an otherwise ambiguous luminance cue to the albedo of a surface (adapted from Knill & Kersten, 1991). In the upper row, the grayscale image shows two objects

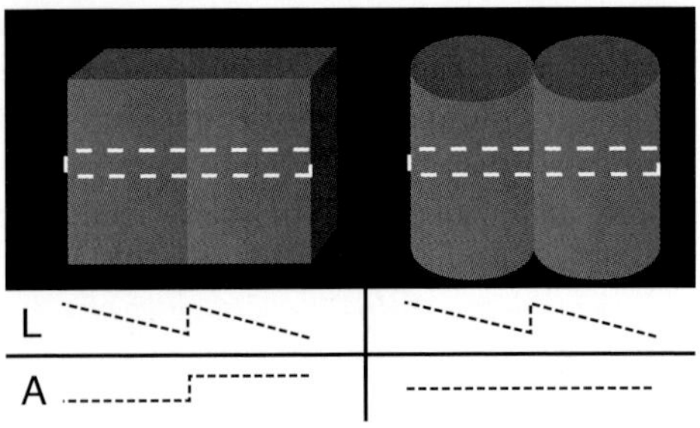


**Figure 3.4** The image depicts two objects with different shapes, yet the luminance profiles within the dotted boxes are identical for both objects, as plotted below the objects in the row labeled "L". The perceived albedo, plotted in the row labeled "A", is different for the different objects.

with different shapes. The observer's task is to decide what the albedo is in a horizontal cross-section across each object (dashed white boxes). Under the image, the rows represent the actual luminance profile of the pixels across each object (labeled "L"), and the perceived albedo profile across each object for a typical observer (labeled "A"). The perceived albedo profiles are due to the different perceived shapes of the objects, indicated by their respective edge cues. In the left object, because the shape looks flat on the front, the luminance difference across the object's center is attributed to variation in albedo. In the right object, the left side of each cylinder is perceived to face the light source more directly; changing albedo is not required to explain the luminance differences across the center of the object.

Figure 3.3G shows the graphical model that characterizes this perceptual-inference problem. The relevant property ($R$) represents the object's albedo/reflectance, the nuisance property ($N$) represents the object's surface shape, the direct cue ($D$) is the luminance, and the auxiliary cue ($A$) is the object's boundary contour that provides direct information about surface shape. Luminance is a function of both surface shape and albedo (and light source intensity and direction, too, but here we assume they are constant). The observer's perceptual task is to estimate the albedo, but the effect that shape has on luminance must be explained away in order to disambiguate the albedo. Because there is auxiliary boundary contour information that provides an independent estimate of the shape, the shape's impact on luminance can be explained away and the albedo unambiguously estimated. The observer requires knowledge of how shape and albedo generate the image data (boundary contour and luminance) to use it for perceptual estimation.

## Size- and Distance-Perception Experiments

The influence of auxiliary distance cues on human size perception has received much attention for more than a half century. However, few studies measuring the influence of size cues on distance perception have been reported, and no experiments have investigated how cues to an object's changing distance influences perception of whether, and to what degree, its size changes.

Holway and Boring (1941) found size constancy (in which perceived size is proportional to object size) was best facilitated by providing many, strong distance cues, though others (Epstein, Park, & Casey, 1961; Gogel, Wist, & Harker, 1963; Ono, 1966) concluded that size constancy was subject to a variety of failures. Epstein et al. (1961) and other authors (Brenner & van Damme, 1999; Gruber & Dinnerstein, 1965; Heinemann & Nachmias, 1965; Ono, Muter, & Mitson, 1974) acknowledge that distance judgments are not always veridical (apparent distances do not always match physical distances), which accounts for some size misperceptions, and specific experimental design choices and task demands often contribute to the nature of the experiment's recorded failure of size constancy (Blessing, Landauer, & Coltheart, 1967; Kaufman & Rock, 1962; Mon-Williams & Tresilian, 1999).

Several studies investigated humans' use of size information for making distance judgments. Granrud, Haake, and Yonas (1985) showed that 7-month-old infants who were allowed to learn the size of different objects by playing with them used the size to judge the distance in postplay test phases. In contrast, 5-month-old infants did not exhibit the use of size information for distance judgments, suggesting the development of knowledge about size and distance occurs as early as 5–6 months old. Yonas, Granrud, and Pettersen (1985) showed that when presented with two objects of different retinal visual angles, infants older than 5 months perceived the larger as nearer, but not 5-month-olds. Yonas, Pettersen, and Granrud (1982) showed that 7-month-old infants' and adults' distance judgments are influenced by familiar-size information associated with faces, but 5-month-olds are insensitive to familiar size. These results suggest that size information can influence distance judgments.

We now describe results from two experiments, one investigates how sensory measurements of depth changes influence judgments of physical object size changes, and a second in which measurements of size influence a depth-dependent action.

The role of auxiliary distance information in size perception was addressed by a recent study. Battaglia et al. (2010) conducted an experiment in which they presented participants with balls that moved in depth and simultaneously either inflated or deflated, and they asked participants to decide "inflation" or "deflation" for each stimulus. The experimenters provided binocular and haptic cues to the ball's distance change to test the effect these auxiliary sensory cues had on size-change perception. They reasoned that because objects do not usually change in size, if participants make use of the auxiliary cues they must have general knowledge of the relationship between size and distance, and not simply exploit a learned association between the auxiliary sensory cues and size-change perception. The results were that in the absence of auxiliary cues, participants relied on prior assumptions that the object was stationary to judge the size change proportional to the image size change, and they made perceptual mistakes in cases when the distance change had a large, opposite effect on image size than the physical size change. But both the binocular and haptic cues were effective in nulling that bias by providing disambiguating distance-change information. Interestingly, binocular cues were more effective than haptic cues, which may reflect observers' weaker "trust" of haptic cues due to possible dissociation from the visual object. They concluded that humans must have knowledge of the relationship between size, distance, image size, and the auxiliary distance cues to make these perceptual judgments.

Figure 3.5 depicts one participant's data in Battaglia e al. (2010)'s experiment; H refers to "haptic" auxiliary cues, B means "binocular" auxiliary cues, a plus sign means the cue was present, and a minus sign means the cue was absent. Notice that in the case with no haptic and no binocular auxiliary cues (labeled H–/B–), those stimuli perceived as "inflating" (gray region) were predicted by whether the image size was growing or shrinking (black, diagonal, dashed line). When haptic and/or binocular cues were available (labeled H+/B–, H–/B+, H+/B+), participants' perception of inflating balls changed to reflect the true physical size change more accurately.

Battaglia, Schrater, and Kersten (2005) conducted an experiment in which participants were asked to intercept a moving ball that varied in size across trials, by positioning their hand at a distance of their choice. The participant's hand was constrained so that it could only move along the line of sight, and the ball moved from left to right, crossing the hand's constraint line at variable distance. The hand's distance placement was considered to be a measure of the participant's percept of the ball's distance. In some trials the participants were allowed preinterception haptic interaction with the ball, which provided an auxiliary cue to the ball's size. By comparing participants' distance judgments in the "haptic auxiliary cue" condition with those in the "no haptic auxiliary cue" condition for trials with identical ball image sizes, experimenters were able to measure participants' abilities to explain away the confounding influence of the ball's physical size on the image size. The distance judgments of an "explaining-away observer" should be less dependent on the physical size than the distance judgments of an observer with no auxiliary information (for one participant, Fig. 3.6). Figure 3.7 summarizes all participants' results, which support the hypothesis that participants explain away the influence of physical size when making distance

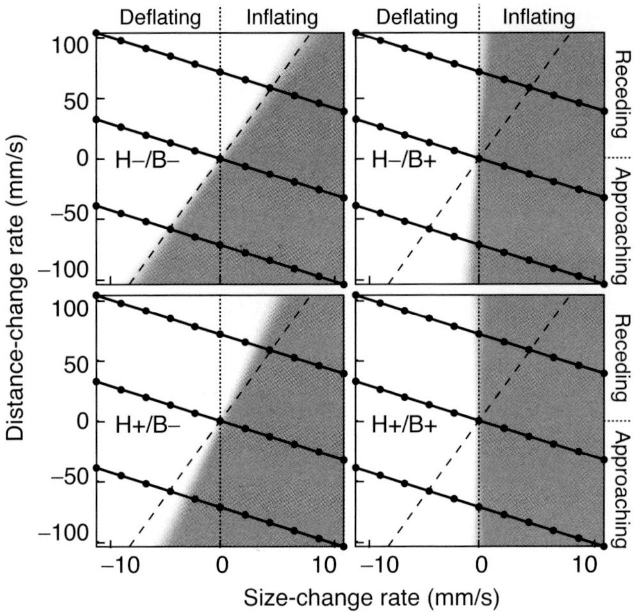


**Figure 3.5** One participant's judgments of balls as inflating (gray) or deflating (white) balls. Each box represents a unique combination of haptic and binocular distance cues (indicated by "H* / B*" on the left side of each box). The black dots represent different size- and distance-change stimulus values. The black diagonal dashed line represents those stimuli whose image size did not change; left of the line indicates shrinking image sizes, and right of the line indicates growing image sizes. The black vertical dotted line indicates the true boundary between inflating and deflating balls. We interpolated between the 50% points of psychometric functions across the solid diagonal lines to estimate the gray/white, inflation/deflation boundaries. When haptic and binocular distance cues are available, the participant's judgments of which stimuli were inflating became more accurate because the confounding influence of distance on image size was explained away by the auxiliary distance cue.

judgments. In particular, Figure 3.7A depicts the correlation between participants' distance judgments and the balls' physical sizes and shows that participants' distance judgments were less dependent on the ball's physical size when auxiliary size cues were available to explain away the size confound. Figure 3.7B shows that interception performance improved as a result of this explaining-away reasoning.

## INFERENCE IN THE PRESENCE OF NUISANCE WORLD PROPERTIES

Until now our discussion has dealt with normative models of perceptual inference, and we have presented *qualitative* evidence that observers use generative knowledge to make perceptual judgments. To model perceptual inference *quantitatively*, a Bayesian observer model is required. We now describe how to use a behavioral experiment to test, and estimate parameters of, such a model.

It is important to realize that for more complex perceptual-inference situations, like discounting and explaining away (Fig. 3.3), the observer requires generative knowledge to interpret input sensations and prior knowledge. An important question is: What generative knowledge does the human observer possess? On the one hand, it seems unlikely that observers know the exact nature and quality of each sensory cue's relationship with the world. On the other hand, human observers' excellent perceptual performance across a wide range of tasks suggests that they use very sophisticated strategies that

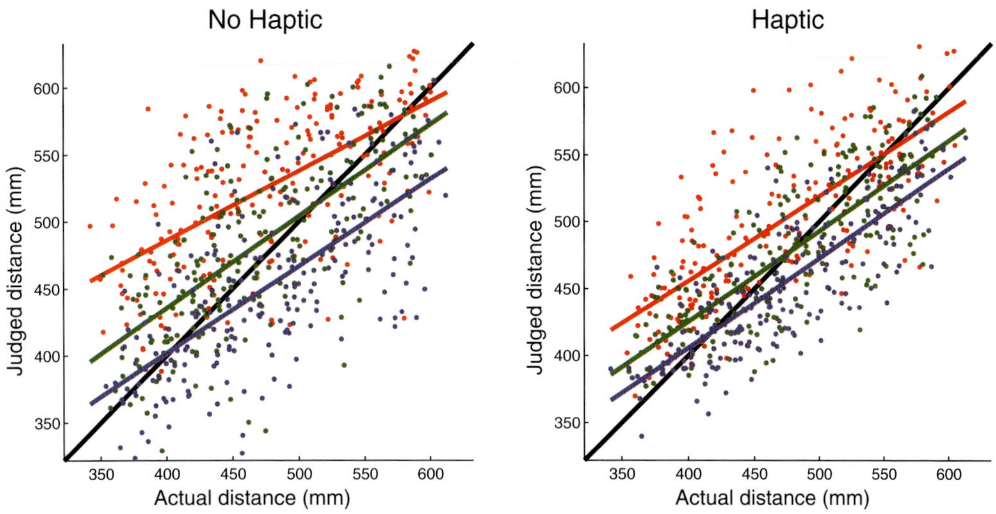


**Figure 3.6** These scatter plots show a typical participant's interception behavior. Each dot represents a single trial's data point; red were smaller balls, green were medium balls, and blue were large balls. The x-axis shows the actual distance of the ball. The y-axis shows the participant's judged distance. The black diagonal line shows the line that indicates perfect judgments. The colored lines are regression fits to the small, medium, and large balls, with color corresponding to the dot colors. The left figure shows the no-auxiliary-haptic-size-cue condition; the right figure shows the condition in which the auxiliary haptic size cue was provided.

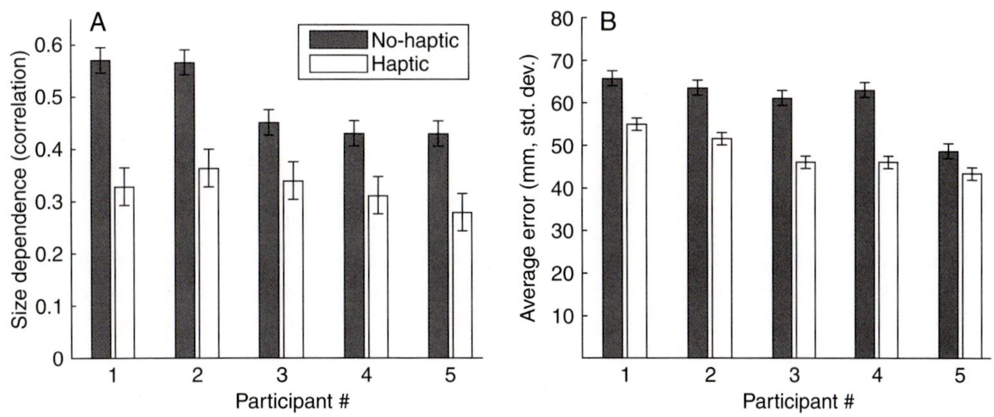


**Figure 3.7** (A) Each pair of bars represents the correlation between distance judgments and ball size for one participant; the gray bars depict the "no-auxiliary-size-cue" condition, and the white bars depict the "haptic-auxiliary-size-cue" condition. All participants' distance judgments are less correlated with the physical size cue when auxiliary information is available to disambiguate the image size cue. (B) Each pair of bars represents participants' average error (standard deviation of distance judgments). Auxiliary cues improved all participants' performance.

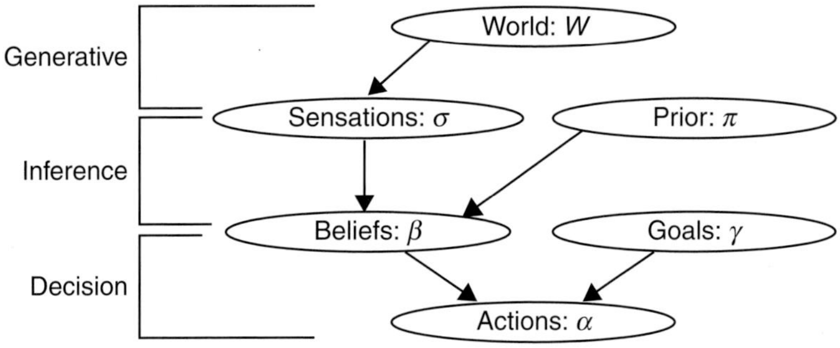


**Figure 3.8** Full psychophysical-observer model. The sensation process is characterized by the sensory generative process in which world properties ($W$) produce sensory input ($\sigma$) in the observer. Perception is characterized by the inference process in which the observer combines sensory cues ($\sigma$) with prior knowledge ($\pi$) to compute beliefs ($\beta$) about the state of the external environment ($W$). Actions are characterized by the decision-making process in which the observer combines beliefs ($\beta$) with goals ($\gamma$) to select actions ($\alpha$) that are predicted to result in highest reward. This model can be formally quantified using the Bayesian decision-theoretic formalism, provided in Eq. 1.5 in Chapter 1.

may include detailed internal knowledge of generative processes. The remainder of this section describes a formal framework to analyze this question.

### Generative Processes versus Knowledge

The distinction between the sensory generative process and an observer's generative knowledge must be recognized when modeling an observer's performance in a psychophysical task. The generative process entails how the world produces sensory cues through physical processes and the statistical regularities of natural scenes that are external to the observer. Generative knowledge is the observer's model, or understanding, of the generative process that is either built in or acquired through experience. For *subjectively* optimal Bayesian inference, the observer uses its generative knowledge in accordance with Bayes' rule for inference. However, for the stronger case of *objectively* optimal Bayesian inference, the generative knowledge also accurately reflects the true generative process.

Figure 3.8 represents a model observer who receives sensory cues from the world (labeled "generative"), integrates prior assumptions with those cues to form perceptual inferences (labeled "inference"), and selects actions based on those inferences and its internal goals (labeled "decision"). Though it does not capture phenomena like attention, sensorimotor feedback, or learning, this framework is very useful for quantifying how a psychophysical observer produces responses based on input stimuli.

The state of the world is represented by the top node and is labeled $W$; the actor's sensory cues are labeled $\sigma$; the actor's prior knowledge is labeled $\pi$; the actor's inferred state of the world, or *beliefs*[1] about the world, are labeled $\beta$; the actor's goals are labeled $\gamma$; and the actor's actions are labeled $\alpha$. The arrow from $W \to \sigma$ represents the sensory generative process; the arrows from $\sigma \to \beta$ and $\pi \to \beta$ represent the perceptual inference process, which is guided by generative knowledge; and the arrows from $\beta \to \alpha$ and $\gamma \to \alpha$ represent the decision process by which the actor chooses actions in response to his or her beliefs about the world and internal goals. The actor has access to sensory cues, $\sigma$; prior knowledge, $\pi$; beliefs about the world, $\beta$; and goals, $\gamma$. Although the actor controls his or her actions, the actual outcome of the actions, $\alpha$, varies with respect to the intended behavior.

[1] The term *belief* is used in a statistical sense, referring to information held by the observer about the external world state.

The experimenter has access to the world state, $W$, and action measurements, $\alpha$.

This modeling framework allows an experimenter to manipulate $W$ in order to study the generative, inference, and decision processes within observers. An ideal-observer model (see Chapter 1) can be used to parameterize the experimentalist's assumptions and hypotheses about the generative, inference, and decision processes for a psychophysical observer, and to compute predicted actions $\alpha$, given $W$. In this way behavioral measurements can be directly compared to model predictions and used to estimate the model's parameter values. When observers' behaviors outperform suboptimal models, these models can be immediately dismissed. Observers' deviations from optimality (see Chapter 8) suggest their use of heuristics, which may be more easily pinpointed by considering the ideal-observer model. Additionally, because of the relationship between human generative knowledge and the true generative process, the estimated *generative knowledge* model parameters can be compared to the estimated *generative process* parameters to assess the quality of the observer's knowledge. Generally ideal-observer predictions allow experimentalists to classify observers into three groups: (1) those who have accurate generative knowledge and make optimal perceptual inferences (objectively optimal observer), (2) those who are suboptimal because they apply inaccurate generative knowledge in a Bayes-consistent manner (subjectively optimal observer), and (3) those who are suboptimal because they do not draw perceptual conclusions in accordance with Bayesian inference rules at all.

This modeling framework also allows the experimenter to ensure a proposed experiment has sufficient power to adequately test a hypothesis. Often there are many assumptions and unknown parameters in a model, and a single experiment is insufficient to distinguish between all possibilities. In this case, multiple tasks may be necessary to estimate them unambiguously. For instance, this is why most experiments include control studies—to isolate certain parameters and reduce the number of parameters each experiment effectively estimates. This framework lets the experimenter simulate the experiment using ideal-observer-model predictions ahead of time to determine whether the experiment is sensitive and selective for distinguishing among individual hypotheses.

### Limitations of Bayes' Nets and Statically Structured Generative Models

While humans incorporate vast contextual information to aid perception (Oliva & Torralba, 2007), Bayes' nets are best suited for representing situations in which several property variables are known to exist, but their state is uncertain. This limits the set of perceptual situations well characterized by Bayes' nets because the structures are predefined, and modifying them is not trivial. For instance, the generative process of a kitchen may not be well modeled by a Bayes' net because some objects may occur only infrequently (e.g., a waffle maker), may have widely varying sets of parts (e.g., overhead lamps can have very different numbers/types of bulbs), and exhibit unique hierarchical and recurrent patterns (e.g., a faucet is typically part of a sink but may instead be part of a refrigerator door). Although theoretically Bayes' nets are able to model such generative processes, they are inefficient because many nodes will never take values. Moreover, an interesting structure that constrains the set of possible scenes is not explicitly or efficiently represented. Nonparametric methods have recently been applied in computer-vision applications to overcome this type of problem and aid visual inference (Sudderth & Jordan, 2009; Sudderth, Torralba, Freeman, & Willsky, 2008). These models use Bayes-net formalism to define abstract relationships among classes of objects and scenes, and nonparametric clusters to characterize specific instances of objects and scenes. This allows the models to share properties across similar objects and scenes while allowing specific instances to have unique and rich properties of their own.

Graph grammars are models that define rules for creating graph instances—in a sense they are a generative process for making generative processes—and may also be used to overcome some of the limitations of Bayes' nets. For example, a graph grammar may specify that each object in a scene must have material and spatial properties, and they generate visual cues as long as they are not occluded by any other object. And a grammar may define how parts are shared across multiple object instances, such as similar cabinet doors/handles across different cabinets in a kitchen. Recently, probabilistic approaches to computer vision have begun achieving success by applying graph grammars to aid object recognition and image segmentation (Aycinena, Kaelbling, & Lozano-Perez, 2008; Han & Zhu, 2009; Zhu, Chen, & Yuille, 2009). In addition, graph grammars have been used to explain cognitive behaviors in a variety of situations (Kemp & Tenenbaum, 2008; Tenenbaum, Griffiths, & Niyogi, 2007).

## CONCLUSION

Human perception entails a sophisticated reasoning strategy that combines sensory measurements with internal knowledge to construct accurate, detailed estimates about the state of the world. Generative knowledge is a useful formalism for characterizing observers' internal knowledge about the relationships among world properties and how they generate sensory cues. An observer can achieve Bayes-optimal perceptual inference if the generative knowledge accurately reflects the true generative process.

The challenges presented in the first section characterize the fundamental difficulties perceptual processing must overcome, and generative knowledge provides a natural solution to each challenge. Specifically, generative knowledge allows prior knowledge and indirect, auxiliary cues to disambiguate perception by ruling out unlikely and inconsistent potential interpretations. Generative knowledge can characterize relationships among world properties to allow vast contextual information to influence perception.

We presented a number of studies that *qualitatively* support discounting and explaining-away behavior in humans. An outstanding question is whether human perception is *quantitatively* consistent with Bayesian explaining away. By using the experimental framework illustrated by Figure 3.8 it will be possible to conduct strong quantitative tests of humans' generative knowledge.

## REFERENCES

Adams, W. J., Graf, E. W., & Ernst, M. O. (2004). Experience can change the "light-from-above" prior. *Nature Neuroscience, 7*, 1057–1058.

Aycinena, M., Kaelbling, L. P., & Lozano-Perez, T. (2008). Learning grammatical models for object recognition. *MIT CSAIL Technical Report*, MIT-CSAIL-TR-2008-011.

Battaglia, P. W., Di Luca, M., Ernst, M. O., Schrater, P. R., Machulla, T., & Kersten, D. (2010). Within- and cross-modal distance information disambiguates visual size perception. *PLoS Computational Biology, 6*(3), e1000697.

Battaglia, P. W., Schrater, P. R., & Kersten, D. (2005). Auxiliary object knowledge influences visually-guided interception behavior. *Proceedings of the 2nd Symposium on Applied Perception, Graphics, and Visualization, ACM International Conference Proceeding Series, 95*, 145–152.

Biederman, I. (1972). Perceiving real-world scenes. *Science, 177*, 77–80.

Blake, R., Sobel, K. V., & James, T. W. (2004). Neural synergy between kinetic vision and touch. *Psychological Science, 15*, 397–402.

Blessing, W. W., Landauer, A. A., & Coltheart, M. (1967). The effect of false perspective cues on distance- and size-judgments: An examination of the invariance hypothesis. *The American Journal of Psychology, 80*, 250–256.

Brenner, E., & van Damme, W. J. M. (1999). Perceived distance, shape and size. *Vision Research, 39*, 975–986.

Epstein, W., Park, J., & Casey, A. (1961). The current status of the size-distance hypotheses. *Psychological Bulletin, 58*, 491–514.

Ernst, M. O., & Banks, M. S. (2002). Humans integrate visual and haptic information in a statistically optimal fashion. *Nature, 415*, 429–433.

Gogel, W. C., Wist, E. R., & Harker, G. S. (1963). A test of the invariance of the ration of perceived size to perceived distance. *The American Journal of Psychology, 76*, 537–553.

Granrud, C. E., Haake, R. J., & Yonas, A. (1985). Infants' sensitivity to familiar size: The effect of memory on spatial perception. *Perception and Psychophysics, 37,* 459–466.

Gruber, H. E., & Dinnerstein, A. J. (1965). The role of knowledge in distance-perception. *The American Journal of Psychology, 78,* 575–581.

Han, F., & Zhu, S. C. (2009). Bottom-up/top-down image parsing with attribute graph grammar. *IEEE Transactions on Pattern Analysis and Machine Intelligence, 31,* 59–73.

Heinemann, E. G., & Nachmias, J. (1965). Accommodation as a cue to distance. *The American Journal of Psychology, 78,* 139–142.

Holway, A. H., & Boring, E. G. (1941). Determinants of apparent visual size with distance variant. *The American Journal of Psychology, 54,* 21–37.

Jacobs, R. A. (1999). Optimal integration of texture and motion cues to depth. *Vision Research, 39,* 3621–3629.

James, T. W., & Blake, R. (2004). Perceiving object motion using vision and touch. *Cognitive, Affective, and Behavioral Neuroscience, 4,* 201–207.

Kaufman, L., & Rock, I. (1962). The Moon Illusion, I: Explanation of this phenomenon was sought through the use of artificial moons seen on the sky. *Science, 136,* 953–961.

Kawato, M. (1999). Internal models for motor control and trajectory planning. *Current Opinion in Neurobiology, 9,* 718–727.

Kemp, C., & Tenenbaum, J. B. (2008). The discovery of structural form. *Proceedings of the National Academy of Sciences, 105,* 10687–10692.

Kersten, D., Mamassian, P., & Yuille, A. (2004). Object perception as Bayesian inference. *Annual Review of Psychology, 55,* 271–304.

Knill, D. C. (1998a) Discriminating planar surface slant from texture: Human and ideal observers compared. *Vision Research, 38,* 1683–1711.

Knill, D. C. (1998b). Surface orientation from texture: Ideal observers, generic observers and the information content of texture cues. *Vision Research, 38,* 1655–1682.

Knill, D. C., & Kersten, D. (1991). Apparent surface curvature affects lightness perception. *Nature, 351,* 228–230.

Knill, D. C., & Pouget, A. (2004). The Bayesian brain: The role of uncertainty in neural coding and computation for perception and action. *Trends in Neuroscience, 27,* 712–719.

Körding, K. P., & Wolpert, D. M. (2006). Bayesian decision theory in sensorimotor control. *Trends in Cognitive Sciences, 10,* 320–326.

Mamassian, P., & Goutcher, R. (2001). Prior knowledge on the illumination position. *Cognition, 81,* B1–B9.

Mamassian, P., & Landy, M. S. (2001). Interaction of visual prior constraints. *Vision Research, 41,* 2653–2668.

Marroquin, J., Mitter, S., & Poggio, T. (1987). Probabilistic solution of ill-posed problems in computational vision. *Journal of the American Statistical Association, 82,* 76–89.

Mon-Williams, M., & Tresilian, J. R. (1999). The size-distance paradox is a cognitive phenomenon. *Experimental Brain Research, 126,* 578–582.

Mumford, D. (1992). On the computational architecture of the neocortex. II. The role of cortico-cortical loops. *Biological Cybernetics, 66,* 241–251.

Oliva, A., & Torralba, A. (2007). The role of context in object recognition. *Trends in Cognitive Sciences, 11,* 520–527.

Ono, H. (1966). Distal and proximal size under reduced and non-reduced viewing conditions. *The American Journal of Psychology, 79,* 234–241.

Ono, H., Muter, P., & Mitson, L. (1974). Size-distance paradox with accommodative micropsia. *Perception and Psychophysics, 15,* 301–307.

Pearl, J. (1988). *Probabilistic reasoning in intelligent systems: Networks of plausible inference.* San Francisco, CA: Morgan Kaufmann.

Rao, R. P., & Ballard, D. H. (1999). Predictive coding in the visual cortex: A functional interpretation of some extra-classical receptive-field effects. *Nature Neuroscience, 2,* 79–87.

Strat, T. M., & Fischler, M. A. (1991). Context-based vision: Recognizing objects using information from both 2-D and 3-D imagery. *IEEE Transactions on Pattern Analysis and Machine Intelligence, 13,* 1050–1065.

Sudderth, E., & Jordan, M. I. (2009). Shared segmentation of natural scenes using dependent Pitman-Yor processes. In D. Koller, D. Schuurmans, Y. Bengio, & L. Bottou (Eds.), *Advances in Neural Information Processing Systems 21* (pp. 1585–1592).

Sudderth, E., Torralba, A., Freeman, W. T., & Willsky, A. (2008). Describing visual scenes using transformed objects and parts. *International Journal of Computer Vision, 1–3,* 291–330.

Tenenbaum, J. B., Griffiths, T. L., & Niyogi, S. (2007). Intuitive theories as grammars for causal inference. In A. Gopnik & L. Schulz (Eds.), *Causal learning: Psychology, philosophy, and computation* (pp. 301–322). Oxford, England: Oxford University Press.

Yonas, A., Granrud, C. E., & Pettersen, L. (1985). Infants' sensitivity to relative size information for distance. *Developmental Psychology, 21*, 161–167.

Yonas, A., Pettersen, L., & Granrud, C. E. (1982). Infants' sensitivity to familiar size as information for distance. *Child Development, 53*, 1285–1290.

Yuille, A., & Kersten, D. (2006). Vision as Bayesian inference: Analysis by synthesis? *Trends in Cognitive Science, 10*, 301–308.

Zhu, L., Chen, Y., & Yuille, A. (2009). Unsupervised learning of probabilistic grammar-Markov models for object categories. *IEEE Transactions on Pattern Analysis and Machine Intelligence, 31*, 114–128.

# CHAPTER 4

## Generative Probabilistic Modeling: Understanding Causal Sensorimotor Integration

*Sethu Vijayakumar, Timothy Hospedales, and Adrian Haith*

### INTRODUCTION

In this chapter, we argue that many aspects of human perception are best explained by adopting a modeling approach in which experimental subjects are assumed to possess a full generative probabilistic model of the task they are faced with, and that they use this model to make inferences about their environment and act optimally given the information available to them. We apply this generative modeling framework in two diverse settings—concurrent sensory and motor adaptation, and multisensory oddity detection—and show, in both cases, that the data are best described by a full generative modeling approach.

Bayesian ideal-observer modeling is an elegant and successful normative approach to understanding human perception. One particular domain in which it has seen much success recently is that of understanding multisensory integration in human perception (see Chapter 1).

Existing applications of this modeling approach have frequently focused on a simple special case where the ideal observer's estimate of an unknown quantity in the environment is a reliability-weighted mean of the individual observed cues. This is all that is needed to understand a wide variety of interesting perceptual phenomena. We argue, however, that the Bayesian-observer approach can be more powerfully and generally applied by clear generative modeling of the perceptual task for each experiment. In other words, this assumes that people have access to a full generative model of their observations and that they use this model to make optimal decisions in performing the task.

This systematic approach effectively provides a "model for modeling" that has some key advantages: (1) It provides the modeler with a clear framework for modeling new tasks beyond simply applying common normative models—such as linear combination—which may not apply for a new scenario and may fail to explain important aspects of human behavior; (2) Human performance can be measured against these clear "optimal" models such that we can draw conclusions about optimality of human perception or reveal architectural limitations of the human perceptual system, which cause it to deviate from optimality.

For a particular perceptual task, the optimal solution requires inference in the true generative model of the task. Here, optimal is defined in the sense that the posterior probability over relevant unknowns in the environment is calculated. Any actions or decisions to be made can then be taken with respect to this posterior and the required loss function (see Chapter 1). As an intuition for the significance of optimality, consider that someone gambling on the state of the real world given this "optimal" posterior is guaranteed not to lose money in the long term to someone gambling with any other distribution, including the posterior from a "wrong" generative model.

To make predictions about human behavior, the modeler must therefore take care to construct a generative model that encompasses all relevant aspects of the task. These models often lead to strong and surprising new predictions, which can be tested experimentally. In this chapter, we illustrate these ideas via two experiments for which we show that it is crucial to consider a complete normative generative model of the data. In these cases, naive application of common simple models fails to even qualitatively explain the data. Rather than conclude that human perception is suboptimal in these ways, we show how a full generative modeling approach can explain the data and provide insight into human behavior.

We first consider the problem of concurrent sensory and motor adaptation. Previous models have assumed that sensory and motor adaptation occur independently from one another, considering one model for sensory adaptation (e.g., Ghahramani, Wolpert, & Jordan, 1997), and another for motor adaptation (e.g., Donchin, Francis, & Shadmehr, 2003). We show that, by considering a full generative model of the joint observations and the disturbances that affect them, a unified model of sensory and motor adaptation can be derived that makes strong and experimentally verifiable predictions about interactions between sensory and motor adaptation (Haith, Jackson, Miall, & Vijayakumar, 2008). Next, we consider the problem of multisensory oddity detection. Common naive normative models of cue combination are not robust, falsely predicting the existence of infinitely many discrepant but still indistinguishable stimuli. A full generative model of the process is required to explain this entire domain of human behavior (Hospedales & Vijayakumar, 2009).

## INTERACTIONS BETWEEN SENSORY AND MOTOR ADAPTATION

Many chapters in this book focus on problems associated with combining multiple, possibly discrepant cues. If, however, two cues are persistently discrepant by the same amount, it is likely that there is a systematic miscalibration of one modality or the other. For example, prism goggles can be worn which shift the entire visual field, introducing a discrepancy between visual and proprioceptive estimates of hand position. Such discrepancies can be eliminated by adapting the senses over time so that they become realigned.

### Previous Models of Sensory Adaptation

If the hand is viewed through prism goggles, a realignment takes place between vision and proprioception with, typically, a shift in the visual estimate of hand position and an opposite shift in the proprioceptive estimate of hand position (Redding & Wallace, 1996). We model sensory adaptation by assuming that the visually and proprioceptively observed hand positions are displaced by some systematic disturbances (i.e., miscalibrations or unknown experimental manipulations), with added Gaussian noise

$$v_t = y_t + r_t^v + \varepsilon_t^v, \tag{4.1}$$

$$p_t = y_t + r_t^p + \varepsilon_t^p. \tag{4.2}$$

Here $v_t$ and $p_t$ are the subject's visual and proprioceptive observations of their hand position. $r_t^v$ and $r_t^p$ are miscalibrations of vision and proprioception, and $\varepsilon_t^v$ and $\varepsilon_t^p$ represent observation noise corrupting each measurement, which we assume to be Gaussian with variance $\sigma_v^2$ and $\sigma_p^2$, respectively. We assume that the subject maintains estimates $\hat{r}_t^v$ and $\hat{r}_t^p$ of each disturbance over time. The subject's visual and proprioceptive estimates of hand position will be given by subtracting the relevant disturbance estimates from their observations, that is,

$$\hat{y}_t^v = p_t - \hat{r}_t^v, \tag{4.3}$$

$$\hat{y}_t^p = p_t - \hat{r}_t^p. \tag{4.4}$$

The maximum likelihood estimate (MLE) of the true hand position $y_t$ is given by

$$\hat{y}_t^{MLE} = \frac{\sigma_p^2}{\sigma_v^2 + \sigma_p^2}\hat{y}_t^v + \frac{\sigma_v^2}{\sigma_v^2 + \sigma_p^2}\hat{y}_t^p. \tag{4.5}$$

This estimate optimally combines the two unimodal estimates into a single estimate, taking into account the relative observation noise in each modality. Ghahramani et al. (1997) proposed that we adapt the estimates of $\hat{r}_t^v$ and $\hat{r}_t^p$ in such a way that the maximum likelihood estimate (MLE) of the actual hand position remains unchanged, which leads to the following update for the disturbance estimates:

$$\hat{r}_{t+1}^v = \hat{r}_t^v + \eta w_p[\hat{y}_t^p - \hat{y}_t^v], \tag{4.6}$$

$$\hat{r}_{t+1}^p = \hat{r}_t^p + \eta w_v[\hat{y}_t^v - \hat{y}_t^p], \tag{4.7}$$

where $\eta$ is some fixed adaptation rate and $w_p$ and $w_v$ are the respective combination weights in Eq. 4.5. From a statistical learning viewpoint, this model can be understood as treating the miscalibrations $\hat{r}_t^v$ and $\hat{r}_t^p$ as unknown *parameters*, which are estimated via an online variant of the standard expectation-maximization algorithm (Bishop, 2006) for parameter estimation in statistical models. The corresponding graphical model is illustrated in Figure 4.1. A crucial prediction of this model is that sensory adaptation will be driven purely by discrepancy between the two senses. This model can successfully account for many features of sensory adaptation, particularly in purely passive contexts such as visual-auditory integration; it has also been proposed as a model for adaptation in visual-proprioceptive integration during active movement (van Beers, Wolpert, & Haggard, 2002).

This model, however, is not quite sufficient on its own to explain adaptation of reaching movements during exposure to shifts in visual feedback. While a recalibration of the visual system will be reflected in reaches toward visual targets, the extent of visual adaptation is always less than the experimentally imposed visual shift. The fact that subjects can nevertheless reach the target successfully implies that they additionally learn a correction to their movements as well as compensating their perceptual estimates of hand and target locations. Simani, McGuire, and Sabes (2007) recently demonstrated that the task performed during exposure affects generalization to reach trials after the visual shift is removed. This difference would not occur if the adaptation were purely sensory in nature.

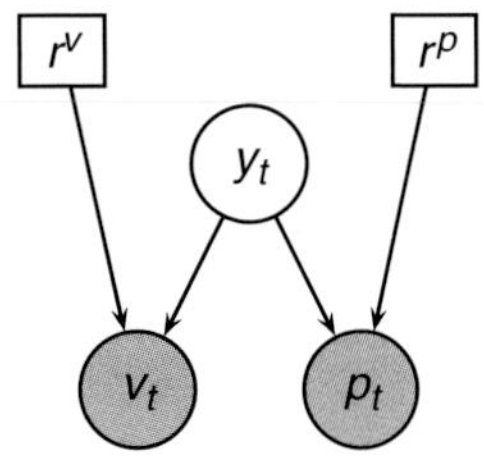


**Figure 4.1** Graphical model for a MLE-based sensory-adaptation model. Shaded circles represent observed random variables. Unshaded circles represent unobserved random variables. Squares represent unknown parameters. Noisy visual and proprioceptive observations, $v_t$ and $p_t$, of unknown hand position $y_t$ are available at each trial/time step. These may be subject to unknown biases $r^v$ and $r^p$ due to miscalibration or experimental manipulation. In the MLE-based model, these unknown biases are treated as parameters of the model which are estimated via online expectation maximization.

Although no explicit model of concurrent sensory and motor adaptation has been previously proposed, it is straightforward to augment the aforementioned sensory-adaptation model with a standard state-space model of motor adaptation. We assume that a motor disturbance affects the relationship between the subject's motor commands and the position of the hand at the end of the movement. Specifically

$$y_t = u_t + r_t^y + \varepsilon_t^y, \tag{4.8}$$

where $u_t$ is the subject's motor command, $r_t^y$ is the motor disturbance acting on the hand, and $\varepsilon_t^y \sim N(0, \sigma_y^2)$ is motor execution noise. Existing state-space models of motor adaptation (e.g., Donchin et al., 2003) typically assume that an estimate of this disturbance is updated according to the error in the hand position midway through the movement. Although the subject does not know the true error in the hand position (since only noisy, corrupted observations of hand position are available), the hand position error can be estimated using the hand position MLE, leading to the following learning rule

$$\hat{r}^y_{t+1} = \hat{r}^y_t + \xi[\hat{y}^*_t - \hat{y}^{MLE}_t], \quad (4.9)$$

where $v^*$ is the visually observed target position, and $\hat{y}^*_t = (v^* - \hat{r}^v_t)$ is the estimated desired hand location, and $\xi$ is some fixed adaptation rate.

This combined model reflects the view that sensory and motor adaptations are distinct processes. The sensory-adaptation component is driven purely by discrepancy between the senses, while the motor-adaptation component only has access to a single, fused estimate of hand position and is driven purely by estimated performance error.

## Bayesian Sensory- and Motor-Adaptation Model

We propose an alternative approach to solving the sensorimotor-adaptation problem. Rather than modeling sensory and motor adaptation independently, we consider a full generative model of how sensory and motor disturbances affect a subject's visual and proprioceptive observations. All three disturbances are now treated as random variables that the subject is attempting to estimate simultaneously. This model is illustrated in Figure 4.2.

The subject generates a motor command $u_t$, which leads to a new hand position $y_t$, perturbed by some unknown motor disturbance $r^y_t$ as well as motor noise $\varepsilon^y_t$, as in Eq. 4.8. This hand position is not directly observed, but noisy and potentially biased visual and proprioceptive observations are available, as described in Eqs. 4.1 and 4.2.

In addition to this statistical model of how actions and observations are affected by the three disturbances, $r^v_t$, $r^y_t$, and $r^p_t$, the subject has some beliefs about how these disturbances evolve over time. These beliefs are characterized by a trial-to-trial disturbance dynamics model given by

$$\mathbf{r}_{t+1} = A\mathbf{r}_t + \eta_t, \quad (4.10)$$

where $A$ is some diagonal matrix and $\eta_t$, is a random drift term with zero mean and diagonal

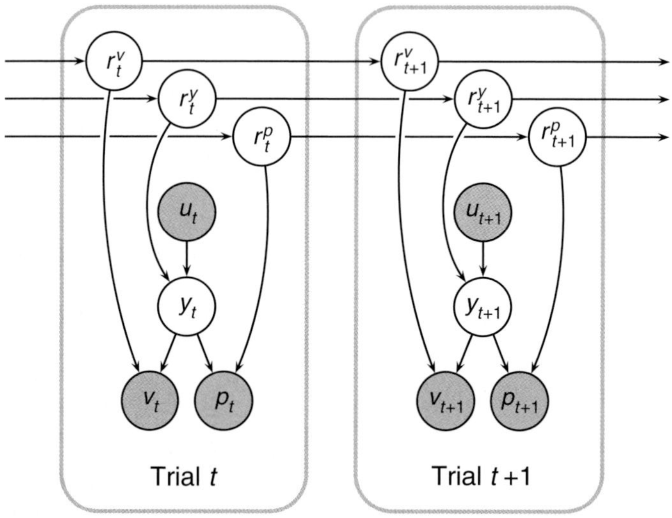


**Figure 4.2** Bayesian sensory- and motor-adaptation model. Shaded circles represent observed random variables (motor command $u_t$; visual and proprioceptive observations $v_t$ and $p_t$). Unshaded circles represent unobserved random variables (hand position $y_t$, and visual and proprioceptive miscalibrations $r^v_t$ and $r^p_t$, and motor disturbance $r^y_t$).

covariance matrix $Q$, that is,

$$\eta_t \sim N(0, Q). \tag{4.11}$$

$A$ and $Q$ are both diagonal to reflect the fact that each disturbance evolves independently. We denote the diagonal elements of $A$ by $\mathbf{a} = (a^v, a^p, a^y)$ and the diagonal of $Q$ by $\mathbf{q} = (q^v, q^p, q^y)$. The vector $\mathbf{a}$ describes the timescales over which each disturbance persists, whereas $\mathbf{q}$ describes the random drift in the disturbance from one trial to the next. These parameters reflect the statistics of the usual fluctuations in sensory calibration errors and motor plant dynamics, which the sensorimotor system must adapt to on an ongoing basis. (Similar assumptions have previously been made elsewhere [Körding, Tenenbaum, & Shadmehr, 2007; Krakauer, Mazzoni, Ghazizadeh, Ravindran, & Shadmehr, 2006]).

We propose that the patterns of adaptation and the sensory after-effects exhibited by subjects correspond to optimal inference of the disturbances $\mathbf{r}_t$ within this full generative model, given the observations on each trial. This is in contrast to alternative models presented earlier in which sensory and motor adaptation are assumed to be mediated by independent processes.

The linear dynamics and Gaussian noise of the observer's model mean that the posterior probability of the disturbances given the observations can be calculated analytically, and it becomes equivalent to a Kalman filter. The latent state tracked by the Kalman filter is the vector of disturbances $\mathbf{r}_t = (r_t^v, r_t^p, r_t^y)^T$, with state dynamics given by Eq. 4.10. The observations $v_t$ and $p_t$ are related to the disturbances via

$$\begin{pmatrix} v_t \\ p_t \end{pmatrix} = \begin{pmatrix} u_t \\ u_t \end{pmatrix} + \begin{pmatrix} 1 & 0 & 1 \\ 0 & 1 & 1 \end{pmatrix} (\mathbf{r}_t + \varepsilon_t), \tag{4.12}$$

where $\varepsilon_t = (\varepsilon_t^v, \varepsilon_t^p, \varepsilon_t^y)^T$. We can write this in a more conventional form as

$$\mathbf{z}_t = H\mathbf{r}_t + H\varepsilon_t \tag{4.13}$$

where $\mathbf{z}_t = (v_t - u_t, \ p_t - u_t)^T$ and $H = \begin{pmatrix} 1 & 0 & 1 \\ 0 & 1 & 1 \end{pmatrix}$. The observation noise covariance is given by

$$R = E\left[(H\varepsilon_t)(H\varepsilon_t)^T\right] = \begin{pmatrix} \sigma_v^2 + \sigma_y^2 & \sigma_y^2 \\ \sigma_y^2 & \sigma_p^2 + \sigma_y^2 \end{pmatrix}, \tag{4.14}$$

where $\sigma_y^2$ is motor execution noise, and $\sigma_v^2$ and $\sigma_p^2$ represent the noise in the subject's visual and proprioceptive estimates as before. The standard Kalman filter update equations can be used to predict how a subject will update estimates of the disturbances following each trial and therefore what actions to select on the next trial, leading to a full prediction of performance from the first trial onward.

### Experiment: Testing Sensory Adaptation during Force-Field Exposure

While the MLE-based model predicts there will be sensory adaptation *only* when there is a discrepancy between the senses, the Bayesian model predicts that there will also be sensory adaptation in response to a motor disturbance (such as an external force applied to the hand). Just as a purely visual disturbance can lead to a multifaceted adaptive response, the Bayesian models predicts that a purely motor disturbance will result in both motor and sensory adaptation, even though there is never any discrepancy between the senses. This occurs because there are three unknown disturbances, but only two observation modalities on each trial. There are therefore many combinations of disturbances that can account for the observations on each trial. Because of the subject's assumptions about how the disturbances vary over time (i.e., Eq. 4.10), explanations that assign credit to all three disturbances are more likely than the true disturbance that was experienced.

We experimentally tested the hypothesis that force-field adaptation would lead to sensory adaptation. We tested 11 subjects who performed a series of trials consisting of reaching movements interleaved with perceptual-alignment tests.

Subjects grasped the handle of a robotic manipulandum with their right hand. The hand was not visible directly, but a cursor displayed via a mirror/flat-screen-monitor setup (Fig. 4.3A) was exactly coplanar and aligned with the handle of the manipulandum. In the movement phase, subjects made an out-and-back reaching movement toward a visual target with their right hand. In the visual localization phase, a visual target was displayed pseudorandomly in one of five positions and the subjects moved their left fingertip to the perceived location of the target. In the proprioceptive localization phase, the right hand was passively moved to a random target location, with no visual cue of its position, and subjects moved their left fingertip to the perceived location of the right hand. Left fingertip positions were recorded using a Polhemus motion tracker. Neither hand was directly visible at any time during the experiment.

Subjects were given 25 baseline trials with zero external force, after which a force field was gradually introduced (Fig. 4.3B). A leftward lateral force $F_x$ was applied to the right hand during the reaching phase. The magnitude of the force was proportional to the forward velocity $\dot{y}$ of the hand, that is,

$$F_x = -a\dot{y}. \tag{4.15}$$

The force was applied only on the outward part of the movement (i.e., only when $\dot{y} > 0$). After steadily incrementing $a$ during 50 adaptation trials, the force field was then kept constant at $a = 0.3N/(cm\ s^{-1})$ for a further 25 postadaptation test trials.

We compared the average performance in the visual and proprioceptive alignment tests before and after adaptation in the velocity-dependent force field. The results are summarized in Figure 4.4A. Most subjects exhibited small but significant shifts in alignment bias in both the visual- and proprioceptive-alignment tests. Two subjects exhibited shifts that were more than two standard deviations away from the average shift and were excluded from the analysis. We found significant lateral shifts in both visual and proprioceptive alignment bias in the direction of the perturbation (both $p < .05$, one-tailed paired t-test). In the $y$-direction, the initial alignment bias was very high. However, there was no significant shift in either modality (Fig. 4.4B),

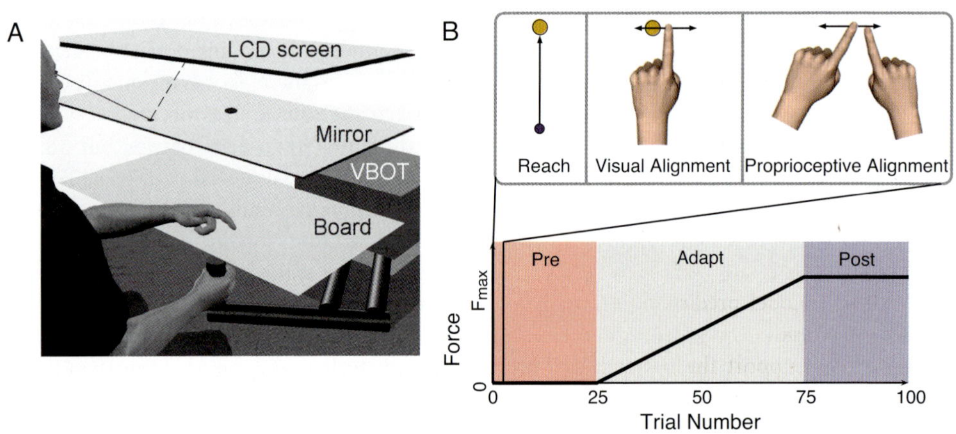


**Figure 4.3** (A) Experimental setup. (B) Subjects made reaching movements in a single direction while perturbed by a force field, the magnitude of which was gradually increased over trials. These reaching movements were interleaved with perceptual alignment tests to measure the extent of sensory recalibration. In these alignment tests, subjects moved their (unseen) left hand to align it as best as possible with either a visual target or their (unseen) right hand.

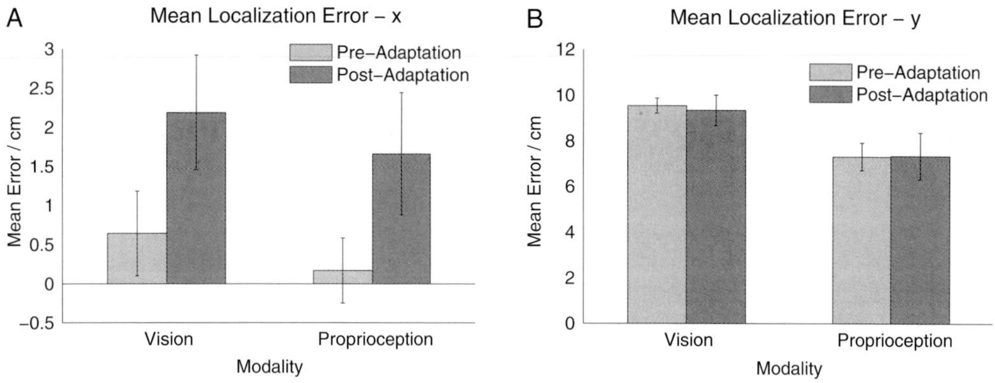


**Figure 4.4** Comparison of visual and proprioceptive alignment biases before versus after adaptation (A) in the direction of and (B) perpendicular to the perturbation.

consistent with the fact that there was no perturbation in this direction.

We assessed subjects' ability to counteract the force during the reach trials by measuring the amount by which subjects missed the target. We quantified this as the perpendicular distance between the furthest point in the trajectory and the straight line passing through both the start position and the target. We fitted the Bayesian and MLE-based models to the data using nonlinear optimization to minimize the squared error between the model and the data across the alignment tests and reach performance. Figure 4.5 shows the averaged data along with the model fits. Both models were able to account similarly well for the trends in reaching performance across trials (Fig. 4.5A). Figures 4.5B and 4.5C show the model fits for the alignment tasks. The Bayesian model is able to account for both the extent of the shift and the time course of this shift during adaptation. Since there was never any sensory discrepancy, the MLE-based model predicted no change in the localization task.

These results support the prediction of the Bayesian model that adaptation to a force field would also lead to sensory adaptation. Alternative models in which sensory and motor adaptation are considered to be independent processes fail to predict this effect, since there is never any discrepancy between the two sensory estimates of hand position. Furthermore, the Bayesian model was able to account accurately for the trends in both reaching performance and alignment-test errors on a trial-to-trial basis, strongly suggesting that the brain uses the principles of Bayesian estimation to guide adaptation.

The brain in this case can be considered to act as an "ideal observer," since it makes the best possible use of all information that it receives through application of an appropriate generative model capturing the dependence of its observations on unknown features of the environment. In the next section, we show how this same general principle can be applied in a different context where information from visual and haptic modalities must be combined to guide decision making in an oddity detection task.

## MULTISENSORY ODDITY DETECTION AS BAYESIAN INFERENCE

Bayesian ideal-observer modeling has been applied extensively and successfully to understand tasks that require integration of two or more cues in the estimation of some real-world stimulus. Much of this work makes common, but simple generative modeling assumptions of independence with Gaussian noise, under which the ideal-observer's strategy for inference in these generative models has the particularly

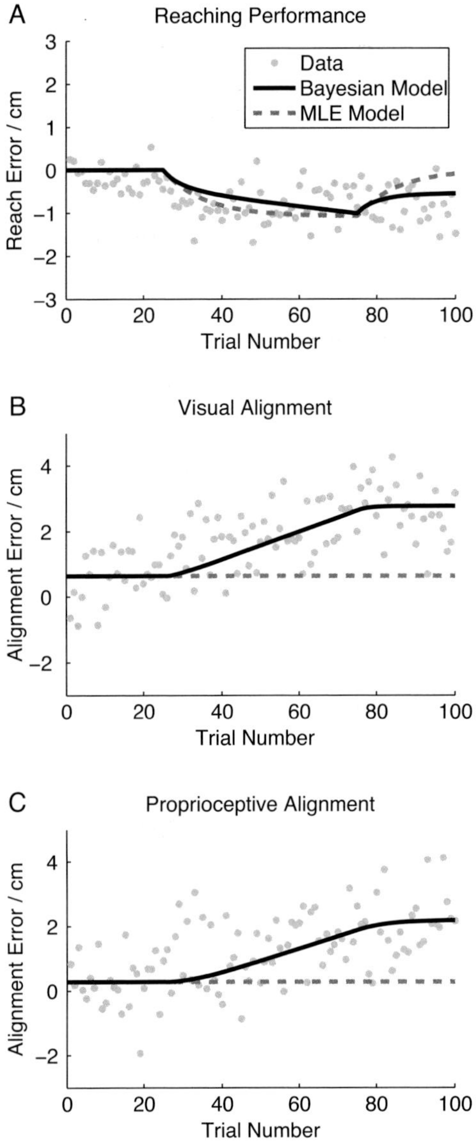


**Figure 4.5** Trial-by-trial reaching and alignment test performance, with model fits. (A) Reaching error. (B) Alignment bias during left-hand-to-visual alignment tests, corresponding to $\hat{r}_t^v$ in the models. (C) Alignment bias during right hand to visual alignment tests, corresponding to $\hat{r}_t^p$ in the models.

simple form of reliability-weighted linear cue combination (see Chapter 1). We will refer to this as maximum likelihood integration (MLI). This approach presumes that the *correspondence* between observations and latent variables (relevant unknown aspects of world state) is obvious and therefore unnecessary to model.

In some cases, experimenters have relaxed this assumption and provided subjects with stimuli where this correspondence (causal structure) was not obvious. That is, it was not obvious which of multiple possible sources caused the observations (Hairston et al., 2003; Shams, Kamitani, & Shimojo, 2000; Shams, Ma, & Beierholm, 2005; Wallace et al., 2004), or which of multiple possible world models was true (Knill, 2007). In these cases, the standard MLI linear-cue-combination approach fails to explain human performance. As we shall see, this seems not to be due to suboptimality of human perception, but mismatch between the experiments and overly simple experimental models.

Under the generative modeling approach proposed in this chapter, we see that uncertain correspondence in a perceptual problem corresponds to uncertain *structure* in the generative model. An ideal Bayesian observer should also infer this uncertain structure. Recently, studies have begun to apply a complete Bayesian-structure-inference perspective (Hospedales & Vijayakumar, 2008) to experiments with correspondence or structure uncertainty and have provided a good explanation for the human perception in these cases (Chapters 2 and 13; Körding, Beierholm et al., 2007).

Here, we consider the challenging modeling problem of *multisensory oddity detection*, in which we shall see that structure uncertainty occurs simultaneously in two different ways. We show how to formalize a generative model of this problem, and how this can explain and unify a pair of experiments (Hillis, Ernst, Banks, & Landy, 2002) where MLI previously failed dramatically.

Next, we briefly review standard MLI ideal-observer modeling for cue combination, and show—by way of theoretical argument as well as a concrete experimental example—why the naive application of mandatory MLI approaches qualitatively fails to explain human multisensory oddity detection.

### Standard Ideal-Observer Modeling for Sensor Fusion

A generative probabilistic model (Bishop, 2006) for a perceptual problem describes the way in which signals are generated by a source, and how they are then observed—including any distorting noise processes. Predictions made by the results of optimal inference in this model can then be compared to experimental results.

Formalized as a generative model, standard cue-combination theory (Fig. 4.6) assumes that multisensory observations $x_m$ in modalities $m$ are generated from some source $y$ in the world, subject to independent noise in the environment and physical sensor apparatus, for example, $x_m \sim N(y, \sigma_m^2)$. Ernst and Banks (2002) asked subjects to make haptic $x_h$ and visual $x_v$ observations of a bar's height $y$ and estimate the true height ($\hat{y}_{h,y}$) in order to compare the sizes of two bars. This requires computing the posterior distribution over height, which under these modeling assumptions is Gaussian $p(y|x_h, x_v; \sigma_h^2, \sigma_v^2) = N(y; \mu_{y|h,v}, \sigma^2_{y|h,v})$, with mean and variance given by Eqs. 4.16–4.17:

$$\mu_{y|h,v} = \frac{\sigma_h^{-2}}{\sigma_h^{-2} + \sigma_v^{-2}} x_h + \frac{\sigma_v^{-2}}{\sigma_h^{-2} + \sigma_v^{-2}} x_v, \tag{4.16}$$

$$\sigma^2_{y|h,v} = \frac{\sigma_h^2 \sigma_v^2}{\sigma_h^2 + \sigma_v^2}. \tag{4.17}$$

Psychophysics experiments (e.g., Alais & Burr, 2004; Battaglia, Jacobs, & Aslin, 2003) typically test multisensory perception for optimality by matching to the ideal-observer performance in two ways. First, the optimal estimate of the true height is $\hat{y}_{h,v} = \mu_{y|h,v}$, so the variance of the human's responses $\hat{y}_{h,v}$ to multisensory stimuli should match the variance of the optimal response $\sigma^2_{y|h,v}$ (Eq. 4.17). Note from Eq. 4.17 that this is always less than the variance of individual observations $\sigma_h^2$, $\sigma_v^2$; hence, it is less than the variance of the unimodal responses $\hat{y}_h$, $\hat{y}_v$. Second, the multisensory response of the

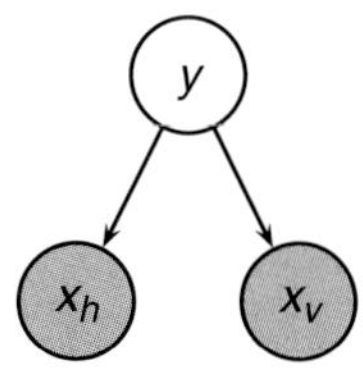


**Figure 4.6** Standard sensor-fusion model. Bar size $y$ is inferred on the basis of haptic and visual observations $x_h$ and $x_v$ (Hillis et al., 2002). Shaded circles indicate observed quantities, and empty circles indicate quantities to estimate.

ideal observer is the precision-weighted mean of the unimodal observations (Eq. 4.16). Therefore, experimentally manipulating the variances $\sigma_h^2$, $\sigma_v^2$ of the individual modalities should produce the appropriate changes in the human perceptual response $\hat{y}_{h,v}$. These quantities can be determined directly in direct-estimation experiments (e.g., Wallace et al., 2004) or indirectly via fitting a psychometric function in two-alternative forced-choice experiments (e.g., Alais & Burr, 2004; Battaglia et al., 2003).

### Oddity Detection

In direct-estimation scenarios, subjects try to make a *continuous estimate* of a particular unknown quantity $y$, such as the height of a bar or spatial stimulus location based on noisy observations $x_m$, such as visual and haptic heights or auditory and visual locations, respectively. In contrast, in the *oddity-detection paradigm*, subjects observe $i = 1 \ldots N$ separate stimuli $x_{m,i} \sim N(y_i, \sigma_m^2)$ and must make a discrete determination of the "odd" stimulus $o$ from among the $N \geq 3$ options $\{y_i\}_{i=1}^N$. Depending on the experimental paradigm, the odd stimulus may be detectable because it is, for example, larger or smaller than the other stimuli.

*Multisensory* oddity detection is a particularly interesting problem to study because it provides novel paradigms for manipulating the oddity. Specifically, the *mandatory* MLI theory of cue combination predicts that a single fused estimate $\hat{y}_{h,v}$ will be made for each multisensory stimulus (Eq. 4.16), and oddity detection will proceed solely based on these estimates. This means that a particular stimulus might be the same as the others when averaged over its modalities of perception (Eq. 4.16), while each individual stimulus modality could simultaneously be radically discrepant. Such stimuli would be known as *perceptual metamers*, meaning that although they would be physically distinct, they would be perceptually indistinguishable under this theory of cue combination. This provides a new and interesting test of Bayesian perception, because if the nervous system was to use solely the fused estimates to detect oddity, then it would not be able to discriminate such metamers. If, on the other hand, the nervous system made an inference about structure in the full generative model of the observations, it could detect such stimuli on the basis of structure (correspondence) oddity. In the following section, we formalize this inference paradigm and look in detail at a pair of experiments that tested oddity detection and found MLI mandatory fusion models unsatisfactory in explaining the data completely.

### Human Multisensory Oddity Detection Performance

Hillis et al. (2002) studied multisensory oddity detection in humans using $N = 3$ options in two conditions: visual-haptic cues for size (across-modal cues) and texture-disparity cues for slant (within-modal cues). We describe this experiment in some detail and will formalize the oddity-detection problem and our solution to it in the context of this experiment. It should be noted that our approach can trivially be generalized to other conditions, such as more modalities of observation and selecting among $N \geq 3$ options.

Three stimuli are presented in two modalities $v$ and $h$ (Fig. 4.7). (To simplify the discussion, we will refer generally to the visual-haptic ($v$-$h$) modalities when discussing concepts which apply to both the visual-haptic and texture-disparity experiments.) Two of the stimuli are instances of a fixed standard stimulus $y_s$ and one is an instance of the (potentially odd) probe stimulus $y_o$. The standard stimuli are always *concordant*, meaning that there is no experimental manipulation across modalities so $y_s = y_{h,s} = y_{v,s}$. The probe stimulus $y_o$ is experimentally manipulated across a wide range of values so that the visual and haptic sources, $y_{v,o}$ and $y_{h,o}$, may or may not be similar to each other or to the standard $y_s$. The subject's task is to detect which of the three stimuli is the probe. If all the stimuli are concordant and the probe is set the same as the standard $y_s = y_o$, then we expect no better than random (33%) success rate (Fig. 4.7A). If all the stimuli are concordant and the probe discrepancy is set very high compared to the standard, then we expect close to 100% success rate (Fig. 4.7B). However, if the probe stimulus is experimentally manipulated to be discordant so that $y_{h,o} \neq y_{v,o}$, then the success rate expected will depend on precisely how the subjects combine their observations of $y_{h,o}$ and $y_{v,o}$ (Fig. 4.7C). The two-dimensional distribution of detection success/error rate as a function of controlled probe values $y_{h,o}, y_{v,o}$ can be measured and used to test different theories of cue combination.

For a single modality, for example, $h$, the error rate distribution for detection of the probe $y_{h,o}$ can be approximated as a one-dimensional Gaussian bump centered at the standard $y_{h,s}$. (If $y_{h,s} = y_{h,o}$ then detection of the odd stimulus will be at chance level; if $y_{h,o} \gg y_{v,o}$ then detection of the odd stimulus will be reliable, etc.) The shape of the two-dimensional performance surface for multimodal probe stimulus detection $p(\text{success}|y_{h,o}, y_{v,o})$ can be modeled as a two-dimensional bump centered at $(y_s, y_s)$. Performance *thresholds* (the equipotentials where $p(\text{success}|y_{h,o}, y_{v,o}) = 66\%$) are computed from the performance surfaces predicted by theory and those of the experimental data. Cue-combination theories are evaluated by the match of their predicted thresholds to the empirical thresholds.

### Basic Cue-Combination Theories

To parameterize models for testing, the observation precisions first need to be determined. Following standard practice for MLI modeling, Hillis et al. (2002) measured the variances of the unimodal error distributions and then used these to predict the combined variance and hence the

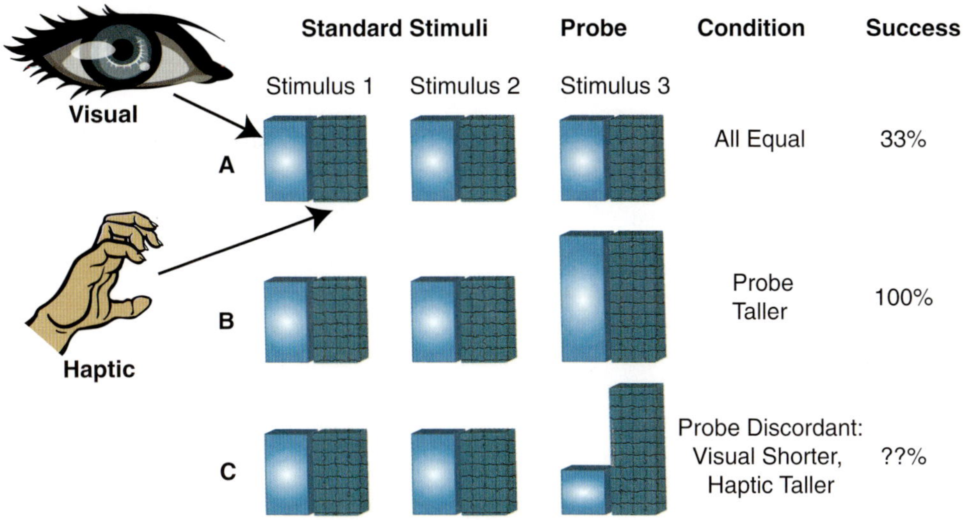


**Figure 4.7** Schematic of visual-haptic height oddity-detection experimental task from Hillis et al. (2002). Subjects must choose the odd probe stimulus based on haptic (textured bars) and visual (plain bars) observation modalities. (A) Probe stimulus is the same as the standard stimuli: Detection is at chance level. (B) Probe stimulus bigger than standard: Detection is reliable. (C) Haptic and visual probe modalities are discordant: Detection rate will depend on cue-combination strategy.

multimodal error distribution under MLI cue-combination theory (Eqs. 4.16–4.17). (In the next section, we will discuss why this approach is not quite ideal for this experiment.)

Specifically, under the MLI theory, the brain would compute a fused estimate $\hat{y}_o$ based on the two observations $x_{h,o}, x_{v,o}$ (Eqs. 4.16–4.17) and then discriminate based on this estimate. In this case, although both cues are now being used, some combinations of cues would produce a metameric probe, that is, physically distinct but perceptually indistinguishable. Specifically, if we parameterize the probe stimuli as $y_{h,o} = y_{h,s} + \Delta y_{h,o}, y_{v,o} = y_{v,s} + \Delta y_{v,o}$, then along the diagonal line through the performance surface where $\Delta y_{h,o} = -(\sigma_v^2/\sigma_h^2)\Delta y_{v,o}$, the fused estimate is on average the same as the standard $\hat{y}_{h,o} = y_s$ and the probe would be undetectable. Performance along the cues-concordant diagonal, however, would be improved compared to the single-cue estimation cases because the combined variance is less than the individual variances ($\sigma^2_{y|h,v} < \sigma_h^2$ and $\sigma^2_{y|h,v} < \sigma_v^2$).

Two variants of the experiment were performed, one for size discrimination across visual and haptic modalities (standard: $y_s = 55$ mm), and one for slant discrimination using texture and stereo disparity cues within vision (standard: $y_s = 0$ deg). Figure 4.8 illustrates the predicted performance surface contours for unimodal models (red lines), the MLI model (green lines), and those observed (dots) by Hillis et al. (2002) for two sample subjects. Contour points closer to the origin $y_s$ indicate better performance.

There are several points to note in Figure 4.8: (1) In the cues-concordant quadrants (1 and 3), the multimodal performance is improved compared to the unimodal performance, as predicted by the MLI theory (magenta points and green lines are inside the red lines in quadrants 1 and 3). (2) Particularly in the intramodal case (Fig. 4.8B), the observed experimental performance is significantly worse than the unimodal performance in the cues-discordant quadrants (2 and 4) (magenta points are outside of the red lines in Fig. 4.8B, quadrants 2 and 4). Note that the green intramodal predicted thresholds in Figure 4.8B are curved, unlike the straight intermodal predicted thresholds in

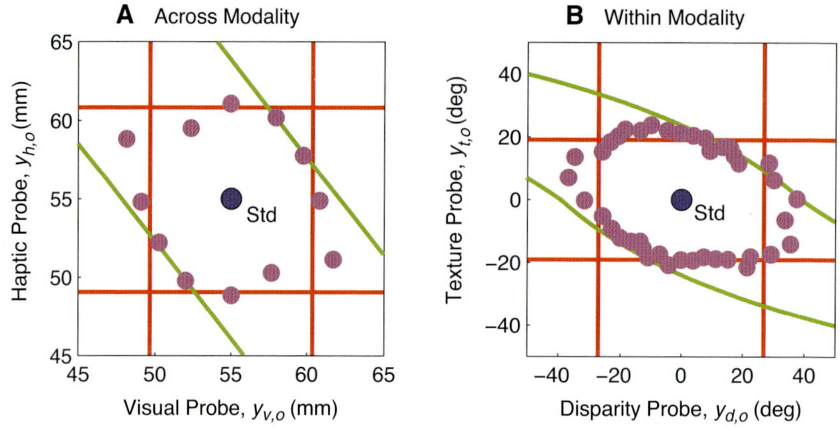


**Figure 4.8** MLI oddity-detection predictions and experimental results. (A) Visual-haptic experiment. (B) Texture-disparity experiment. Red lines: Observed unimodal discrimination thresholds. Green lines: Discrimination-threshold predictions assuming mandatory fusion. Magenta points: Discrimination threshold observed experimentally for two sample subjects from Hillis et al. (2002).

Figure 4.8A. This is due to the use of a slightly more complicated model than described here, which reflects the fact that the variance of the slant cue $\sigma_s^2$ itself depends on the current slant $y_s$ (see Hillis et al., 2002, for details). The essential insights remain the same, however.

Hillis et al. concluded that mandatory fusion applied within (Fig. 4.8B) but not between (Fig. 4.8A) the senses, in part because poor performance in the cues-discordant quadrants 2 and 4 was noted to be less prominent in the intermodal case. They hypothesized that the discrepancy between the observed limited region of poor performance in the intramodal cues-discordant quadrants 2 and 4, and the MLI predicted infinite region of nondiscriminability could be due to a separate texture consistency mechanism ultimately enabling the discrimination in quadrants 2 and 4 (Hillis et al., 2002).

Nevertheless, the classical unifying theory of ideal-observer maximum-likelihood combination retains a strong *qualitative* discrepancy with the experimental results (Fig. 4.8, green lines and points) in both experiments. It does not predict good performance in the cues-concordant quadrants 1 and 3 as well as a *limited* region of poor performance in the cues-discordant quadrants 2 and 4. In the next sections, we will show how an alternative unifying approach, exploiting a complete generative model of the oddity-detection problem, including the associated structure uncertainty, can explain both of these experiments quantitatively and intuitively.

## Modeling Oddity Detection

The classical MLI approach to sensor fusion has failed as a means to understand human performance in this multisensory oddity-detection problem. Let us step back and reconsider the match between the problem and its generative model. There are two key components of this problem that are not modeled by the classical approach (Fig. 4.6): the discrete model-selection nature of the problem, and the variable structure component of the problem.

The task posed—"*Is stimulus 1, 2 or 3 the odd one out?*"—is actually no longer simply an estimation of a combined stimulus $\hat{y}_{h,v}$. This estimation is involved in solving the task, but ultimately the task effectively asks subjects to make a *probabilistic model selection* (Mackay, 2003) between three models. To understand the model-selection interpretation intuitively, consider the following reasoning process: I have experienced three noisy multisensory observations. I do not know the true values of these three stimuli, but I know they come from two categories, standard and probe. Which of the following is more plausible:

1. Multisensory stimuli two and three come from one category, and stimulus one comes from another.
2. Stimuli one and three come from one category, and stimulus two comes from a different category.
3. Stimuli one and two come from one category, and stimulus three comes from another.

With this in mind, to take a Bayesian ideal-observer point of view on this experiment, the experimental task is clearly to estimate which of three distinct *models* is the best one for the data. That is, the experiment effectively asks which model in an entire set of models best explains the data, rather than asking the value of some variable within a model. The ideal-observer should *integrate over the distribution of unknown stimulus values* $y_s$ and $y_o$ (since subjects are not directly asked about these) in determining the most plausible model (assignment of oddity).

The second key aspect of this task which must be included in any full generative model of this problem is that oddity can be entailed in the probe stimulus not only by its combined difference from the standard, but by discrepancy within the probe stimulus. In this case (similar to other recent multisensory perception experiments with variable causal structure: Hairston et al., 2003; Shams et al., 2000, 2005; Wallace et al., 2004), the variable structure can effectively "give away" the probe. We introduced the approach needed to solve this type of problem in multisensory perception as *structure inference* (Hospedales & Vijayakumar, 2008). Körding, Beierholm et al. (2007) carried out a detailed analysis of the experiments of Hairston et al. (2003) and Wallace et al. (2004) and showed how the structure inference approach was necessary to explain the results, but they termed the procedure *causal inference* (see Chapter 2).

### Formalizing Optimal Oddity Detection

A generative-model Bayesian network formalization of the oddity-detection task for the three multisensory observations $\{x_{h,i}, x_{v,i}\}_{i=1}^{3}$ is shown in Figure 4.9, where the aim is to determine which observation is the odd probe. The graph on the left indicates that the four observations composing the other two standard stimuli are all related to the standard stimulus value $y_s$. The graph on the right indicates that the probe visual-haptic observations are independent of the standard but *might* be related via their common parent, the latent probe stimulus of value $y_o$. The latent variable $C$ switches whether the probe observations have a common cause in the generative model. The prior probability of common causation is given

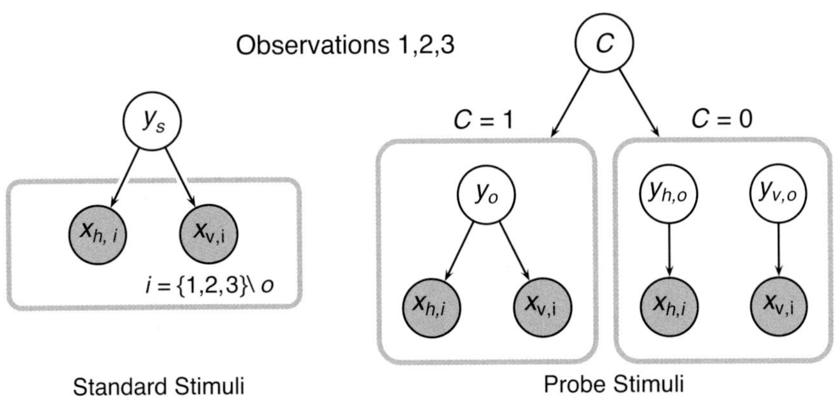


**Figure 4.9** Graphical model for oddity detection via structure inference. A subject observes three multisensory stimuli, $x_{h,i}$ and $x_{v,i}$, $i = 1,2,3$. The three options for assigning oddity correspond to three possible models indexed by $o = 1,2,3$. The uncertain causal structure of the probe stimulus is now represented by $C$, which is computed in the process of evaluating the likelihood of each model $o$.

by the new parameter $\pi_c$, so $p(C=1)=\pi_c$ and $p(C=0)=1-\pi_c$. Under the hypotheses of common causal structure $C=1$, we assume that the two observations $x_{h,o}$, $x_{v,o}$ were produced from a single latent variable $y_s$. Alternately, if $C=0$, we assume separate sources $y_{h,o}$ and $y_{v,o}$ were responsible for each. An ideal Bayesian observer in this task should integrate over both the unknown stimulus values and the causal structure $C$ (i.e., whether we are feeling and seeing the same thing).

The three different possible models are given by the different probe hypotheses $o=1,2,3$, which separate the standard and probe stimuli into different clusters. We represent this clustering in terms of the *set difference operator* "\." For example, $o=3$ would mean that stimuli $\{1,2,3\}\backslash 3=\{1,2\}$ are drawn from the standard $y_s$, and therefore observations $\{x_{h,1},x_{v,1},x_{h,2},x_{v,2}\}$ (Fig. 4.9, left) should be similar to each other—and potentially dissimilar to odd probe observations $\{x_{h,3},x_{v,3}\}$ (Fig. 4.9, right), which were generated independently. The ideal Bayesian observer would base its estimation of oddity on the marginal likelihood of each stimulus/model $o$ being odd, $p(o|\{x_{h,i},x_{v,i}\}_{i=1}^3\theta)\propto p(\{x_{h,i},x_{v,i}\}_{i=1}^3|o,\theta)p(o|\theta)$:

$$p(\{x_{h,i},x_{v,i}\}_{i=1}^3|o,\theta)$$

$$=p_s(\{x_{h,i},x_{v,i}\}_{i\in\{1,2,3\}\backslash o}|o,\theta)p_o(x_{h,o},x_{v,o}|o,\theta),$$

$$p_s(\{x_{h,i},x_{v,i}\}_{i\in\{1,2,3\}\backslash o}|o,\theta)$$

$$=\int\prod_{i\in\{1,2,3\}\backslash o}\prod_{j=h,v}N(x_{j,i}|y_s,\theta)N(y_s|\theta)dy_s,$$

$$p_o(x_{h,o},x_{v,o}|o,\theta)=\int\prod_{j=h,v}N(x_{j,o}|y_o,\theta)N(y_o|\theta)$$

$$\times\pi_c dy_o+\iint\prod_{j=h,v}N(x_{j,o}|y_{j,o},\theta)N(y_{j,o}|\theta)$$

$$\times(1-\pi_c)dy_{h,o}dy_{v,o}. \tag{4.18}$$

The marginal likelihood factors into a product of standard $p_s$ and probe $p_o$ parts, which may be decomposed into integrals of Gaussian products, which are simple to evaluate analytically (see Hospedales & Vijayakumar, 2009, for more details). This procedure evaluates how likely each stimulus $o$ is to be odd, accounting for the uncertainty in stimulus values $y$ (integrals) and the uncertain causality of the probe data $C$ (sum). Here, $\theta$ summarizes all the fixed model parameters, for example, the observation variances $\sigma_h^2$ and $\sigma_v^2$.

### Results

To evaluate our multisensory oddity-detection model, we assume no prior preference for which stimulus is odd ($p(o)$ uniform) and therefore estimate the probe based on the likelihood, $\hat{o}=\arg\max_o p(\{x_{h,i},x_{v,i}\}_{i=1}^3|o,\theta)$. Evaluating the detection success rate for a range of probe values $y_{v,o}$ and $y_{h,o}$, we can then compare the 66% performance thresholds of the model's success rate $p_m(\hat{o}_{\text{correct}}|y_s,y_{h,o},y_{v,o})$ against the human success rate $p_e(\hat{o}_{\text{correct}}|y_s,y_{h,o},y_{v,o})$ as reported by Hillis et al. (2002). To set the various model parameters: The prior variance $\sigma_y^2$ is fixed globally to an arbitrary large value so as to be fairly uninformative; the prior mean $\mu_y$ is assumed known; the unimodal variances $\sigma_h^2$ and $\sigma_v^2$ and so forth are determined a priori for each experiment and subject by fitting to the unimodal data as in Hillis et al. (2002); and only $\pi_c$ is fit to the data for each multisensory experiment, with $\pi_c=0.935$ and 0.99 for the across and within-modality cases, respectively (see Hospedales & Vijayakumar, 2009, for further details).

***Detection Threshold Contours*** Figures 4.10A and 4.10B illustrate the across- and within-modality results, respectively, for the two sample subjects from Figure 4.8. The experimental data (dots) are shown along with the global performance of the model across the whole input space (grayscale background, with white indicating 100% success) and the 66% performance contour (blue lines). The human experimental measurements broadly define a region of nondetection centered about the standard stimuli and slanted along the cues-discordant line and stretched slightly outside the bounds of the inner unimodal threshold rectangle. The extent of the nondetection region along this line is increased somewhat in the

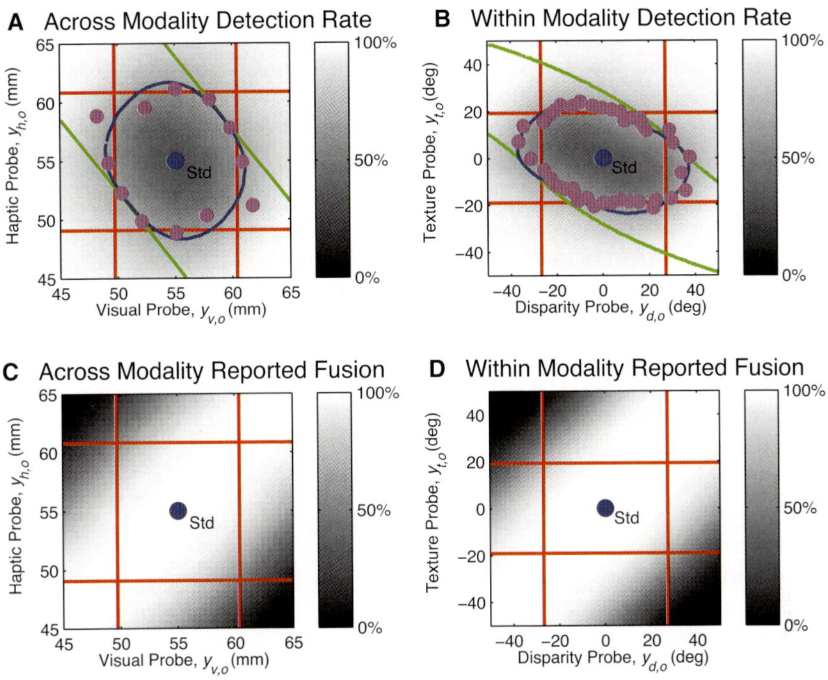


**Figure 4.10** Oddity-detection predictions of the structure-inference approach. (A and B) Oddity-detection-rate predictions for the ideal Bayesian observer (grayscale background) using a variable-structure model (Fig. 4.9). Oddity-detection contours of our model (blue lines) and human (magenta points) are overlaid with the MLI prediction (green lines); chance = 33%. (C and D) Fusion report rates for the ideal observer using the variable-structure model. Across-modality conditions are reported in (A) and (C) and within-modality conditions are reported in (B) and (D).

within-modality case as compared to the across-modality case (Hillis et al., 2002). Recall that the only free parameter varying between these experiments is the common-causation prior $\pi_c$, (a larger $\pi_c$ leads to a longer band of nondetection), which would be expected to vary between pairs of cue modalities.

The MLI model makes the qualitative error of predicting infinite bands of indiscriminability (Fig. 4.10, green lines). In contrast, our Bayesian model provides an accurate quantitative fit to the data (Fig. 4.10, blue lines).

To gain some intuition into these results, consider the normalized distribution of the data (Eq. 4.18) under each model. For example, for $o = 3$, the probability mass in the standard part $p_s$ lies bunched on a four-dimensional line through the standard (where $x_{h,1} = x_{v,1} = x_{h,2} = x_{v,2}$). The probability mass in the probe part $p_o$ is a mixture between a simple model ($C = 1$) around $x_{h,3} = x_{v,3}$, and a more complex model ($C = 0$), spread more uniformly over the space. Therefore, model $o = 3$ will be likely for multisensory observations involving a set of similar pairs $i = 1$, $i = 2$ and a third pair $i = 3$, which is either different from the first set or different from each other.

***Perception of Fusion*** Another benefit of the full generative modeling of this problem is that it also yields a perceptual inference for the fusion (common multisensory source) of the probe $p(C|\{x_{h,i}, x_{v,i}\}_{i=1}^{3})$. This is shown in Figures 4.10C and 4.10D and corresponds to the predicted human answer to the question "*Do you think the odd visual and haptic observations are caused by the same object, or have they become discordant?*" This question was not asked systematically (Hillis et al., 2002), but they did note that subjects sometimes reported oddity detection by way of noticing the discordance of cues, which is in line with the strategy that falls out of inference with our model.

Along the cues-concordant line, the model has sensibly inferred fusion (Fig. 4.10C and D, quadrants 1 and 3). In these regions, the model can effectively detect the probe (Fig. 4.10A and B, quadrants 1 and 3), and the fused probe estimate $\hat{y}_o$ is different from the standard probe estimate $\hat{y}_s$. Considering instead trials moving away from the standard along the cues-discordant line, the model eventually infers fission (Fig. 4.10C and D, quadrants 2 and 4). The model infers the probe stimuli correctly in these regions (Fig 4.10A and B, quadrants 2 and 4) where the mandatory fusion models cannot (Fig. 4.10a, b, quadrants 2 and 4, green lines) because the probe and standard estimates would be the same $\hat{y}_o = \hat{y}_s$. The strength of discrepancy between the cues required before the fission is inferred depends on the variance of the observations ($\sigma_h^2$ and $\sigma_v^2$) and the strength of the fusion prior $\pi_c$, which will vary depending on the particular subject, combination of modalities, and task.

### Discussion

We have developed a Bayesian ideal-observer model for multisensory oddity detection and tested it by reexamining the experiments of Hillis et al. (2002). In those experiments, the standard maximum-likelihood-integration ideal-observer approach failed with drastic qualitative discrepancy compared to human performance; however, we argue that this was due to simple MLI being an inappropriate model rather than a failure of ideal-observer modeling or human suboptimality. The more complete Bayesian ideal-observer model developed here represents the full generative model of the experimental task. This required modeling the multisensory oddity-detection problem as a full model-selection problem with potentially variable probe structure. The Bayesian ideal-observer provides an accurate quantitative explanation of the data with only one free parameter, $\pi_c$, which represents a clearly interpretable quantity: prior probability of common causation. Moreover, our interpretation of the problem is satisfying in that it models explicitly and generatively the unknown discrete index $o$ of the odd object: a quantity that the brain is clearly computing since it is the goal of the task.

***Generative Modeling Assumptions*** We have consciously made a stronger assumption than MLI does about how much the human subject knows about the experiment, notably that probe stimulus was possibly discordant. The justification for this is that the subjects were instructed to detect oddity by any means, for which both interstimuli and within-stimulus intercue discrepancy are reasonable indicators. We therefore expect that perceptual circuitry dealing with oddity detection should allow for both kinds of oddity, and as such we model both. Moreover, as discussed in the Introduction, from a normative point of view on generative modeling and ideal observers, we should start with the assumption that the subject has—or learns over the session—a good generative model of the problem; and we were able to model the data without altering this assumption. Of course, it makes more sense for the perceptual system to allow for intermodal discrepancy (because we regularly see and touch different things simultaneously) than intramodal discrepancy as in the texture-disparity case. Nevertheless, this second unintuitive assumption allowed us to make a much better model of the experiment. Exactly why intramodal discrepancy should be permitted and how it is resolved by the perceptual system are open research questions, but we speculate that this could imply some sharing of perceptual integration circuitry between different cue pairs.

***Alternative Oddity Models*** A simple estimator for unimodal three-alternative oddity task is the "triangle rule" (Macmillan & Creelman, 2005). This measures the distances between all three-point combinations, discards the two points with minimum distance between them, and nominates the third point as odd. Note that this simple rule does not provide an acceptable alternative model of the *multisensory* oddity detection scenario studied here because it still does not address the uncertain correspondence between multisensory observations. Specifically, if the multisensory observations were considered to be fused first (Eq. 4.16), metameric discordant probe observations would still occur—and these cannot be detected by this rule, again producing an infinite band of nondetectability (Fig. 4.8, green lines). In contrast, if the rule were applied directly to the multisensory observations in two dimensions, there would be no room for fusion effects, and detection would be good throughout, in contrast to the tendency toward fusion illustrated by the human data (Fig. 4.8, magenta dots).

***Generative Modeling and Structure Inference***
The theory and practice of generative modeling for inference problems is extensively studied in other related fields, for example, artificial intelligence (Bishop, 2006). In this context, generative modeling of uncertain causal structure in inference tasks goes back to Bayesian multinets (Geiger & Heckerman, 1996). Today, this theory is applied, for example, in building artificial-intelligence systems to explicitly understand "who said what" in multiparty conversations (Hospedales & Vijayakumar, 2008).

***Robust Cue Combination*** A variety of recent studies have investigated the limits of multisensory cue combination and have reported "robust" combination, that is, fusion when the cues are similar and fission when the cues are dissimilar (Bresciani, Dammeier, & Ernst, 2006; Ernst, 2005; Körding, Beierholm et al., 2007; Roach, Heron, & McGraw, 2006; Shams et al., 2005; Wallace et al., 2004). Some authors have tried to understand robust combination by simply defining a correlated joint prior $p(y_h, y_v)$ over the multisensory sources like $y_h$ and $y_v$ (Bresciani et al., 2006; Ernst, 2005, 2007; Roach et al., 2006). These are in general special cases of the full generative approach introduced here (and the equivalent models for other experimental paradigms, e.g., Körding, Beierholm et al., 2007). In the correlated-prior approach, the uncertain structure $C$ is not represented, and the joint prior over latents is defined as $\sum_C p(y_{h,o}, y_{v,o}|C,\theta)p(C|\theta)$. See Chapter 2 for more details. In our case this would be unsatisfactory because the perceptual system would then not represent causal structure, which subjects do infer explicitly in the work of Hillis et al. (2002) and other related experiments (Wallace et al., 2004). Another reason for the perceptual system to represent and infer causal structure explicitly is that it may be of intrinsic interest. For example, in an audio-visual context, explicit knowledge of structure corresponds to knowledge of "who said what" in a conversation (for example, see Hospedales & Vijayakumar, 2008).

## CONCLUSIONS

In this chapter, we have argued that the normative modeling approach of choice for perceptual research should be generative modeling of the perceptual task for each experiment. In this chapter, we have illustrated two sets of experiments in which striking results in human perception can only be explained by full generative models of the respective tasks. These were in domains as diverse as multisensory integration for oddity detection (Hospedales & Vijayakumar, 2009), and visual-proprioceptive integration for sensorimotor adaptation (Haith et al., 2008). The nature of the generative models is quite different in each of these cases: For multisensory integration we considered models in which the unknown variables to be estimated are discrete variables describing the dependency between observations. For sensorimotor learning, we considered a model with continuous, time-varying unknown variables that describe the various possible sources of systematic error affecting each sensory observation. The success of these two contrasting models supports the quite general principle—that the experimental results can only be properly explained by considering a complete generative model of the subject's observations.

In our view, there are two key areas for future research: perceptual learning and physiological implementation. Chapter 9 of this volume introduces some current research progress in perceptual learning. This encompasses questions such as: How do people learn appropriate generative models and parameters for particular tasks? Are there limits to the types of learnable distributions (e.g., Gaussian, unimodal) and the complexity of learnable models? In online learning, how can the brain adapt parameters online rapidly from trial to trial? How does the brain know when to adapt an existing model or set of parameters versus creating a new one for a new task? Chapter 21 of this volume introduces some current research progress in physiological implementation. This encompasses questions such as: How could these models be computed by biological machinery? Does the brain carry out the exact ideal-observer computations like those we describe here, or is it using heuristics that offer a good approximation in the circumstances considered here. Insofar as human performance falls short of ideal-observer performance in particular experiments, what can this tell us about the architecture of the brain?

## ACKNOWLEDGMENTS

T. M. H. and A. M. H. were supported by the UK EPSRC/MRC Neuroinformatics Doctoral Training Center (Neuroinformatics DTC) at the University of Edinburgh. S. V. is supported through a fellowship of the Royal Academy of Engineering in Learning Robotics, cosponsored by Microsoft Research and partly funded through the EU FP6 SENSOPAC and FP7 STIFF projects. We thank Carl Jackson and Chris Miall for assistance with the sensorimotor adaptation experiments.

## REFERENCES

Alais, D., & Burr, D. (2004). The ventriloquist effect results from near-optimal bimodal integration. *Current Biology, 14*, 257–262.

Battaglia, P. W., Jacobs, R. A., & Aslin, R. N. (2003). Bayesian integration of visual and auditory signals for spatial localization. *Journal of the Optical Society of America A: Optics, Image Science, and Vision, 20*, 1391–1397.

Bishop, C. M. (2006). *Pattern recognition and machine learning.* New York, NY: Springer.

Bresciani, J-P., Dammeier, F., & Ernst, M. O. (2006). Vision and touch are automatically integrated for the perception of sequences of events. *Journal of Vision, 6*, 554–564.

Donchin, O., Francis, J. T., & Shadmehr, R. (2003). Quantifying generalization from trial-by-trial behavior of adaptive systems that learn with basis functions: Theory and experiments in human motor control. *Journal of Neuroscience, 23*, 9032–9045.

Ernst, M. O. (2005). A Bayesian view on multimodal cue integration. In G. Knoblich, M. Grosjean, I. Thornton, & M. Shiffrar (Eds.), *Human body perception from the inside out* (pp. 105–131). Oxford, England: Oxford University Press.

Ernst, M. O. (2007). Learning to integrate arbitrary signals from vision and touch. *Journal of Vision, 7(5):7*, 1–14.

Ernst, M. O., & Banks, M. S. (2002). Humans integrate visual and haptic information in a statistically optimal fashion. *Nature, 415*, 429–433.

Geiger, D., & Heckerman, D. (1996). Knowledge representation and inference in similarity networks and bayesian multinets. *Artificial Intelligence, 82*, 45–74.

Ghahramani, Z., Wolpert, D. M. & Jordan, M. I. (1997). Computational models for sensorimotor integration. In P. G. Morasso & V. Sanguineti (Eds.), *Self-organization, computational maps and motor control* (pp. 117–147). Amsterdam, The Netherlands: North-Holland.

Hairston, W. D., Wallace, M. T., Vaughan, J. W., Stein, B. E., Norris, J. L., & Schirillo, J. A. (2003). Visual localization ability influences cross-modal bias. *Journal of Cognitive Neuroscience, 15*, 20–29.

Haith, A., Jackson, C., Miall, C., & Vijayakumar, S. (2009). Unifying the sensory and motor components of sensorimotor adaptation. In D. Koller, D. Schuurmans, Y. Bengio, & L. Bottou (Eds.), *Advances in Neural Information Processing Systems 21*, 593–600.

Hillis, J. M., Ernst, M. O., Banks, M. S., & Landy, M. S. (2002). Combining sensory information: Mandatory fusion within, but not between, senses. *Science, 298*, 1627–1630.

Hospedales, T., & Vijayakumar, S. (2008). Structure inference for Bayesian multisensory scene understanding. *IEEE Transactions on Pattern Analysis and Machine Intelligence, 30*, 2140–2157.

Hospedales, T., & Vijayakumar, S. (2009). Multisensory oddity detection as Bayesian inference. *PLoS ONE, 4*, e4205.

Knill, D. C. (2007). Robust cue integration: A Bayesian model and evidence from cue-conflict studies with stereoscopic and figure cues to slant. *Journal of Vision, 7(7):5*, 1–24.

Körding, K. P., Beierholm, U., Ma, W. J., Quartz, S., Tenenbaum, J. B., & Shams, L. (2007). Causal inference in multisensory perception. *PLoS ONE, 2*, e943.

Körding, K. P., Tenenbaum, J. B., & Shadmehr, R. (2007). The dynamics of memory as a consequence of optimal adaptation to a changing body. *Nature Neuroscience, 10*, 779–786.

Krakauer, J. W., Mazzoni, P., Ghazizadeh, A., Ravindran, R., & Shadmehr, R. (2006). Generalization of motor learning depends on the history of prior action. *PLoS Biology*, 4e316.

MacKay, D. (2003). *Information theory, inference, and learning algorithms.* Cambridge, England: Cambridge University Press.

Macmillan, N. A., & Creelman, C. D. (2005). *Detection theory: A user's guide.* Hillsdale, NJ: Lawrence Erlbaum Associates.

Redding, G. M., & Wallace, B. (1996). Adaptive spatial alignment and strategic perceptual-motor control. *Journal of Experimental Psychology, 22*, 379–394.

Roach, N. W., Heron, J., & McGraw, P. V. (2006). Resolving multisensory conflict: A strategy for balancing the costs and benefits of audio-visual integration. *Proceedings Biological Sciences, 273*, 2159–2168.

Shams, L., Kamitani, Y., & Shimojo, S. (2000). Illusions: What you see is what you hear. *Nature, 408*, 788.

Shams, L., Ma, W. J., & Beierholm, U. (2005). Sound-induced flash illusion as an optimal percept. *Neuroreport, 16*, 1923–1927.

Simani, M. C., McGuire, L. M., & Sabes, P. N. (2007). Visual-shift adaptation is composed of separable sensory and task-dependent effects. *Journal of Neurophysiology, 98*, 2827–2841.

van Beers, R. J., Wolpert, D. M., & Haggard, P. (2002). When feeling is more important than seeing in sensorimotor adaptation. *Current Biology, 12*, 834–837.

Wallace, M. T., Roberson, G. E., Hairston, W. D., Stein, B. E., Vaughan, J. W., & Schirillo, J. A. (2004). Unifying multisensory signals across time and space. *Experimental Brain Research, 158*, 252–258.

# CHAPTER 5

# Modeling Cue Integration in Cluttered Environments

*Maneesh Sahani and Louise Whiteley*

## INTRODUCTION

A complex, cluttered environment is replete with cues, and deciding which of them go together can be at least as great a challenge as properly integrating the ones that do. Although human observers are often imperfect in such settings, they usually outperform machine-perception algorithms on tasks such as demarcating and identifying objects seen against a cluttered background, or following a conversation in a noisy crowd. The failure to build machines capable of matching human performance may be seen as a sign that the field of perceptual studies has not yet found the right way in which to analyze such complex situations. Indeed, one of the biggest challenges for making a successful analysis of perception and cue integration in complex contexts comes right at the outset in setting up an appropriate model. In this chapter we will take some modest strides toward building new cue-integration models with the expressive power necessary to capture at least some of these complex settings.

Setting up an appropriate model is, of course, only the first step. Solving the problems of grouping and integration efficiently is still challenging. Indeed, the apparent imperfections of human observers suggest that the problem is, in fact, very difficult in a fundamental sense. Here, we will quantify this difficulty in terms of the algorithmic complexity of drawing exact inferences within our model, which requires resources in terms of computational hardware or time that grow unfeasibly large for even moderate problem sizes. Thus, the actual process of inference will require approximation in many real-world settings. Accompanying our model, we will introduce one very simple such approximation here.

The structure of model we choose will be based deliberately, but loosely, on the sort of spatial "feature maps" that are seen in neural systems, particularly those involved in vision. This neuromorphic structure is important for at least two reasons. First, and most obviously, it might allow for connections to be built between perceptual modeling of behavior and the underlying neural function. Second, and perhaps more subtly, the structure of any approximation will very likely be determined by the structure of the representations used. Thus, even to describe human behavior we may very well have to construct our models along neurally plausible lines to properly capture the form of approximations to optimality necessary in complex scenarios. Indeed, we have argued elsewhere (Whiteley, 2008) that the phenomenon of visual attention may be understood as a mechanism that has evolved to refine perceptual approximations within a model such as the one described here.

### Integrating Two Independent Cues

The simplest probabilistic formulation of cue integration begins by identifying a physical *attribute* or feature of the environment that an observer might wish to estimate from sensory data. Let us call this attribute $a$. It might be the size or location of an object, its slant or reflectance, its material or chemical composition, or its relationship to other objects in the environment. The observer now gathers sensory data, which we call $\mathbf{s}$ (the bold symbol representing a vector, or more generally a set). In their raw form these data are extremely numerous—they include the activity of billions of sensory receptors in the eye, ear, nose, and throughout the body. For the purposes of analysis, however, these data are usually reduced to a smaller set of, often scalar, *cues*: $c_i$. These are functions of the sensory input $\mathbf{s}$, and together carry much or all of the information about the attribute that was present in the sensory data—in a sense, they act much like *sufficient statistics* in the theory of statistical inference.[1]

It is important to realize that the computation required to obtain a cue $c$ from the sensory activity $\mathbf{s}$ might be rather involved. For example, the projected aspect ratio of an object might be a cue carrying information about its slant. That aspect ratio is not sensed directly by any of the observer's sensory receptors but must be computed from the retinal image by a part of the observer's sensory system that is able to extract the boundary of the object. In many cases, this computation of cues from the sensory input appears to introduce "internal noise" to the cue value. There are other cues for slant, for example, the gradient in apparent size of texture elements along a surface, and these may be computed by different parts of the sensory system. Existing probabilistic analyses of situations where multiple cues carry information about a particular feature have often focused on cues that convey *independent* information about the value of the external attribute. In probabilistic terms, the distributions of the cue values are independent given the attribute value:

$$P(c_1, c_2|a) = P(c_1|a)P(c_2|a), \tag{5.1}$$

where these distributions capture both essential variation in the value of the cue due to uncontrolled aspects of the world, as well as the internal "noise" added by the nervous system. Then, armed with knowledge of the background or "prior" distribution of the attribute value, $P(a)$, cue integration proceeds by Bayes' rule:

$$P(a|c_1, c_2) = \frac{P(c_1, c_2|a)P(a)}{\int da\, P(c_1, c_2|a)P(a)} \propto P(c_1|a)P(c_2|a)P(a). \tag{5.2}$$

This yields the familiar multiplicative form of cue combination, and if the likelihoods[2] $P(c_1|a)$ and $P(c_2|a)$, and the prior $P(a)$ are all Gaussian in form, then the mean of the integrated estimate will be a linear combination of the mean estimates derived from each cue alone.

This simple framework has been successfully used to describe a great deal of human behavior. It has also been extended in many ways, a number of which are discussed at length in the other chapters of this book. Here, we will review two extensions that lay the groundwork for the more elaborately structured model that we will develop in the next section.

### Linked Attributes

In the first case, consider the situation where the computed value of a cue depends on more than one aspect of the external environment—that is, there are two separate attributes, $a_1$ and $a_2$, that must both be taken into account to determine the value of a single cue. For example, the apparent aspect ratio of a surface depends not only on its slant but also on its true shape. Thus, a more complete analysis of this situation would require that we consider both attributes $a_1$, the slant as before, and $a_2$ the veridical aspect ratio. The distribution for $c_1$ then depends on both, and, specifically, the prior on shapes $a_2$ may have

[1] These definitions—of *attribute* as a physical property or feature of the environment that is to be estimated and *cue* as a function of the sensory input that carries information about that property—will be used throughout this chapter to formalize the probabilistic setting.

[2] The probability $P(c|a)$ viewed as a function of $a$ for fixed $c$ is known as a likelihood function.

a substantial impact on the effective likelihood function $P(c_1|a_1)$:

$$P(c_1|a_1) = \int da_2 P(c_1|a_1, a_2)P(a_2). \quad (5.3)$$

This influence on the interpretation of cues due to priors over the attributes in the environment is discussed extensively in Chapter 9. The situation is far from uncommon: Color cues depend on both the reflectance of a surface and the color of the illuminant; spectral cues to sound location depend on both the position and spectrum of the source; otolithic cues to attitude depend on both head orientation and linear acceleration (this final example being of considerable importance to airplane pilots during takeoff).

### Binding Uncertainty

In the second case, the observer might extract two cues from the sensory input but be unsure whether they provide information about the same external attribute. This situation occurs most commonly when the two cues might have been derived from information about different objects. A foundational yet simple example, considered in Chapter 2, is when both visual and acoustic information about location are available, but it is not known whether the light and sound originated from the same place. In this case, the observer might consider the two possibilities separately. That is, estimates are formed simultaneously under two *models*, $m_1$ and $m_2$, each associated with a prior probability of its being the true situation. In the first, there is only one object in one location, and both cues depend on it:

$$\begin{aligned} &P(c_1, c_2, a_1|m_1) \\ &\quad = P(c_1|a_1, m_1)P(c_2|a_1, m_1)P(a_1|m_1). \quad (5.4) \end{aligned}$$

In the second, each cue derives from a different source and therefore a different location.

$$\begin{aligned} P(c_1, c_2, a_1, a_2|m_2) &= P(c_1|a_1, m_2) \\ &\quad \times P(c_2|a_2, m_2)P(a_1|m_2)P(a_2|m_2). \quad (5.5) \end{aligned}$$

Inference about the location of the light source would then be performed by averaging over the two possible models:

$$\begin{aligned} &P(a_1|c_1, c_2) \\ &\quad \propto P(c_1, c_2|a_1, m_1)P(a_1|m_1)P(m_1) \\ &\quad + \int da_2\, P(c_1|a_1, m_2)P(c_2|a_2, m_2) \\ &\quad \times P(a_1, a_2|m_2)P(m_2). \quad (5.6) \end{aligned}$$

Again, this same formal structure applies in more than one situation. Examples include inference about the direction of object motion, where local motion cues might be assigned to one or more (possibly transparent) objects; and a host of auditory grouping phenomena, where sound energy must be sorted into auditory streams.

## MULTIPLE OBJECTS AND CLUTTER

A typical real-world environment contains many objects. Each of these is described by a number of different attributes or features, and in each case a number of different potential sensory cues provide information about the objects and their attributes. Extracting cues, and sorting out which provide information about which attributes, may be challenging. Furthermore, the attributes of one object may influence the interpretation of cues to another. An extreme if common example is the color of a light source, which affects the interpretation of reflectance cues for all of the surfaces around it. Perhaps less obviously, and yet possibly even more common, aspects of the form of objects that are placed close to one another, particularly in the visual periphery, may be difficult to resolve even if a single object under the same viewing conditions would be easily recognized. This phenomenon is known as "crowding" (e.g., Levi, 2008). We will refer to environments in which this sort of cue interference takes place as "cluttered" (Baldassi, Megna, & Burr, 2006; van den Berg, Cornelissen, & Roerdink, 2009).

At first glance, it might seem that the model-averaging approach described above

(Eqs. 5.4–5.6) could be extended to describe inference with respect to an arbitrary number of objects. For instance, one might first specify a prior over the number of objects $N_{obj}$ present in the scene, where we define an "object" rather loosely as a source of attributes that generate cues which need integrating. Conditioned on the number of objects one might then specify a distribution over the attributes, and conditioned on those a distribution over cues. In principle, the cues may provide information about a single attribute value associated with a single object (although we would not know which one); or they may provide simultaneous information about more than one attribute, as in the aspect ratio example described earlier; or indeed may provide simultaneous information about particular attributes for more than one object.

There are, however, a number of difficulties that would be encountered in attempting this approach:

1. First, and as in the two-source example, the most natural way to approach inference within such a model structure would be to integrate cues separately for each possible number of objects, and then average the results of inference weighted by the probability of each model. While not unreasonable when there are only two possibilities, this evaluation and comparison of multiple discrete hypotheses seems both behaviorally and neurally implausible when many different numbers of objects must be considered.
2. Second, closer examination of the model $m_2$ in our multimodal example reveals that it does not just specify that there were two objects present. It also assigns the visual cue to one object's location attribute, and the auditory cue to the other's (that is, $c_1$ depends on $a_1$ and $c_2$ on $a_2$). In this simple case nothing would have been added by also considering the symmetric alternative where object 2 was the light source and object 1 the origin of the sound, but in the general case the misassignment of cues to object attributes may have substantial impact. Thus, either we must specify a separate model for each possible assignment of observed cues to objects, or we must consider all such assignments within a model of a given size. In either case, the computational resources needed to consider all possible cue-attribute assignments grows combinatorially in $N_{obj}$.
3. This situation grows yet more difficult if we attempt to model the interference effects of clutter, for this would require that we consider not only the assignment of cues to objects but also all the potential linkages between attributes that might influence the interpretation of the cues.
4. Finally, this representation does not make explicit the information needed to work out the correct association of cues. Visual cues, for example, are most likely to be grouped together—and to interfere—if they originate from the same region of space, and auditory cues are more likely to be grouped together if their onsets are simultaneous. In its simplest form, this model has no way of encoding such spatial or temporal information, and uncertainty about that information, alongside the cues.

In fact, this final point provides a basis on which to formulate an alternative model structure. We argue that a model of cue combination in complex scenarios must be described in terms of a distribution of attribute values along a suitable dimension, rather than in terms of discrete cue and attribute values. While much of the development that follows would apply to any sensory process—and indeed we will apply it to the multimodal location example—we focus our development on vision, where the distributions are expressed in terms of spatial location.

## Sensory Maps

In the visual domain, objects, their attributes in the real world, the sensory input originating from these attributes, and the low- or midlevel cues extracted from that sensory input are all distributed over visual space. It is therefore natural to replace the discrete attribute and cue values of the combinatorial model with functions of space. We will refer to these functions as "maps," which resonates with experimental evidence for the continuous, map-like quality of neural representations over space. Each map must represent both the presence, and the values, of attributes and cues at each possible location. Since a cluttered environment may contain spatially overlapping objects that possess multiple different attribute values, a simple function that indicates an attribute value at each point in space would be insufficient. For example, the estimated direction of local motion at a point in visual space may be an important cue to the movement of an extended object. However, a single function giving local motion direction would be unable to express the potential absence or indeed simultaneous presence of more than one local motion vector (as might occur for transparent objects; Sahani & Dayan, 2003). Instead, each feature map is a function of both location and attribute (when modeling physical features in the environment) or of location and cue (when modeling internal feature representations) value. The value of the function indicates the "strength" of the attribute or cue with that value at that location. Exactly what we mean by "strength" depends on the cue or attribute under consideration. For a local motion cue, the "strength" may correspond to motion energy extracted from the visual input at a point in space. For a color attribute associated with the reflectance of a physical surface, the "strength" may be the color saturation, and what we have called the attribute value may be the hue. In other settings, there may be no graded "strength" variable. In this case, the feature map may be represented as a sum of Dirac deltas (or a binary-valued function if discretized). In many cases, the true attribute map will be sparse, with only a few values exhibiting any strength at the few locations where objects are present. Cue maps, on the other hand, may often be dense—even when there is no attribute at a particular location, noise is likely to lead to non-zero cue values at each point in space.

It may be valuable at this point to review the roles of the variables involved in the model. The attribute functions represent the veridical value of object attributes at different points in space. Examples might include surface reflectance properties, depth, slant, and veridical motion. These attributes combine to generate sensory input, and this sensory input forms the basis for the computation of the cue (or sensory feature) maps. Examples of these latter maps would be luminance and color-opponent information, binocular disparity, orientation, and local (aperture-viewed) motion. Each of these cue maps can be derived via local computations on the sensory information carried in retinal images, and each provides an inferential "cue" to the value of the corresponding attribute at corresponding points in space. Other types of cue involve nonlocal computation; for example, computing the apparent aspect ratio requires integration across an object's boundaries. These "high-level" cues are difficult to handle within the framework we are developing, and they will be considered only briefly in the final section.

In our discussion of simple cue integration, the perceived location of a flash or sound was a cue just like any other. In our new formulation, space plays a special role. Each sensory map provides information about the location of its associated cues. Thus, a flash of light might result in a luminance cue map with a single "bump" at the corresponding point in space. Information from these different maps must then be combined, with the encoded locations providing a strong signal as to which cues are most likely to go together. In some cases, this integration might be relatively involved. For example, by combining information about orientation and local motion energy across a region of space, one may estimate veridical local motion, resolving the so-called aperture problem. This might allow generalization of motion results such as those of Weiss, Simoncelli, and Adelson (2002) to cluttered environments with multiple moving objects (Weiss, 1998).

### Structuring the Prior

In the scheme we have sketched, attributes and cues have both been replaced by map functions. But what should we do about the distribution over the number of objects and their locations? Certainly, we could continue to use a "nested" prior as in the multiple-model case, in which the distribution is expressed hierarchically—first, a distribution over the number of objects;

then, conditioned on that number, a distribution over their locations. However, it is possible to structure this prior in a way that is more appropriate to the structure of the proposed attribute and sensory-cue maps. In this view, the priors over the number of objects and their locations are combined into a single distribution, known as a *spatial point process*—a probability distribution over sets of points in space. The number of points in a set drawn from this distribution would correspond to the number of objects, whereas the points themselves correspond to the object locations. Indeed, it is often convenient to represent a draw from a spatial point process as a sum of Dirac delta functions, and this would bring the object representation into essentially the same form as that of the attributes and cues. In practice, we will simulate models in which space has been discretized, and thus the prior will express a probability distribution over a binary vector.

### Approximation

The sensory map representation was chosen to make models of cue combination in cluttered scenes with multiple objects easier to express and analyze. Could it also resolve the combinatorial issues we raised when discussing the hierarchical object-based representation? Unfortunately, these problems are fundamental to the problem of grouping cues, and simply recasting the model does not allow us to escape them. The representation provides a framework within which it is easier to see how to make approximations (although see work by Lücke & Sahani, 2008, for an example of the opposite approach, where a model expressed in terms of maps is approximated by iterating a small number of possible contributory objects). This point is difficult to discuss in depth at the abstract level we have used up to now, but it will be looked at in more detail later, once we have developed a more concrete (if simplified) mathematical model.

## THE MODEL

The previous section has outlined a general but still very abstract scheme for the representation of object locations, attributes, and spatially-distributed cues in complex environments with multiple objects and cluttered cues. In this section, we will implement this scheme within a simple discretized model. While this will allow us to simulate some of the essential features of multiobject cue integration, our goal here is not to develop the best possible model within the framework—that is a matter for future research. Instead, we will keep the model (and the accompanying approximation) as simple as possible, with a view to illustrating the representational and modeling capabilities of the framework.

The model rests on a simple "grid world" consisting of a single, discretized spatial dimension ($\mathbf{x}$) and two discretized feature dimensions labeled $\alpha$ and $\beta$. For illustrative purposes, we may think of these as corresponding to orientation ($\alpha$) and color ($\beta$). Figure 5.1 illustrates a single state of the grid world and what the two "attribute maps" that describe the grid world would look like for this state. Four spatial locations, labeled $x_1$, $x_2$, $x_3$, and $x_4$, each take one value of orientation and one value of color, indicated by the gray entries in the orientation feature map; $a^{\alpha}(\mathbf{x}, \alpha)$, and color feature map; $a^{\beta}(\mathbf{x}, \beta)$. Grayscale values indicate the strength of the attribute, so for orientation this corresponds to contrast and for color this corresponds to luminance. In Figure 5.1 all contrasts and luminances are equal, as indicated by the shared gray level of the "on" entries in the maps.

Later we describe a simple mathematical model for how states of the grid world produce noisy observations (corresponding to noisy sensory-cue maps), and how inverse inference works back from these observations to an approximate posterior belief about the state of the world that caused them. We then show how simulated judgments made from this posterior mimic behavioral results observed in two different experiments.

Figure 5.2 illustrates the generation of noisy observations (i.e., sensory cues) in the model. The prior over objects is sparse, so that only a small number of objects—and therefore attributes—are expected to be present at any

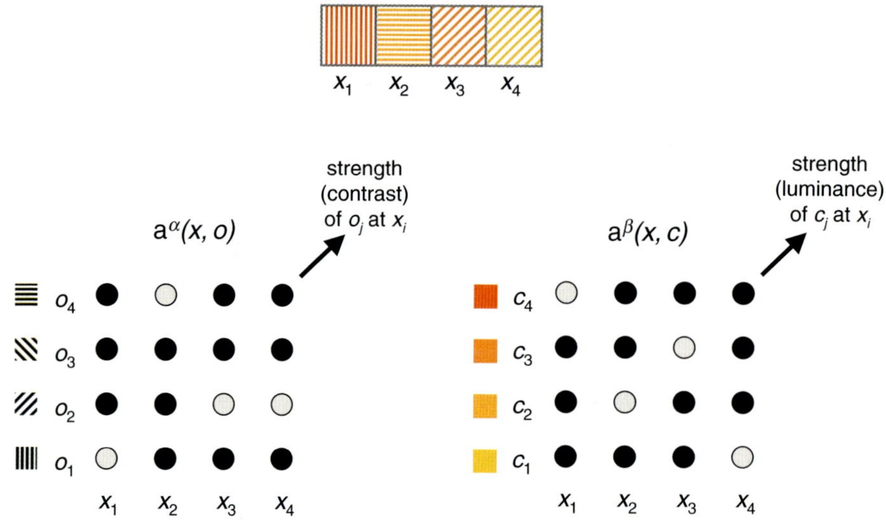


**Figure 5.1** "Grid world" setting for simulations. Illustrates the simple "grid world" in which the simulations take place. The picture at the top represents a state of the environment, with oriented colored patches at each of four locations. The two arrays below represent the orientation $\mathbf{a}^\alpha$ and color $\mathbf{a}^\beta$ attribute maps corresponding to this state. The gray level of each circle in the attribute map indicates the "strength" with which each feature value ($o$ or $c$) is present at the corresponding location (for example, contrast for orientation and luminance for color).

one time. The location, orientation, and color of the objects present is encoded in a binary vector $\mathbf{u}$. Each "1" element in this vector corresponds to an object with a particular location and pair of attribute values, as depicted in the three-dimensional grid at the left of the figure—the vector in the mathematical model is formed by unwrapping this three-dimensional grid into a long vector of pixels. Two rectangular projection matrices, $\mathbf{P}^\alpha$ and $\mathbf{P}^\beta$, can then be used to obtain two two-dimensional representations, one for each feature type, as shown in the next panel of the figure. The corresponding rasterized vectors indicate the spatial locations of non-zero orientation values ($\mathbf{u}^\alpha$) and color values ($\mathbf{u}^\beta$):

$$\mathbf{u}^\alpha = \mathbf{P}^\alpha \mathbf{u}\,, \qquad \mathbf{u}^\beta = \mathbf{P}^\beta \mathbf{u}\,. \tag{5.7}$$

The binary vectors $\mathbf{u}^\alpha$ and $\mathbf{u}^\beta$ thus indicate the *location* of the peaks in the attribute map functions. The *amplitudes* of these peaks—that is, the strength of the corresponding features—are each drawn independently from a zero-mean Gaussian distribution. Equivalently, we can view the attribute maps themselves[3] as drawn from zero-mean multivariate normal distributions with diagonal covariances $\mathrm{U}^\alpha$ and $\mathrm{U}^\beta$, whose diagonal elements are given by the vectors $\mathbf{u}^\alpha$ and $\mathbf{u}^\beta$:

$$\mathbf{a}^\alpha \sim N(\mathbf{0}, \mathrm{U}^\alpha) \quad \text{with} \quad \mathrm{U}^\alpha = \mathrm{diag}[\mathbf{u}^\alpha], \qquad \mathbf{a}^\beta \sim N(\mathbf{0}, \mathrm{U}^\beta) \quad \text{with} \quad \mathrm{U}^\beta = \mathrm{diag}[\mathbf{u}^\beta]. \tag{5.8}$$

(The symbol $\sim$ means "is distributed according to" and $N(\mu, \Sigma)$ is a normal or Gaussian distribution with mean $\mu$ and (co)variance $\Sigma$.) Thus, where there is no object with the corresponding attribute value—that is, where there is a "0" entry in $\mathbf{u}^\alpha$ or $\mathbf{u}^\beta$—the value of the corresponding attribute map is zero, as generated by a zero-mean, zero-variance Gaussian. However, when there is such an object—that is, there is a "1" entry in $\mathbf{u}^\alpha$ or $\mathbf{u}^\beta$—then the attribute value is drawn from a zero-mean Gaussian with a variance of 1, thus

[3] In this discretized model, feature maps have of course become feature vectors, but we continue to use the same terminology because the effects of interest are the same.

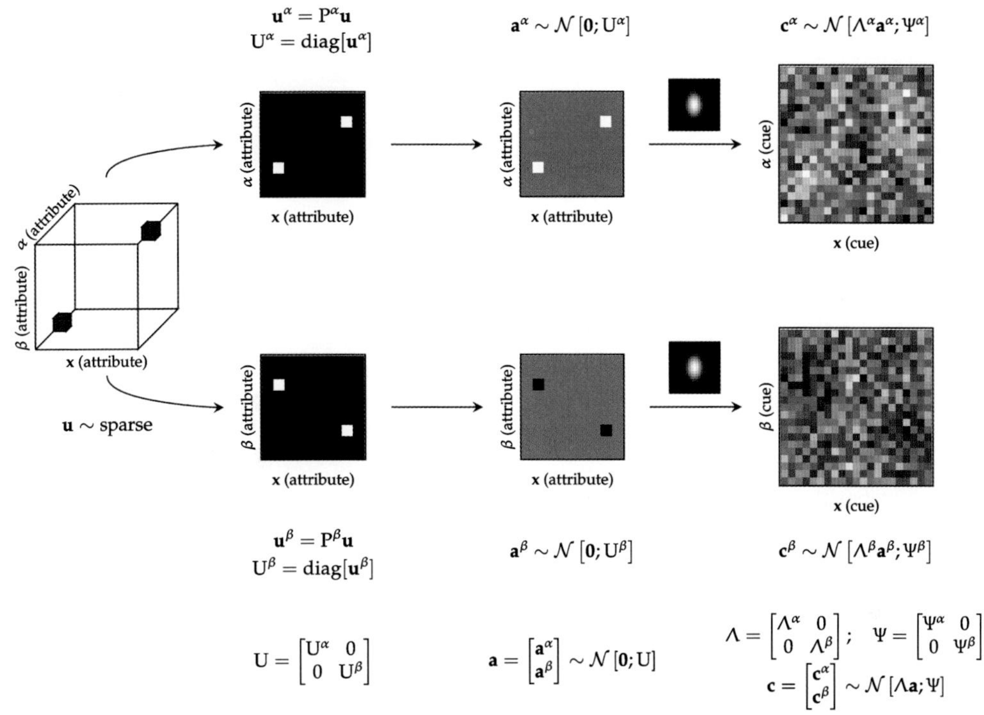


**Figure 5.2** The generative model for "grid world." This schematic illustrates the generation of noisy observations or sensory data, **c**, from an underlying state of the world, **u**, in the simple grid world in which simulations take place. The white squares in $\mathbf{u}^\alpha$ and $\mathbf{u}^\beta$ indicate which feature-location pairs are "on," and the strength of these features (for example, contrast for orientation and luminance for color) is generated from a zero-mean Gaussian distribution, producing attribute maps $\mathbf{a}^\alpha$ and $\mathbf{a}^\beta$. In the figure, gray indicates zero strength, and black and white indicate the extremes of an opponent axis (for example, a blue-yellow axis for color). To generate noisy observed cues, $\mathbf{a}^\alpha$ and $\mathbf{a}^\beta$ are multiplied by Gaussian weight matrices, $\Lambda^\alpha$ and $\Lambda^\beta$, which smear out the attribute map entries. One component of $\Lambda$ is illustrated above the arrows that join **a** to **c**, and the matrix consists of one such component centered on each location-feature pair. Independent Gaussian noise, $\Psi$, then corrupts the cues $\mathbf{c}^\alpha$ and $\mathbf{c}^\beta$, representing the combined influence of various internal noise sources.

generating a range of attribute strengths. Note that because the Gaussian is zero mean, high feature strengths may be represented by high positive or high negative values. This accords with neurally inspired representations of features in terms of a pair of opposing axes—for example, a blue-yellow axis for color or a positive-negative polarity axis for orientation contrast.

The third panel in Figure 5.2 shows an example of attribute feature maps drawn from this distribution, $\mathbf{a}^\alpha$ and $\mathbf{a}^\beta$, where now gray represents 0. The relationship between these and the corresponding cue feature maps **c** is modeled very simply. Each attribute vector is multiplied by a corresponding weight matrix $\Lambda$, whose effect is to convolve the attribute map with a kernel. The Gaussian shape of this kernel, as shown above the arrows linking **a** to **c** in Figure 5.2, is inspired by the typical form of a neuronal receptive field and has the effect of smearing out the sparse entries of **a**. These cue maps are also affected by internal noise, which we model as an independent normally-distributed perturbation with a (diagonal) covariance matrix $\Psi$. Thus, the mapping from attribute to cue maps can be written:

$$\mathbf{c}^\alpha \sim N(\Lambda^\alpha \mathbf{a}^\alpha, \Psi^\alpha),$$
$$\mathbf{c}^\beta \sim N(\Lambda^\beta \mathbf{a}^\beta, \Psi^\beta). \tag{5.9}$$

An example of observations, or sensory cues, generated by this process is shown in the rightmost panel of Figure 5.2. The cue space is taken to be higher dimensional (here represented by a finer discretization) than the attribute space. This transformation from a state of the world, **a**, to noisy observations, **c**, can be thought of as representing all the sources of stochasticity that render perceptual inference necessarily probabilistic—including noise in the external world, unreliable neural firing, and coarse response properties. It also mixes attribute values from nearby points in the same cue values, thus providing a very simple model of cue interference in a cluttered scene.

Having set up the model, we can write it more compactly by concatenating the two feature dimensions. First, attribute vectors are generated from binary feature-location vectors through zero-mean Gaussians:

$$\mathbf{a} = \begin{bmatrix} \mathbf{a}^{\alpha} \\ \mathbf{a}^{\beta} \end{bmatrix} \sim N(\mathbf{0}, \mathrm{U}) \quad \text{with}$$

$$\mathrm{U} = \begin{bmatrix} \mathrm{U}^{\alpha} & 0 \\ 0 & \mathrm{U}^{\beta} \end{bmatrix}. \tag{5.10}$$

Second, observed cues are generated from the attribute functions, which are passed through a weight matrix to form the mean of a Gaussian with diagonal noise:

$$\mathbf{c} = \begin{bmatrix} \mathbf{c}^{\alpha} \\ \mathbf{c}^{\beta} \end{bmatrix} \sim N(\Lambda\mathbf{a}, \Psi) \quad \text{with}$$

$$\Lambda = \begin{bmatrix} \Lambda^{\alpha} & 0 \\ 0 & \Lambda^{\beta} \end{bmatrix}, \Psi = \begin{bmatrix} \Psi^{\alpha} & 0 \\ 0 & \Psi^{\beta} \end{bmatrix}. \tag{5.11}$$

These equations represent a "generative model" for noisy cue observations, expressed as an indirect prior on attribute feature maps $p(\mathbf{a}) = \int d\mathbf{u}\, p(\mathbf{a}|\mathbf{u}) p_0(\mathbf{u})$, where $p_0$ is the sparse prior; and a simple likelihood term $p(\mathbf{c}|\mathbf{a})$. Perceptual inference involves inverting the generative model by Bayes' rule, to compute a posterior belief about the true attribute map given the noisy cues it generated:

$$p(\mathbf{a}|\mathbf{c}) \propto p(\mathbf{c}|\mathbf{a}) p(\mathbf{a}) \tag{5.12}$$

$$\propto p(\mathbf{c}|\mathbf{a}) \int d\mathbf{u}\; p(\mathbf{a}|\mathbf{u}) p_0(\mathbf{u}). \tag{5.13}$$

Written in this way, the operation seems no more difficult than that of Eq. 5.2. Indeed, it might seem simpler because the vector form obscures both the presence of multiple cues and attributes, as well as the binding problem, thus subsuming both simple cue combination (Eq. 5.2) and the two extensions discussed in the Introduction to this chapter (Eqs. 5.3 and 5.6). Has the map-based formulation really resolved the computational difficulties of the combinatorial representation?

The answer, of course, is no. These combinatorial difficulties are fundamental to the multiobject problem. In the map formulation they manifest themselves in the difficulty of computing the integral over **u** (or the sum over its values in a discretized setting). The point-process prior embodies knowledge about the sparse distribution of objects made up of spatially colocated features, and thus it may be highly structured. For example, in the simple discrete model, it may take the form of a mixture of sparse distributions each with a fixed number of objects present. Each setting of the object vector **u** induces a different Gaussian distribution of attribute vectors, and so the net prior distribution on **a** is a mixture of Gaussians. If the binary vector **u** is $n$ entries long, it has $2^n$ possible settings, giving a mixture of $2^n$ Gaussians—summing over each of these is indeed intractable.

So what *have* we gained? In fact, we have gained two important things. First, by expressing all features as functions of space, we have avoided the need for an explicit search over all possible assignments of cues to objects—an operation that had added a further layer of combinatorial complexity to the nonspatial model. Second, as we will see in the next section, the current framework lends itself to a straightforward approximation, and thus provides a substrate for addressing the problem of approximation that has prevented Bayesian modelling from approaching cue combination in complex, real-world scenarios.

## APPROXIMATE INFERENCE

Many probabilistic models used in machine perception, or as the bases for models of biological perception, have led to intractable problems of inference. As a result, probabilists have devoted substantial effort to finding reliable, fast, and accurate approximations to the exact inferential operation. Many different schemes of approximation have been proposed, each with its own advantages and disadvantages. In many cases, the theoretical basis for the approximations may be as involved as the development of the underlying models themselves—or, indeed, more so. Because our goal in this chapter is to illustrate the potential of our modelling approach rather than to develop it optimally with regard to a particular problem, we will develop an approximation that is particularly simple but not particularly accurate. It is related, albeit distantly, to a family of powerful state-of-the-art approximation algorithms known as expectation propagation, or EP (Minka, 2001). A full application of EP with iterative refinement of the approximation may, in fact, be as good a deterministic approximation as would be available within the grid-world model. Our noniterative, simple version of this approach provides a didactically helpful and conceptually transparent example.

Our approach is to ignore the correlations in the prior, exploiting the Gaussian properties of the generative model to arrive at a Gaussian approximation. We start by noting that, conditioned on the value of $\mathbf{u}$, $\mathbf{a}$ and $\mathbf{c}$ are jointly Gaussian with zero-mean:

$$p\left(\begin{bmatrix}\mathbf{a}\\ \mathbf{c}\end{bmatrix}\middle|\,\mathbf{u}\right) = p(\mathbf{c}|\mathbf{a})p(\mathbf{a}|\mathbf{u}) = N(\Lambda\mathbf{a},\Psi)N(\mathbf{0},\mathrm{U}) = N\left(\mathbf{0},\begin{bmatrix}\mathrm{U} & \mathrm{U}\Lambda^{\mathrm{T}}\\ \Lambda\mathrm{U} & \Lambda\mathrm{U}\Lambda^{\mathrm{T}}+\Psi\end{bmatrix}\right). \tag{5.14}$$

We could, in principle, find $p(\mathbf{a}|\mathbf{c})$ from the joint distribution over $\mathbf{a}$ and $\mathbf{c}$ obtained by integrating Eq. 5.14 with respect to the prior distribution on $\mathbf{u}$. This integral, however, is the exponentially large mixture of zero-mean Gaussians we described earlier, with one Gaussian for each possible setting of $\mathbf{u}$:

$$p\left(\begin{bmatrix}\mathbf{a}\\ \mathbf{c}\end{bmatrix}\right) = \sum_{\mathbf{u}} p_0(\mathbf{u})\,p\left(\begin{bmatrix}\mathbf{a}\\ \mathbf{c}\end{bmatrix}\middle|\,\mathbf{u}\right), \tag{5.15}$$

and is, of course, intractable—it requires summing over too many possible combinations of variables. We therefore approximate the joint posterior by minimizing the Kullback-Leibler (KL) divergence between the true joint distribution above and a Gaussian approximation, $q(\cdot)$. This optimal approximating distribution also has a zero mean, and it can be found simply by replacing the covariance matrix U in the conditional distribution (Eq. 5.14) with its average under the prior. We write this average covariance matrix as $\bar{U}_0$, giving:

$$q\left(\begin{bmatrix}\mathbf{a}\\ \mathbf{c}\end{bmatrix}\right) = \underset{\tilde{q}\in N}{\operatorname{argmin}}\,\mathbf{KL}\left[\sum_{\mathbf{u}} p_0(\mathbf{u})\mathrm{N}\left(\mathbf{0},\begin{bmatrix}\mathrm{U} & \mathrm{U}\Lambda^{\mathrm{T}}\\ \Lambda\mathrm{U} & \Lambda\mathrm{U}\Lambda^{\mathrm{T}}+\Psi\end{bmatrix}\right)\middle\|\,\tilde{q}(\cdot)\right] = N\left(\mathbf{0},\begin{bmatrix}\bar{\mathrm{U}}_0 & \bar{\mathrm{U}}_0\Lambda^{\mathrm{T}}\\ \Lambda\bar{\mathrm{U}}_0 & \Lambda\bar{\mathrm{U}}_0\Lambda^{\mathrm{T}}+\Psi\end{bmatrix}\right). \tag{5.16}$$

The covariance matrix U is diagonal, with “1” entries on the diagonal indicating the presence of a particular feature-location combination, and “0” entries elsewhere. The *average* of each diagonal element under the prior will thus be a number between 0 and 1 equal to the marginal prior probability of generating that particular feature-location combination (i.e., the probability of the relevant entry on the diagonal of $\bar{\mathrm{U}}_0$ being “on”).

Eq. 5.16 is a joint normal distribution over $\mathbf{a}$ and $\mathbf{c}$. To obtain the posterior distribution needed to model perceptual inference, we must transform this into a conditional distribution on $\mathbf{a}$ given $\mathbf{c}$. This calculation is omitted here for conciseness, but is a standard operation of probabilistic calculus that can be found in tables of probabilistic identities.[4] The resulting posterior distribution is

$$q(\mathbf{a}|\mathbf{c}) = N\left(\bar{\text{U}}_0\Lambda^{\text{T}}\left(\Lambda\bar{\text{U}}_0\Lambda^{\text{T}}+\Psi\right)^{-1}\mathbf{c}, \bar{\text{U}}_0 - \bar{\text{U}}_0\Lambda^{\text{T}}\left(\Lambda\bar{\text{U}}_0\Lambda^{\text{T}}+\Psi\right)^{-1}\Lambda\bar{\text{U}}_0\right). \quad (5.17)$$

We must emphasize again at this point that Eq. 5.17 is far from being an optimal approximation to Eq. 5.13. Nonetheless, we will use it below to successfully model behavior in a perceptual experiment involving very brief presentations of visual stimuli in which features are sometimes incorrectly bound. In the final section, we will briefly discuss the possibility that exactly this sort of crude approximation may underlie rapid inattentive perception, which is prone to perceptual errors, whereas more elaborate attentive processes may depend on refining the form of the approximation to match the particular stimulus or task.

## MODELING BEHAVIOR

We now turn to the question of how the framework developed here may be used to model data from two different behavioral experiments, both of which involve the combination of cues from multiple sources. As has been the case throughout the chapter, our goal here is purely didactic. The same data can be, and indeed have been, modeled just as successfully using simpler frameworks—these simpler frameworks were, however, tailored specifically to the particular experimental settings. By showing that similar results can be obtained from a more generic framework that can in principle be extended to highly complex scenarios beyond the scope of tailored, object-centered models, we hope both to illustrate its power and to draw useful parallels between apparently disparate phenomena.

[4]The specific result we require is that if $\begin{bmatrix}\mathbf{x}\\ \mathbf{y}\end{bmatrix} \sim N\left(\mathbf{0}, \begin{bmatrix} A & C \\ C^{\text{T}} & B\end{bmatrix}\right)$ then $\mathbf{x}|\mathbf{y} \sim N\left(CB^{-1}\mathbf{y}, A - CB^{-1}C^{\text{T}}\right)$.

### Localizing Simple Cues

The first experiment we look at concerns a version of the "ventriloquist" effect. When presented simultaneously with a flash of light and a short burst of sound, observers often mislocate the source of the sound in a way that seems to be influenced by the location of the light. This phenomenon was studied by Körding et al. (2007), who argued that the way in which the size of the effect falls off with the separation between the light and sound sources made it unlikely that this was a simple case of observers invariably combining visual and auditory cues to location. Instead, they developed a simple binding model of the type described in the introduction to this chapter, in which an ideal observer estimated the source of the sound, taking into account two possibilities: one, that the sound and light came from the same source, and two, that each originated independently of the other. The estimated location of the sound was then derived from the cues by weighting the effects of both models (Eq. 5.6).

The map-based framework that we have developed in the preceding sections may also be used to model these data, and in this section we will explore how. In fact, the model we will require here is considerably simpler than the one that we have laid out to this point, as we have no need to consider multiple different values of visual or auditory attributes. Each flash of light and burst of sound looks and sounds the same as any other. Thus, the only variable that we need keep track of is space. In this version of the model, then, the binary vector $\mathbf{u}$ extends only over space. A value of "1" indicates that a source (either visual, auditory, or both) is present at the corresponding location. In the simulations that follow, we choose a simple independent prior on the elements of $\mathbf{u}$. As there is only one possible value for each attribute, the attribute-specific vectors, $\mathbf{u}^{\alpha}$ and $\mathbf{u}^{\beta}$, are identical to $\mathbf{u}$ in this case (that is, the projection matrices $\text{P}^{\alpha}$ and $\text{P}^{\beta}$ are both identity matrices). The attribute maps, $\mathbf{a}^{\alpha}$ and $\mathbf{a}^{\beta}$, have the same dimensionality as $\mathbf{u}$ and indicate the "strength" (here, brightness or loudness) of the corresponding feature.

To simulate the experiment within this model, we construct attribute maps that contain exactly one source each, positioned in the same way as the visual and auditory stimuli in the original experiment (see Fig. 5.3). Körding et al. used five possible locations for the light and the sound, and so the dimension, $D$, of the attribute map vectors is taken to be 5. As the brightness and loudness of the stimuli used in the experiment did not vary, we can set the strength of a feature that is present to "1" without losing generality. Thus, the simulated attribute maps resemble source maps $\mathbf{u}$. The difference is that although two sources, and therefore two "1"s, might be needed in the source vector $\mathbf{u}$, only one of these will appear in each of the corresponding visual and auditory attribute location vectors. The attribute value for the other source will be "0." These attribute maps are then used to generate noisy cue maps as in the full model, now using one-dimensional Gaussian weights in the matrices $\Lambda^\alpha$ and $\Lambda^\beta$. The difference in accuracy between the auditory and visual localization systems is reflected in both different Gaussian extents within the weight matrices and different degrees of noise (set by $\Psi^\alpha$ and $\Psi^\beta$) in the cue maps.

We then simulate the observer's inferential process as follows. Based on the noisy cue maps we construct a separate (marginal) posterior distribution over each attribute map, without specific reference to the structure of the experiment. That is, we do not assume during inference that $\mathbf{u}$ has either one or two non-zero entries, nor that $\mathbf{a}^\alpha$ and $\mathbf{a}^\beta$ each contain exactly one non-zero attribute. The posterior is thus given by

$$\begin{aligned} p(\mathbf{a}^\alpha|\mathbf{c}^\alpha, \mathbf{c}^\beta) &\propto p(\mathbf{c}^\alpha, \mathbf{c}^\beta, \mathbf{a}^\alpha) \\ &= \sum_{\mathbf{u}\in\{0,1\}^D} p(\mathbf{u})p(\mathbf{c}^\alpha, \mathbf{c}^\beta, \mathbf{a}^\alpha|\mathbf{u}) \\ &= \sum_{\mathbf{u}\in\{0,1\}^D} p(\mathbf{u})p(\mathbf{c}^\alpha|\mathbf{u})p(\mathbf{c}^\beta|\mathbf{u})p(\mathbf{a}^\alpha|\mathbf{c}^\alpha, \mathbf{u}), \end{aligned} \tag{5.18}$$

with the corresponding expression for $\mathbf{a}^\beta$. For each setting of $\mathbf{u}$, the conditional distributions of both the attribute and cue maps are Gaussian, and so the summand is straightforward to evaluate. Writing $N(\mathbf{x}; \mu, \Sigma)$ for the multivariate normal pdf with mean $\mu$ and covariance matrix $\Sigma$ as before, but now evaluated at $\mathbf{x}$,

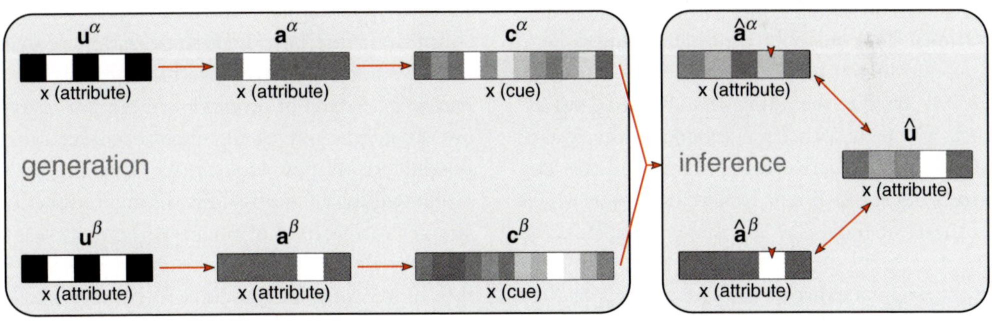


**Figure 5.3** Visual and auditory stimuli: example observations and inference. The left panel illustrates *generation* of one simulated example of attribute and cue maps, each a function of space ($x$) alone, with the sound source at position 2 and light at position 4. Feature-presence maps ($\mathbf{u}$) both reflect both sources, but for each feature (sound, $\alpha$, or light, $\beta$) only one source has a nonzero attribute value ($\mathbf{a}$). Cue maps ($\mathbf{c}$) are more densely sampled and noisy. The auditory cue ($\mathbf{c}^\alpha$) is more extensively smeared and more noisy than the visual. Red arrows show the flow of dependence. The right panel illustrates *inference* of attribute and source maps given the cues. The shaded maps represent the mean of the inferred distributions over each corresponding variable, where in each case the other two variables have been integrated or summed over (e.g., Eq. 5.19). Bidirectional red arrows reflect the interdependence of the estimates. Red arrowheads over the mean estimated attribute maps indicate the locations of the maxima, which correspond to the simulated reported locations. Thus, in this simulation, the sound source was mislocalized toward the position of the light.

we have:

$$p(\mathbf{a}^\alpha|\mathbf{c}^\alpha, \mathbf{c}^\beta) = \sum_{\mathbf{u}\in\{0,1\}^D} \pi(\mathbf{u}) N(\mathbf{a}^\alpha; \Sigma_a^\alpha (\Lambda^\alpha)^{\mathrm{T}} (\Psi^\alpha)^{-1} \mathbf{c}^\alpha, \Sigma_a^\alpha), \tag{5.19}$$

with $(\Sigma_a^\alpha)^{-1} = (\Lambda^\alpha)^{\mathrm{T}}(\Psi^\alpha)^{-1}\Lambda^\alpha + U^{-1}$, $\pi(\mathbf{u}) = p(\mathbf{u}) \cdot N(\mathbf{c}^\alpha; \mathbf{0}, \Lambda^\alpha U(\Lambda^\alpha)^{\mathrm{T}} + \Psi^\alpha) \cdot N(\mathbf{c}^\beta; \mathbf{0}, \Lambda^\beta U(\Lambda^\beta)^{\mathrm{T}} + \Psi^\beta)$ and $U = \mathrm{diag}[\mathbf{u}]$ as before. Thus, the posterior distribution over the attribute map is given by a mixture of $2^D$ (here 32) Gaussians. In this case, the small number of possible locations (and the fact that all lights and all sounds are identical) means that exact computation of this posterior is possible, and so we will not need to invoke the approximation scheme for these data.

We now have a modeling choice to make. How should this posterior distribution be translated into a reported location for the sound? Or, in other words, how should a probabilistic "neural" representation of the likely state of the world be translated into a perceptual decision? The best justified approach would be to define a "cost" associated with each possible answer, and then choose the report that minimizes the expected cost under the calculated posterior. However, the form of the cost function is not obvious. Two possible candidates might be a zero-one match-based cost, where the penalty for any error is the same; or a "squared-error" cost, where the penalty is related to the square of the distance between the report and the true source location. But it is hard to know which of these, or indeed of the many other possible cost functions, observers might have employed in the original experiment—particularly as they were given no feedback about performance. We therefore choose a simple cost function suited to the form of the model. We can easily find the mean of the posterior distribution on the attribute map: It is simply the average of the means of the Gaussians within the mixture, weighted by the proportions $\pi(\mathbf{u})$. We thus take the reported location to be that associated with the peak of this mean function.

Figure 5.4A shows the distribution of reported locations in the experimental data of Körding et al., as well as the distribution recovered from the simple binding model reported in the same study. The simulated distribution of reported locations resulting from our map-based model appears in Figure 5.4B. Both models reproduce the essential features of the behavioral data. One such feature that is difficult to capture in a simple cue-combination model is the way in which the relative bias in the reported sound location falls off as the true separation between the light and sound is increased. This is much easier to explain with a multiple-object model, as pointed out by Körding et al. (see Fig. 5.4C). In essence, the chance of mistakenly thinking that there was a single common source for both light and sound is reduced for larger separations, thus reducing the extent of the bias. The results from our model also display this feature (Fig. 5.4D).

As we said at the outset of this section, our goal in developing a model for these data was purely didactic. In this one experiment we do not expect the predictions of this type of model to differ substantially from those of the simple multiple-objects model. The difference, of course, is in potential. Our cues and attributes are spatial maps rather than scalar location variables. This means the inferential model takes on a generic form, without specific reference to the fact that the experiment involved a single sound and light. (We did assume that there were only five possible source locations, although this was only a matter of convenience. Similar results are obtained carrying out inference over more possible locations.) As such, we have implicitly integrated over the possibility of any number of sources (up to five) of each type being present. In these data the difference in the results of this more complex model will be very small, because these other alternatives carry very little posterior probability. In principle, however, a similar model can be used with no changes to handle a much more crowded environment.

Finally, before moving on to model a second experiment, it is worth reviewing some of the modeling choices we have made. First, we used a simple independent prior on the source locations ($p(\mathbf{u})$) with a high appearance probability. The experiment itself did not accord with this prior, and it is unlikely that observers' general

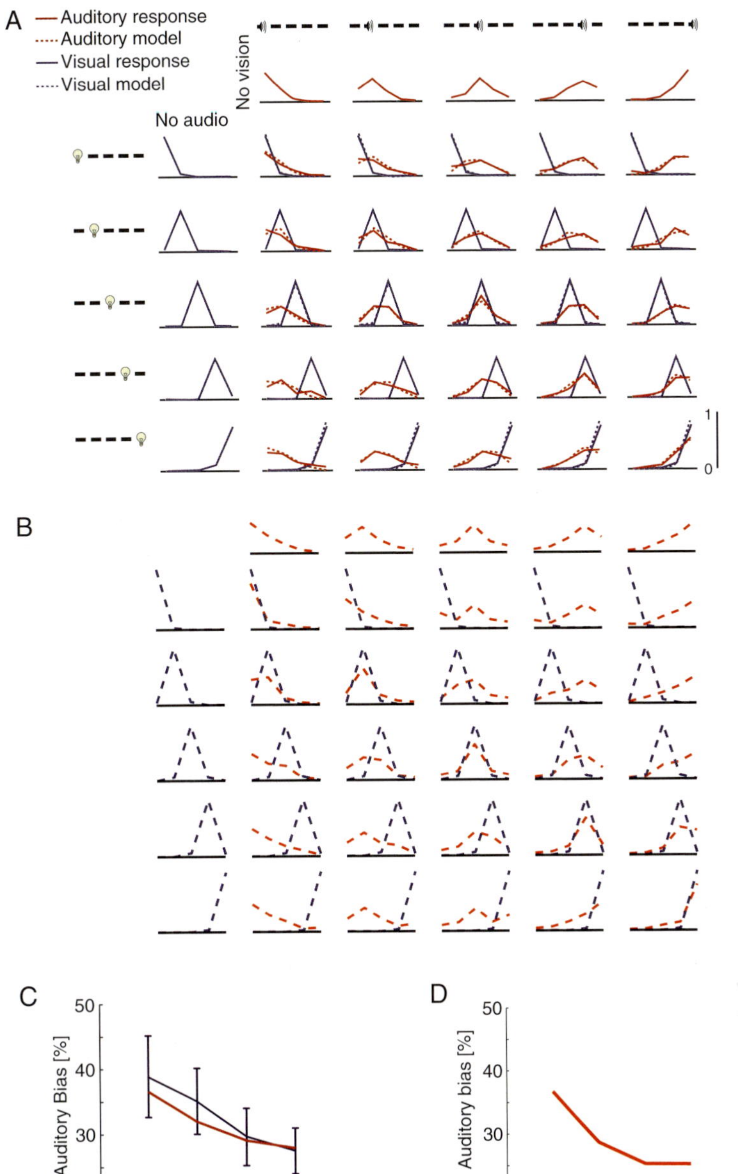


**Figure 5.4** Combining visual and auditory stimuli. (A) (Fig. 2c of Körding et al., 2007). Observers were asked to indicate at which of five possible locations they saw a light or heard a sound. Each graph represents one configuration of true light and sound source locations: The sound source location in each column (and its absence in the left-most column) is indicated by the diagrams at the top; the light source location in each row (and its absence in the top row) is indicated by the diagrams on the left. Solid lines show the distribution of observers' responses across the five alternatives in each case — reported sound source locations in red, and light locations in blue. Dotted lines show the corresponding distributions for a simple binding model simulated by Körding et al. (B) The corresponding distributions, arranged and colored in the same way, generated by simulations of the map-based model developed here. (C) (From Fig. 2e of Körding et al., 2007). The average auditory bias, defined as the (signed) error in location of the sound source divided by the (signed) displacement between sound and light sources, and shown as a function of the distance between the sound and light sources. Experimental data are in blue and the prediction of the binding model in red. (D) The predicted bias as a function of sound and light separation for the map-based model developed here.

experience would either. A more structured prior might therefore be preferable from a modeling standpoint, although determining the appropriate form would itself be something of a challenge—indeed, this is the far broader problem of characterizing prior expectations about the structure of real-world scenes. Second, the Gaussian distribution on attribute values, conditioned on the presence of the source, is a general form that does not closely match the particular set-up of the experiment. In fact, about two-thirds of the objects in the experiment are associated with a 0 value of either loudness or luminance. The model, on the other hand, expects that most objects will exhibit both audible and visible attributes. It is thus arguable that a more appropriate model of this task would include a conditional distribution over attribute values that is sparse, even when a corresponding object is present. Finally, as pointed out earlier, there are a number of ways in which the posterior distribution over attribute maps may be reduced to a single answer in the simulated experiment—that is, there are many possible cost functions that could be employed in computing a perceptual decision. In each case, one can see how to structure the model to reflect the experiment more accurately, and possibly the observers' broader experience. However, the simple version we have described suffices to show how the general framework may be applied.

### Localizing Misbindings

A similar approach may be taken to model a related but slightly more elaborate experiment due to Hazeltine, Prinzmetal, and Elliott (1997), in which the reported location of an object was conditioned on the misbinding of two visual features. The study of visual feature misbinding or "illusory conjunctions" dates to an experiment of Treisman and Schmidt (1982), who noted that observers asked to recall a briefly glimpsed display of colored letters would often report having seen one letter with the color of another. Despite some controversy (Donk, 1999, 2001; Prinzmetal, Diedrichsen, & Ivry, 2001) a number of related experiments have elicited errors in binding judgments in a number of different ways (see, e.g., Ashby, Prinzmetal, Ivry, & Maddox, 1996; Cohen & Ivry, 1989; Prinzmetal, Presti, & Posner, 1986; as well as Hazeltine et al., 1997). In the experiment we seek to model, observers briefly viewed a horizontal array of colored letters, followed by a masking display. They were asked to report the location of the green letter by pointing at the screen, and then to say whether that green letter was an "O." In half the trials, the green letter was indeed an O, in a quarter an O of another color appeared somewhere else in the display, and in the remaining quarter no Os were present. Hazeltine et al. were interested in trials where the green letter was misidentified as an O while an O of another color was present, and found that the reported location of the green letter was displaced toward the location of the actual O, suggestive of an illusory conjunction in space (see Fig. 5.6A). A second experiment yielded similar results when the roles of letter identity and color were reversed—subjects reporting the location of the letter O and then whether it was green—showing that the role of the two feature dimensions was symmetric.

The model depends on the same sort of "grid world" as before, this time exploiting two different feature dimensions as well as location, and thus requiring the approximation developed earlier. We consider three objects placed close together in the center of a field with nine possible locations,[5] each with a different combination of nine possible feature values. The simulation is illustrated in Figure 5.5, where the three different feature conjunctions are represented by the three white entries in each of the two $\mathbf{u}$ matrices at the far left. In this case the number of possible source configurations is $2^{9\times9\times9}$ and exact inference is clearly intractable, despite the modest size of the model. Therefore, inference was performed approximately, with posterior distributions over both feature maps, $\mathbf{a}^{\alpha}$ and $\mathbf{a}^{\beta}$, being inferred according to Eq. 5.17. The means of these posteriors (equal to the modes, $\hat{\mathbf{a}}_{\alpha}$ and $\hat{\mathbf{a}}_{\beta}$, as the distribution is Gaussian) were used to make judgments. A particular discretized

[5] Hazeltine et al. used an array of five letters, but we can obtain similar results using the smaller, three-object array.

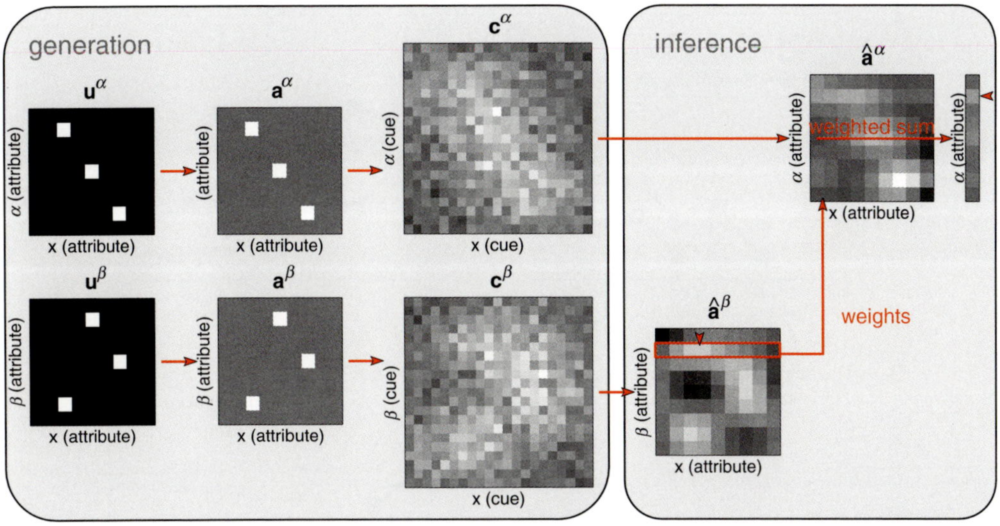


**Figure 5.5** Illusory conjunctions: example observations and inference. The left panel illustrates *generation* of one simulated example of attribute and cue maps. The attribute maps indicate three letters in the display, each with a unique combination of color ($\beta$) and letter identity ($\alpha$), which generate smeared and noisy cue maps as in Figure 5.2. The right panel illustrates *inference* of attribute maps, reported location and binding, given the noisy cues. Mean attribute maps ($\hat{\mathbf{a}}$) are estimated under the approximation of Eq. 5.17. The red box over $\hat{\mathbf{a}}^\beta$ indicates the instructed color to be located ("green"); the red arrowhead indicates the reported location (thresholded center-of-mass). The marginal false color map to the right of $\hat{\mathbf{a}}^\alpha$ shows the summed attribute strength, weighted by the values of $\hat{\mathbf{a}}^\beta$ within the red box. The red arrowhead indicates the reported letter identity. In this simulation the green letter was mislocalized toward the left and misassociated with the identity of the leftmost letter.

value of $\beta$ (corresponding to "the letter is green" in the experiment) was taken to identify the target. We modeled the reported location of this target as the center of mass along the location dimension, $x$, for that target value (i.e., in a restricted region of the feature map, as indicated by the red horizontal box in $\hat{\mathbf{a}}^\beta$). Each location within the $\alpha$ feature map (each column of $\hat{\mathbf{a}}^\alpha$) was then weighted accorded to its value in the restricted region of the $\beta$ map. We then summed the weighted map over space to obtain a marginal distribution over $\alpha$, from which the highest mean feature strength could be selected. This perceived feature value was compared to the target value of $\alpha$ (corresponding to "Is the green letter an O?") to yield a binary yes or no response.

We found the same displacement effect as reported by Hazeltine et al., illustrated in Figure 5.6. The plots in Figure 5.6 include data from trials where the target value of $\beta$ was *not* colocated with the target value of $\alpha$—that is, the green letter was not an O—and show the reported locations of the (green) target for both correct rejections (where the observer correctly says that the green letter was not an O; white circles) and false positives (where the observer incorrectly reports that the green letter *was* an O; black squares). The abscissae of the graphs are oriented so that the "distracter" letter (the O) was located to the right of the target on the plot, and so there is an attraction toward the location of the distracter when the observer incorrectly judges that both target feature values came from the same object. Thus, once again the simple model—this time with a simple approximation—is able to capture the essential features of the behavioral data.

## FINAL THOUGHTS

In this chapter we have laid out one approach to describing the inferential problem encountered

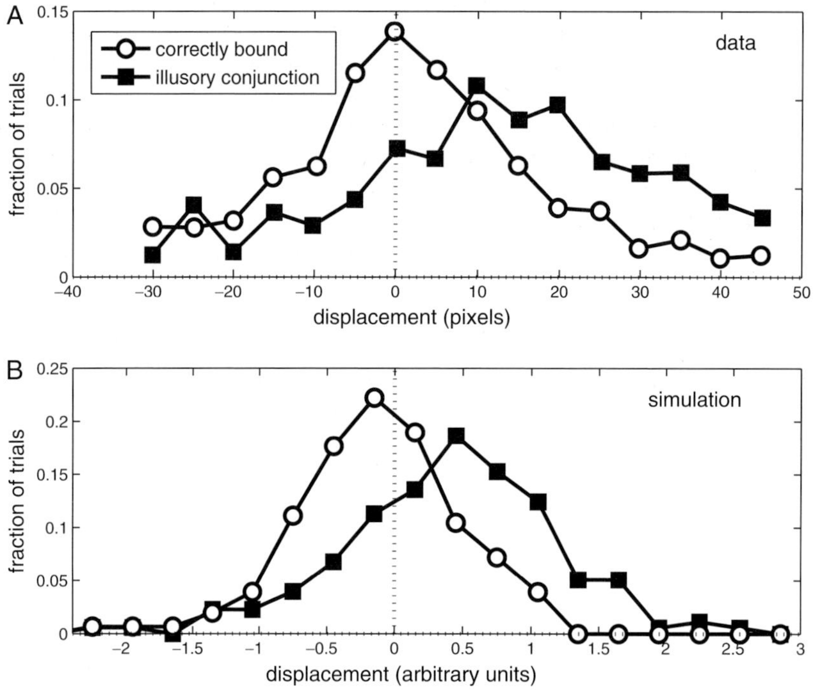


**Figure 5.6** Localization of illusory conjunctions. (A) Results from Hazeltine et al. (1997), replotted from their Figure 1. Observers were asked to locate the green letter, and then say whether it was the letter O—trials shown here are those in which the green letter was not an O, but where an O of another color was present in the display (at +28 pixels). Graphs show binned histograms of reported locations when observers incorrectly identified the green letter as an O (black squares) and when they correctly reported that it was not an O (white circles). The distribution of reported locations of misbound letters is displaced toward the location of the "distractor" O. (B) Results of the map-based model simulation, sorted and binned as in A. The distractor is at position 2. Responses are less dispersed, but a bias in reported locations associated with misbinding is evident.

when integrating multiple different cues that may arise from many different objects. By switching representations from a set of discrete single-valued cues to a spatial representation based on attribute and cue "maps," we were able to naturally model observers' behavior in some simple multiobject and multicue settings, and provide a natural, tractable approach to approximation within these settings.

While effective in these simple cases, the framework is still far from providing a complete description of perceptual inference and integration in cluttered scenes. A first shortcoming is that the model is tuned to a particular level of analysis, corresponding to what is often termed "midlevel" perception, but cues must be integrated at all levels of perception. Second, while the framework makes it easier to phrase grouping and integration questions at this middle level, it cannot resolve the fundamental intractabilities associated with answering these questions. Thus, the identification of good approximate algorithms, and possibly of approximations that adapt to the task context, is an active area of research.

### Object-Based (High-Level) Cues

The framework we have developed here works best when the cues used for inference are inherently localized in space (in the visual case) or with respect to some other dimension important for determining grouping. We pointed out that this is not true of all possible cues. For example, finding the apparent aspect ratio of an object requires a nonlocal computation over the object's boundary, and the resulting cue value is not uniquely identified with any particular position. However, while such nonlocality is difficult to fit into the precise formulation we have developed, by itself it would not prove a fundamental obstacle to extension.

A more significant distinction may be drawn, on the other hand, between "high-level" cues, which can only be identified once a scene has *already* been parsed into objects but which then provide information about the properties of those objects; and "midlevel" ones. Midlevel cues require only presegmentation computations on the sensory image and provide information that is helpful for the segmentation process itself as well as for the determination of object properties. As can be seen in the other chapters of this book, the integration of these high-level cues often seems to follow principles similar to those that characterize integration at the lower levels. Despite this, the dependence of high-level cues on object segmentation makes it difficult to analyze them in parallel with *pre*segmentation cues. A model that incorporated both would be most naturally structured hierarchically, with the extraction and integration of high-level cues performed using the output of the midlevel processing modeled here. This is not to say that high-level cues cannot be integrated with midlevel ones, but that such integration is likely to occur either by the propagation of midlevel information to the higher levels or by constraint-based message passing between layers.

### Approximation and Attention

We have argued that the combinatorial complexity of cue integration in a cluttered environment compels both human observers and machine-based algorithms to rely on approximations to optimal inference. The exact signatures of such approximation in behavior are not easy to tease out. In one sense, they should show up as suboptimality in perception. But while humans certainly appear to make "mistakes" in perception, it is difficult to know whether these "mistakes" arise from a mismatch between the stimulus and the observer's expectations, from a mismatch between the observer's goals and the expectations of the experimenter, or from a genuine suboptimality of processing. On the other hand, one possible signature of this approximation process may come not from "mistakes" as such, but from the phenomenon of sensory attention.

One way in which human observers appear to be suboptimal is in their inability to process or "attend" to all aspects of a cluttered scene at once. Intriguingly, attention has often been linked to the problem of feature integration, and some of the largest behavioral and neural effects of attention are seen when scenes are crowded. Sensory attention is often described as a response to a limitation of some resource. In such accounts, however, the questions of precisely what the resource *is*, and why it should be limited, often go unanswered.

The sort of analysis we have described here may suggest an answer to this question, as explored by Whiteley (2008) in her Ph.D. thesis (see also Whiteley & Sahani, invited submission under review). In this view, the limited resource is *computational*: It is the capacity to perform inference within combinatorially complex settings. To do so optimally would require either physical resources or time that would grow combinatorially in the number of possible objects that must be considered. Faced with limited physical systems and with the need to perceive and act rapidly, observers have evolved to approximate. However, a single fixed approximation of the sort that was considered here may not be ideal. A more refined approach would be to tailor the approximation to the job at hand: that is, to adjust it according to both the current sensory environment and the current task set. Indeed, a number of different approximations may be attempted, one after the other, to achieve a sort of serial search. We argue that this process of adapting the approximation can be thought of as the effect of, and reason for, sensory attention.

## REFERENCES

Ashby, F. G., Prinzmetal, W., Ivry, R., & Maddox, W. T. (1996). A formal theory of feature binding in object perception. *Psychological Review 103*, 165–192.

Baldassi, S., Megna, N., & Burr, D. C. (2006). Visual clutter causes high-magnitude errors. *PLoS Biology, 4*(3), e56.

Cohen, A., & Ivry, R. (1989). Illusory conjunctions inside and outside the focus of attention. *Journal of Experimental Psychology: Human Perception and Performance, 15*, 650–663.

Donk, M. (1999). Illusory conjunctions are an illusion: The effects of target-nontarget similarity on conjunction and feature errors. *Journal of Experimental Psychology: Human Perception and Performance, 25*, 1207–1233.

Donk, M. (2001). Illusory conjunctions die hard: A reply to Prinzmetal Diedrichsen, and Ivry (2001). *Journal of Experimental Psychology: Human Perception and Performance, 27*, 542–546.

Hazeltine, R. E., Prinzmetal, W., & Elliott, W. (1997). If it's not there where is it? Locating illusory conjunctions. *Journal of Experimental Psychology: Human Perception and Performance, 23*, 263–277.

Körding, K. P., Beierholm, U., Ma, W. J., Quartz, S., Tenenbaum, J. B., & Shams, L. (2007). Causal inference in multisensory perception. *PLoS ONE, 2*(9), e943.

Levi, D. M. (2008). Crowding–an essential bottleneck for object recognition: A mini-review. *Vision Research, 48*, 635–654.

Lücke, J., & Sahani, M. (2008). Maximal causes for non-linear component extraction. *Journal of Machine Learning Research, 9*, 1227–1267.

Minka, T. (2001). Expectation propagation for approximate Bayesian inference. In J. A. Breese & D. Koller (Eds.), *Uncertainty in artificial intelligence, 17* (pp. 362–369). Washington, DC: Morgan Kaufman.

Prinzmetal, W., Diedrichsen, J., & Ivry, R. (2001). Illusory conjunctions are alive and well: A reply to Donk (1999). *Journal of Experimental Psychology: Human Perception and Performance, 27*, 538–541.

Prinzmetal, W., Presti, D. E., & Posner, M. I (1986). Does attention affect visual feature integration? *Journal of Experimental Psychology: Human Perception and Performance 12*, 361–369.

Sahani, M., & Dayan, P. (2003). Doubly distributional population codes: Simultaneous representation of uncertainty and multiplicity. *Neural Computation, 15*, 2255–2279.

Treisman, A., & Schmidt, H. (1982). Illusory conjunctions in the perception of objects. *Cognitive Psychology, 14*, 107–141.

van den Berg, R., Cornelissen, F. W., & Roerdink, J. B. T. M. (2009). A crowding model of visual clutter. *Journal of Vision, 9*(4):24, 1–11.

Weiss, Y. (1998). *Bayesian motion estimation and segmentation* (Unpublished doctoral dissertation). Massachusetts Institute of Technology, Cambridge.

Weiss, Y., Simoncelli, E. P., & Adelson, E. H. (2002). Motion illusions as optimal percepts. *Nature Neuroscience, 5*, 598–604.

Whiteley, L. (2008). *Uncertainty reward, and attention in the Bayesian brain* (Unpublished doctoral dissertation). University College London, England.

Whiteley, L., & Sahani, M. (invited submission under review). Attention in a Bayesian framework.

# CHAPTER 6

# Recruitment of New Visual Cues for Perceptual Appearance

*Benjamin T. Backus*

## INTRODUCTION

Can the adult visual system recruit—that is, learn to use—new visual cues for the purpose of constructing visual appearances? How can one test whether cue recruitment occurs? And what inferences can we draw from these tests about the purposes and operation of visual perception?

We begin the chapter with discussion of perception and appearance, to provide the background necessary for testing whether changes in appearance occur. "Cue theory" is the framework assumed by most modern students of perception, but it is nevertheless useful to review Egon Brunswik's (1956) description of cue theory for his definition of important concepts (such as ecological validity) and various distinctions (such as between the measurement and utilization of a cue). Next we address some of the problems that made cue recruitment difficult to study in the past, such as the problem of establishing that a change in behavior is caused by a change in how things look. We then describe a theoretically sensible method to quantify cue recruitment, give some examples, briefly relate cue recruitment to the animal and computer learning literatures, and finally discuss some of the interesting conceptual issues that arise during consideration of the topic.

The term *visual perception* has been used in many ways. Our first task must therefore be to clarify our goal: We want to know whether, through training, a specific signal that was not previously effective for controlling some attribute of appearance becomes effective. We will not be concerned here with learning that affects visually guided behaviors generally, which would include such diverse phenomena as visual-motor recalibration (as occurs when wearing prism glasses) and changes in declarative knowledge (learning the color of a fruit). Instead, this chapter specifically reviews recent work on the unconscious, automatic processes by which our minds construct those mental representations that are consciously known to us, when our eyes are open, as "the way things look." These *attributes of visual appearance* include apparent size, shape, color, surface pattern, distance, motion path, and so on.

The problem of whether new cues can be recruited is worth investigating if one believes two things: (1) that visual appearance *mediates* some behaviors, and (2) that the construction of appearance is in some sense a near-optimal process. The motivation to understand how subjective appearance is constructed derives from (1), while our suspicion that new cues can be recruited derives from (2), as discussed in the next section, "Visual Appearance and Optimality."

Regarding (1), it is safe to say that some visually guided behaviors are mediated by representations that do not reach conscious awareness (e.g., Farah, 1990; Williams & Mattingley, 2004). However, it seems also safe to say that many overt behaviors and cognitive acts are mediated by representations that correspond closely to—and perhaps are one and the same as—the representations of which we become aware when our eyes are open. Obvious uses for consciously accessible visual representations include, at least: learning about the properties of objects in the environment (Barlow, 1990); describing things to other people; and choosing a course of action when one is not under time pressure, for example, "Which side of the mountain should I climb?" (Clark, 2001). We therefore take it as meaningful to ask how particular *attributes* of appearance are constructed. We assume that these attributes make manifest, within a visual percept, a visually derived estimate of some property or properties of an object or scene, which the organism might wish to use.

We examine the effect of a new visual cue on appearance by asking: Can the new cue come to control a perceptual attribute, that is, some aspect of how a stimulus looks? To answer this question one must be specific as to which perceptual attribute is supposedly influenced by the new cue. It is not sufficient to demonstrate that the observers' responses are contingent on the value of the new cue. Instead, one must argue persuasively that an experimentally targeted perceptual attribute has come to depend on some visually measured signal that it did not previously depend upon.

To have a new effect on appearance, a cue's meaning must be learned, presumably from other cues that already specify that meaning. Thus, the learning is associative. As a result, classical (Pavlovian) conditioning procedures offer a flexible tool to test for cue recruitment. Clear demonstrations of cue recruitment in the associative learning literature are rare, but they do exist. For example, the mapping between two-dimensional (2D) images and three-dimensional (3D) representations that they evoke when animated can be trained (Sinha & Poggio, 1996; Wallach, O'Connell, & Neisser, 1953), and the perceived distance to the photographic image of a U.S. coin depends on whether the image depicts a small coin or a large one (which is presumably learned; Epstein, 1965). Several other studies are noted later (see section on "Conceptual Issues"). In any case, it seems clear that the visual system's mapping between signals and percepts can change with experience, such that new cues are learned and used during visual perception. We do not yet know how generally cue recruitment occurs, so establishing a framework within which to study the question is as important as demonstrating a few new examples of it.

## CUE THEORY

Before giving a cue theory, we must define what a "cue" is. Like *visual perception* the word *cue* has been used in many ways. We will not mean "cue" in the sense of an explicit symbol that tells the observer where, when, or what to attend to in a difficult detection or recognition task (as in Posner's cueing of attention to spatial location). Furthermore, a visual signal (i.e., a statistic computable from the optic array or other sensory input) will not be a "cue" by virtue of its perceptual effect, but rather by virtue of being dependent upon, and thus informative about, a property of the world. Thus, the system "fails to use a cue" if it fails to make use of a predictive signal from the environment, and an informative signal is still a cue regardless of whether the perceptual system utilizes it to construct appearance. Binocular disparity is a depth cue, period. This cue is not utilized by all observers.

Conversely, a signal that affects appearance may or may not be a cue. Occasionally the perceptual system uses a signal to construct appearance as though the signal were informative when in fact it is not (see Chapter 1, also Chapter 14 in which Landy et al. discuss the visual system's reliance on confounded signals, dubbed "pseudocues"). If an irrelevant signal participates in the construction of a perceptual attribute, we will say that the signal is "treated by the system as though it were a cue" but not that it *is* a cue. In sum, whether a signal is a cue depends on the statistical properties of the environment, not on cognitive mechanisms. Informally we will sometimes also use the word *cue* to speak of a signal within the perceptual system, constructed by it from the sense data, but properly this would be a *cue measurement*.

In cue theories, the visual system's task is taken to be the construction of useful representations of the immediate environment. To do this the visual system must utilize a cue appropriately: It must use the cue according to its *ecological validity* (Fig. 6.1). Brunswik (1956) considered this to be the correlation between a property of the world and a cue available to be measured, and a modern Bayesian would speak in terms of how well one knows the property, given a measurement of the cue (see Chapter 15). In the laboratory an "artificial cue" can be created by putting some signal into correlation with cues that are informative in the natural environment (and trusted by the perceptual system for that reason). This new "cue" may (or may not) be recruited by the perceptual system for purposes of constructing appearance.

Figure 6.1 illustrates this possibility using Brunswik's "lens model" (Brunswik, 1956; Stewart, 2001; Vicente, 2003). Here, a property of the world $\boldsymbol{x}$ causes various effects $a - e$ within the optic array that are measured by the visual system, $a'$–$e'$, and used to estimate the property, $\boldsymbol{y}$. The analogy between perception and a convex lens derives from the nature of the perceptual act in which one (property) gives rise to many (cues) that are combined back into one (attribute of appearance), that is reminiscent of the divergence and regathering and focusing of light from a point source by a lens. In Figure 6.1, an experimental "new cue" $e$ is made to vary with cues $a$, $b$, and $d$ that are already trusted, and the question is whether $e$ will be recruited, that is, whether it will come to affect appearance in a manner similar to the trusted cues. ($c$ is a signal that does not have ecological validity for $\boldsymbol{x}$ and is not utilized to construct $\boldsymbol{y}$.)

## VISUAL APPEARANCE, OPTIMALITY, AND CUE RECRUITMENT

For cue combination to work, the world must be sufficiently stable so that cues' meanings can be learned at one time and exploited at another. Many cues have been reliable indicators of scene properties throughout evolutionary history. Dynamic occlusion and crossed binocular disparity have always been reliable indicators

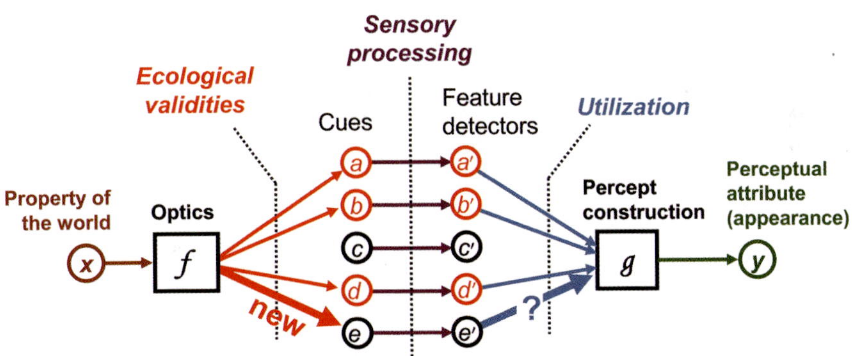


**Figure 6.1** Lens Model and cue recruitment. In Brunswik's lens model, a goal of the perceptual system is to construct an internal representation ($\boldsymbol{y}$) that captures a property of the world ($\boldsymbol{x}$). $\boldsymbol{x}$ can be known from its covariation with cues ($a$, $b$, $d$) that are extracted from the optic array by the visual system ($a'$, $b'$, $d'$) and then utilized to build $\boldsymbol{y}$. Cues are said to have high or low "ecological validity" depending on whether their correlation with the world property is high or low, respectively. $c$ is a signal that has no ecological validity for $\boldsymbol{x}$ and, accordingly, $c'$ is not utilized to construct $\boldsymbol{y}$. Some new signal ($e$) may become a cue (gain ecological validity) when the environment changes. The only way for the system to know that $e$ has become a cue for $\boldsymbol{x}$ is by measuring patterns of activity across $e'$ and the other cues that are already utilized (trusted) to construct $\boldsymbol{y}$. Any change in the utilization (recruitment) of $e'$ must be in consequence of learning that measures its correlation with $a'$, $b'$, and/or $d'$, from which follows Brunswik's prediction of classical (Pavlovian) conditioning: pairing $e$ with $\boldsymbol{x}$ will cause $e'$ to covary with $a'$, $b'$, and $d'$, and potentially cause $e'$ to evoke a similar perceptual response.

of an object's nearness relative to surrounding objects, for example. The ability to measure these cues could therefore develop in phylogenetic time. In some species, utilization depends on exposure to the cues during development, but this can presumably be considered a cost-effective developmental strategy rather than a specific adaptation of the organism to its particular environment, because all natural environments contain these cues and almost all members of these species learn to use them.

On the other hand, some cues may not be universally present, or they may gain ecological validity at some point during the organism's life. The regularity with which this happens in representative environments of our own is not known. Exploitable new contingencies certainly do arise in our interactions with the modern world, and they do contribute to learned perceptual responses, but whether they contribute to visual appearance per se is less clear. The odd feeling of disequilibrium that one has when stepping onto a broken (stationary) escalator, for example, is revealing of a particular learned association (Reynolds & Bronstein, 2003) that is specific to modern environments. This is learning that affects visually guided behavior but that may or may not affect appearances.

If the construction of appearance is near optimal, then the visual system will exploit whatever valid cues are available (e.g., Kersten, Mamassian, & Yuille, 2004). Whether any given cue should be learned is much more difficult to say, because whether a new cue *should* be learned depends on the probability that it is simply in temporary agreement with trusted cues by coincidence, and this, again, is something that occurs with unknown frequency in natural environments.

However, even if we cannot determine which predisposition for learning would lead to the most accurate use of visual cues in natural situations, we can at least see that it might be sensible for the visual system to retain an ability to learn the meanings of new cues into adulthood. Can one train the adult perceptual system to interpret new cues automatically, the way it interprets cues that have long been trusted? If the organism's environment changes, such that some property of the world can be reliably inferred from a signal—a cue—that did not previously have ecological validity and was therefore not effective psychologically during construction of that property's appearance, will the system learn to use the cue?

A *cue-recruitment experiment* can be used to answer this question (Haijiang, Saunders, Stone, & Backus, 2006). Since a cue's ecological validity can only be known from its pattern of correlation with other cues, a cue-recruitment experiment consists of putting some new signal into correlation with long-trusted cues and then testing whether the system treats the new cue as having a meaning similar to that of the long-trusted cues.

## USE OF PERCEPTUALLY BISTABLE STIMULI TO STUDY EFFECTS OF CUES ON APPEARANCE

After training in a cue-recruitment experiment, we might ask an observer about some aspect of appearance and notice that the observer's answers have come to depend on our new cue. How can we rule out the possibilities that observers have, during training, either (1) developed an explicit hypothesis (declarative knowledge) about the meaning of the new cue that they use to answer our questions about appearance, or (2) developed an unconscious cue-contingent feeling about how to respond that controls the observers' responses, quite independently of appearance?

The first possibility would be illustrated by a hypothetical cue-recruitment experiment in which color is made into a cue for distance and either learned or not learned. During training, the experimenter might cause distant objects to be red and near objects to be blue (with distance specified by size, occlusion, stereopsis, perspective, etc.). Suppose the experimenter then discovers, during subsequent testing, that the color of the object affects the observer's estimate of distance, in a manner that agrees with the meaning of color during training. The problem is that the observer might have noticed the correlation during training and used this explicit knowledge to help estimate distance. Indeed, the observer might literally find it impossible to ignore apparent color (which is a different perceptual attribute than apparent distance) while making the distance estimate. One could not be certain that the new color cue truly affected apparent distance, as opposed to having a new effect during a postperceptual decision about how to answer the experimenter's question about distance.

*Perceptually bistable stimuli* prove to be a useful tool here. Because these stimuli *always* appear to the observer in exactly one of two easily distinguished forms, it is trivial for observers to follow an experimenter's instruction to report which one they see. The two forms must be sufficiently distinct that observers know which one they are experiencing (a condition that is implied when we describe a stimulus as perceptually bistable, but worth noting explicitly). A strong incentive, such as paying the subject to say he or she sees one form, could create sufficient postperceptual bias to distort reporting, but this is easy to avoid. The point is that for these stimuli, the *visual system* makes a binary choice about some attribute of appearance. Observers do not feel they are guessing (as they do when judging threshold-level differences between stimuli) but simply, and effortlessly, reporting what they see. When looking at surface curvature in the hollow mask illusion, for example, an observer can report whether the mask appears concave or convex (see Fig. 9.1). This attribute of appearance can be put into correlation with some new cue during training, and, if the new cue has a biasing effect on responding, we can attribute this effect to a preperceptual change in the visual system.

Figure 6.2 illustrates this point with rotating Necker-cube stimuli, similar to the stimuli in the experiments to be described shortly. Before training, a "new visual cue" has no effect on the apparent rotation direction of the cube. During training, stereo and occlusion cues are used that specify the direction of rotation on each trial, forcing one or the other perceptual interpretation. Two values of the new cue (designated − and +) are presented in correlation with the two directions of rotation. The test of cue recruitment is whether, after training, the new cue is effective on its own at disambiguating perceived rotation, with more (+) trials than (−) trials being seen to rotate rightward.

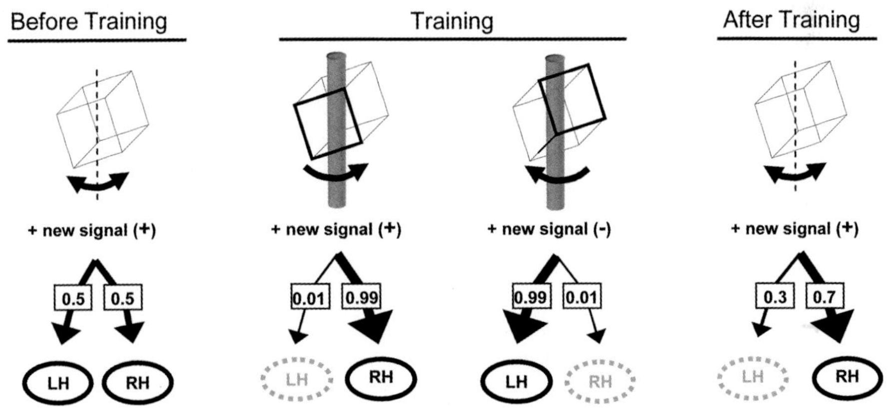


**Figure 6.2** Experimental paradigm to study cue recruitment. Before training, an ambiguous stimulus was equipotential, and a new signal had no effect. During training, stereo and occlusion cues specified the direction of rotation on each trial, and two values of the new signal (–) and (+) were presented in correlation with the two directions of rotation. After training, the new signal disambiguated the rotation. (Ovals: LH = left-handed perceived rotation; RH = right-handed perceived rotation. Typical probabilities for each of these perceptual outcomes are shown in the boxes.) (Reproduced from Haijiang et al., 2006. Copyright 2006. National Academy of Sciences, USA.)

It should be noted that perceptual rivalry is a different phenomenon from perceptual bistability. To exploit bistability in a cue-recruitment experiment, it is best to use short-duration stimuli that do *not* change their appearance during a given trial. It is the stimulus' potential to be seen in either of two ways that is important rather than the fact that it changes appearance with prolonged viewing. Short-duration stimuli are more representative of ordinary stimuli for perception. Thus, despite a vast literature on perceptual rivalry, it is actually more important for understanding perception that we explain single perceptual decisions than rivalry during continuous viewing.

## MEASUREMENT OF CUE EFFECTIVENESS VIA PROBIT ANALYSIS

This section describes how to measure the effectiveness of a cue using probit analysis (e.g., Finney, 1971), which is naturally suited to quantifying (and measuring changes of) the probabilistic outcomes of binary perceptual decisions. Dosher, Sperling, and Wurst (1986) used probit analysis to quantify the relative effectiveness of three visual cues—binocular disparity, perspective, and proximity luminance covariance—that biased the apparent direction of rotation of a Necker cube. When the "strength of evidence" from each cue was described as a z-score—also known as probit units or normal equivalent deviations (NEDs; Gaddum, 1933)—their effects were found to be additive. Thus, it made sense to think of the perceptual outcome on any given trial as the result of a *noisy binary decision* in which each cue contributed some units of belief in favor of one or the other outcome.

Backus (2009) described two methods by which the use of probit analysis can be formally justified within a theoretical framework of Bayesian inference: the Mixture of Bernoulli Experts, and a model based on the more familiar log-odds approach. In both of these approaches, cues provide evidence that moves the value of a scalar decision variable up or down relative to a criterion. Probit analysis applies because there is normally distributed noise in the decision variable, attributable to variability in the measurements of the cues and to internal process noise. The decision is probabilistic because the value of the decision variable changes from trial to trial, even for a fixed stimulus, and the probability of seeing a given stimulus one way rather than the other is given by the area under the normal curve to the right of the decision criterion (for that stimulus). The decision is optimal in that the system chooses the most likely interpretation on every trial, which is determined by the location of the decision variable relative to the criterion.

These models differ from "probability-matching" models (e.g., Mamassian & Goutcher, 2005), which are optimal only up to the estimation of posterior probability. In probability-matching models the system flips an appropriately biased coin at the decision-making stage. Thus, in the probit models a 70% rate of seeing one form (and thus 30% seeing the other) indicates that the posterior probability was greater than 0.5 on 70% of trials. In probability-matching models, a 70% rate of seeing indicates that the posterior probability was 70%.

It is not clear whether these models can be distinguished experimentally. A probit model, however, is theoretically convenient because it allows the quantification of a cue's effect, that is, the amount of evidence it provides, in units of uncertainty (NEDs). As effects come to be understood, the noise is reduced and effect sizes relative to the noise increase.

To measure a cue's effect on a binary perceptual decision using probit analysis, one can simply convert percent seen, for each of the two values of the new cue, to a z-score (inverse cumulative normal) and take the difference. This will give the effect $d^*$ of the new cue in units of (normally distributed) decision noise. For example, if the Necker cube appears to rotate rightward on 70% of (+) trials and 10% of (−) trials, then the differential effect of the cue is $d^* = \text{cdf}^{-1}(0.7) - \text{cdf}^{-1}(0.1) = 0.52 - (-1.28) = 1.80$ NEDs, for an average effect of 0.9 NEDs in each of the two stimuli.

More generally, one can use maximum-likelihood methods to fit a general linear model.

This method is especially useful if some conditions resulted in 0% or 100% seeing, because the direct approach above would require calculating $\text{cdf}^{-1}(0)$ or $\text{cdf}^{-1}(1)$, which is infinite. The result is a set of model coefficients $\{a_i\}$ that gives a best fit of the probit model to the data:

$$\mathbf{M} = a_0 + a_1 x_1 + a_2 x_2 + \ldots + a_n x_n + \boldsymbol{\varepsilon}, \quad (6.1)$$

where $\boldsymbol{\varepsilon}$ is a random variable with standard-normal distribution, $a_0$ captures overall bias, and $x_i$ is the value of the $i$th cue under experimenter control. $x_i$ would typically be $+1$ or $-1$ in the case of a cue with two values, or real-valued in the case of a stimulus property that takes on multiple, graded values during the experiment, corresponding to "cue strength." This equation describes how the decision variable $\mathbf{M}$ is computed by the visual system on each trial of the experiment, with $\mathbf{M} < 0$ resulting in one perceptual choice and $\mathbf{M} \geq 0$ resulting in the other.

One can think of each term in Eq. 6.1 as contributing a signed *subjective reliability* to the visual system's belief about the state of the binary-valued stimulus property. Because these subjective reliabilities add linearly to $\mathbf{M}$, and because each one can be decomposed into a product of estimated ecological validity for the cue and certainty about that estimate (a weighting), we may call them the *moments* of the respective cues (Backus, 2009). By analogy, a moment in classical mechanics is the product of a tangential force and lever-arm length.

It is important to understand the noise term $\boldsymbol{\varepsilon}$ in Eq. 6.1. This term combines both external noise, caused by unmodeled effects from trial-to-trial variation in the physical stimulus, and internal noise, caused by unmodeled variation in the effects of endogenous processes that contribute to the perceptual disambiguation. When one of these effects is understood, it can be taken out of the noise term and given its own term on the right side of Eq. 6.1. In that case, it is important to note, the standard-normal noise in the model becomes smaller relative to the cue moments. Thus, the moments, measured in NEDs, will grow not because the cue has acquired a greater absolute subjective reliability but because it is larger relative to residual unexplained trial-to-trial variation in $\mathbf{M}$.

## CUE RECRUITMENT: AN EXAMPLE OF LEARNED DEPTH BIASES

Two new cues upon which a Necker cube's apparent direction of rotation can be made to depend are the cube's position relative to a fixation mark (the POSN cue) and its direction of translation (TRANSL, with the entire cube moving upward or downward as it rotates right or left). By contrast, a sound cue (SOUND) that consisted of a low- versus high-pitched two-tone sound sequence was not recruited (Haijiang et al., 2006).

Figure 6.3 depicts stimuli for two values of the POSN cue (TOP and BOTTOM). The small square represents a fixation mark. A small dot

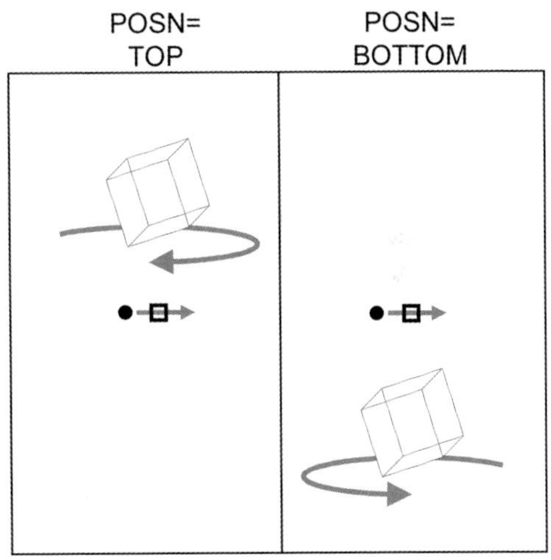


**Figure 6.3** Stimuli. Wire-frame (Necker) cube stimuli. This stimulus is perceptually bistable and appears to rotate either left or right about a vertical axis. Two values of the POSN cue are shown, TOP and BOTTOM. The small square at the middle of the display represents a fixation box. A small dot moved either left or right through the fixation box on each trial (determined by random choice) and the observer pressed a button to indicate whether it moved in the same direction as the front or the back of the cube.

moved through the fixation mark as part of a response-mapping procedure, the purpose of which was to decorrelate the observer's responses from rotation direction and from position. On each trial, the dot moved with equal probability either rightward or leftward. The observer's task was to press the "2" key on a numeric keypad if the dot moved the same direction as the *front* of the cube (both moving rightward or both moving leftward), or to press the "8" key if the dot moved the same direction as the *back* of the cube (the front and back of a rotating cube move in opposite directions, so the dot always moved with either the front or the back of the cube).

Data from three groups (POSN, TRANSL, SOUND) with eight observers each are shown in Figure 6.4, reproduced from Haijiang et al. (2006). Each session in this experiment started with a block of 80 training trials, followed by sequences of 10 training plus one test trial until 440–470 trials had been run. Test trials were presented monocularly and contained no disambiguating cues (other than the new cue of POSN, TRANSL, or SOUND) and feedback was given on training trials. Subsequent experiments showed that the feedback was not important and that small amounts of disparity can be added to test trials without significantly changing the results (Backus & Haijiang, 2007). The data in Figure 6.4 show that POSN was rapidly recruited, TRANSL was slowly recruited, and SOUND was not recruited.

To determine whether these effects were due, at least in part, to long-term learning

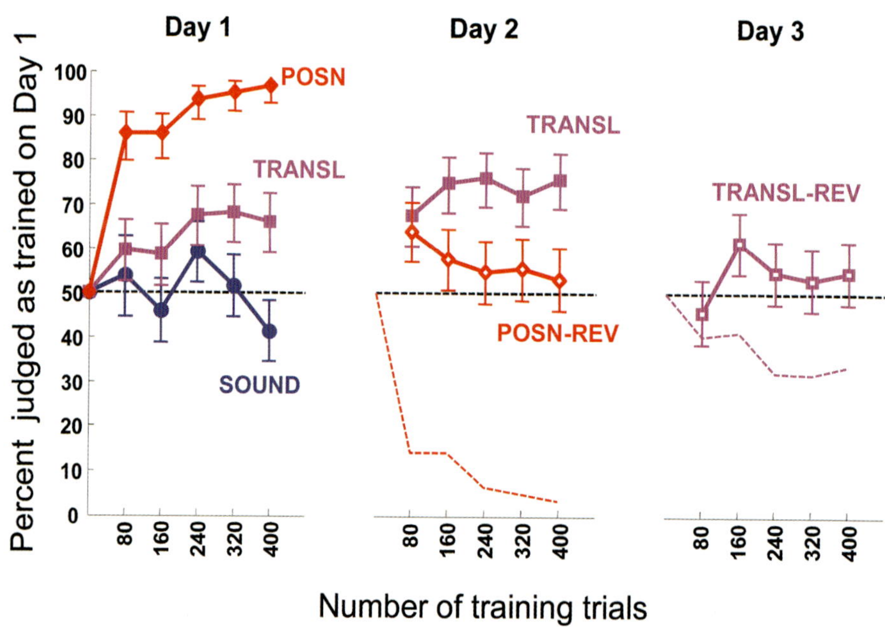


**Figure 6.4** Time course of learning in three experiments. The experiments measured learning for three cues, respectively: POSN (position cue), TRANSL (translation cue), and SOUND (sound cue). Each data point is based on 7–8 test trials per observer (62–64 judgments per data point). Error bars are 67% confidence intervals for binomially distributed data. Data were included only for those observers who completed all sessions of their experiment (eight different observers per experiment). Cue contingency was reversed on Day 2 in the POSN experiment (POSN-REV) and on Day 3 in the TRANSL experiment (TRANSL-REV). The dashed curves replot the data from Day 1 of the POSN and TRANSL experiments, respectively, reflected about the 50% line. New observers, if run in the POSN-REV and TRANSL-REV conditions, would be expected to produce data along these dashed curves. (Reproduced from Haijiang et al., 2006. Copyright 2006. National Academy of Sciences, USA.)

(as opposed to a short-term cue-contingent priming effect), observers in the TRANSL condition were trained (and tested) for a second day, on which the effect increased. On Day 3 (for TRANSL) or Day 2 (for POSN) the meaning of the cue was reversed. For example, those observers who were trained to see rightward rotation when POSN was TOP now saw training trials in which leftward rotation was at TOP and rightward rotation at BOTTOM. The dashed line shows the predicted data in case observers were in the same state at the start of Day 3 (or 2) as they were at the start of Day 1. This prediction is just a reflection of the Day 1 data. Instead of learning the reversed correlation, observers unlearned what they had learned before, and the new cue was ineffective by the end of the session.

Interestingly, the learning in this case appears to be primarily a learned bias to see rotation in a single direction at a specific *retinal* location, not a specific location relative to the head or environment (Backus & Haijiang, 2007; Harrison & Backus, 2010).

## CUE RECRUITMENT AND THE ANIMAL-LEARNING LITERATURE

The work of Ivan Pavlov (1927) had an enormous influence on virtually all aspects of psychology, including, in the first half of the 20th century, perception. Modern theories of perception no longer refer to his work, but in the 1930s and 1940s they did, because it had long been assumed that perception required learning by association (Berkeley, 1709). Brunswik (1956) was explicit about this connection to Pavlov, and Hebb (1949) believed it necessary to find a neurophysiological explanation as to how perceptual learning by association could occur. Experimentally, however, Pavlov's basic paradigm did not prove effective and by the 1950s many perceptual scientists had given up the search for associative learning in perception (Drever, 1960; Gibson & Gibson, 1955). Only recently, with the success of Bayesian approaches to cue integration (as described by many chapters in this volume), has it seemed theoretically necessary to reexamine this area. If the environment changes such that a new cue becomes available, there is no obvious way to learn the new cue's meaning other than by association (Haijiang et al., 2006; Hochberg & Krantz, 2004).

### Classical (Pavlovian) Conditioning

The terms *classical conditioning* and its synonym *Pavlovian conditioning* actually have several meanings. They can refer to an experimental procedure that may or may not cause learning, or to the learning itself if it occurs, or to a set of theoretical ideas about the neural mechanisms by which the learning is implemented. In the experimental procedure, some stimulus $S_1$ evokes a response $R$. Another stimulus $S_2$ does not. $S_1$ and $S_2$ are then presented in correlation for some period of training, and learning is then measured by the extent to which $S_2$ now evokes $R$. Associative learning was understood to be of great importance for three centuries before Pavlov, but Pavlov's formulation made it possible to study associative learning in its simplest form under controlled laboratory conditions.

In the case of visual perception, $S_1$ and $S_2$ may be sensory cues (such as $a$ and $e$ in Fig. 6.1) and $R$ may be a perceptual response (**y** in Fig. 6.1). We still do not know how useful the application of this idea will be in visual perception, but it is possible with hindsight to see several reasons why it would be difficult to observe. First, many perceptual mechanisms are self-calibrating, as is appropriate under an assumption that outputs should be normalized over time (e.g., Barlow & Földiák, 1989; Clifford & Wenderoth, 1999; Gibson, 1937) to improve resolution or compensate for drift. This self-correction leads to a negative contingent adaptation after-effect (such as a motion after-effect that is contingent on retinal location, binocular disparity, color, etc.). By contrast, learning to utilize a new signal that correlates with trusted cues predicts a positive after-effect, so it would be masked by mechanisms that implement self-calibration. Second, the meanings of visual cues may be very stable within the environment—in which case new cues ought not to be learned by adults.

Instead, the cost of being open to learning new cues would be borne during evolution (Geisler & Diehl, 2002) and childhood. It will therefore be important to compare rates of cue recruitment in children and adults, and eventually to measure the rates at which new visual cues change or become available during a person's lifetime.

### Incremental Learning and Counterconditioning

*Incremental learning* occurs if repeated exposure to paired stimuli on training trials causes a strengthening in the response (or increased probability of response) to trained cues. In its ideal form this increase occurs in multiple steps and is monotonic with training, as Pavlov observed for the volume of saliva secreted by dogs presented with tones, after pairing tones with food. Incremental learning is of theoretical importance in part because it can be described by simple learning equations such as the Rescorla-Wagner equation (1972) that could describe incremental growth in a hypothetical internal variable representing the strength of association. In practice, individual animals often change their behavior in an all-or-none fashion that leads one to question the generality with which incremental learning actually occurs (Gallistel, Fairhurst, & Balsam, 2004).

Cue recruitment does appear to be incremental, though it must be stated with caveats. For the recruitment of position as a cue to 3D rotation direction, initial acquisition of the learning is usually very rapid, followed by a plateau, and sometimes a partial decline by the end of the session. Where one sees clear indications of incremental learning is during counterconditioning, after the contingency between position and 3D rotation direction is reversed. An observer who is strongly trained in the first session will show a gradual reduction in effect during subsequent sessions; an observer who is strongly trained in the first block of a single session will show gradual reduction in effect during subsequent blocks within that session.

Figure 6.5 illustrates the incremental nature of counterconditioning with position trained as a cue for 3D rotation direction. Different individuals responded differently on the first block of the session, and their reverse learning occurred at different rates. It seems fair to say, however, that reverse learning occurred incrementally, as one might expect from a slow change in belief over time.

### The Absence of "Learning to Learn"

If the meaning of a cue changes rapidly, the system has two options: It can ignore the cue for its being inconsistent and unreliable in the long run, or it can track the changes to exploit its consistent meaning at short time scales. When contingency is periodically reversed, animals sometimes acquire behavior that reflects the new contingency at a rate that increases with the number of reversals. This behavior has been called "reversal learning" or "learning to learn" and is seen even in honeybees (Giurfa, 2003; Komischke, Giurfa, Lachnit, & Malun, 2002). A straightforward prediction for cue recruitment is that the acquisition rate will go up across successive reversals of a signal's contingency.

What does the visual system do? Figure 6.6 shows that the "learning to learn" prediction was not borne out for position as a cue to 3D rotation. Instead, the visual system chose to stop tracking changes in contingency. This absence of "learning to learn" may tell us something about the actual stabilities of newly discovered cues in natural environments; the visual system may be using a good strategy when it stops tracking changes in the meaning of a cue. For honeybees, the true ecological validity of flower color or scent as a cue to the presence of sugar changes dramatically over time, but the ecological validities of visual signals for the scene parameters that are manifest in visual percepts might ordinarily change little. Indeed, our visual systems may construct appearances that represent certain properties of the world (e.g., object size) but not others (e.g., food flavor) *because* those properties tend to be ones that can be inferred in relatively stable and therefore unconscious ways, using visual cues.

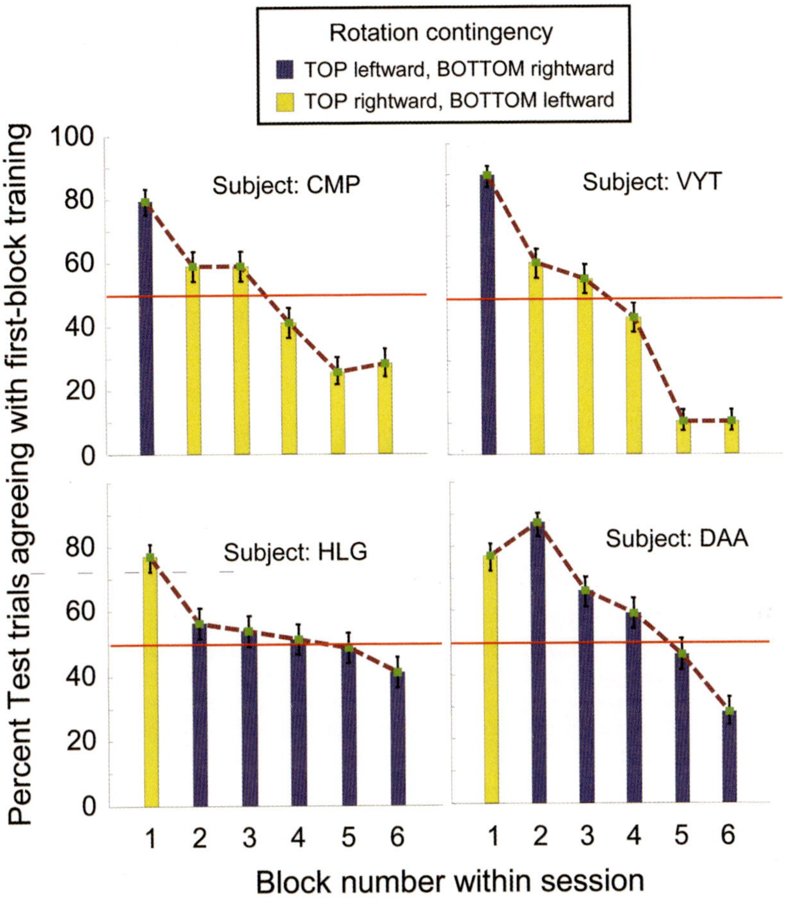


**Figure 6.5** Counterconditioning within a single session demonstrates incremental learning. The four graphs are data from four observers. Four hundred eighty trials per session were divided into six blocks of 80 trials each (40 training and 40 test). In the first block in training trials, the POSN cue specified rotation in one direction at the TOP position and the other direction at the BOTTOM position; this contingency was reversed for the training trials in blocks 2–6, as shown by the change in bar color (from yellow to blue or blue to yellow). All four observers show rapid acquisition in the first block followed by a slow acquisition of the new reversed contingency in subsequent blocks.

## CONDITIONAL INDEPENDENCE OF CUES

When the system learns a new cue, what assumptions does it make about what the new cue indicates? In other words, how does the learning generalize to new situations? At one extreme, the system might believe that the new cue is to be trusted only in the presence of multiple additional signals that were also present during training (learning conditioned on the presence of other cues). At the other extreme, it might believe that the cue has fixed meaning, regardless of whether other cues are present. In a given situation there will be a correct inference to make about the cue's generality, but the system has no way to know which inference is correct, so the extent of generalization tells us how the system is set up to learn (and thus perhaps what is normally the right thing to do). In this section we look at an investigation from Backus (2009) that addresses this issue.

Specifically, in this section we will ask whether the visual system, when it recruits a new cue,

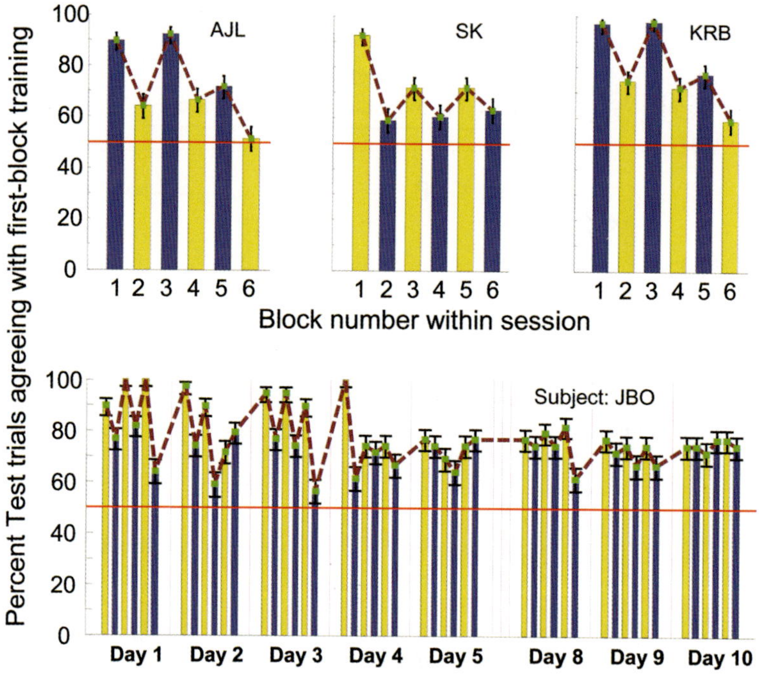


**Figure 6.6** Absence of "learning to learn." The four graphs are data from four observers, plotted in the same manner as Figure 6.5. The fourth observer (bottom graph) repeated the experiment for a total of eight sessions. In this experiment, the contingency between POSN and rotation direction was reversed after each block. Observers' visual systems did not discover and track this rapid alternation, but rather stiffened and stopped tracking the changes in contingency. As with Figure 6.5, learning in the first block was more rapid than learning in subsequent blocks.

treats the new cue as though its value depends directly on (and is therefore directly informative about) a property of the world. The alternative is that the visual system could treat the new cue as though its value depends on (and is therefore informative about) the value of the long-trusted cues with which it covaried during training. Behavior of the former sort would reflect the assumptions of a *naive-Bayes classifier* (Lewis, 1998) because the new cue is assumed conditionally independent of the long-trusted cues from which the new cue's meaning was inferred.

Conditional independence predicts that the new cue will be equally effective regardless of whether the long-trusted cues are also present within the test display. The new cue's subjective reliability (as measured in NEDs for example) should not depend on the values of the other cues, or indeed, whether they are even present in the display. Thus, the presence of long-trusted cues should neither facilitate nor diminish the new cue's effect on appearance. Alternatively, if there is an interaction, it could be that the new cue is believed by the system to be informative about the value of the long-trusted cues; in that case removing the long-trusted cues from the display would increase the effect of the new cue, because the value of the long-trusted cue could then be known only from the new cue, not also from the stimulus.

In Figure 6.7, causal Bayes nets are used to illustrate two possible changes in belief that might occur during cue recruitment. Before the experiment (left graph) the system implicitly believes that some internal state variable **T** depends on a property **A** of the world. This makes **T** informative about the state of **A** and so **T** is trusted as a cue for inferring the state of **A**. When a second internal variable

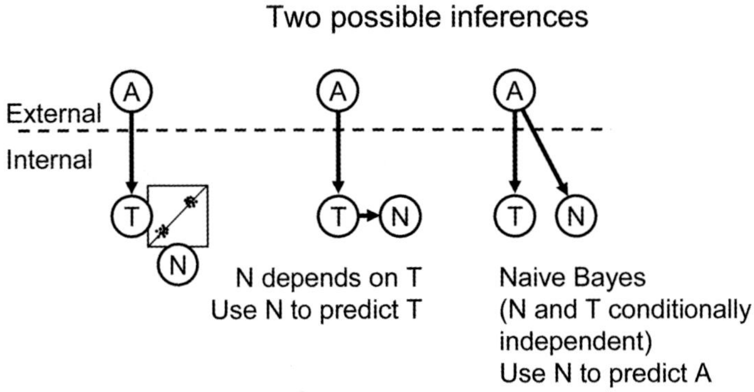


**Figure 6.7** Causal Bayes' net depiction of change in belief during cue recruitment. **A** is a property of the world, and **T** and **N** are internal state variables that represent measured cues. (Left) Only **T** is believed to depend on **A**, but a new cue **N** is put into correlation with **T** during training. (Middle) One way to explain why training causes **N** to be recruited as a cue for **A** is that after training, **N** is believed to depend on **T**. (Right) Another explanation is that after training **N** is believed to depend on **A**, reflecting an assumption of conditional independence between **T** and **N**.

**N** is put experimentally into covariation with **T** (symbolized for two-point training by the scatterplot icon), **N** is recruited as a cue for inferring the state of **A**.

The middle and right diagrams of Figure 6.7 show two inferences about the cause of variation in **N** that could explain the system's new use of **N** to estimate **A**. In the middle graph, **N** depends on **T**, so **N** and **T** are not conditionally independent. **N** is directly informative about **T**, but only indirectly informative about **A**. We might therefore expect **N** to have a larger impact on the system's inferences about **A** when the stimulus does not support separate direct measurement of **T**. In the right graph, **N** depends on **A**. Now $P(\mathbf{N}|\mathbf{A}, \mathbf{T}) = P(\mathbf{N}|\mathbf{A})$, that is, **T** and **N** are independent when conditioned on **A**. As a result, **A** can be estimated from **N** at least as well as **T** can be estimated from **N** (since the latter estimation must be done via **A**), and we expect experimental manipulation of **N** to have equal impact on inferences about **A** whether or not **T** can be measured in the stimulus.

The experimental test of these propositions was done in six observers (Backus, 2009). As before, anaglyph displays showed brief (2 sec) movies of a spotted Necker cube that rotated about a vertical axis. Observers received no feedback on either training trials or test trials. Training trials contained natural binocular disparity for the simulated object (27 arcmin front-to-back disparity) as well as an occlusion cue (the vertical pole shown in the middle panels of Fig. 6.2). These two cues controlled apparent rotation direction on training trials. Each observer saw 960 trials over two sessions, with training and test trials presented in alternation. Test trials were either monocular, or else binocular with a disparitiy that was −4/6, −1/6, +1/6, or +4/6 of the normal disparity for a right-rotating cube.

To model apparent rotation direction using Eq. 6.1, we took into account four factors: a prior, noise, a trusted cue (binocular disparity), and the newly recruited POSN cue. The perceptual decision on each trial depended on all four factors. Figure 6.8 shows data from 320 binocular test trials and 160 monocular test trials collected in two sessions from each of six observers. The percentage of trials with rightward apparent rotation is the ordinate. The ordinate therefore estimates the fraction of trials on which the hypothetical decision variable exceeded criterion, that is, $P(\mathbf{M} > 0)$ for **M** in Eq. 6.1.

Disparity (for the binocular stimuli) is the abscissa. Response at the TOP position is plotted as blue circles (binocular) or a light blue line

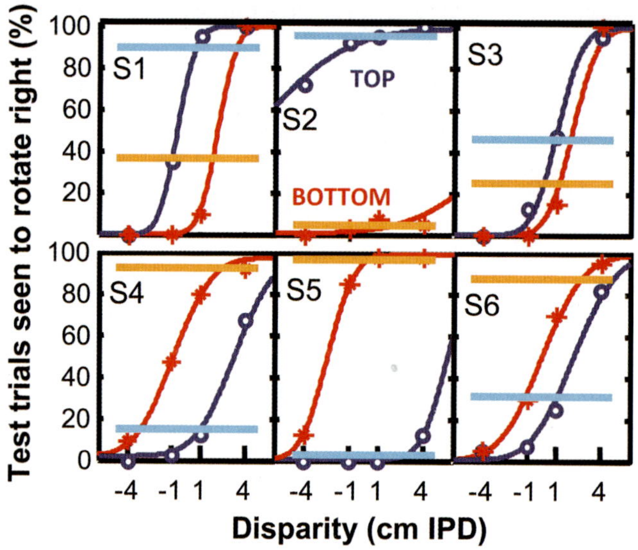


**Figure 6.8** Test trial data for six observers. The percentage of trials in which the cube was seen to rotate rightward is plotted as a function of POSN on monocular trials (light blue, orange horizontal segments) or as a function of POSN and disparity (blue circles and red stars). The abscissa plots the binocular disparity between rightward- and leftward-moving parts of the cube's image in centimeters of interpupillary distance (cm IPD); naturally occurring disparity is therefore ~6.2 cm (typical for the actual separation of the eyes). The ordinate plots the percentage of trials (out of 40 monocular trials or 20 binocular trials) in which the cube was seen to rotate rightward. Blue circles and red stars represent data for cubes that were shown above and below fixation, respectively. The blue and red curves are cumulative Gaussians fitted to maximize the likelihood of the data. Observers who showed a large effect of POSN on binocular trials tended to show a large effect of POSN on monocular trials.

segment (monocular). The percentage appearing to rotate rightward at the BOTTOM position is plotted as red stars (binocular) or an orange line segment (monocular). Both disparity and POSN were effective as cues for all observers, and there were significant individual differences in both cues' effectiveness.

We assumed that for a given observer the prior ($m_0$) was the same on all trials, and that the noise ($\boldsymbol{\varepsilon}$) was drawn from a standard normal distribution on each trial. $\boldsymbol{\varepsilon}$ was assumed to be the same for monocular and binocular stimuli. The terms $m_1$ and $m_2$ correspond to the POSN and disparity cues, respectively. For each observer $m_1$ takes on two values, $\pm a$, that we can write as $ax_1$ where $x_1$ is $-1$ or $+1$ and $a$ is a model parameter chosen to maximize the likelihood of the data. The moment of the POSN cue is $a$ and we plot the effect of the cue as $2a$ so that its size will correspond to the full effect of the POSN cue across the two positions. $m_2$ was assumed to be linearly related to disparity: $m_2 = bx_2$ where $x_2$ is disparity $(-4, -1, 1, 4)$ and $b$ is chosen to maximize the likelihood of the data. The model is now described by

$$\mathbf{M} = m_0 + ax_1 + bx_2 + \boldsymbol{\varepsilon}, \tag{6.2}$$

with $\boldsymbol{\varepsilon}$ distributed as standard normal, so we can apply probit analysis. To compute $2a$ on monocular test trials, $b$ was set to 0. In addition, fits were better when the cumulative Gaussians in Figure 6.8 were forced to asymptote not at 0% and 100% but rather at $\lambda/2$ and $100 - \lambda/2$, where $\lambda$ was the percentage lapse rate, estimated as twice the error rate for training trials.

Figure 6.9 plots the effect of POSN in binocular stimuli as a function of its effect in monocular stimuli for each of the six observers. The diagonal line with unit slope is the prediction

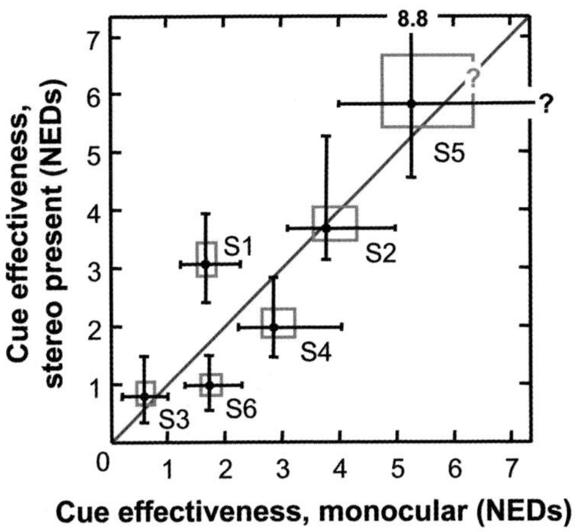


**Figure 6.9** Comparison of POSN cue effectiveness in monocular and binocular stimuli. The data from the six observers (S1–S6) in Figure 6.8 are replotted as cue moments (d*) for the POSN cue. Gray boxes show 50% confidence intervals and black bars show 95% confidence intervals, computed using a bootstrap procedure that resampled data and fitted a probit model as in Figure 6.8. The data show that the POSN cue had very different effects in different observers, but that it had approximately the same effect in a given observer whether or not binocular disparity was also present as a cue in the stimulus. Confidence intervals for observer S5 could not be reliably estimated from the data.

for a system that interprets the new POSN cue as though it is conditionally independent of the long-trusted binocular disparity cue. Boxes show 50% confidence intervals and bars show 95% confidence intervals. Two individuals (S1 and S6) deviated from the prediction with statistical significance ($p < 0.05$) assuming bivariate normal error, but deviations from this line are not systematic and the fit appears to be quite good, considered at the population level. Additional details of the data are described in Backus (2009).

That the data fell along the prediction line suggests that cue recruitment, as a form of perceptual learning, occurred under the naive-Bayes assumption. There were unsystematic but individually reliable deviations from the prediction, showing that individual visual systems do not implement this strategy exactly.

## CONCEPTUAL ISSUES

### Nature of the "Reward" Signal

A common conceptual error is that conditioning (whether classical or operant) requires the use of stimuli that reward or punish. When training an animal, reinforcers (rewards and punishments) are useful; operationally they are simply signals that cause an increase or decrease in some behavior. Evidently the hedonic nature of some signals allows them to act as reinforcers, but a more general view is that the animal's state of knowledge is updated when a learning algorithm encounters certain critical patterns in neural activity to which it is attuned. One such pattern may be correlated activity between a signal (a new cue) and trusted cues, which could in principle be sufficient to cause learning, provided the correlation was detected by the system. This learning can be considered a change in the animal's representation of contingency between various signals (Rescorla, 1988), and functionally it could serve to enhance achievement; using the new cue might normally be the right thing to do when such a pattern of correlation is encountered.

Interestingly, this general approach was taken by Hebb (1949), who thought that percepts should be treated as responses, and who provided a framework for understanding the neural basis by which these responses are learned through association. He did not restrict learning to cases in which a muscular or glandular behavior was rewarded or punished, writing that his theory was "not an 'S–R' psychology, if R means a *muscular* response. The connections serve rather to establish autonomous central activities, which then are the basis for further learning" (p. xix).

### Superstitious Learning

Test trials may be important for learning in our experiments. From a Bayesian point of view, this would be odd: Test trials contain the new cue but do not contain any information about the meaning of the new cue. Instead, one must appeal to other notions: that the system "practices" using the new cue on test trials, or that it gets into the habit of using the new cue, or that there is a cost to learning that is not borne by the system unless the new cue is needed. This need would be evidenced by the fact that on some trials (namely test trials) the new cue is the only one available to disambiguate the stimulus.

Skinner (1948) described laboratory pigeons that learned peculiar behaviors even when food rewards were unconnected to their behavior. A bird that received food at regular intervals might learn to circle leftward or peck a particular location in its cage, presumably because the behavior was by chance followed by food on one or two occasions. Analogously one might suppose that successful disambiguation of an ambiguous stimulus causes the system to resolve ambiguous stimuli similarly on future trials, for surely the perceptual system values the resolution of ambiguity. In this sense, learning to use the position cue in consequence of its value on test trials that happen to be seen one way or the other constitutes superstitious learning.

It may be sensible as a heuristic approach for the system to learn this way. Natural stimuli are complicated, so it is probably the case that very few natural stimuli have good interpretations that are not the correct interpretation. In that case, finding a good interpretation would normally constitute finding the correct interpretation, and the learner would be justified in remembering which signals were present so as to exploit them to resolve the stimulus more quickly when those signals are present in the future.

### Contributors to Subjective Reliability: Ecological Validity, Measurement Noise, and Utilization

A cue's subjective reliability is measured by the extent to which the system uses it during the construction of a perceptual attribute. We can identify three conceptually distinct phenomena that should, in principle, contribute to its subjective reliability. In the Brunswikian tradition, Stewart and Lusk (1994) distinguish between "reliability of information acquisition" and "reliability of information processing" when an organism estimates a property of the world from a cue. The former describes the transmission of information that occurs during measurement of the cue by the system, whereas the latter describes whether the system makes appropriate use of the measured cue. This distinction is similar to that between intrinsic noise and efficiency (Pelli & Farell, 1999). Both are distinct from the cue's ecological validity (correlation with the property in the world) prior to measurement by the system. All three of these steps are present as processing stages (marked by the dotted lines) in Figure 6.1.

Ecological validity prior to measurement and reliability of information acquisition (error in cue measurement) are together responsible for spread in the likelihood function of the measured cue. In other words, the pattern of neural activity evoked by a property of the world at a given instant depends probabilistically on both how good the cue is and on how well the cue is measured by the system. The system's ability to infer the property of the world is then further limited by the reliability of additional information processing, that is, how efficiently the system uses the measured cue during the construction of appearance. For additional discussion, see Backus (2009).

### Cue Recruitment versus Learning to Discriminate

Gibson (1963) defined "perceptual learning" as follows:

> Any relatively permanent and consistent change in the perception of a stimulus array following practice or experience with this array will be considered perceptual learning.

This definition matches the generic meaning of the words *perceptual learning*. However, many researchers have defined perceptual learning as improvement in the ability to discriminate physically similar stimuli (Dosher & Lu, 1999; Fahle, 2002; Fahle & Morgan, 1996; Fine & Jacobs, 2002; Gibson & Pick, 2000; Gibson & Gibson, 1955; Sagi & Tanne, 1994). This is an incorrect restriction of meaning that is not theoretically justified. Perceptual learning rightfully encompasses cue recruitment and perceptual recalibration, in addition to improvement in the discrimination of similar stimuli.

Current textbooks do discuss effects that are presumably the result of learned associations. As noted earlier, Epstein (1965) demonstrated implicit knowledge of familiar objects' sizes. Jacobs and Fine (1999) demonstrated that stimulus height could be learned as an ancillary cue (Landy, Maloney, Johnston, & Young, 1995) that controlled the relative weights assigned by the system to preexisting depth cues. These forms of learning are qualitatively different from learning to discriminate. They consist of learning contingency between signals and properties of the world, rather than improvement in the resolution with which signals can be measured or represented internally. Additional distinctions between cue recruitment and learning to discriminate are described by Haijiang et al. (2006).

### Time Scale of the Learning

The data shown in the figures of this chapter are from test trials that were intermixed with training trials during experimental sessions. The learning is therefore a mixture of short- and long-term effects (Backus & Haijiang, 2007; Haijiang et al., 2006). Averaged data from a single session cannot determine how long the learning lasts. If the learning lasts only for a few trials, one might rather call it "priming"—which is not to call it un-useful (see, for example, Maloney, Dal Martello, Sahm, & Spillmann, 2005; Yu & Cohen, 2008). Data were collected across several sessions, or several blocks within a session, for many of the experiments in studies that have been mentioned in this chapter. These data show that initial and later learning are different. Typically there is additional learning on additional days, and less learning after cues are reversed in meaning, as compared to initial learning (see Figs. 6.4, 6.5, and 6.6). Such effects demonstrate a long-term component to the learning that may be properly called "cue recruitment" rather than priming.

## CONCLUSIONS

The visual system constructs visual appearances to represent various properties of visible objects. "Cue theory" is the old name for the currently accepted framework for understanding appearance: Objects give rise to informative patterns in the optic array that can be described with simple (low-dimensional) statistics; these patterns or "cues" are then measured by the visual system and used to recover the properties of the objects. To be optimal the visual system must make full use of the available cues, which predicts that the system should recruit a new cue if the environment changes such that the cue becomes a reliable indicator of a represented object property. New cues are in fact recruited by the system, but study of this phenomenon has only just begun.

"Visual appearances" are mental representations of visually acquired information that admit to conscious introspection. Not all visually guided behavior is mediated by appearance, so there are limits to what can be learned about visual perception if one fails to determine the extent to which a visually guided behavior under study is mediated by appearance. The contributions of different cues to the appearance of a perceptually bistable stimulus can be quantified in a theoretically meaningful way by probit analysis. Perceptually bistable stimuli are a particularly useful tool for studying cue recruitment and cue combination during the construction of appearance. Whether cue recruitment will prove conceptually useful in the long run to understanding perception remains to be seen.

Cue-combination experiments suggest that, by default, the system assumes that a newly discovered cue is conditionally independent from long-trusted cues that inform about the same object property. However, the unwillingness of the visual system to track reversals in the meaning of a new cue suggests that visual perception is designed to construct representations from visual signals whose meanings do not change much over time.

## ACKNOWLEDGMENTS

The author thanks his colleague and former student, Qi Haijiang, for collaboration and for collecting data, including the previously unpublished data in Figures 6.5 and 6.6.

Dr. Haijiang's doctoral dissertation describes additional work on cue recruitment and is available from the University of Pennsylvania, Department of Bioengineering. The work in this chapter was funded by grants from the National Institutes of Health (R01 EY 013988), the National Science Foundation (BCS-0810944), and the Human Frontier Science Program (RPG 3/2006).

## REFERENCES


Backus, B. T. (2009). The mixture of Bernoulli experts: A theory to quantify reliance on cues in dichotomous perceptual decisions. *Journal of Vision, 9,* 6 1–19.

Backus, B. T., & Haijiang, Q. (2007). Competition between newly recruited and pre-existing visual cues during the construction of visual appearance. *Vision Research, 47,* 919–924.

Barlow, H. (1990). Conditions for versatile learning, Helmholtz's unconscious inference, and the task of perception. *Vision Research, 30,* 1561–1571.

Barlow, H. B., & Földiák, P. (1989). Adaptation and decorrelation in the cortex. In R. M. Durbin, C. Miall, & G. J. Mitchison (Eds.), *The computing neuron* (pp. 54–72). Wokingham, England: Addison-Wesley.

Berkeley, G. (1709). *An essay towards a new theory of vision.* Indianapolis, IN: Bobbs-Merrill.

Brunswik, E. (1956). *Perception and the representative design of psychological experiments.* Berkeley, CA: University of California Press.

Clark, A. (2001). Visual experience and motor action: Are the bonds too tight? *The Philosophical Review, 110,* 495–519.

Clifford, C. W., & Wenderoth, P. (1999). Adaptation to temporal modulation can enhance differential speed sensitivity. *Vision Research, 39,* 4324–4332.

Dosher, B. A., & Lu, Z. L. (1999). Mechanisms of perceptual learning. *Vision Research, 39,* 3197–3221.

Dosher, B. A., Sperling, G., & Wurst, S. A. (1986). Tradeoffs between stereopsis and proximity luminance covariance as determinants of perceived 3D structure. *Vision Research, 26,* 973–990.

Drever, J. (1960). Perceptual learning. *Annual Review of Psychology, 11,* 131–160.

Epstein, W. (1965). Nonrelational judgments of size and distance. *American Journal of Psychology, 78,* 120–123.

Fahle, M. (2002). Introduction. In M. Fahle & T. Poggio (Eds.), *Perceptual learning* (pp. ix–xii). Cambridge, MA: MIT Press.

Fahle, M., & Morgan, M. (1996). No transfer of perceptual learning between similar stimuli in the same retinal position. *Current Biology, 6,* 292–297.

Farah, M. (1990). *Visual agnosia.* Cambridge, MA: MIT Press.

Fine, I., & Jacobs, R. A. (2002). Comparing perceptual learning tasks: A review. *Journal of Vision, 2,* 190–203.

Finney, D. J. (1971). *Probit analysis.* Cambridge, England: Cambridge University Press.

Gaddum, J. H. (1933). *Reports on biological standards. III. Methods of biological assay depending on a quantal response.* London, England: H.M. Stationary Office.

Gallistel, C. R., Fairhurst, S., & Balsam, P. (2004). The learning curve: Implications of a quantitative analysis. *Proceedings of the National Academy of Sciences USA, 101,* 13124–13131.

Geisler, W. S., & Diehl, R. L. (2002). Bayesian natural selection and the evolution of perceptual systems. *Philosophical Transactions of the Royal Society of London B: Biological Sciences, 357,* 419–448.

Gibson, E. J. (1963). Perceptual learning. *Annual Review of Psychology, 14,* 29–56.

Gibson, E. J., & Pick, A. D. (2000). *An ecological approach to perceptual learning and development.* New York, NY: Oxford University Press.

Gibson, J. J. (1937). Adaptation with negative after-effect. *Psychological Review, 44,* 222–244.

Gibson, J. J., & Gibson, E. J. (1955). Perceptual learning: Differentiation or enrichment? *Psychological Review, 62,* 32–41.

Giurfa, M. (2003). Cognitive neuroethology: Dissecting non-elemental learning in a honeybee brain. *Current Opinion in Neurobiology, 13,* 726–735.

Haijiang, Q., Saunders, J. A., Stone, R. W., & Backus, B. T. (2006). Demonstration of cue recruitment: Change in visual appearance by means of Pavlovian conditioning. *Proceedings of the National Academy of Science USA, 103,* 483–488.

Harrison, S. J., & Backus, B. T. (2010). Disambiguating Necker cube rotation using a location cue: What types of spatial location signal can the visual system learn? *Journal of Vision, 10*(6):23, 1–15.

Hebb, D. O. (1949). *Organization of behavior.* New York, NY: Wiley.

Hochberg, J. E., & Krantz, D. (2004). Brunswik and Bayes: A review of The Essential Brunswik: Beginnings, Explications, Applications, by Kenneth R. Hammond, Thomas R. Stewart, New York: Oxford University Press, 2001. *Contemporary Psychology: APA Review of Books, 49,* 785–787.

Jacobs, R. A., & Fine, I. (1999). Experience-dependent integration of texture and motion cues to depth. *Vision Research, 39,* 4062–4075.

Kersten, D., Mamassian, P., & Yuille, A. (2004). Object perception as Bayesian inference. *Annual Review of Psychology, 55,* 271–304.

Komischke, B., Giurfa, M., Lachnit, H., & Malun, D. (2002). Successive olfactory reversal learning in honeybees. *Learning and Memory, 9,* 122–129.

Landy, M. S., Maloney, L. T., Johnston, E. B., & Young, M. (1995). Measurement and modeling of depth cue combination: In defense of weak fusion. *Vision Research, 35,* 389–412.

Lewis, D. D. (1998). *Naive Bayes at forty: The independence assumption in information retrieval.* In C. Nedellec & C. Rouveirol (Eds.), *Proceedings 10th European Conference on Machine Learning, Lecture Notes in Computer Science, Vol. 1398* (pp. 4–15). New York: Springer.

Maloney, L. T., Dal Martello, M. F., Sahm, C., & Spillmann, L. (2005). Past trials influence perception of ambiguous motion quartets through pattern completion. *Proceedings of the National Academy of Science USA, 102,* 3164–3169.

Mamassian, P., & Goutcher, R. (2005). Temporal dynamics in bistable perception. *Journal of Vision, 5,* 361–375.

Pavlov, I. P. (1927). *Conditioned reflexes.* Oxford, England: Oxford University Press.

Pelli, D. G., & Farell, B. (1999). Why use noise? *Journal of the Optical Society of America A, 16,* 647–653.

Rescorla, R. A. (1988). Pavlovian conditioning. It's not what you think it is. *The American Psychologist, 43,* 151–160.

Rescorla, R. A., & Wagner, A. R. (1972). A theory of Pavlovian conditioning: Variation in the effectiveness of reinforcement and non-reinforcement. In A. H. Black & W. F. Prokasy (Eds.), *Classical conditioning II: Current theory and research* (pp. 64–99). New York, NY: Appleton Century Crofts.

Reynolds, R. F., & Bronstein, A. M. (2003). The broken escalator phenomenon. Aftereffect of walking onto a moving platform. *Experimental Brain Research, 151,* 301–308.

Sagi, D., & Tanne, D. (1994). Perceptual learning: Learning to see. *Current Opinion in Neurobiology, 4,* 195–199.

Sinha, P., & Poggio, T. (1996). I think I know that face . . . [letter]. *Nature, 384,* 404.

Skinner, B. F. (1948). "Superstition" in the pigeon. *Journal of Experimental Psychology, 38,* 168–172.

Stewart, T. R. (2001). The lens model equation. In K. R. Hammond & T. R. Stewart (Eds.), *The essential Brunswik* (pp. 357–362). New York, NY: Oxford University Press.

Stewart, T. R., & Lusk, C. M. (1994). 7 components of judgmental forecasting skill–Implications for research and the improvement of forecasts. *Journal of Forecasting, 13,* 579–599.

Vicente, K. J. (2003). Beyond the lens model and direct perception: Toward a broader ecological psychology. *Ecological Psychology, 15,* 241–267.

Wallach, H., O'Connell, D. N., & Neisser, U. (1953). The memory effect of visual perception of three-dimensional form. *Journal of Experimental Psychology, 45,* 360–368.

Williams, M. A., & Mattingley, J. B. (2004). Unconscious perception of non-threatening facial emotion in parietal extinction. *Experimental Brain Research, 154,* 403–406.

Yu, A. J., & Cohen, J. D. (2008). Sequential effects: Superstition or rational behavior? *Advances in Neural Information Processing Systems, 21,* 1873–1880.

# CHAPTER 7

## Combining Image Signals before Three-Dimensional Reconstruction: The Intrinsic Constraint Model of Cue Integration

*Fulvio Domini and Corrado Caudek*

Bayesian probability theory provides a normative framework for describing how prior knowledge and information from multiple cues can be combined to make perceptual inferences (Knill & Richards, 1996; Körding, 2007). Landy, Banks, and Knill (Chapter 1) describe a particular instantiation of the Bayesian normative model, which gives rise to linear models to maximize reliability. In this chapter, we will focus only on this particular version of Bayesian cue combination. It has been linear cue integration, in fact, that has motivated the largest amount of empirical investigation to characterize how primate observers combine information from multiple cues (e.g., Angelaki, Gu, & DeAngelis, 2009; Drewing & Ernst, 2006; Gu, DeAngelis, & Angelaki, 2008; Helbig & Ernst, 2007; Nardini, Jones, Bedford, & Braddick, 2008).

One application of the models in which the cues are combined linearly with weights proportional to the reliability of individual cues (see Chapters 1 and 2) concerns the case in which a world property causes two (or more) direct cues (see Fig. 2.1, left panel). In these circumstances, linear cue combination is meaningful. There are other cases, however, in which the relation between the world's property and the image cues is indirect, that is, it is mediated by "nuisance" parameters not specified by optical information.

To provide a concrete example, let us consider the relationship between surface orientation, on the one hand, and disparity and velocity information, on the other. The orientation of a planar surface is usually described in terms of two parameters: slant ($\sigma$) and tilt ($\tau$). $\sigma$ is the angle between the surface normal and the line of sight; $\tau$ is the angle between the projection of the surface normal onto the image plane and the horizontal axis. Whereas $\tau$ is *fully* specified by either the disparity field or the velocity field, the recovery of $\sigma$ requires knowledge of parameters that are not specified by optical information. The recovery of $\sigma$ from disparity requires knowledge of the viewing distance ($z_f$) and the recovery of $\sigma$ from velocity requires knowledge of the relative rotation between the object and the observer ($\omega$).

What is important for the present discussion is that the application of the linear models for maximum reliability is faced with different problems when recovering $\tau$ or $\sigma$. The application of the model is straightforward when recovering $\tau$, but it is more problematic when recovering $\sigma$. In this second case, in fact, it must assume unbiased estimates of the "nuisance" parameters $z_f$ and $\omega$.

In the present chapter, we will examine the possibility that the visual system is unable to generate unbiased estimates of world properties from any single depth cue (see Chapter 1 in this volume). In terms of the aforementioned example, this possibility corresponds to the recovery of $\sigma$ when unbiased estimates of the parameters $z_f$ and $\omega$ are not available. If the single-cue estimates of the world properties are indeed biased, then we can envisage two consequences. First, the model in which the cues are combined linearly with weights proportional to the reliability of individual cues can no longer be used. If the estimates of the world properties are biased, in fact, it is meaningless to maximize reliability. Second, we need to rethink our understanding of the goal of the visual system. Is the goal of the visual system to recover an undistorted depth map of the spatial layout and of the objects within it? Or is the goal of the visual system to guarantee a successful interaction between the observer and the environment without recovering metric three-dimensional (3D) information?

By questioning the necessity of an unbiased metric representation, we can develop a normative model with a different objective. Here, we will propose a normative model in which the recovery of 3D information follows two successive stages of processing. In the first stage of processing, the *affine* depth map is estimated *locally*. In the second stage of processing, the recovered local estimates are integrated in a global representation and are opportunely scaled (e.g., by taking into consideration extraretinal information and the properties of the whole visual scene).

In this chapter, we will only focus on the first processing stage. We will hypothesize that, in this stage of processing, the goal of the system is to estimate the *scaled* depth map (not the metric depth map). A scaled depth map is related to the metric depth map through an unknown scaling constant $k$. Note that the problem of recovering the scaled depth map is isomorphic to the multimodal integration problem of estimating the spatial localization of a target. In both cases, in fact, the sensory data are sufficient for generating an *unbiased* estimator of the world property.

For the sake of simplicity, here we will discuss only two depth cues: disparity and velocity. In the first part of this chapter, we will show that (1) retinal disparities and retinal velocities are sufficient to guarantee *unbiased* estimates of the scaled depth map, and (2) by optimally combining these two cues (a process which we term *intrinsic constraint*, or IC), we can maximize the reliability of the solution. In the second part of this chapter, we will present a methodology for testing the hypothesized combination process and we will discuss the available empirical results.

## LINEAR COMBINATION OF DEPTH ESTIMATES

Features on the surface of a 3D object project to slightly different locations in the two retinal images. The differences between these projections specify binocular disparities and provide information about the 3D arrangement of distal features. In turn, the relative motion between the observer and the distal object induces retinal velocities. The magnitudes of these velocities depend on the 3D locations of the distal features and are informative about the 3D structure of the distal object. In the following, we will show how the linear model of cue combination can be applied to the problem of depth estimation from these two depth cues. Then, we will discuss the limits of such an approach.

### Retinal Disparities

If an object is small enough, then the relationship between retinal disparities and the 3D location of the projecting features can be characterized by a simple equation. Let us term $d_i$ the horizontal disparity of the $i^{th}$ feature point. Assume that the object is placed at a fixation distance $z_f$ from the observer and that $z_i$ is the relative depth of the $i^{th}$ feature point with respect to the fixation point $F$ (Fig. 7.1). For an object subtending a small visual angle, Eq. 7.1 defines the relationship among the *image signals* $\mathbf{d} = (d_1, \ldots, d_n)$, the *depth map* $\mathbf{z} = (z_1, \ldots, z_n)$, and the *scene parameters* $\mathbf{p_d} = (z_f)$:

$$d_i \approx IOD\frac{z_i}{z_f^2} + \varepsilon_{d_i}, \tag{7.1}$$

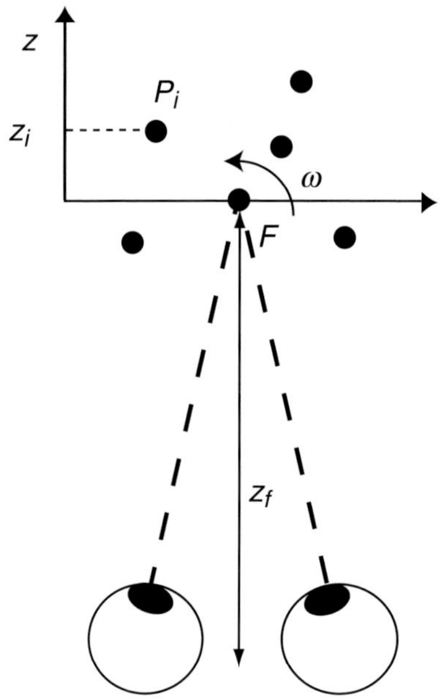


**Figure 7.1** Schematic representation of a binocular observer viewing an object composed of the feature points $P_i$. The observer fixates a point $F$ located at an exocentric distance $z_f$. We term $z_i$ the depth of each point $P_i$ relative to the fixation point. The instantaneous angular velocity about a vertical axis centered at $F$ is indicated by $\omega$.

where *IOD* is the observer's interocular distance and $\varepsilon_{d_i}$ is a Gaussian random variable representing the noise in the disparity measurements.

### Retinal Velocities

Let us term $v_i$ the retinal velocity of the $i^{th}$ feature point. If the observer translates horizontally by $T_x$ while fixating the object, or the object rotates about a vertical axis centered at the fixation point $F$, then the pattern of retinal velocities is

$$v_i \approx \omega \frac{z_i}{z_f} + \varepsilon_{v_i}. \tag{7.2}$$

If the observer moves about an otherwise stationary object, then $\omega = T_x/z_f$. $\varepsilon_{v_i}$ is a Gaussian random variable representing the noise in the velocity measurements. The *scene parameters* are $\mathbf{p_v} = (z_f, T_x)$.

### Maximum A Posteriori Estimation of Depth

Suppose that we are interested in estimating the depth $\mathbf{z}$ from the image signals $\mathbf{d}$ and $\mathbf{v}$. According to Bayesian cue integration, an estimate of $\mathbf{z}$ is provided by the mode of the posterior distribution

$$p(\mathbf{z}|\mathbf{d}, \mathbf{v}) = \frac{p(\mathbf{d}, \mathbf{v}|\mathbf{z})p(\mathbf{z})}{p(\mathbf{d}, \mathbf{v})}, \tag{7.3}$$

where $p(\mathbf{d}, \mathbf{v}|\mathbf{z})$ is the likelihood function, $p(\mathbf{z})$ is the prior, and $p(\mathbf{d}, \mathbf{v})$ is a constant term. To find the maximum a posteriori (MAP) estimate, we need to specify both the likelihood function $p(\mathbf{d}, \mathbf{v}|\mathbf{z})$ and the prior $p(\mathbf{z})$. Let us focus on the former.

The likelihood function can be specified in different ways, depending on the assumptions that are made about the underlying mechanisms that are responsible for the processing of disparity and velocity information. The linear case of Bayesian cue integration described in Chapter 1 is a particular instantiation of the Bayesian normative model. If we assume a strictly modular architecture, with stereo and velocity processing modules providing independent estimates of the depth map, then the likelihood function of Eq. 7.3 can be written as follows:

$$p(\mathbf{d}, \mathbf{v}|\mathbf{z}) = p(\mathbf{d}|\mathbf{z}; \mathbf{p_d})p(\mathbf{v}|\mathbf{z}; \mathbf{p_v}), \tag{7.4}$$

where $\mathbf{p_d}$ and $\mathbf{p_v}$ are the scene parameters and $p(\mathbf{d}|\mathbf{z}; \mathbf{p_d})$ and $p(\mathbf{d}|\mathbf{z}; \mathbf{p_v})$ are Gaussian functions peaked at the veridical depth value $\mathbf{z_0}$. As stated in Chapter 1 (Eqs. 1.1–1.3), for Gaussian distributions and for flat prior distributions, the MAP estimate is found through a weighted linear combination of the depth estimates computed separately for each distinct signal.

### Independent Modules and Estimates of 3D Properties

The model of linear cue combination described in Chapter 1 has been developed under the assumption that an unbiased estimate of a world property (e.g., depth) can be derived from each cue separately. Only if we make this assumption, in fact, does it make sense to look for the combination rule that minimizes the variance of the combined estimate. Suppose, instead, that each distinct cue generates a biased estimate of the world property. In such circumstances, rather than the minimum-variance estimator, it would make sense to look for a combination rule that minimizes the bias of the final estimate. But how can this goal be reached? There is no simple answer to this question. And the reliabilities of the cues do not help. In fact, the most biased estimate may also be the most reliable. From these considerations, it is easy to conclude that the linear model of cue combination must assume unbiased estimates from single cues and it cannot be applied if this assumption is violated.

It is of tantamount importance, therefore, to understand whether the human visual system can obtain unbiased estimates of world properties from single cues or from multiple cues. Let us start from the first case.

### Depth Estimates from Motion-Only Stimuli

The recovery of the veridical Euclidean 3D structure from retinal motion requires the analysis of both the first-order and second-order temporal properties of the optic flow (Koenderink, 1986; Longuet-Higgins & Prazdny, 1980). Several studies, however, have shown that the visual system is only sensitive to first-order temporal information (i.e., to retinal velocities): Performance in 3D tasks does not improve when second-order temporal properties (i.e., retinal accelerations) are provided (Hogervorst & Eagle, 2000; Todd & Bressan, 1990).

Two-frame random-dot cinematograms elicit a vivid percept of a specific 3D shape in a manner similar to multiple-frame random-dot cinematograms. A computer vision program, however, can extract the metric 3D structure from the latter case, but it would fail in giving any metric 3D interpretation to the former. If only the first-order temporal properties are analyzed, in fact, retinal motion is ambiguous: Infinite combinations of depth maps $\mathbf{z}$ and parameters $\mathbf{p}_v = (z_f, \omega)$ give rise to the same velocity field $\mathbf{v}$ (Eq. 7.2).

In spite of this ambiguity, a unique perceptual solution is found, with little variability within and across observers. Domini and Caudek (1999, 2003a, 2003b) showed that visual performance can be accounted for by the same maximum-likelihood estimator, regardless of whether observers are presented with ambiguous (first-order) or unambiguous (second-order) information.

If the perceptual solution depends on the first-order properties of the optic flow, then the perceptual response cannot be veridical. Domini and Caudek, in fact, found that perceived slant does not depend on simulated slant, but only on the gradient of the velocity field. When observers were shown different velocity gradients produced by a planar surface with a constant slant, they perceived different 3D orientations. When observers were shown the projections of surfaces with different slants, but projecting the same velocity gradient, they perceived a constant slant. The same pattern of results was also found for the perception of relative depth.

In conclusion, a large body of empirical evidence suggests that the perceptual analysis of the optic flow does not generate unbiased estimates of slant or depth. The psychophysical literature, therefore, suggests that the term $p(\mathbf{v}|\mathbf{z};\, \mathbf{p}_v)$ of the likelihood function of Eq. 7.4 does not peak at the veridical depth value.

### Depth Estimates from Stereo-Only Stimuli

To specify metric depth, disparity must be scaled by the viewing distance $z_f$ (e.g., Longuet-Higgins, 1981; Mayhew & Longuet-Higgins, 1982). The vast majority of experiments on depth perception from binocular disparity, however, have revealed systematic failures of shape constancy (for a discussion, see Todd & Norman, 2003). Some of these experiments have been conducted in the laboratory with computer-generated displays (Bradshaw, Glennerster, & Rogers, 1996; Brenner & Landy, 1999; Brenner & van Damme, 1999; Collett, Schwarz, & Sobel, 1991; Glennerster, Rogers, & Bradshaw, 1996, 1998; Johnston, 1991; Johnston, Cumming, & Landy, 1994; Norman & Todd, 1998; Tittle, Todd, Perotti, & Norman, 1995; Todd, Oomes, Koenderink, & Kappers, 2001), whereas other studies have been carried out by using real objects in fully illuminated natural environments (Baird & Biersdorf, 1967; Battro, Netto, & Rozestrasten, 1976; Bradshaw, Parton, & Glennerster, 2000; Cuijpers, Kappers, & Koenderink, 2000a, 2000b; Gilinsky, 1951; Harway, 1963; Hecht, van Doorn, & Koenderink, 1999; Koenderink, van Doorn, Kappers, & Todd, 2002; Koenderink, van Doorn, & Lappin, 2000; Loomis, Da Silva, Fujita, & Fukusima, 1992; Loomis & Philbeck, 1999; Norman, Lappin, & Norman, 2000; Norman, Todd, Perotti, & Tittle, 1996; Thouless, 1931; Toye, 1986; Wagner, 1985). In both cases, the psychophysical literature provides no evidence that human observers can estimate $z_f$ veridically. In turn, this means that the function $p(\mathbf{d}|\mathbf{z}; \mathbf{p}_d)$ of Eq. 7.4 does not peak at the veridical depth value.

### Interpretations of the Distortions of Perceived 3D Shape

The psychophysical literature suggests that "observers' judgments of 3D metric structure can be systematically distorted and often exhibit large failures of constancy over changes in viewing distance and/or orientation" (Todd & Norman, 2003, p. 43). These findings have been interpreted in different ways by visual researchers.

According to one interpretation, these findings do not provide conclusive evidence that the visual system fails to recover the correct metric structure of distal objects. This interpretation stems from the acknowledgment of the inherent limitations of the experimental settings used within the laboratory. The limitations of computer-generated displays for the study of cue integration are the result of the unavoidable presence of cues to flatness and cue conflict. The notion of "cues to flatness" was introduced by Young, Landy, and Maloney (1993). They pointed out that cues manipulated in a computer simulation are always accompanied by "other, extraneous cues (vergence, accommodation, motion parallax if the head is free to move, prior knowledge) all of which may signal that the display is flat (which, in fact, it is)" (Johnston et al., 1994, p. 2270). When the cues manipulated by the experimenter are of low quality, "more weight is given to these extraneous cues, resulting in a display which appears flattened" (see also Atkins, Jacobs, & Knill, 2003). The consequences of cue conflict have been recently illustrated by Watt, Akeley, Ernst, and Banks (2005). Watt et al. pointed out that some of the biases in perceived 3D scene structure in typical displays may be due, in some circumstances, to a cue conflict between two-dimensional (2D) geometrically correct projections and inappropriate focus cues, such as accommodation and the gradient of retinal blur. It has also been noticed, moreover, that there are other experimental situations in which observers seem quite good at making metric judgments, so the finding that people are poor at metric depth judgments is not universal (Buckley & Frisby, 1993; Durgin, Proffitt, Olson, & Reinke, 1995; Frisby, Buckley, & Duke, 1996; Frisby, Buckley, & Horsman, 1995). Finally, it has been argued that, in more natural situations, many cues to three-dimensional shape will be available, and accurate perception of depth will follow from the integration of a number of sources of information (Bradshaw et al., 2000; Landy, Maloney, Johnston, & Young, 1995).

Other researchers (e.g., Braunstein, 1994; Domini & Caudek, 2003a; Glennerster et al., 1996; Hecht et al., 1999; Tittle et al., 1995; Todd, 2004) consider the large failures of constancy of 3D metric structure over changes in viewing distance and/or orientation to be an important empirical finding that needs to be addressed by any theory of cue combination. If estimates of specific world properties from single cues are biased, it is obvious that an averaging model does not suffice (in other words, the goal of minimizing variance makes no sense). In such circumstances, how can the information provided by different cues be combined? In the next section, we will try to provide an answer to such a question.

## AN ALTERNATIVE APPROACH

### Maximization of the Direct Information about 3D Shape

The purpose of our alternative approach, called the *intrinsic constraint* (IC) model, is to maximize the signal-to-noise ratio (SNR) of the direct information about 3D shape. Often (but not always), this also maximizes the discriminability of stimuli with different values of depth. To maximize the SNR, we propose that information provided by different cues is combined *before* imposing a metric interpretation on each signal individually. In a successive stage of processing, then, some form of metric scaling can be applied to this composite signal (Tassinari, Domini, & Caudek, 2008).

The family of depth maps $kz_i$ resulting from a linear scaling of the $z_i$ depth map is called *affine* (e.g., Koenderink & van Doorn, 1991; Todd et al., 2001). Figure 7.2 shows three structures that belong to the same affine family. Affine transformations do not alter properties such as depth order, relative depth between pairs of points, and parallelism.

Eqs. 7.1 and 7.2 reveal that binocular disparities and retinal velocities directly specify the affine structure of local surfaces, since

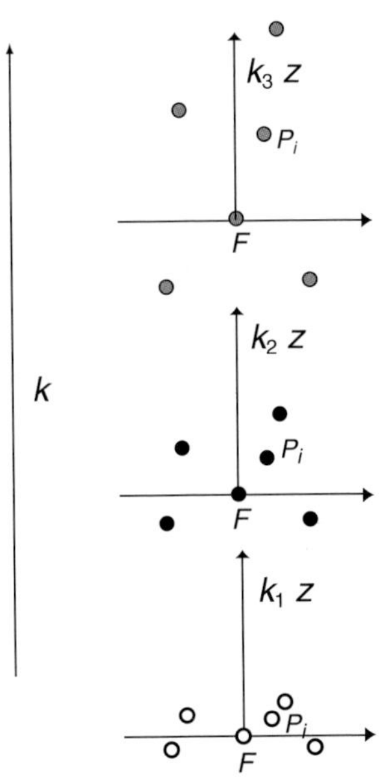


**Figure 7.2** The three panels represent three *x-z* views of a configuration of points. The three configurations share the same affine structure and are affine transformations of the configuration of points represented in Figure 7.1. The stretch factors applied to the configuration of points of Figure 7.1 are indicated by $k_1 < k_2 < k_3$.

both image signals are proportional to the depth map $z_i$. This is illustrated in Figure 7.3 (left panels), where we plot the disparity and velocity values projected by the 3D structure of Figure 7.1. Figure 7.3 also reports the error bars representing one standard deviation of the measurement noise. Note from Figure 7.3 that the reliability of the affine structure depends on both the magnitude of image noise and the values of the disparity and velocity signals.

The notion of the signal-to-noise ratio is crucial to the IC model. To clarify this point, consider a thought experiment in which observers are asked to judge whether a point $P_i$ is in front or behind the fixation point $F$. To provide such a judgment, an observer may rely on disparity information. In fact, she only needs to establish whether the relative disparity $d_i$ of the point $P_i$ is positive or negative (see Fig. 7.3, top left panel). Suppose that the point $P_i$ is in front of $F$. In the absence of noise, $d_i$ will be positive. Since image signals are perturbed by measurement noise, however, sometimes $d_i$ will take on a positive value (as it would in absence of noise) and sometimes will take on a negative value. The frequency of the sign reversal for $d_i$ depends on the ratio between the modulus of the expected value of the image signal, $|E(d_i)|$, and the standard deviation of the measurement noise, $\sigma_d$.

In Figure 7.3 (central panels), we plotted the signal-to-noise ratios of the disparity measurements[1]

$$SNR_d = \frac{E(d_i)}{\sigma_d} \tag{7.5}$$

and the signal-to-noise ratios of the velocity measurements

$$SNR_v = \frac{E(v_i)}{\sigma_v}. \tag{7.6}$$

[1]Even though the standard deviations of the measurement noise may change with signal intensity, we assume that this change is negligible within a local image region. We therefore chose not to add an index $i$ to $\sigma_v$ and $\sigma_d$. The issue of Weber's law in relation to the IC model will be discussed in the section, "IC Model, Fechnerian Scaling, and Weber's Law.

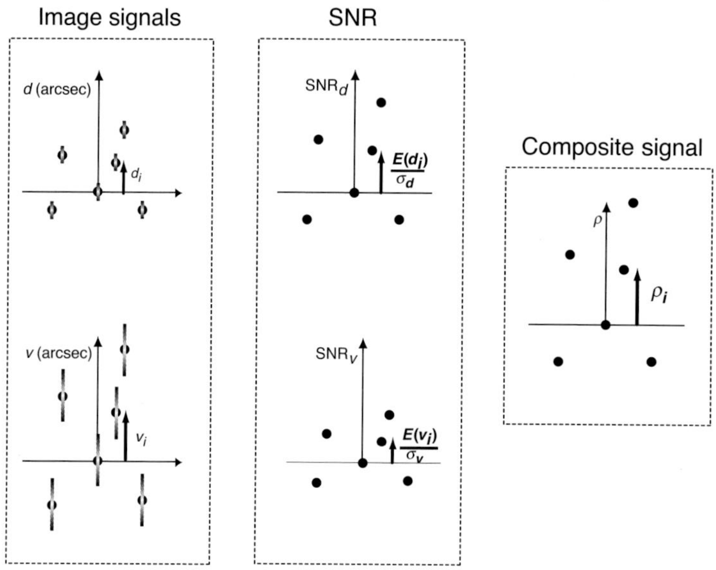


**Figure 7.3** (Left) Hypothetical disparity ($d_i$) and velocity ($v_i$) values projected by the six points belonging to the configuration of Figure 7.1. Suppose that the image is corrupted by Gaussian noise. The gray bars indicate ± one standard deviation of multiple measurements of the image signals. (Middle) Signal-to-noise ratios (SNRs) of the disparity and velocity signals computed by dividing the expected value of the disparity $[E(d_i)]$ and velocity $[E(v_i)]$ measurements by the standard deviation of the disparity ($\sigma_d$) and velocity ($\sigma_v$) noise. (Right) The SNR of the composite signal resulting from the combination of the velocity and disparity signals with the optimal combination rule of Eq. 7.7. Since the IC model generates a composite signal $r_i$ affected by Gaussian noise with zero mean and unitary variance, the expected value $\rho_i = E(r_i)$ provides a direct measure of the SNR.

In the example of Figure 7.3, the affine structure defined by disparity signals is more reliable than the affine structure defined by velocity signals: The SNR is larger in the former than in the latter case.

The IC theory of cue integration postulates that the visual system combines raw signals before depth reconstruction through a combination rule that maximizes the reliability of the affine estimate. By so doing, IC also maximizes the SNR of the affine solution.

### The Combination Rule of the IC Model

The linear model of cue combination and IC are not different ways of combining the same elements. They differ not only because they propose different combination rules but also because they combine different elements. Linear cue combination produces a weighted combination of depth estimates derived from single cues; IC produces a weighted combination of image signals. The purpose of linear cue combination is to minimize the variance of the integrated depth estimate; the purpose of IC is to maximize the SNR of a composite image signal.

According to IC, disparity and velocity signals are combined through a weighted sum

$$r_i = w_d d_i + w_v v_i, \tag{7.7}$$

where the weight for the disparity signal is $w_d \propto |E(d_i)|/\sigma_d^2$ and the weight for the velocity signal is $w_v \propto |E(v_i)|/\sigma_v^2$. $E(d_i)$ and $E(v_i)$ denote the expected values over repeated observations, that is, the disparity and velocity signal without measurement errors. With such a choice of weights, the linear combination of disparity and velocity signals takes on the maximum SNR (see Domini & Caudek, 2010; MacKenzie, Murray, & Wilcox, 2008; Tassinari et al., 2008).

Domini, Caudek, and Tassinari (2006) showed that the weights of Eq. 7.7 can be estimated by a principal component analysis (PCA) carried out on the disparity ($d_i$) and velocity ($v_i$) signals scaled by the standard deviation of their measurement noise. The resulting scores on the first principal component correspond to the $r_i$ values of Eq. 7.7. In general, $r_i = \rho_i + \varepsilon_r$, with $\varepsilon_r \sim N(0, 1)$ and $E(r_i) = \rho_i$. Note that the weight $w_d$ in Eq. 7.7 estimated by the PCA is the same for all disparity values $d_i$ and similarly for velocity weight $w_v$ and velocity values $v_i$.

Figure 7.3 (right panel) shows the composite signal resulting from the combination of the velocity and disparity signals with the optimal combination rule of Eq. 7.7. Note that the SNR of the composite signal is larger than the SNR of the velocity-only signal and the SNR of the disparity-only signal.

The IC model hypothesizes that perceived depth $z'$ is a monotonic function of the combined signal $\rho$ (see Fig. 7.4):

$$z' = f(\rho). \tag{7.8}$$

As a consequence, IC predicts that two stimuli having the same SNR ($\rho$) should be perceived to be matched in depth.

## Relationship between $\rho$ and Simulated Depth

In the following sections, the predictions of the IC model will be expressed in terms of simulated depth. Thus, it is important to specify the relationship between $\rho$ and simulated depth.

Let us consider a point **P**, which generates the disparity and velocity signals $d_C$ and $v_C$, respectively. If $d_C$ and $v_C$ are combined according to Eq. 7.7, and if the weights are chosen so as to obtain a noise distribution with unitary variance, then $r_C$ will be equal to the square root of the sum of the squared SNRs of the two signals:

$$r_C = \rho_C + \varepsilon_1 = \sqrt{\frac{E(d_C)^2}{\sigma_d^2} + \frac{E(v_C)^2}{\sigma_v^2}} + \varepsilon_1. \tag{7.9}$$

We can thus think of $\rho_C$ as the length of a vector with components $(E(d_C)/\sigma_d)$ and $(E(v_C)\sigma_v)$ (Fig. 7.5, left panel).

The combined-cue stimulus can be represented within the depth space as a vector having components $z_d$ and $z_v$ (the simulated depth magnitudes for the disparity-only and motion-only stimuli)—see Figure 7.5, right panel. If we

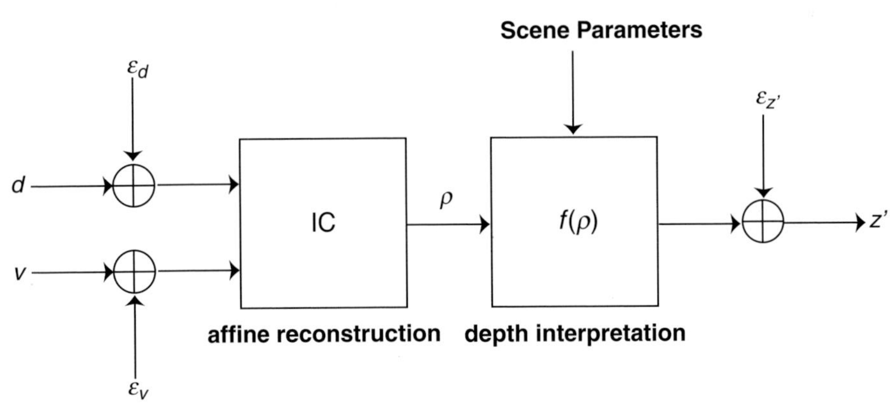


**Figure 7.4** Block diagram of the IC model. The disparity signal $d$ and velocity signal $v$, affected by noise $\varepsilon_d$ and $\varepsilon_v$, are combined in a first stage of processing by a combination rule that produces the best estimate of the affine structure ($\rho$). In a second stage, the affine structure is scaled by a function $f(\rho)$ that depends on the scene parameters. The scaling provides a metric interpretation $z'$ corrupted by noise $\varepsilon'_z$. In this chapter, we do not discuss the consequences of this further source of noise. For an in-depth discussion, see Domini & Caudek (2010).

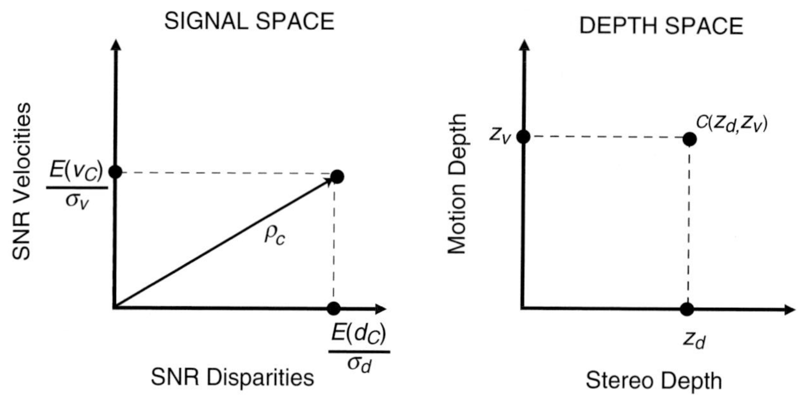


**Figure 7.5** (Left) On the vertical and horizontal axes are shown the signal-to-noise ratios (SNRs) of the velocity ($v_C$) and disparity ($d_C$) signals, respectively. The disparity and velocity signals are combined through the IC combination rule. The SNR of the combined signal, $\rho_C$, is equal to the square root of the sum of the squared SNRs of the disparity ($E(d_C)/\sigma_d$) and velocity ($E(v_C)/\sigma_v$) signals. The combined signal can therefore be represented as a vector having ($E(d_C)/\sigma_d$) as $x$-component and ($E(v_C)/\sigma_v$) as $y$-component. (Right) The disparity and velocity signals are generated by the image projection of the simulated depths $z_d$ and $z_v$, respectively. Within the depth-space, the combined stimulus $C$ can be represented as a vector having $z_d$ as $x$-component and $z_v$ as $y$-component.

wish to formulate the predictions of the IC model in terms of simulated depth values, therefore, it is necessary to express Eq. 7.9 accordingly. Let us write Eqs. 7.1 and 7.2 as $d_C = k_d z_d + \varepsilon_d$ and $v_C = k_v z_v + \varepsilon_v$, where $k_d$ and $k_v$ are proportionality constants depending on the simulated parameters $z_f$ and $\omega$. The SNRs of the disparity and velocity signals can be written as

$$\frac{E(d_C)}{\sigma_d} = k_{d_s} z_d \tag{7.10}$$

and

$$\frac{E(v_C)}{\sigma_v} = k_{v_s} z_v. \tag{7.11}$$

where $k_{d_s} = k_d/\sigma_d$ and $k_{v_s} = k_v/\sigma_v$. The absolute value of the composite signal $\rho_C$ will therefore be equal to

$$|\rho_C| = \sqrt{(k_{d_s} z_d)^2 + (k_{v_s} z_v)^2}. \tag{7.12}$$

Now, consider the particular case of disparity and velocity signals produced by the same simulated depth $z_C$. Suppose also that the two signals have the same SNR.[2] In such circumstances, the constants $k_{d_x}$ and $k_{v_s}$ of Eqs. 7.10–7.12 must take on the same value, which we will denote with $k_S$. Then

$$\frac{E(d_C)}{\sigma_d} = \frac{E(v_C)}{\sigma_v} = k_S z_C \tag{7.13}$$

and

$$\rho_C = \sqrt{k_S^2 + k_S^2} z_C = \sqrt{2} k_S z_C. \tag{7.14}$$

The previous equations reveal a fundamental aspect of IC. If disparity-only and velocity-only stimuli are equated in terms of their SNRs, then we can expect both of the following:

1. The SNRs of the two stimuli are related to the simulated depth $z_C$ through the same proportionality constant $k_S$.
2. The SNR of the composite signal $\rho_C$ is related to the simulated depth $z_C$ through the proportionality constant $\sqrt{2} k_S$.

[2]This can be achieved, for example, by manipulating the scene parameters $z_f$ and $\omega$.

## EMPIRICAL TEST OF THE IC MODEL

The IC model makes predictions about both perceived depth and the variances of the observers' judgments. Both aspects will be examined in turn, with reference to the experimental technique proposed by Domini et al. (2006).

Domini et al. (2006) simulated random-dot half-cylinders. A static binocular view of these cylinders only provided disparity information (disparity-only stimulus). In another experimental condition, the cylinders rotated back and forth about the horizontal axis, while no binocular disparity was present (velocity-only stimulus). In a third experimental condition, both stereo and motion information were presented in the display (combined-cue condition).

In a 2AFC task, observers were asked to report which of two successfully presented stimuli had the largest perceived front-to-back depth. In each trial, the *comparison* stimulus was kept fixed, whereas the relative depth of the *test* stimulus was varied according to a staircase procedure. We computed both the point of subjective equality (PSE; i.e., the simulated depth of the test stimulus that elicited the same perceived depth as the comparison stimulus) and the just noticeable difference (JND). The experiment had two main parts.

Part 1: Perceptual depth match for single-cue stimuli. Domini et al. (2006) generated a pair of motion-only and disparity-only stimuli by keeping constant the distal depth extent used to generate the images (25 mm). For each observer, the magnitude of angular velocity $\omega$ was manipulated until the two stimuli were perceived to have the same depth (see Domini & Caudek, 2003a).[3]

[3] A disparity-only stimulus simulating 25 mm of distal depth does not, in general, appear to be as deep as a velocity-only stimulus display simulating the same distal depth amount. Perceived depth from motion, in fact, depends on the first-order properties of the velocity field, not on the distal depth magnitudes; perceived depth from disparity, in turn, depends on the perceptual estimate of the fixation distance.

Part 2: Perceptual depth match for single-cue and combined-cue stimuli. In part 2 of the experiment, observers were asked to discriminate between the perceived depth magnitudes of two stimuli in three different experimental conditions. In condition COND1, observers were asked to discriminate between a disparity-only stimulus (or a velocity-only stimulus) and a disparity-velocity stimulus. The simulated depth extent of the disparity-velocity stimulus was kept fixed at 25 mm, whereas the depth of the single-cue stimulus was varied according to a staircase procedure. In condition COND2, observers were also asked to discriminate between a disparity-only stimulus (or a velocity-only stimulus) and a disparity-velocity stimulus. In this case, however, the depth of the single-cue stimulus was kept fixed at 25 mm, whereas the depth of the disparity-velocity stimulus was varied. Finally, in condition COND3, observers were asked to discriminate between two disparity-velocity stimuli. The depth of one stimulus was kept fixed at 25 mm, whereas the depth of the other was varied according to a staircase procedure.[4]

### Depth Matches

According to IC, when only one cue is informative about 3D shape, $\rho$ is equal to the SNR of that cue. In the following discussion, the subscripts $d$, $v$, and $C$ will denote the disparity-only stimulus, the velocity-only stimulus, and the disparity-velocity stimulus, respectively. In the left panel of Figure 7.6, two single-cue stimuli are represented by two vectors: The vector parallel to the horizontal axis represents a disparity-only stimulus and the vector parallel to the vertical axis represents a velocity-only stimulus. In Figure 7.6, these vectors have the same length ($\rho_d = \rho_v$). This indicates that the two stimuli have the same SNR.

The right panel of Figure 7.6 represents the simulated depth magnitudes of the two single-cue stimuli. Here, we consider the case in which

[4] The angular rotation $\omega$ used to generate the motion-only and disparity-velocity stimuli took on the value that had been determined, for each observer, in part 1 of the experiment.

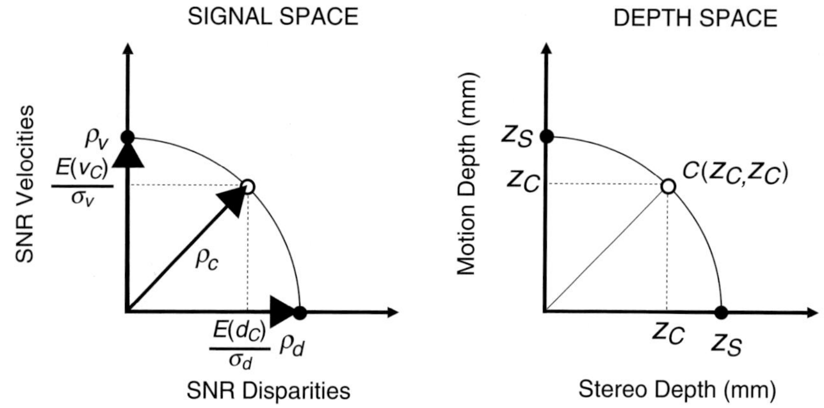


**Figure 7.6** Predictions of the IC model for depth-matched stimuli. The predictions are formulated both within the signal space (left) and within the depth space (right). (Left) The vertical and horizontal vectors represent the velocity-only and disparity-only stimuli coded as hypothesized by the IC model. If only binocular disparities are present, then the vector identifying the combined signal coincides with the horizontal axis. If only retinal velocities are present, then the vector coding the image signal coincides with the vertical axis. As explained in the text, we assume that the single-cue signals are perceptually matched in depth. According to IC, therefore, the vector coding the disparity-only stimulus ($\rho_d$) has the same length as the vector coding the velocity-only stimulus ($\rho_v$). The combined-cue stimulus is represented by a vector having $(E(d_C)/\sigma_d)$ as $x$-component and $(E(v_C)/\sigma_v)$ as $y$-component. IC predicts that the combined-cue stimulus is perceived to be matched in depth to the single-cue stimuli when $\rho_C$ has the same length as $\rho_d$ and $\rho_v$. Note that, in order to obtain $|\rho_C| = |\rho_d| = |\rho_v|$, the components of the combined-cue vector must be smaller than the SNR of the single-cue stimuli. Note that researchers usually distinguish between the case in which a cue is absent and the case in which a cue is present, but it has a value of zero. These two cases are thought to lead to different perceptual solutions. According to IC, instead, they produce the same output. (Right) Simulated depths for the single-cue and combined-cue stimuli. For the experimental conditions described in the text, both single-cue stimuli simulate the same amount $z_S$ of depth. In such circumstances, IC predicts a perceptual depth match between single-cue and combined-cue stimuli when $|C(z_C, z_C)| = z_S$. For obtaining a perceptual depth match, IC predicts that the simulated depth of the combined-cue stimulus ($z_C$) must therefore be $\sqrt{2}$ smaller than the simulated depth of the single-cue stimuli ($z_S$).

$z_d = z_v = z_S$. The IC model hypothesizes that perceived depth $z'$ is a monotonic function of the combined signal $\rho$ (Eq. 7.8). In the present case, $\rho_d = \rho_v$ and, therefore, the two single-cue stimuli should be perceived as having the same amount of depth (see section on "Empirical Results for Discrimination Thresholds").

According to IC, a perceptual depth match between a disparity-only stimulus and a disparity-velocity stimulus occurs when $\rho_d = \rho_C$. Likewise, a perceptual depth match between a velocity-only stimulus and a disparity-velocity stimulus occurs when $\rho_v = \rho_C$. Any mixture of signals defining a point on the circle of Figure 7.6 (left panel) should elicit the same amount of perceived depth.

To better illustrate the predictions of the IC model, let us consider the case of two single-cue stimuli having the same SNR. In such circumstances, by Eqs. 7.13 and 7.14, we have

$$\rho_d = \frac{E(d_S)}{\sigma_d} = k_S z_S, \tag{7.15}$$

$$\rho_v = \frac{E(v_S)}{\sigma_v} = k_S z_S, \tag{7.16}$$

and

$$\rho_C = k_C z_C = \sqrt{2} k_S z_C. \tag{7.17}$$

We can thus conclude that, within the signal space, the disparity-velocity stimulus can be represented by a vector with 45° orientation (Fig. 7.6, left panel).

The IC model deals with the combination of image signals. But image signals have a counterpart within the domain of simulated depth. In the depth space, the vector identifying the disparity-velocity stimulus will also be oriented at 45°, since the stereo-only and disparity-only stimuli are defined by the same amount of simulated depth $z_C$ (Fig. 7.6, right panel).

In part 1 of the experiment of Domini et al. (2006), a disparity-only stimulus was judged to be perceptually matched in depth to a motion-only stimulus. The two stimuli, moreover, were generated by the same amount $z_S$ of distal depth. In these circumstances, according to Eqs. 7.15–7.17, we should expect the following:

1. The two single-cue stimuli have the same SNR.
2. The disparity-velocity stimulus resulting from combining the two single-cue stimuli should have a SNR larger by a factor of $\sqrt{2}$ than the SNR of the single-cue stimuli. As a consequence, at the point of subjective equality, the simulated depth $z_C$ of the disparity-velocity stimulus should be smaller by a factor of $\sqrt{2}$ than the simulated depth $z_S$ of each of the single-cue stimuli.

To test these predictions, Domini et al. (2006) asked observers to discriminate the perceived depth extents of two stimuli in three different conditions. In condition COND1 (where the simulated depth of the disparity-velocity stimulus was kept fixed at 25 mm and the simulated depth of the disparity-only or velocity-only stimulus was varied within a staircase procedure), IC predicts that a perceptual depth match should be found when the single-cue stimulus takes on a value equal to $\sqrt{2} \times 25$ mm. In condition COND2 (where the simulated depth of the disparity-only or velocity-only stimulus was kept fixed at 25 mm and the simulated depth of the disparity-velocity stimulus was varied within a staircase procedure), IC predicts that a perceptual depth match should be found when the disparity-velocity stimulus takes on a value equal to $25/\sqrt{2}$ mm. Finally, in condition COND3, there are no reasons to expect any bias in the perceptual depth matches.

Figure 7.7 (left panels) shows the predictions of the IC model together with the mean PSE value of eight observers in each of the three conditions (right panel). It is easy to see the good match between the quantitative predictions of the IC model (with no free parameters) and the empirical data.

## Thresholds

The linear model of cue integration is usually tested by measuring the depth-discrimination thresholds for single-cue and combined-cue

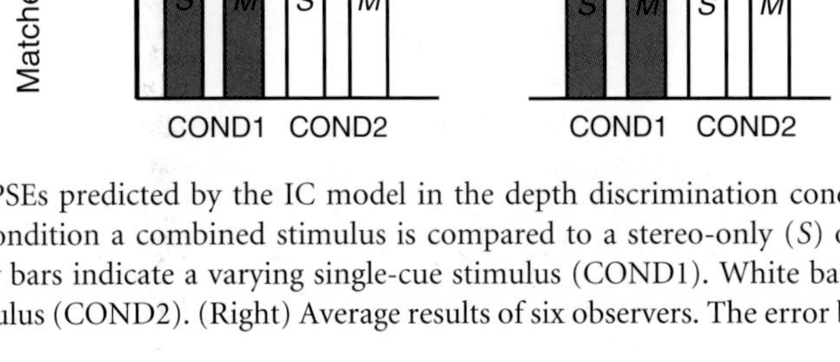


**Figure 7.7** (Left) PSEs predicted by the IC model in the depth discrimination conditions COND1 and COND2. In each condition a combined stimulus is compared to a stereo-only ($S$) or motion-only ($M$) stimulus. Dark gray bars indicate a varying single-cue stimulus (COND1). White bars indicate a varying combined-cue stimulus (COND2). (Right) Average results of six observers. The error bars represent ± one standard error.

stimuli. In the present context, we define the threshold (or JND) as the depth increment that yields correct performance on 84% of the depth-discrimination trials.

The linear model of cue integration interprets the JND as the standard deviation of the putatively Gaussian noise that corrupts each estimate of depth. The strength of linear cue integration lies in its ability to account for the relation existing between the JNDs found in single-cue and combined-cue depth-discrimination experiments.

Domini et al. (2006) showed the following:

1. IC makes the same predictions as linear cue integration within the stimulus conditions in which linear cue integration has been tested.
2. IC accounts for the relation between the JNDs within stimulus conditions in which linear cue integration fails.

In the following discussion, we will illustrate these two points.

According to IC, a composite signal is a Gaussian random variable with mean $\rho$ and standard deviation of 1 (Eq. 7.9). If two composite signals $s_1$ and $s_2$ both have unitary variance, then they will be discriminated with 84% accuracy when their expected values $\rho_1$ and $\rho_2$ differ by an amount equal to $\sqrt{2}$. This is true regardless of the number of signals on which $\rho$ has been computed.[5]

To increase $\rho$ by the amount $\Delta\rho$, simulated depth must be increased by $\Delta z$. Let us consider the relation between $\Delta\rho$ and $\Delta z$ for the three cases in which $\rho$ is defined by disparity-only, velocity-only, and disparity-velocity signals. We shall restrict the present discussion only to the case in which the two stimuli that must be discriminated have the same SNR. From Equations 7.15–7.17 we have:

$$\Delta\rho_d = k_S \Delta z_S, \tag{7.18}$$

$$\Delta\rho_v = k_S \Delta z_S, \tag{7.19}$$

[5]This value may be larger if additional noise is introduced in further stages of processing (Fig. 7.4). However, even with two sources of noise, as hypothesized in Figure 7.4, the conclusions of the present discussion do not change.

and

$$\Delta\rho_C = \sqrt{2} k_S \Delta z_C. \tag{7.20}$$

Let us suppose that, in a discrimination task, the simulated depth of one stimulus is kept constant, whereas simulated depth of the other stimulus is varied through a staircase procedure. According to IC, regardless of the mixture of stimuli defining $\rho$, correct performance on 84% of the discrimination trials should be obtained when the $\rho$ magnitudes of two stimuli differ by an amount equal to $\Delta\rho = \sqrt{2}$ (Fig. 7.8, left panel). It follows that Eqs. 7.18 and 7.19 can both be written as

$$\sqrt{2} = k_S JND_S, \tag{7.21}$$

and Eq. 7.20 becomes

$$\sqrt{2} = k_S JND_C, \tag{7.22}$$

where $JND_S$ and $JND_C$ are the just noticeable differences for the single-cue stimulus and the combined-cue stimulus, respectively (Fig. 7.8a, right panel).

The predictions of IC for the three conditions of Domini et al. (2006) are reported next.

***Depth Comparison between Fixed Combined-Cue Stimuli and Varying Single-Cue Stimuli (COND1)*** According to IC, 84%-correct performance in depth discrimination is obtained when the $\rho$ value of the single-cue stimulus differs by $\sqrt{2}$ from the $\rho$ value of the combined-cue stimulus[6] (see Fig. 7.8, left panel). This occurs if $JND_S = \sqrt{2}/k_S$ (see Eq. 7.21 and Fig. 7.8, right panel). The same can be said about the comparison between a velocity-only stimulus and the combined-cue stimulus, since disparity-only and velocity-only stimuli have the same SNR (see Eq. 7.21).

[6]This should be true regardless of whether the comparison (fixed) stimulus is defined by a single cue or by multiple cues.

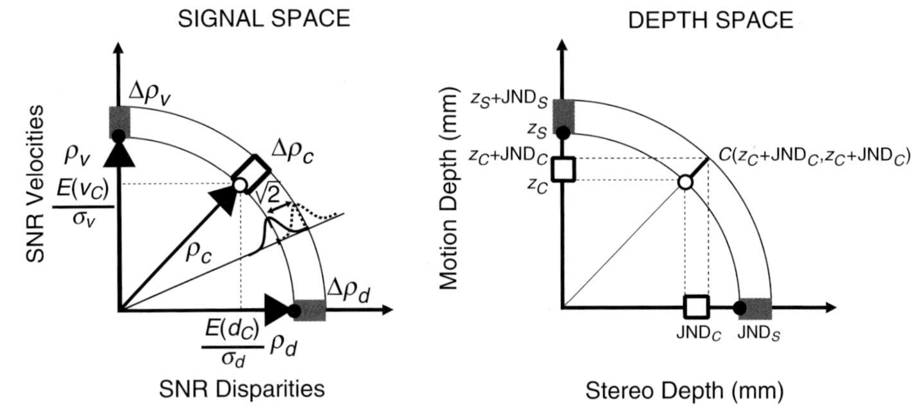


**Figure 7.8** Predictions of IC for the just-noticeable differences (JNDs). (Left) Predictions formulated within the signal space. For perceptually matched stimuli, the SNRs $\rho_d$, $\rho_v$, and $\rho_C$ of the single-cue and combined-cue stimuli take on the same values. According to IC, two signals can be discriminated with 84% accuracy if their SNRs differ by an amount equal to $\sqrt{2}$. The SNR increments that yield 84%-correct performance for discrimination among single-cue and combined-cue stimuli are termed $\Delta\rho_v$, $\Delta\rho_d$, and $\Delta\rho_C$. (Right) Predictions formulated within the depth space. The depth increments that yield 84%-correct performance for discrimination among single-cue and combined-cue stimuli are termed $\mathrm{JND}_S$ and $\mathrm{JND}_C$. According to IC, if two single-cue stimuli simulating the same depth appear to be perceptually matched, then they will have the same $\mathrm{JND}_S$. If this is the case, then the just-noticeable depth increment for the combined stimulus ($\mathrm{JND}_C$) will be $\sqrt{2}$ smaller than the for the single-cue stimuli ($\mathrm{JND}_S$).

***Depth Comparison between Fixed Single-Cue Stimuli and Varying Combined-Cue Stimuli (COND2)*** By following the same pattern of reasoning as the earlier argument, IC predicts a correct performance on 84% of the discrimination trials when $\rho$ of the combined-cue stimulus differs by $\sqrt{2}$ from $\rho$ of the single-cue stimulus (Fig. 7.8, left panel). This occurs if $JND_C = 1/k_S$ (see Eq. 7.22 and Fig. 7.8, right panel). Note that $JND_C = JND_S/\sqrt{2}$. It follows that, in COND1, the discrimination threshold should be larger by a factor $\sqrt{2}$ than in COND2.

***Depth Comparison between Combined-Cue Stimuli (COND3)*** According to IC, condition COND3 is equivalent to COND2, since correct performance in 84% of discrimination trials should be observed when $\rho$ of the varying (combined-cue) stimulus differs by $\sqrt{2}$ from $\rho$ of the fixed (combined-cue) stimulus. This occurs if $JND_C = 1/k_S$ (see Eq. 7.22) or $JND_C = JND_S/\sqrt{2}$. The thresholds measured in conditions COND2 and COND3, therefore, should be equal.

***Empirical Results for Discrimination Thresholds*** The predictions of IC are shown on the left panel of Figure 7.9, together with the averaged results of six observers (Domini et al., 2006). It is easy to see that the empirical data are consistent with the predictions of the model.

## EMPIRICAL TEST OF LINEAR CUE COMBINATION

Next we discuss the predictions of linear cue combination for the three experimental conditions of Domini et al. (2006).

### Depth Matches

Linear cue combination rests on the assumption of unbiased depth estimates. From this it follows that test and comparison stimuli should appear to be matched in depth when they are both the 2D projection of the same 3D depth magnitude. This is expected to be true, regardless of whether observers perform

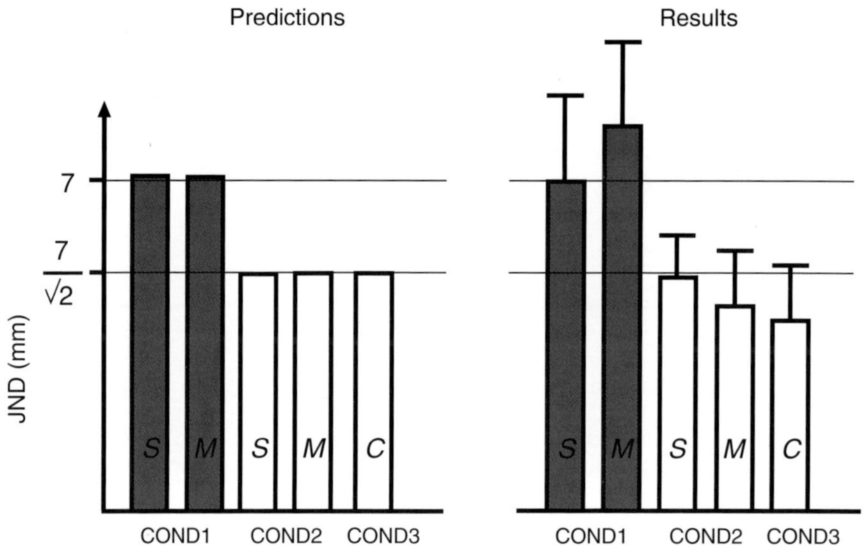


**Figure 7.9** (Left) JNDs predicted by the IC model in the depth discrimination conditions COND1, COND2, and COND3. In each condition a combined stimulus is compared to a stereo-only ($S$), motion-only ($M$) or combined ($C$) stimulus. Dark gray bars indicate a varying single-cue stimulus (COND1). White bars indicate a varying combined-cue stimulus (COND2, COND3). (Right) Average results of six observers. The error bars represent ± one standard error.

the depth-discrimination task in conditions COND1, COND2, or COND3.[7]

### Just Noticeable Differences

According to linear cue combination, discrimination thresholds should not differ across conditions COND1 and COND2. In both cases, in fact, observers compare one depth estimate obtained from a combined-cue stimulus and one depth estimate obtained from a single-cue stimulus (in the bottom panels of Figure 7.10, these estimates are represented by Gaussian distributions centered at the PSEs).

Linear cue combination also predicts that the variance of the observers' judgments made with single-cue stimuli should be larger than the variance of the observers' judgments made with combined-cue stimuli. The slope of the psychometric function in condition COND3 (depth discrimination between two combined-cue stimuli), therefore, should be larger than the slope of the psychometric function in conditions COND1 and COND2 (depth discrimination between single-cue and combined-cue stimuli)—see the right panel of Figure 7.10.

The empirical results reported in the right panel of Figure 7.9, however, clearly show that these predictions are not met.

## THE "CUE-PROMOTION" HYPOTHESIS

Richards (1985) proved that two binocular views of three moving points uniquely specify the Euclidean depth map. Through the solution of a system of linear equations, in fact, it is possible to specify the likelihood function $p(\mathbf{d},\mathbf{v}|\mathbf{z})$ peaked at the true depth map, without the need of knowing the nuisance parameters $z_f$ and $\omega$ (see Eqs. 7.1–7.2). In the following discussion, we will examine the implications of the "promotion" hypothesis for linear cue combination.

[7] If any bias is found in depth-discrimination performance, then this bias is attributed to the presence of unmodeled cues (such as cues to flatness) or to the presence of a prior. The limit of this account is that it does not allow us to make any a priori predictions about what will be observed in any specific stimulus situation.

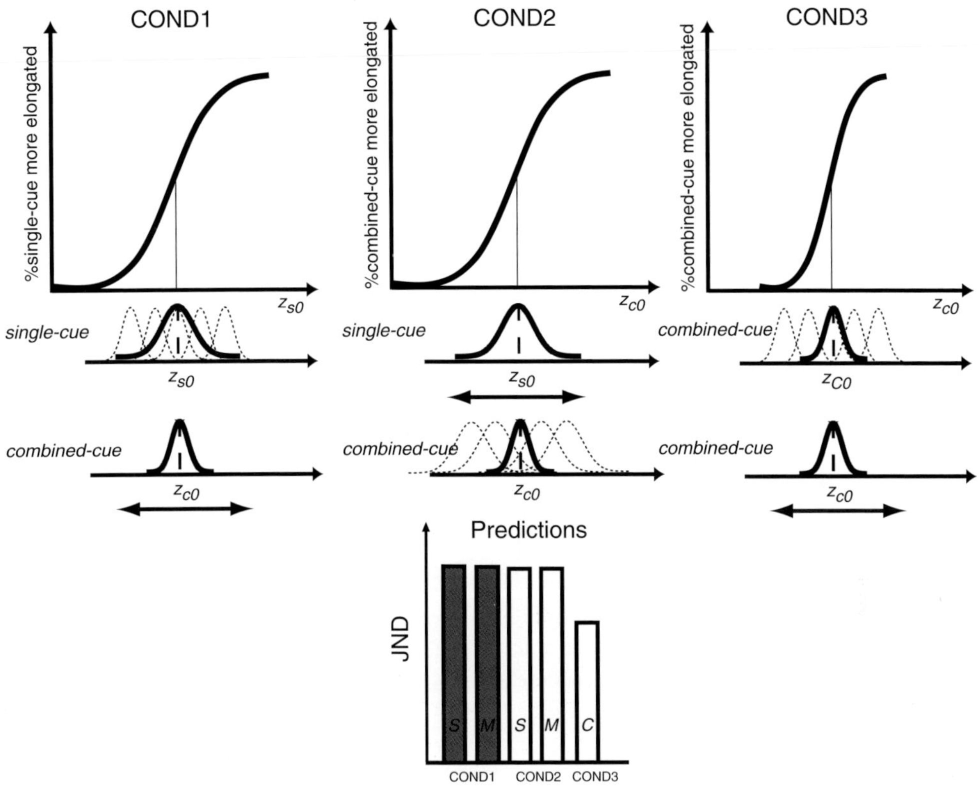


**Figure 7.10** (Top) Expected psychometric functions for the linear model of cue combination in the depth-discrimination experiment COND1 (left), COND2 (center), and COND3 (right). (Center) Expected Gaussian functions modeling the noise of the depth estimates. Solid lines represent fixed stimuli, whereas dotted lines represent stimuli that are varied according to a staircase procedure. (Bottom) JNDs predicted by the linear model in the depth-discrimination conditions COND1, COND2, and COND3. *S* and *M* indicate the type of single-cue stimulus. Dark gray bars indicate a varying single-cue stimulus (COND1). White bars indicate a varying combined-cue stimulus (COND2, COND3).

In a typical cue-combination experiment, a researcher measures the variance of observers' performance from single-cue and from combined-cue stimuli. For simplicity's sake, Eqs. 7.1 and 7.2 can be rewritten as:

$$d \approx k_d z + \varepsilon_d, \tag{7.23}$$

and

$$v \approx k_v z + \varepsilon_v, \tag{7.24}$$

where $k_d = IOD/z_f^2$ and $k_v = \omega/z_f$.

A depth estimate ($z'$) can thus be recovered from each signal as

$$z'_d = \frac{d}{k_d} \tag{7.25}$$

and

$$z'_v = \frac{v}{k_v}. \tag{7.26}$$

The standard deviations of these depth estimates are equal to

$$\sigma_{z'_d} = \frac{\sigma_d}{k_d} \tag{7.27}$$

and

$$\sigma_{z'_v} = \frac{\sigma_v}{k_v}, \qquad (7.28)$$

where $\sigma_d$ and $\sigma_v$ are the standard deviations of the noise of the disparity and velocity signals, respectively.

The optimal rule of cue combination states that:

$$\sigma^2_{z'_C} = \frac{\sigma^2_{z'_d}\sigma^2_{z'_v}}{\sigma^2_{z'_d} + \sigma^2_{z'_v}}, \qquad (7.29)$$

where $\sigma^2_{z'_d}$ and $\sigma^2_{z'_v}$ can be estimated from the discrimination performance with disparity-only and velocity-only stimuli, respectively, and $\sigma^2_{z'_C}$ can be estimated from the discrimination performance with disparity-velocity stimuli. Eq. 7.29 holds only if, for both single-cue and combined-cue stimuli, the depth estimates are computed by scaling the image signals with the correct constants $k_d$ and $k_v$.

According to the "promotion" hypothesis, if both signals are present, then the disparity and velocity signals are indeed scaled by the correct constants $k_d$ and $k_v$, respectively. From the psychophysical literature we know, however, that depth judgments elicited by single-cue stimuli are biased. In other words, for single-cue stimuli, $z'$ is computed by scaling the disparity and velocity signals by wrong constants. Let us call these "wrong" constants $k_{d_s}$ and $k_{v_s}$, respectively. Thus,

$$\sigma_{z_{d_s}} = \frac{\sigma_d}{k_{d_s}} \neq \sigma_{z_d} \qquad (7.30)$$

and

$$\sigma_{z_{v_s}} = \frac{\sigma_v}{k_{v_s}} \neq \sigma_{z_v}, \qquad (7.31)$$

since $k_{d_s} \neq k_d$ and $k_{v_s} \neq k_v$. Hence,

$$\frac{\sigma^2_{z_{d_s}}\sigma^2_{z_{v_s}}}{\sigma^2_{z_{d_s}} + \sigma^2_{z_{v_s}}} \neq \sigma^2_{z_C}. \qquad (7.32)$$

In conclusion, if promotion takes place, then we should expect both of the following:

1. With combined-cue stimuli, depth judgments are more accurate than with single-cue stimuli.
2. The JNDs estimated from discrimination performance with single-cue and combined-cue stimuli do not satisfy Eq. 7.29. This conclusion relies on the assumption that noise is added after scaling and thus is detectable in a single-cue experiment. Conversely, if noise is added before scaling, then the JNDs measured in the combined-cue experiments will satisfy Eq. 7.29, that is, the reliabilities will be additive in stimulus units.

### Empirical Test for the First Prediction of the "Cue-Promotion" Hypothesis

In a first experiment, Domini et al. (2006) tested the cue-promotion hypothesis by asking observers to provide absolute metric judgements about a stimulus made up of three vertical lines arranged in depth. The central line was simulated to be in front of two flanking lines. Observers indicated whether the relative depth between the central line and the two flanking lines was larger or smaller than the horizontal distance between the central line and one of the flanking lines. The simulated depth of the stimuli was varied through a staircase procedure. The PSE was the simulated depth for which the horizontal and the depth dimensions of the stimulus appeared to be matched.

In part 1 of the experiment, single-cue stimuli were used (disparity-only or velocity-only stimuli). For each observer, we found the angular rotation and the viewing distance for which observers' judgments were veridical. At the PSE, the horizontal and the depth dimensions of the stimulus appeared to be matched while also simulating the same relative depth. These results are shown in Figure 7.11 (left panel). The observers' settings at the PSE are coded as the ratio between the simulated distances along the depth and horizontal dimensions. Thus, a value of 1 indicates veridical performance, values smaller than 1 indicate depth overestimation, and values larger than 1 indicate depth underestimation.

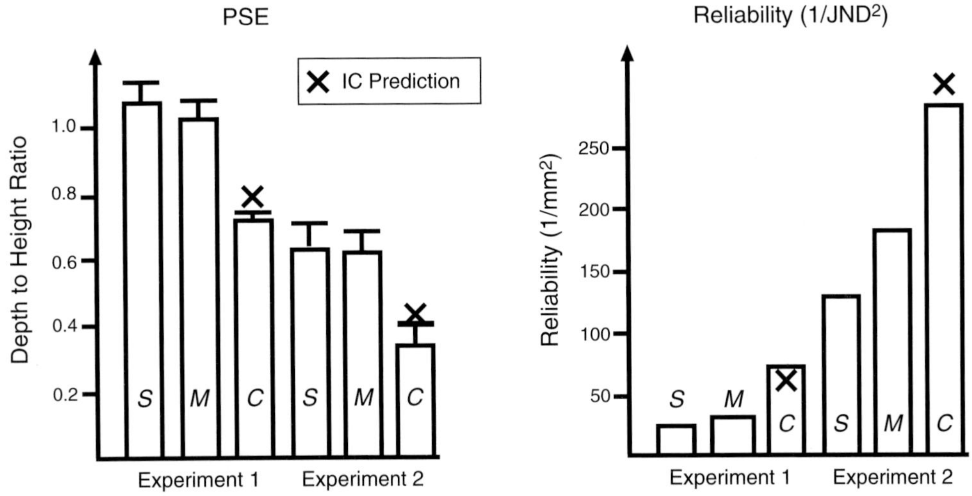


**Figure 7.11** Results of Domini, Caudek, and Tassinari (2006). (Left) Empirical (vertical bars) and predicted (×) depth-to-height ratios. *S*, *M*, and *C* indicate stereo-only, motion-only, and combined-cue stimuli, respectively. The error bars represent ± one standard error. (Right) Empirical (vertical bars) and predicted (open circles) reliabilities.

In part 2 of the experiment, the methodology and the task were the same as in part 1, but combined-cue stimuli were used. The results are shown in Figure 7.11 (left panel). As predicted by IC, in part 2 depth was overestimated.

In a second experiment, we modified the viewing parameters (viewing distance for the disparity signals and angular rotation for the velocity signals), so that perceived depth from each single-cue stimulus was overestimated (see Fig. 7.11, left panel). Then we asked the critical question: What happens when the two single-cue stimuli are combined? In Experiment 2, we found that the amount of depth perceived from combined-cue stimuli was overestimated by an even larger amount than in Expt. 1.

In conclusion, the results of Domini et al. (2006) are incompatible with the first prediction of the cue-promotion hypothesis: Perceptual performance was veridical for judgments made with single-cue stimuli, but it was clearly biased for judgments made with combined-cue stimuli. Note that, in contrast to linear cue combination, IC can predict, from the results found with the single-cue stimuli, the magnitude of depth overestimation found with the combined-cue stimuli.

### Empirical Test for the Second Prediction of the Cue-Promotion Hypothesis

The second prediction of the cue-promotion hypothesis was tested by Domini et al. (2006) by measuring the discrimination thresholds of motion-only, stereo-only, and stereo-motion stimuli. The discrimination thresholds are shown in Figure 7.11 (right panel) as the inverse of the squared JNDs (reliabilities). If Eq. 7.29 holds, then, according to IC, the reliability of the combined-cue stimuli should be equal to the sum of the reliabilities of the single-cue stimuli (Domini et al., 2006; Tassinari et al., 2008). The right panel of Figure 7.11 shows that this was indeed the case. Also, the second prediction of the cue-promotion hypothesis was thus falsified (Eq. 7.32).

It might be argued that the perceptual biases of Domini et al. (2006) are the effects of unmodeled cues (e.g., cue-to-flatness) or that they might depend on a prior to flatness. According to this interpretation, in fact, we should expect that single-cue stimuli elicit a smaller amount of perceived depth than combined cue stimuli. If this were the case, however, we should also expect that the relation among the JNDs would not comply with Eq. 7.29. The results shown in Figure 7.11, however, do not support this alternative explanation.

## SOME CAVEATS ABOUT THE IC MODEL

According to IC, image signals are combined so as to produce the most precise estimate of the affine structure. By assuming that measurement noise is (fairly) constant within a small patch, we showed that this goal can be achieved through a PCA on the image signals scaled by the standard deviation of the image noise (Domini et al., 2006). But is the assumption of constant noise reasonable? Several empirical studies show, on the contrary, that noise varies with signal intensity. In the following section, we address this possible criticism.

### IC Model, Fechnerian Scaling, and Weber's Law

MacKenzie and colleagues (2008) pointed out that "IC has similarities to Fechnerian theories of sensory scaling, in that it predicts that perceived depth can be meaningfully measured in terms of Just-Noticeable Differences (JND's)" (p. 4). By assuming that JNDs remain constant, MacKenzie et al. found that a simple sum of JNDs does not predict the resulting change in sensory magnitudes.

This experiment was also carried out by Domini and Caudek (2010), who estimated six successive JNDs from a common starting point, for both disparity-only and velocity-only stimuli. In the first part of the experiment, a staircase procedure was used to determine the PSE of a stereo-only stimulus that appeared to be perceptually matched to a motion-only stimulus. In a second part of the experiment, two independent psychophysical scales (motion-based and stereo-based) were generated by adding successive JNDs to the common starting point. By comparing the apparent depths associated with corresponding points of these two psychophysical scales, Domini and Caudek (2010) concluded that the separation between two objects measured in JNDs does in fact predict their separation in depth.

MacKenzie et al. (2008) based their conclusion on the hypothesis that IC assumes that signal noise is constant. It was this assumption that justified the method that they used to count the number of JNDs separating two sensory magnitudes. On the basis of this assumption, they concluded that IC fails to account the empirical data.

Domini and Caudek (2010) adopted a different method for counting JNDs, a method that does not rely on the assumption of constant noise. By so doing, Domini and Caudek (2010) found that perceived depth can indeed be meaningfully measured in terms of JNDs, as predicted by IC. The results of the two studies can thus be reconciled by saying that IC only requires constant noise in a small neighborhood; it does not require constant noise over large variations of the signal intensity.

There is a specific relation between signal and noise, however, that would falsify the IC model: IC would be falsified if depth perception were governed by Weber's law. According to Weber's Law, in fact, the ratio of the increment threshold to the pedestal intensity is a constant. But does Weber's law holds in the domain of depth perception? If Weber's law were true, then, in the experiment described in the previous section, observers would perceive the same amount of depth at any successive step of the (motion-based and stereo-based) psychophysical scales. But they did not. In general, all the data that we have collected in the domain of depth perception do not comply with Weber's law: if Weber's law were true, then the IC model would not fit any empirical data.

### Local and Global Processing

IC is a model for the local analysis of the image signals; it is not a model for the global analysis of the visual scene. If only a local region of the retinal image is considered, the image signals vary by a small amount and, consequently, the noise variation is negligible. At the local level, therefore, IC generates an accurate estimate of affine structure.

Accurate local estimates, however, do not exclude global inconsistencies. Rather than being a problem for the IC model, this possibility would confirm our previous results. Domini, Caudek, and Richman (1998), for example, found that their stimuli were still perceived as consistent global 3D shapes, even though the biases in local slant perception did not cancel out by spatial integration. This result (among others) indicates that the properties of perceived global 3D shape cannot be completely accounted for by a local analysis. Since the scope of IC is restricted to local processing, IC does not account for all the aspects of global 3D shape perception from multiple cues.

## CONCLUSIONS

The problem of explaining visually guided behavior has been traditionally approached by assuming that the visual system estimates the metric properties of the 3D layout of the environment and of the shapes of objects within it. In the present chapter, we question this approach. Some researchers speculate, indeed, that our interaction with the environment does not require the recovery of a metric representation: Visually guided behavior may not require an internal representation of external space but, rather, it may be based on more concrete representations directly linked with the sensory channels (Bradshaw et al., 2000; Gårding, Porrill, Mayhew, & Frisby, 1995; Glennerster et al., 1996; Morasso & Sanguineti, 1997; Todd, 2004). The input patterns may be mapped in a task-dependent way into output patterns without requiring the full specification of the Euclidean depth map of the spatial layout. For example, it has been shown that the behavior of a fly, its ability to land or take off, or to pursue another fly, can be explained by an algorithm that does not require metric knowledge (e.g., Poggio & Reichardt, 1976, 1981; Wehrhahn, Poggio, & Bülthoff, 1982). Since it does not rely on unreliable estimates of "nuisance parameters," such an approach may prove to be more advantageous for an organism's interactions with its environment.

We argue that the existence of perceptual distortions, even under full-cue conditions (Baird & Biersdorf, 1967; Battro et al., 1976; Bhalla & Proffitt, 1999; Bradshaw et al., 2000; Cuijpers et al., 2000a, 2000b; Hecht et al., 1999; Koenderink et al., 2000, 2002; Loomis et al., 1992; Loomis & Philbeck, 1999; Norman, Crabtree, Clayton, & Norman, 2005; Norman et al., 1996, 2000; Toye, 1986; Wagner, 1985; Wu, Ooi, & He, 2004), is not surprising, since a biological system does not need to estimate the full metric representation of the visual scene in order to interact with it. For humans, exact metric estimates are necessary only within a limited reaching space, where objects need to be successfully grasped and manipulated. Within this space, the scene parameters that relate image signals to 3D properties vary by a very small range. Biomechanical constraints, in fact, limit the grasping distance to a range of, say, 50–70 centimeters; we do not grasp objects that are too close or too far away. Moreover, the self-motion of the observer is also confined to a small range of velocities; when we grasp an object, we seldom move very fast or stay perfectly still. Within these stimulus conditions, variations of the retinal signals mostly reflect variations in the 3D structure of the objects. Going back to the discussion of the perceptual interpretation of disparity and velocity signals, these considerations imply that the "nuisance" parameters $z_f$ and $\omega$ are fairly constant. As a consequence, variations in retinal disparities or velocities can be attributed, for the most part, to variations of depth.

The previous considerations are very speculative. Nevertheless, they suggest a plausible alternative to the "inverse-geometry" approach to 3D shape perception. According to the inverse-geometry approach, the nuisance parameters (such as $z_f$ and $\omega$) must be estimated so as to recover a metric depth estimate from each cue individually. These metric depth estimates are then combined. Contrary to this approach, we propose that the image signals are combined before assigning any depth interpretation.

We have shown that the combination of image signals hypothesized by the IC model yields the most precise estimate of the local depth-map up to a scaling factor. We hypothesize that, in very constrained situations and for very specific tasks (such as grasping), the estimated affine structure may be appropriately scaled, when metric knowledge is required. In all other situations, we hypothesize that the perceptual representation of 3D shape is based solely on the affine properties of 3D structure that can be determined reliably from visual information. The data that we have discussed are consistent with such view.

We can propose a very loose analogy. The distinction between IC and linear cue combination, in a way, parallels the distinction between the feature-based approach (e.g., Goldstein, Harmon, & Lesk, 1971; Kaya & Kobayashi, 1972) and the appearance-based approach (e.g., Turk & Pentland, 1991) in the face-recognition literature. The feature-based approach seeks to extract distinctive features (e.g., the eyes, nose, mouth, and chin) that are invariant under general viewing conditions. The appearance-based approach, conversely, compares the target to stored templates which are defined only in terms of image (i.e., 2D) properties. Similarly to the feature-based approach, the explanatory power of linear cue combination lies on the recovery of "features" not specified by sensory information (i.e., the depth map). Similarly to the appearance-based approach, IC capitalizes on the available sensory information; IC tries to understand how far we can go (in predicting visual performance) by relying only on retinal information.

The IC model specifies the first stage of 3D shape processing; it specifies the input used by the visual system and the kind of 3D information that is locally extracted. The IC model has been found to be consistent with the psychophysical data collected in reduced-stimulus conditions. However, in such conditions extraretinal information also plays a role. For example, we know that depth from stereo is scaled by vergence information (e.g., Mon-Williams, Tresilian, & Roberts, 2000; Trotter, Celebrini, Stricanne, Thorpe, & Imbert, 1992). How can we reconcile these findings with the fact that IC is a purely retinal model? According to our proposal, extraretinal information is not used to estimate the "missing parameters" (such as $\omega$ and $z_f$), but rather to scale the vector $\rho$ in a second stage of processing (Eq. 7.8). We should therefore expect to find different results, for the same disparity and velocity values, for example, when extraretinal information is varied. In its current formulation, however, the IC model does not account for these effects.

In a richer visual scene, furthermore, both global and local information are provided. Linear perspective, vertical disparities, the presence of a ground plane, and so on specify mutual relations between points located far apart from each other (i.e., those requiring a shift of the fixation point). Local affine information may thus be somehow rescaled so as to take into consideration these mutual constraints (e.g., Bian, Braunstein, & Andersen, 2005, 2006; Ni, Braunstein, & Andersen, 2005, 2007; Zhong & Braunstein, 2004). In its current formulation, again, the IC model does not account for these effects.

In conclusion, future research should identify the tasks and stimulus conditions in which visual performance can be accounted for by a purely retinal model of local processing, and those in which the global properties of the whole visual scene must be taken into account. Moreover, future research should also establish whether there are tasks and stimulus conditions in which a retinal model does not suffice and perceptual performance can be explained only by assuming a veridical recovery of the metric 3D properties of distal objects.

## REFERENCES

Angelaki, D. E., Gu, Y., & DeAngelis, G. C. (2009). Multisensory integration: Psychophysics, neurophysiology, and computation. *Current Opinion in Neurobiology, 19*, 452–458.

Atkins, J. E., Jacobs, R. A., & Knill, D. C. (2003). Experience-dependent visual cue recalibration based on discrepancies between visual and haptic percepts. *Vision Research, 43*, 2603–2613.

Baird, J. C., & Biersdorf, W. R. (1967). Quantitative functions for size and distance judgments. *Perception and Psychophysics, 2*, 161–166.

Battro, A. M., Netto, S. P., & Rozestraten, R. J. A. (1976). Riemannian geometries of variable curvature in visual space: Visual alleys, horopters, and triangles in big open fields. *Perception, 5*, 9–23.

Bhalla, M., & Proffitt, D. R. (1999). Visual-motor recalibration in geographical slant perception. *Journal of Experimental Psychology: Human Perception and Performance, 25,* 1–21.

Bian, Z., Braunstein, M. L., & Andersen, G. J. (2005). The ground dominance effect in the perception of 3D layout. *Perception and Psychophysics, 67,* 815–828.

Bian, Z., Braunstein, M. L., & Andersen, G. J. (2006). The ground dominance effect in the perception of relative distance in 3D scenes is mainly due to characteristics of the ground surface. *Perception and Psychophysics, 68,* 1297–1309.

Bradshaw, M. F., Glennerster, A., & Rogers, B. J. (1996). The effect of display size on disparity scaling from differential perspective and vergence cues. *Vision Research, 36,* 1255–1264.

Bradshaw, M. F., Parton, A. D., & Glennerster, A. (2000) The task-dependent use of binocular disparity and motion parallax information. *Vision Research, 40,* 3725–3734.

Braunstein, M. L. (1994). Decoding principles, heuristics and inference in visual perception. In G. Jansson, S. S. Bergstrom, & W. Epstein (Eds.), *Perceiving events and objects* (pp. 436–446). Hillsdale, NJ: Erlbaum.

Brenner, E., & Landy, M. S. (1999). Interaction between the perceived shape of two objects. *Vision Research, 39,* 3834–3848.

Brenner, E., & van Damme, W. J. (1999). Perceived distance, shape and size. *Vision Research, 39,* 975–986.

Buckley, D., & Frisby, J. P. (1993). Interaction of stereo, texture and outline cues in the shape perception of three-dimensional ridges. *Vision Research, 33,* 919–933.

Collett, T. S., Schwarz, U., & Sobel, E. C. (1991). The interaction of oculomotor cues and stimulus size in stereoscopic depth constancy. *Perception, 20,* 733–754.

Cuijpers, R. H., Kappers, A. M. L., & Koenderink, J. J. (2000a). Investigati on of visual space using an exocentric pointing task. *Perception and Psychophysics, 62,* 1556–1571.

Cuijpers, R. H., Kappers, A. M. L., & Koenderink, J. J. (2000b). Large systematic deviations in visual parallelism. *Perception, 29,* 1467–1482.

Domini, F., & Caudek, C. (1999). Perceiving surface slant from deformation of optic flow. *Journal of Experimental Psychology: Human Perception and Performance, 25,* 426–444.

Domini, F., & Caudek, C. (2003a). 3-D structure perceived from dynamic information: A new theory. *Trends in Cognitive Sciences, 7,* 444–449.

Domini, F., & Caudek, C. (2003b). Perception of slant and angular velocity from a linear velocity field: modeling and psychophysics. *Vision Research, 43,* 1753–1764.

Domini, F., & Caudek, C. (2010). Matching perceived depth from disparity and from velocity: Modeling and psychophysics. *Acta Psychologica, 133*(1), 81–89.

Domini, F., Caudek, C., & Richman, S. (1998). Distortions of depth-order relations and parallelism in structure from motion. *Perception and Psychophysics, 60,* 1164–1174.

Domini, F., Caudek, C., & Tassinari, H. (2006). Stereo and motion information are not independently processed by the visual system. *Vision Research, 46,* 1707–1723.

Drewing, K., & Ernst, M. O. (2006). Integration of force and position cues to haptic shape. *Cognitive Brain Research, 1078,* 92–100.

Durgin, F. H., Proffitt, D. R., Olson, T. J., & Reinke, K. S. (1995). Comparing depth from motion with depth from binocular disparity. *Journal of Experimental Psychology: Human Perception and Performance, 21,* 679–699.

Frisby, J. P., Buckley, D., & Duke, P. A. (1996). Evidence for good recovery of lengths of real objects seen with natural stereo viewing. *Perception, 25,* 129–154.

Frisby, J. P., Buckley, D., & Horsman, J. M. (1995). Interaction of stereo, texture, and outline cues during the pinhole viewing of real ridge-shaped objects and stereograms of ridges. *Perception, 24,* 181–198.

Gårding, J., Porrill, J., Mayhew, J. E. W., & Frisby, J. P. (1995). Stereopsis, vertical disparity and relief transformations. *Vision Research, 35,* 703–722.

Gilinsky, A. S. (1951). Perceived size and distance in visual space. *Psychological Review, 58,* 460–482.

Glennerster, A., Rogers, B. J., & Bradshaw, M. F. (1996). Stereoscopic depth constancy depends on the subject's task. *Vision Research, 36,* 3441–3456.

Glennerster, A., Rogers, B. J., & Bradshaw, M. F. (1998). Cues to viewing distance for stereoscopic depth constancy. *Perception, 27,* 1357–1365.

Goldstein, A. J., Harmon, L. D., & Lesk, A. B. (1971). Identification of human faces. *Proceedings of the IEEE, 59,* 748–760.

Gu, Y., DeAngelis, G. C., Angelaki, D. E. (2008). Neural correlates of multisensory cue integration in macaque MSTd. *Nature Neuroscience, 11*, 1201–1210.

Harway, N. I. (1963). Judgment of distance in children and adults. *Journal of Experimental Psychology, 65*, 385–390.

Hecht, H., van Doorn, A., & Koenderink, J. J. (1999). Compression of visual space in natural scenes and in their photographic counter-parts. *Perception and Psychophysics, 61*, 1269–1286.

Helbig, H. B., & Ernst, M. O. (2007). Optimal integration of shape information from vision and touch. *Experimental Brain Research, 179*, 595–606.

Hogervorst, M. A., & Eagle, R. A. (2000). The role of perspective effects and accelerations in perceived three-dimensional structure-from- motion. *Journal of Experimental Psychology: Human Perception and Performance, 26*, 934–955.

Johnston, E. B. (1991). Systematic distortions of shape from stereopsis. *Vision Research, 31*, 1351–1360.

Johnston, E. B., Cumming, B. G., & Landy, M. S. (1994). Integration of stereopsis and motion shape cues. *Vision Research, 34*, 2259–2275.

Kaya, Y., & Kobayashi, K. (1972). A basic study on human face recognition. In S. Watanabe (Ed.), *Frontiers of pattern recognition* (pp. 265–289). New York, NY: Academic Press.

Knill, D. C., & Richards, W. (Eds.). (1996). *Perception as bayesian inference.* Cambridge, England: Cambridge University Press.

Koenderink, J. J. (1986). Optic flow. *Vision Research, 26*, 161–180.

Koenderink, J. J., & van Doorn, A. J. (1991). Affine structure from motion. *Journal of the Optical Society of America A, 8*, 377–385.

Koenderink, J. J., van Doorn, A. J., Kappers, A. M. L., & Todd, J. T. (2002). Pappus in optical space. *Perception and Psychophysics, 64*, 380–391.

Koenderink, J. J., van Doorn, A. J., & Lappin, J. S. (2000). Direct measurement of the curvature of visual space. *Perception, 29*, 69–79.

Körding, K. (2007). Decision Theory: What "should" the nervous system do? *Science, 318*, 606–610.

Landy, M. S., Maloney, L. T., Johnston, E. B., & Young, M. J. (1995). Measurement and modeling of depth cue combination: in defense of weak fusion. *Vision Research, 35*, 389–412.

Longuet-Higgins, H. C. (1981). A computer algorithm for reconstructing a scene from two projections, *Nature, 293*, 133–135.

Longuet-Higgins, H. C., & Prazdny, K. (1980). The interpretation of a moving retinal image. *Proceedings of the Royal Society of London B: Bioogical Sciences, 208*, 385–397.

Loomis, J. M., Da Silva, J. A., Fujita, N., & Fukusima, S. S. (1992). Visual space perception and visually directed action. *Journal of Experimental Psychology: Human Perception and Performance, 18*, 906–921.

Loomis, J. M., & Philbeck, J. W. (1999). Is the anisotropy of perceived 3-D shape invariant across scale? *Perception and Psychophysics, 61*, 397–402.

Mayhew, J. E. W., & Longuet-Higgins, H. C. (1982). A computational model of binocular depth perception. *Nature, 297*, 376–379.

MacKenzie, K. J., Murray, R. F., & Wilcox, L. M. (2008). The intrinsic constraint approach to cue combination: An empirical and theoretical evaluation. *Journal of Vision, 8*(8), 1–10.

Mon-Williams, M., Tresilian, J. R., & Roberts, A. (2000). Vergence provides veridical depth perception from horizontal retinal image disparities. *Experimental Brain Research, 133*, 407–413.

Morasso, P., & Sanguineti, V. (Eds.). (1997). *Self-organization, computational maps and motor control.* New York, NY: Elsevier.

Nardini, M., Jones, P., Bedford, R., & Braddick, O. (2008). Development of cue integration in human navigation. *Current Biology, 18*, 689–693.

Ni, R., Braunstein, M. L., & Andersen, G. J. (2005). Distance perception from motion parallax and ground contact. *Visual Cognition, 12*, 1235–1254.

Ni, R., Braunstein, M. L., & Andersen, G. J. (2007). Scene layout from ground contact, occlusion, and motion parallax. *Visual Cognition, 15*, 46–68.

Norman, J. F., Crabtree, C. E., Clayton, A. M., & Norman, H. F. (2005). The perception of distances and spatial relationships in natural outdoor environments. *Perception, 34*, 1315–1324.

Norman, J. F., Lappin, J. S., & Norman, H. F. (2000). The perception of length on curved and flat surfaces. *Perception and Psychophysics, 62*, 1133–1145.

Norman, J. F., & Todd, J. T. (1998). Stereoscopic discrimination of interval and ordinal depth relations on smooth surfaces and in empty space. *Perception, 27,* 257–272.

Norman, J. F., Todd, J. T., Perotti, V. J., & Tittle, J. S. (1996). The visual perception of three-dimensional length. *Journal of Experimental Psychology: Human Perception & Performance, 22,* 173–186.

Poggio, T., & Reichardt W. (1976). Nonlinear interactions underlying visual orientation behavior of the fly. *Cold Spring Harbor Symposia on Quantitative Biology, 40,* 635–645.

Poggio, T., & W. Reichardt (1981). Visual fixation and tracking by flies: Mathematical properties of simple control systems. *Biological Cybernetics, 40,* 101–112.

Richards, W. (1985). Structure from stereo and motion. *Journal of the Optical Society of America A, 2,* 343–349.

Tassinari, H., Domini, F., & Caudek, C. (2008). The intrinsic constraint model for stereo-motion integration. *Perception, 37,* 79–95.

Thouless, R. H. (1931). Phenomenal regression to the real object. I. *British Journal of Psychology, 21,* 339–359.

Tittle, J. S., Todd, J. T., Perotti, V. J., & Norman, J. F. (1995). Systematic distortion of perceived three-dimensional structure from motion and binocular stereopsis. *Journal of Experimental Psychology: Human Perception and Performance, 21,* 663–678.

Todd, J. T. (2004). The visual perception of 3D shape. *Trends in Cognitive Sciences, 8,* 115–121.

Todd, J. T., & Bressan, P. (1990). The perception of 3-dimensional affine structure from minimal apparent motion sequences. *Perception and Psychophysics, 48,* 419–430.

Todd, J. T., Oomes, A. H. J., Koenderink, J. J., & Kappers, A. M. L. (2001). On the affine structure of perceptual space. *Psychological Science, 12,* 191–196.

Todd., J. T., & Norman, J. F. (2003). The visual perception of 3-D shape from multiple cues: Are observers capable of perceiving metric structure? *Perception and Psychophysics, 65,* 31–47.

Toye, R. C. (1986). The effect of viewing position on the perceived layout of space. *Perception and Psychophysics, 40,* 85–92.

Trotter, Y., Celebrini, C., Stricanne, B., Thorpe, S., & Imbert, M. (1992). Modulation of neural stereoscopic processing in primate area V1 by the viewing distance. *Science, 257,* 1279–1281.

Turk, M., & Pentland, A. (1991). Eigenfaces for recognition. *Journal of Cognitive Neuroscience, 3,* 71–86.

Wagner, M. (1985). The metric of visual space. *Perception and Psychophysics, 38,* 483–495.

Watt, S. J., Akeley, K., Ernst, M. O., & Banks, M. S. (2005). Focus cues affect perceived depth. *Journal of Vision, 5,* 834–862.

Wehrhahn, C., Poggio, T., & Bülthoff, H. H. (1982). Tracking and chasing in houseflies (Musca). An analysis of 3-D flight trajectories. *Biological Cybernetics, 45,* 123–130.

Wu, B., Ooi, T. L., He, Z. J. (2004). Perceiving distance accurately by a directional process of integrating ground information. *Nature, 428,* 73–77.

Young, M. J., Landy, M. S., & Maloney, L. T. (1993). A perturbation analysis of depth perception from combinations of texture and motion cues. *Vision Research, 33,* 2685–2696.

Zhong, H., & Braunstein, M. L. (2004). Effect of background motion on the perceived shape of a 3D object shape. *Vision Research, 44,* 2505–2513.

# CHAPTER 8

## Cue Combination: Beyond Optimality

*Pedro Rosas and Felix A. Wichmann*

The last two decades have seen impressive progress toward understanding cue combination in human observers on different levels: theoretically, psychophysically, and on the level of the putative neural implementation. Many examples of this progress can be found in the chapters of this book. In this chapter we briefly introduce the robust-weak-fusion model, which offers an exceptionally clear and elegant framework within which to understand empirical studies on cue combination (for a more extensive introduction, see Chapter 1). Research on cue combination is an area in the cognitive neurosciences where *quantitative* models and predictions are the norm rather than the exception—and this is certainly a development we, the authors, welcome wholeheartedly. What we view critically, however, is the strong emphasis on so-called optimal cue combination. Optimal in the context of human cue combination typically refers to the minimum-variance unbiased estimator for multiple sources of information, corresponding to maximum-likelihood estimation when the probability distribution of the estimates based on each cue are Gaussian, independent, and the prior of the observer is uniform (noninformative) (Ernst & Banks, 2002). The central aim of this chapter is to spell out our worries regarding both the term *optimality* as well as against the use of the minimum-variance unbiased estimator as the statistical tool to go from the reliability of a cue to its weight in robust weak fusion.

### THE ROBUST WEAK FUSION FRAMEWORK FOR CUE COMBINATION

Cue combination in the psychophysical literature has been greatly influenced by machine vision. Machine vision is driven predominantly by normative approaches to analyze visual input in order to guide the behavior of artificial devices (compare with David Marr's computational level, "an analysis of the problem as an information-processing task"; Marr, 1982, p. 19). In machine vision the problem of cue combination is subsumed under the heading of *sensor fusion*, which is cast as an estimation problem within statistical decision theory. Here, the value of the parameter of interest, for example, the depth of an object, is estimated based on the information obtained from different sensors, each one of these potentially containing noise or measurement error (McKendall, 1990; McKendall & Mintz, 1992). Clark and Yuille (1990) in their influential book on artificial sensory systems distinguished two fundamentally different model-classes for sensor fusion: *strong-fusion* and *weak-fusion* models. The critical difference between them concerns the assumption of independence of the information derived from the available sensors. In strong fusion the information from different sensors interacts in order to obtain a single depth estimate, whereas in weak fusion the estimates obtained from each sensor are independent.

The final estimate in weak fusion is obtained by combining the individual estimates.

In human depth-cue combination both types of models have been proposed (for a review see Parker, Cumming, Johnston, & Hurlbert, 1995; Yuille & Bülthoff, 1996). At least initially weak fusion was associated with linear, and strong fusion with nonlinear cue combination (e.g., Curran & Johnston, 1994). Currently, the de-facto standard model is that of Maloney and Landy (1989) treating depth-cue combination as *robust weak fusion* of depth cues. In this formulation, the depth percept is constructed from a weighted linear combination of cues (weak fusion). However, a strongly discrepant depth estimate—compared with the estimates based on other cues—is given reduced weight in the final combination (robustness). For large cue differences, often termed *cue conflict*, the model thus exhibits nonlinear cue-combination behavior, whereas it is linear for small cue discrepancies thought to arise in the natural environment. Maloney and Landy (1989) and Landy, Maloney, and Young (1991) thus advise experimenters to introduce only small discrepancies between their cues when studying cue combination in order to avoid having the linear cue combination be contaminated by the nonlinearities stemming from the brain's application of robust statistics. Maloney and Landy refer to this experimental approach as *perturbation analysis.*[1]

Within the robust-weak-fusion framework the results obtained with a few, highly discrepant cues are thus interpreted as stemming from robust down-weighting: *Visual capture* in Rock and Victor (1964) or Cutting and Millard's failure to find "synergies of information" in their data (Cutting & Millard, 1984, p. 214) are the result of the large conflicts introduced between the cues in these studies: The cue-combination system does not operate in its "normal" linear cue-combination mode but changes its operation to a highly nonlinear "robust" cue-combination mode, simply ignoring the very discrepant cues. The robust-weak-fusion framework thus not only inspired many perturbation-analysis studies but also allowed the hitherto diverse literature to be unified.

### Reliability-Sensitive Weak Fusion

Perhaps the most insightful aspect of weak fusion was to link the weight of a cue to its *reliability*—from a normative point of view it is useful to reduce the variability of the estimate of a parameter. In the original proposal by Maloney and Landy (1989) reliability was suggested to be estimated using "ancillary measures" providing "information relevant to predict the performance" (p. 1159). Thus, (robust) reliability-sensitive weak fusion requires two independent pieces of information from each cue: the value, for example, "sensor A says distance to target is equal to 173 cm" and its reliability, for example, "sensor A's distance estimate should not be relied upon too much, the 95% confidence interval extends from 55 cm to 456 cm."

Psychophysically, there is ample evidence that the overt behavior of an observer estimating distance is sensitive to the reliability of the cues (Ellard, Goodale, & Timney, 1984; Goodale, Ellard, & Booth, 1990). Since the influential paper by Landy, Maloney, Johnston, and Young (1995), there are literally dozens of cue-combination experiments, from depth estimation to multisensory integration, showing that cue weight in cue combination increases with the reliability of the cue. The reliability of visual cues, for example, has been manipulated by changing their geometrical properties as in the study of Young, Landy, and Maloney (1993) in which the circular shapes of the texture cue were randomly changed into ellipses, or by introducing visual noise in the stimuli, as in the study of Ernst and Banks (2002) in which the disparity of the random dots used in their stimulus was changed to introduce "noise" in the stereo cue. In our own

[1] Continuous nonlinearities are approximately linear over suitably small regions of their domain—a way to "linearize" a nonlinear system is thus to probe it with small stimulus changes only; compare the impressive success of linear early-spatial-vision models at predicting (low-contrast) *detection* data with their equally impressive failure to predict (high-contrast) *discrimination* data. Thus, there may arise the problem that perturbation analysis yields data consistent with linear cue combination even in nonlinear systems.

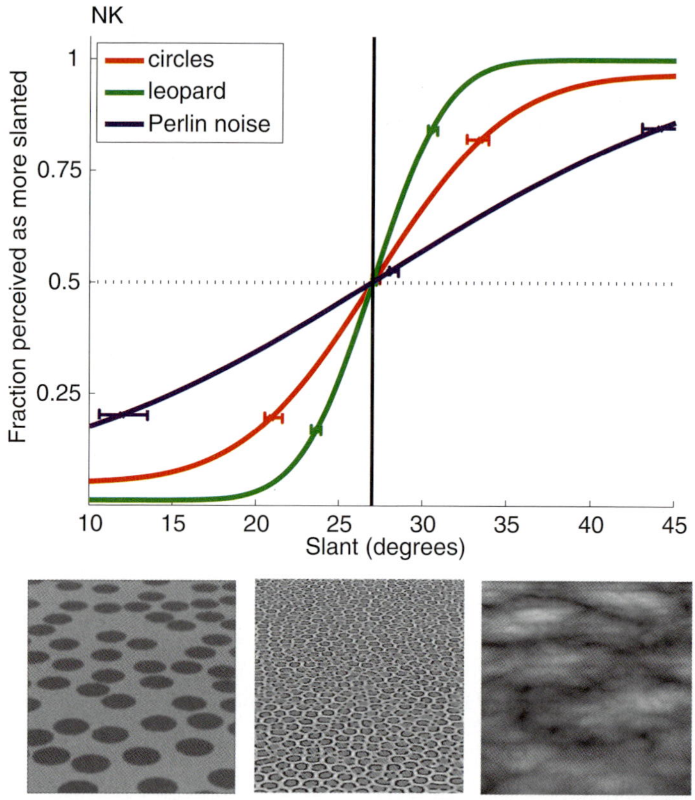


**Figure 8.1** Texture type affects slant discrimination: The top panel shows the psychometric functions for discrimination of slant for three texture types for one observer (NK). Error bars represent 68% confidence intervals derived using a parametric bootstrap procedure (Wichmann & Hill, 2001a, 2001b). The bottom panel shows the three texture types used to obtain the data; from left to right: *circles*, *leopard-skin-like*, and *Perlin noise* (Perlin, 1985). For this observer the task was easiest when the texture leopard was mapped onto the slanted planes and was most difficult for *Perlin noise*.

studies of cue combination in depth perception, we have used the classic slant-from-texture paradigm introduced by James Gibson. Texture is a monocular cue that Gibson argued to be of general importance in vision (Gibson, 1950). In Rosas, Wichmann, and Wagemans (2004) we showed that the texture type used in slant discrimination affected performance, allowing us to define a set of texture types ordered according to their psychophysical effectiveness for slant from texture (see Fig. 8.1 for example textures). Such an empirically obtained rank order *should* represent a set of different reliabilities for the texture cue, at least in the (weak) fusion framework. At the same time we believe that exchanging one texture for another to manipulate the reliability of the texture cue is a more "natural" experimental protocol than to try and alter the individual textures. We tested whether cue combination is sensitive to the texture reliability associated with different texture types by combining visual cues (texture and motion; Rosas, Wichmann, & Wagemans, 2007) and visual and haptic cues (texture and touch; Rosas, Ernst, Wagemans, & Wichmann, 2005). We have found that in general human observers are indeed sensitive to the reliability of the texture type.

### The Minimum-Variance Unbiased Estimator

Consider the specific case in which the cues (in human vision) or sensors (in machine vision) are independent, and their reliabilities (internal noises) are normally distributed, uncorrelated, and the priors are uniform (noninformative). If these rather strict conditions are met, then the simple average of the estimates weighted by the inverse of the cues' (sensors') variances corresponds to the minimum-variance unbiased estimator (Landy et al., 1995). Landy and colleagues (1995) argued that such a scenario may be plausible in human cue combination and Jacobs (1999) first tested it for visual cues and found data to be at least consistent with it. Ernst and Banks (2002) tested it for two sensory modalities and again found the data to be consistent with the predictions of minimum-variance unbiased estimation. They concluded that human observers do indeed combine cues optimally—in the psychophysical cue-combination literature minimum-variance unbiased-estimation combination is termed "optimal," and it is frequently argued that humans combine cues "optimally."

We would like to stress that "optimal" cue combination is but one special case of reliability-sensitive cue combination. In fact, there are results consistent with reliability-sensitive cue reweighting that do not match the precise predictions of the optimal cue combination, not least our own (Rosas et al., 2005, 2007) but also, for example, Zalevski, Henning, and Hill (2007).

More fundamentally, we would like to argue that the variance is not a good measure of the reliability of a cue, thus calling the minimum-variance unbiased estimator "optimal" is an unfortunate choice—optimality implies a teleological correctness that the minimum-variance unbiased estimator cannot deliver. All moment-based summary statistics—mean, variance, skewness, kurtosis, and so forth—of a probability distribution are highly sensitive to outliers; a single wild data value can exert an arbitrarily large effect on them (see, e.g., Hoaglin, Mosteller, & Tukey, 1983). In addition, for skewed distributions the variance is not necessarily a particularly meaningful summary statistic, and for leptokurtic distributions such as the Laplace or the Student's $t$-distribution with low degrees of freedom, the variance is "inflated" compared to that of a Gaussian distribution roughly appearing equally reliable ("chi-by-eye"[2] or if dispersion is measured by nonparametric confidence intervals). For heavy-tailed distributions, defined not to have a finite variance, it is obvious that the minimum-variance unbiased estimator is not an "optimal" choice: It simply ignores all estimates with a heavy-tailed reliability. Figure 8.2 illustrates this point. (Knill [2003] has a related discussion about the shape of the probability densities and their influence on cue combination in the context of mixture models of prior constraints in depth perception.)

It is somewhat peculiar, we think, that the weak-fusion model was augmented with the term *robust* to deal with outliers and errors naturally occurring in biological systems—non-Gaussian data—but that nonrobustness is brought back through the back door by the reliance on a moment-based estimate of reliability. Of greater concern, according to current cue-combination terminology, any human observer *not* ignoring the cue on the right in the bottom panel of Figure 8.2 is suboptimal; any observer moving his or her combined estimate further toward the middle in the middle panel of Figure 8.2, ditto. We beg to differ: Sensitivity to the reliability of cues is obviously good and necessary, equating reliability simply with the variance of the underlying density, however, is not.

## OPTIMALITY—EVOLUTIONARY PERSPECTIVE AND STATISTICAL IMPLICATIONS

Given a set of environmental conditions and enough time, only those organisms capable of proper sensory-motor processing will reproduce and hence survive as a species. Thus, the natural selection inherent in evolution can be seen as an

[2] "They deem a fit acceptable if a graph of data and model 'looks good.' This approach is known as *chi-by-eye*" (Press, Teukolsky, Vetterling, & Flannery, 1992, p. 657).

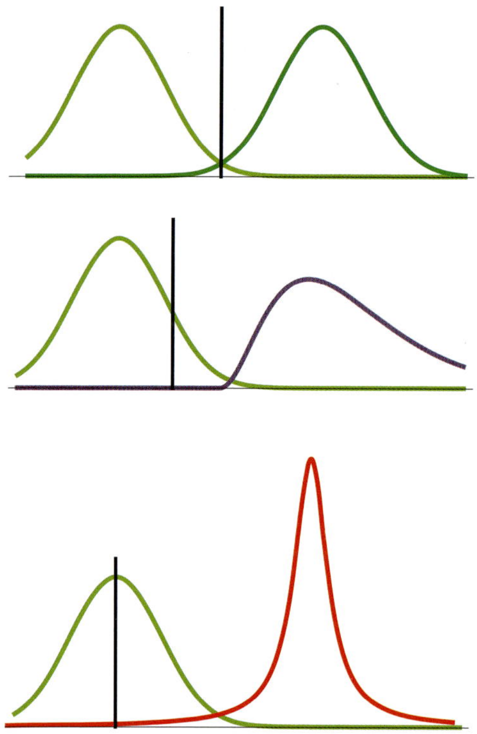

**Figure 8.2** "Optimal" cue combination? Example of minimum-variance unbiased estimates for two cues in cue combination using different distributions for the reliability (arbitrary units on horizontal axis). On each plot the distribution on the left remains a normal distribution with a variance of 1.0 units, while the distributions on the right, from top to bottom, are as follows: a normal distribution with a variance of 1.0 units; a gamma distribution with variance of 2.6 units and skewness of 1.1; and a Cauchy distribution with an indeterminate (infinite) variance. In each panel we show—as a vertical line—the "optimal" estimate obtained using the weighted average of the modes of the distributions inversely weighted by their variances. The top panel shows the commonly assumed all-Gaussian scenario leading to a "sensible" estimate; the middle panel illustrates the failure of the minimum-variance unbiased estimator to deal with skewed distributions. The bottom panel illustrates the failure of the minimum-variance unbiased estimator to deal with heavy-tailed distributions.

optimization process (certainly in the *economical* sense of balancing benefits and costs, e.g., Krebs & Davies, 1987). For example, inspired by evolution, genetic algorithms are employed in multiobjective optimization problems (Schaffer, 1985). Thus, it is not necessarily surprising to observe that behavior tends to be very well adapted to its environment—particularly if the tasks and stimuli provided in the laboratory are representative of natural conditions, like tasks involving hand-eye-coordination movements, such as in, for example, Trommershaeuser, Maloney, and Landy (2003, 2008), or estimating size by grasping as in Ernst and Banks (2002). In animal behavior research (optimal) adaptation is *axiomatic*: Researchers try and find the variables or dimensions an animal is (optimally) adapted to, rather than trying to prove that it is (optimally) adapted (Krebs & Davies, 1987). Similarly, it may be beneficial to study those cases where behavior is suboptimal in the minimum-variance-unbiased-estimator sense and start asking what the observers may have optimized or under what conditions, for example, form of non-Gaussian density, the observed behavior could be termed *optimal.*

Given the importance of "correct" cue combination during everyday life, we *expect* human observers to tend to be very good in psychophysical cue-combination tasks. This very good performance poses a statistical problem, though. Enough statistical power is needed to differentiate optimal from suboptimal combination strategies, and possibly different strategies for different observers. Consider, for example, our data depicted in Figure 8.3. Here we show the thresholds predicted and measured for slant discrimination of a plane when using a visual cue (texture) and a haptic cue (freely exploring the plane with one index finger for 1000 ms). The texture-only and haptic-only discrimination thresholds were measured and used to predict the thresholds for combined cues assuming minimum-variance unbiased estimation. Because each measured data point is based on full psychometric functions fitted to at least 500 trials, the threshold differences were assessed using at least 1000 trials. Looking at the data

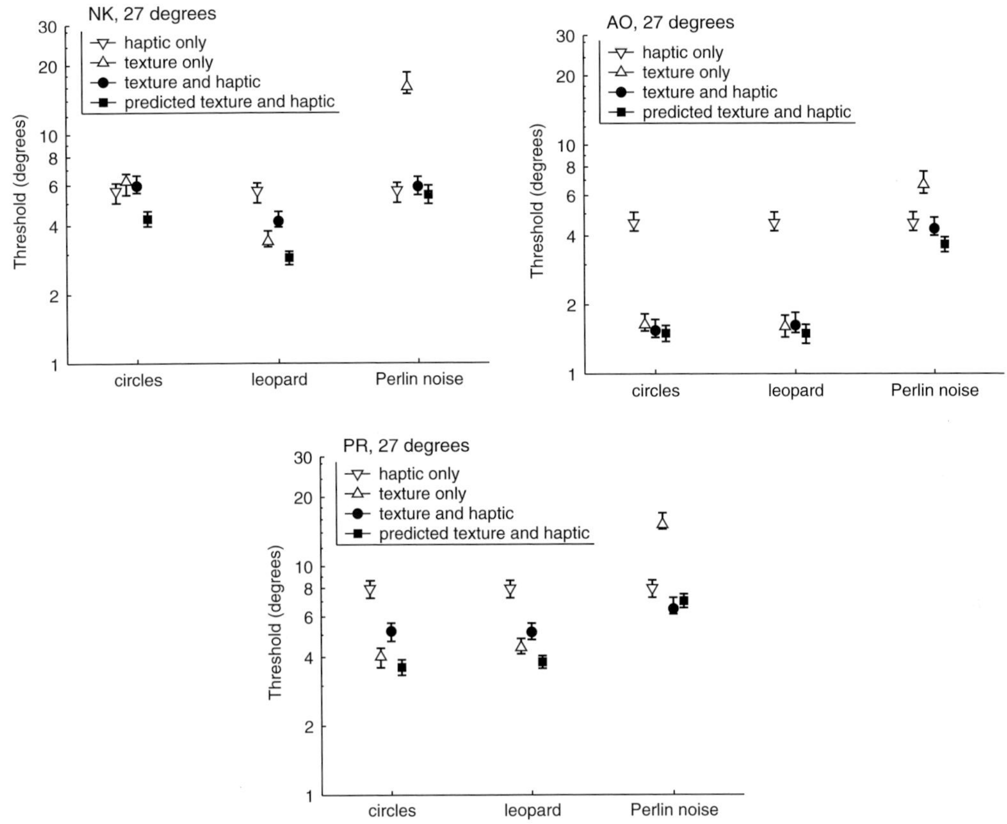


**Figure 8.3** Measured and predicted thresholds for slant discrimination based on visual (texture) and haptic information. Thresholds are defined as the difference between the stimulus judged 84% of the trials as more slanted and the PSE. Each panel shows data for one subject. Open downward-pointing triangles (Haptic-only), open upward-pointing triangles (texture-only), and filled circles (combined cues, texture and haptic) show measured, empirical thresholds. Each measured threshold was obtained from a psychometric function fitting between 500–700 trials. Filled squares show the combined texture and haptic thresholds if the observers were to combine the single-cue estimates (open symbols) using the minimum-variance unbiased estimation rule (see Chapter 1). (Data published in Rosas, Ernst, Wagemans, & Wichmann, 2005.)

for subject AO and the Perlin noise texture—shown in the middle panel of Figure 8.3—we see that the difference between visual-haptic performance and predicted variance-minimizing performance is very small, but statistically significant; however, in the bottom panel the data for subject PR and texture Perlin Noise do not reject minimum-variance unbiased estimation.

Had we collected fewer data for subject AO, the confidence intervals would have been larger (roughly scaling by $\sqrt{N}$ if $N$ is the number of trials), and we may have been led to "accept" the minimum-variance unbiased estimator as a good model for our data—this is, of course, trivially true. The opposite is trivially true, too: In psychology two conditions or observers are never *exactly* the same, thus collecting thousands or millions of trials will *always* find statistically significant differences between everything and everybody. The key is to find differences that are not only statistically significant but have an interesting effect size, that is, that the failures from one's predictions are large.

Our point may initially appear obvious, perhaps even trivial. But it implies that it may be difficult to reject "optimal" cue combination because we expect observers to be very good, that is, perform close to the "optimal" observer. Consequently there may only be a small range of number of trials $N$ where we have enough power to reject the Null Hypothesis ("optimal" cue combination is typically treated as such) without falling prey to the accusation that because $N$ is unusually large, the rejection itself is trivial. In our own data we believe to have shown such interesting, nontrivial failures of the optimal cue-combination model (Rosas et al., 2005, 2007).

## CONCLUSIONS

Robust weak fusion provides a fruitful and powerful framework within which to think about cue combination. It even allowed research to progress beyond looking for a finite set of rules of combination to search for factors that (dynamically) affect the weights of the cues. Greenwald, Knill, and Saunders (2005), for example, reported that binocular cues dominate monocular cues in a motor task because they were available sooner in their experiments, thus affecting a larger proportion of the movement. Related to learning, Atkins, Fiser, and Jacobs (2001) reported that the cue influence on a visuohaptic task changed after training using feedback indicating which was the informative cue for the task at hand. As a final example, Ernst (2007) showed that subjects can be trained to integrate cues that are not related in the real world for a given task.

However, we would like to argue that calling the minimum-variance unbiased estimator "optimal" is an unfortunate choice—optimality implies a teleological correctness that the minimum-variance unbiased estimator cannot deliver. Thus, we think, the term hinders rather than helps the field. Second, we suggest that cue combination is clearly sensitive to the reliability of cues, but that this sensitivity is taken all too frequently as evidence for "optimality" in the minimum-variance-unbiased-estimator sense. Closer inspection of cue-combination data—our own as well as some examples in the literature—show that the data are often at best *consistent* with this notion (and sometimes not even that). Consistency, however, is weak evidence and we feel that at least some of the cue-combination literature may have a tendency for *verification* (affirmative null-hypothesis testing) instead of explicitly attempting *falsification*. We argue that "nonoptimal" behavior (in the minimum-variance-unbiased-estimator sense) should be welcomed and treated as a powerful means to gain a more general view of cue combination, studying, for example, under what circumstances apparently statistically optimal behavior may result from a simpler heuristic cue-combination rule that yields "nonoptimal" cue combination under different circumstances. Do we use nonparametric estimates of reliability? Can we infer the underlying (non-Gaussian) distributions from our data? Can we test whether observers are truly Bayesian, that is, integrate over the posterior rather than relying on a point estimate such as the maximum a posteriori estimator? These, we believe, are some of the fruitful questions for further research.

## REFERENCES

Atkins, J. E., Fiser, J., & Jacobs, R. A. (2001). Experience-dependent visual cue integration based on consistencies between visual and haptic percepts. *Vision Research, 41*, 449–461.

Clark, J. J., & Yuille, A. L. (1990). *Data fusion for sensory information processing systems*. Boston, MA: Kluwer Academic Publishers.

Curran, W., & Johnston, A. (1994). Integration of shading and texture cues: Testing the linear model. *Vision Research, 34*, 1863–1874.

Cutting, J. E., & Millard, R. T. (1984). Three gradients and the perception of flat and curved surfaces. *Journal of Experimental Psychology: General, 113*, 198–216.

Ellard, C. G., Goodale, M. A., & Timney, B. (1984). Distance estimation in the mongolian gerbil: The role of dynamic depth cues. *Behavioural Brain Research, 14*, 29–39.

Ernst, M. O. (2007). Learning to integrate arbitrary signals from vision and touch. *Journal of Vision, 7*(5):7, 1–14.

Ernst, M. O., & Banks, M. S. (2002). Humans integrate visual and haptic information in a statistically optimal fashion. *Nature, 415*, 429–433.

Gibson, J. J. (1950). The perception of visual surfaces. *American Journal of Psychology, 63*, 367–384.

Goodale, M. A., Ellard, C. G., & Booth, L. (1990). The role of image size and retinal motion in the computation of absolute distance by the mongolian gerbil (meriones unguiculatus). *Vision Research, 30*, 399–413.

Greenwald, H. S., Knill, D. C., & Saunders, J. A. (2005). Integrating visual cues for motor control: A matter of time. *Vision Research, 45*, 1975–1989.

Hoaglin, D. C., Mosteller, F., & Tukey, J. W. (1983). *Understanding robust and exploratory data analysis.* New York, NY: John Wiley and Sons.

Jacobs, R. A. (1999). Optimal integration of texture and motion cues to depth. *Vision Research, 39*, 3621–3629.

Knill, D. C. (2003). Mixture models and the probabilistic structure of depth cues. *Vision Research, 43*, 831–854.

Krebs, J. R., & Davies, N. B. (1987). *An introduction to behavioural ecology* (2nd ed.). New York, NY: Blackwell Scientific Publications.

Landy, M. S., Maloney, L. T., Johnston, E. B., & Young, M. (1995). Measurement and modeling of depth cue combination: In defense of weak fusion. *Vision Research, 35*, 389–412.

Landy, M. S., Maloney, L. T., & Young, M. J. (1991). Psychophysical estimation of the human depth combination rule. In P. S. Schenker (Ed.), *Sensor fusion III: 3-D perception and recognition. Proceedings of the SPIE, 1383*, 247–254. Bellingham, WA: SPIE.

Maloney, L. T., & Landy, M. S. (1989). A statistical framework for robust fusion of depth information. In W. A. Pearlman (Ed.), *Visual communications and image processing IV, Proceedings of the SPIE, 1199*, 1154–1163. Bellingham, WA: SPIE.

Marr, D. (1982). *Vision.* San Francisco, CA: Freeman.

McKendall, R. (1990). Statistical decision theory for sensor fusion. In *Proceedings of the 1990 DARPA Image Understanding Workshop* (pp. 861–866). San Mateo, CA: Morgan Kaufmann Publishers, Inc.

McKendall, R., & Mintz, M. (1992). Robust sensor fusion with statistical decision theory. In M. A. Abidi & R. Gonzalez (Eds.), *Data fusion in robotics and machine intelligence* (pp. 211–244). Boston, MA: Academic Press.

Parker, A. J., Cumming, B. G., Johnston, E. B., & Hurlbert, A. C. (1995). Multiple cues for three-dimensional shape. In M. S. Gazzaniga (Ed.), *The cognitive neurosciences* (pp. 351–364). Cambridge, MA: The MIT Press.

Perlin, K. (1985). An image synthesizer. *Computer Graphics, 19*, 287–296.

Press, W., Teukolsky, S., Vetterling, W., & Flannery, B. (1992). *Numerical recipes in C* (2nd ed.). Cambridge, England: Cambridge University Press.

Rock, I., & Victor, J. (1964). Vision and touch: An experimentally created conflict between the two senses. *Science, 143*, 594–596.

Rosas, P., Ernst, M. O., Wagemans, J., & Wichmann, F. A. (2005). Texture and haptic cues in slant discrimination: Reliability-based cue weighting without statistically optimal cue combination. *Journal of the Optical Society of America A, 22*, 801–809.

Rosas, P., Wichmann, F. A., & Wagemans, J. (2004). Some observations on the effects of slant and texture type on slant-from-texture. *Vision Research, 44*, 1511–1535.

Rosas, P., Wichmann, F. A., & Wagemans, J. (2007). Texture and object motion in slant discrimination: Failure of reliability-based weighting of cues may be evidence for strong fusion. *Journal of Vision, 7(6):3*, 1–21.

Schaffer, J. D. (1985). Multiple objective optimization with vector evaluated genetic algorithms. In *Proceedings of the 1st International Conference on Genetic Algorithms* (pp. 93–100). Hillsdale, NJ: L. Erlbaum Associates Inc.

Trommershaeuser, J., Maloney, L., & Landy, M. (2003). Statistical decision theory and trade-offs in the control of motor response. *Spatial Vision, 16*, 255–275.

Trommershaeuser, J., Maloney, L., & Landy, M. (2008). Decision making, movement planning and statistical decision theory. *Trends in Cognitive Sciences, 12*, 291–297.

Wichmann, F. A., & Hill, N. J. (2001a). The psychometric function: I. Fitting, sampling, and goodness of fit. *Perception and Psychophysics, 63*, 1293–1313.

Wichmann, F. A., & Hill, N. J. (2001b). The psychometric function: II. Bootstrap-based confidence intervals and sampling. *Perception and Psychophysics, 63*, 1314–1329.

Young, M. J., Landy, M. S., & Maloney, L. T. (1993). A perturbation analysis of depth perception from combinations of texture and motion cues. *Vision Research, 33,* 2685–2696.

Yuille, A. L., & Bülthoff, H. H. (1996). Bayesian decision theory and psychophysics. In D, C, Knill & W. Richards (Eds.), *Bayesian approaches to perception* (pp. 123–161). Cambridge, England: Cambridge University Press.

Zalevski, A. M., Henning, G. B., & Hill, N. J. (2007). Cue combination and the effect of horizontal disparity and perspective on stereoacuity. *Spatial Vision, 20,* 107–138.

# SECTION II

## Introduction to Section II: Behavioral Studies

Section II introduces a wide range of behavioral paradigms applied to the study of cue combination. These chapters test critical aspects of the models introduced in the first section. Section II consists of three parts. The first three chapters focus on linear cue combination. The next two chapters analyze examples of nonlinear cue combination. The last two chapters focus on learning as well as the experimental demonstration of limits of the models introduced in Section I.

This section starts with three chapters that test variants of the basic linear Bayesian cue-combination model. Seydell, Knill, and Trommershäuser give an overview of behavioral evidence that demonstrates how humans use prior information in cue integration. Burr, Binda, and Gori discuss applications of the linear cue-integration model to the combination of visual, auditory, and haptic sensory signals and the development of sensory cue integration. Banks, Burge, and Held suggest that the statistics of the natural world lead to prior distributions that allow both a Bayesian ideal and human observer to estimate depth from cues one might expect to be incapable of providing information about metric depth: occlusion and blur.

The next two chapters analyze cue-integration scenarios in which the ideal cue-integration scheme is nonlinear. Ernst and DiLuca discuss situations in which the observer must determine whether cues should be integrated, leading to nonlinear effects. This chapter also gives an introduction into cue calibration (as typically studied in adaptation experiments), that is, into the problem of how the brain determines which cue is correct and which cue needs to be recalibrated. Shams and Beierholm discuss several experiments in cross-modal cue integration along with causal-inference models that predict nonlinear cue-integration effects.

The last two chapters analyze learning effects in cue integration. Landy, Ho, Serwe, Trommershäuser, and Maloney discuss cues to texture and shape and introduce the concept of "pseudocues," that is, cues that confound the property being estimated with other, irrelevant scene properties. Finally, Michel, Brouwer, Jacobs, and Knill discuss sensory cue integration in the context of two information-integration problems. The first study analyzes how the nervous system learns which cues are relevant. The second study requires subjects to combine a currently viewed cue with a remembered, but no longer visible cue in the context of a visuomotor-control task.

# CHAPTER 9

# Priors and Learning in Cue Integration

*Anna Seydell, David C. Knill, and Julia Trommershäuser*

In his *Handbuch der physiologischen Optik*, Hermann von Helmholtz (1866) stated that "reminiscences of previous experiences act in conjunction with present sensations to produce a perceptual image which imposes itself on our faculty of perception with overwhelming power, without our being conscious of how much of it is due to memory and how much to present perception" (p. 436). Helmholtz's statement is an early recognition of the important role that prior knowledge about the world plays in perception—a fundamental part of Bayesian models of perception. "Present sensations" refers to what is typically called the likelihood function $P(d|s)$, the probability of observing a set of sensory data $d$ conditioned on a possible scene $s$ we might be viewing. "Memory" captures what in the Bayesian framework is referred to as the prior $P(s)$, the probability of a given scene $s$ prior to (or independent of) collecting any sensory data. A striking example of how prior knowledge biases perception is the so-called hollow-face illusion (Gregory, 1973; for an illustration, see Fig. 9.1), in which the observer looks at the inside of a facial mask and perceives a convex face. Despite sensory data to the contrary, the concave mask is perceived as convex because our prior belief about faces is that they are convex, with the nose pointing outward. While in the case of the hollow-face illusion prior knowledge biases our perception to deviate from the true stimulus, relying on prior knowledge usually improves our estimate of what the real state of the world is, because the available (sensory) data are noisy, unreliable, insufficient, or biased.

In this chapter we review the role of prior knowledge for the integration of sensory information and discuss how priors can be modified by experience. As we will see, prior knowledge affects perception at different levels. First, it often serves as an additional cue at the level of cue integration (see section "Prior Knowledge as an Additional Cue"). Second, prior knowledge of statistical regularities in the world is also important for interpreting cues, because it can provide information needed to disambiguate sensory information and thus determines the shape of the likelihood function, as we discuss in the section "Mixture Models." Third, prior knowledge is also effective at a higher cognitive level, where it determines whether and how cues are integrated; examples for this kind of prior are given in the section "Causal Models" (see also Chapters 2 and 13). We will conclude the chapter by discussing where prior knowledge comes from and how flexible it is.

## WHY IS PRIOR KNOWLEDGE IMPORTANT?

As introduced in Chapter 1, Bayes' rule states that

$$P(s|d) = \frac{P(d|s)P(s)}{P(d)}, \tag{9.1}$$

with $P(s|d)$ denoting the posterior, $P(d|s)$ the likelihood function, $P(s)$ the prior, and $P(d)$ a normalization factor. In general, Bayes' rule

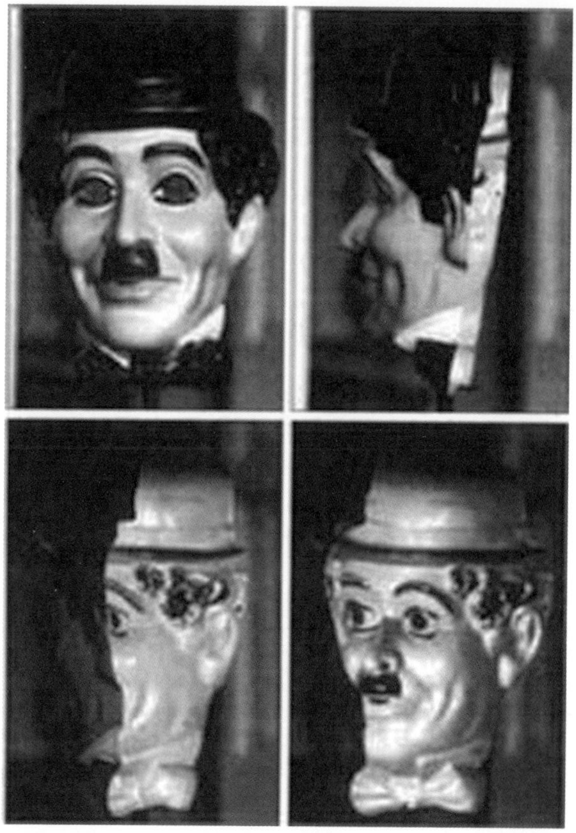

**Figure 9.1** The hollow-face illusion. The upper two panels show the front and side view of the convex side of the mask, in which the hat is black. The lower two panels (white hat) show the inside of the mask. Even though it is concave, the percept is that of a convex face. The illusion holds even if the mask is rotating right in front of the viewer (as opposed to shown in a picture), despite the fact that there are ample cues, such as binocular disparities and the fact that the side view of the convex face makes it obvious that the side with the white hat cannot be convex, indicating that the side with the white hat has to be concave. (Figure reprinted from Gregory, 1997, Fig. 1.)

provides a way to update an existing belief in the presence of newly observed sensory information. Imagine you want to know the weight of an apple, but you do not have a kitchen scale. You pick it up and estimate its felt weight to be about 200 g, but you do not trust your felt weight judgment. You know that your felt weight judgments vary considerably, and what feels like 200 g to you could in fact weigh 203 g or 195 g, or even 250 g, though that is much less likely. These considerations reflect the shape of the likelihood function $P(d|s)$, here P(felt weight = 200 g | true weight), determined by the reliability of the sensory signal (Fig. 9.2A). In addition to the felt weight, you have another source of information about the weight of apples, namely, your prior knowledge about apple weight. This takes the form of a prior probability density function over different weights. For example, of all the apples you weighed previously, the majority may have weighed 170 g or close to that, and your prior on apple weight might look as shown in Figure 9.2B. (It has indeed been shown that the fruit weight distribution of apples follows a normal distribution; see Zhang, Thiele, & Rowe, 1995.) To obtain a representation of your probabilistic knowledge about the weight of the apple you are holding, given the current

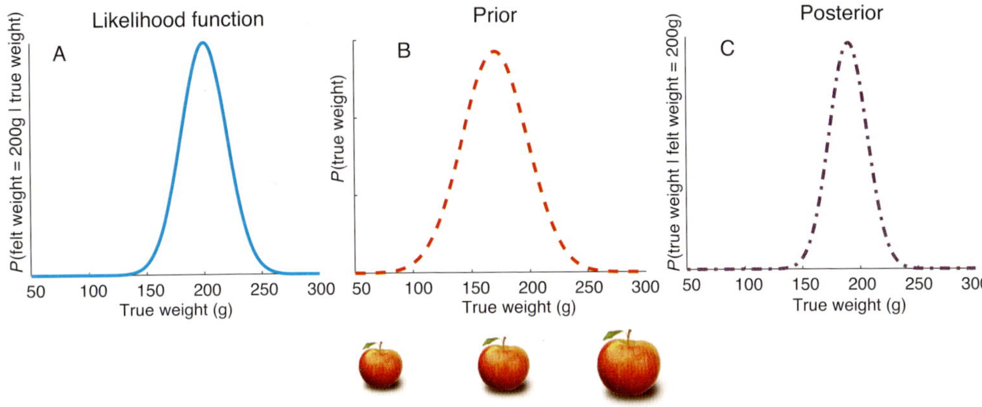


**Figure 9.2** Reducing uncertainty by using prior knowledge. Likelihood function (A) and prior (B) are multiplied and renormalized to obtain the posterior (C). If, as here, prior and likelihood functions are Gaussians, the peak of the posterior lies in between those of the prior and the likelihood function, closer to the peak of the one with lower variance. The variance of the posterior is lower than the variances of likelihood function and prior.

sensory data—the posterior probability density function—you simply multiply the likelihood function and the prior and normalize the result so that it integrates to 1. The result is shown in Figure 9.2C. The maximum is between the felt weight and the most likely prior weight, and the distribution is narrower than the likelihood function and the prior. You have thus reduced your uncertainty about the apple's weight by taking into account prior knowledge. This demonstrates that taking into account prior knowledge can improve data-based estimates.

Applied to modeling human perception, the importance of quantifying prior knowledge using Bayes' rule becomes clear when we recognize the ambiguity inherent in sensory data. In vision, for example, three-dimensional scenes project to two-dimensional images. Any single two-dimensional image is geometrically consistent with many possible three-dimensional interpretations. Knowledge of what configurations are most likely in our world is central to disambiguating image information about three-dimensional scenes. Another example comes from the domain of color perception. The spectral distribution of light energy reflected from surfaces is a function of the spectral distribution of the light sources illuminating them, the spectral reflectance functions of surfaces, their reflectance properties (how they reflect light as a function of incident illumination angle), and their shapes. Prior knowledge about all of these scene properties plays a crucial role in generating color constancy, the ability of the human visual system to perceive an object as having the same color despite different illuminations (Brainard & Freeman, 1997; Brainard et al., 2006).

Prior assumptions about scenes successfully account for a number of visual illusions, and Bayesian models incorporating quantitative priors have recently been able to account for several perceptual effects previously attributed to other, more mechanistic factors. A good example is provided by motion perception. It is well known that the perceived speed of moving stimuli depends on their contrast; low-contrast stimuli appear to move more slowly than high-contrast stimuli (Stone & Thompson, 1992). Weiss, Simoncelli, and Adelson (2002) succeeded in modeling human speed judgments as a combination of noisy speed judgments derived from the visual input and a prior on movement speed that preferred slow motion. Since the reliability of sensory motion signals decreases as stimulus contrast decreases, the relative influence of the slow-motion prior on perceived speed increases. Beyond accounting for the basic speed effect, the model also accounted for well-known biases in the perceived direction of certain plaid stimuli as well as effects of contrast on other pattern-motion percepts.

## PRIOR KNOWLEDGE AND THREE-DIMENSIONAL VISUAL PERCEPTION

A fundamental problem visual perception has to overcome and does successfully overcome every day is that the image falling on the retina is two dimensional, whereas the world we are interacting with is three dimensional. Part of the solution to this problem is that we have two retinas and that the images falling on the two retinas are slightly different because the retinas are in slightly different places. This can easily be demonstrated by holding up a finger at arm's length, closing the left eye, and aligning the finger with some landmark farther away. When the right eye is closed and the left eye is opened, it becomes apparent that finger and landmark are not aligned from the left eye's point of view. These systematic differences between the location of an object's image on the left and right retinas, called binocular disparities, serve as a cue to depth. The fact that we still have a three-dimensional impression of the world when looking at it with only one eye suggests that there are additional visual cues to depth, so-called monocular depth cues (Fig. 9.3). We will next give some examples of monocular depth cues and point out which prior assumptions are needed to interpret them.

### Inferring Distance from Retinal Image Size

One of the monocular cues to depth is the retinal image size of an object. If the object is close to the viewer, its projection on the retina will be bigger than when it is far away. Nevertheless, retinal image size alone is not a cue to depth. The image of a bird flying 10 m above you can have the same size on your retina as a plane flying much higher. In other words, if you see an object through an aperture, it is hard to estimate how far away it is and what its true size is, and sometimes, the perceptual system will be wrong about the final estimate—a weather balloon flying at moderate height might be mistaken for a giant UFO flying high above. To infer distance from retinal image size, prior knowledge or assumptions about the real size of the viewed object have to be made.

### Inferring Shape from Shading

Another example of a monocular cue to depth that requires a prior to become useful is shading. When looking at Figure 9.3A, most people interpret the stimulus as a bump, even though all that is "really there" is a circular area whose

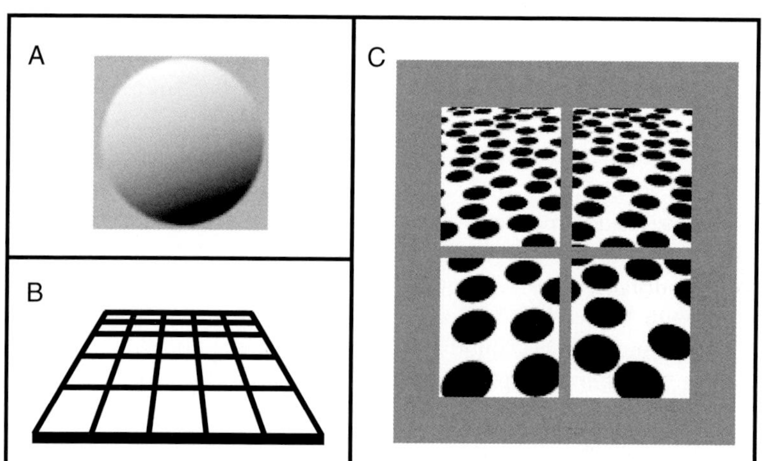


**Figure 9.3** Examples of monocular depth cues. (A) Shading; (B) foreshortening; (C) texture density gradient, size gradient, foreshortening.

luminance gradually changes from white at the top left to black at the lower right. The reason that we perceive a bump is that we have learned to use shading as a cue to object shape. And indeed, a bump on a uniformly painted matte surface illuminated from the upper left would look much like Figure 9.3A. It is important to note that it is not true that any bump under any illumination would look like this. Try looking at the same stimulus with the book held upside down. Does it still look like a bump? For most observers, it does not; instead, it looks like a dent. Why does our perception of the stimulus change when it is turned upside down? The reason is that shading is a cue to shape only if the location of the light source(s) is known or assumed, and for reasons that are still argued about (Mamassian & Goutcher, 2001; Sun & Perona, 1998), humans assume that objects are illuminated from the upper left. It is this prior assumption that disambiguates the stimulus. If not for the light-from-above prior (and the assumption that the surface is uniformly colored and matte), the stimulus could just as well be a dent illuminated from the lower right. There is, in fact, an unlimited number of alternative interpretations of the stimulus. For example, the luminance gradient we see could be partly due to shading and partly due to changes in surface albedo, but humans have a preference to interpret albedo as uniform. Without such prior assumptions, the stimulus interpretation is ambiguous, and shading cannot be used as a particularly reliable cue to shape.

### Inferring Three-Dimensional Orientation from Perspective Distortions

Another important monocular cue to depth, foreshortening, is illustrated in Figure 9.3B. It is related to the retinal image size cue. For example, the retinal distance between parallel lines receding in depth becomes smaller, and the upper end of a square will project to a shorter line on the retina than the lower end when the top is slanted away from the viewer. In Figure 9.3B, the distance between lines becomes smaller toward the upper end of the stimulus, and our prior assumption that the lines are parallels forming a grid of squares (one could call that a regularity or homogeneity prior) leads us to attribute this foreshortening to changes in depth. Different priors will lead to different stimulus interpretations, and without a prior, the stimulus is ambiguous.

### Inferring Three-Dimensional Orientation from the Texture Density Gradient

The texture density gradient of the surface shown in Figure 9.3C makes the surface appear slanted away from the viewer, because we have a strong prior on texture homogeneity—assuming that the texture elements are distributed uniformly across the surface and that they are on average the same size—and on isotropy—that the texture has no orientation bias (e.g., the texture elements are circles). These assumptions are necessary to make density, size, and shape gradients as well as texture foreshortening (reflected in the aspect ratios of the texture elements) reliable cues to surface orientation and shape. The assumptions of texture homogeneity and isotropy make us attribute the higher texture density and the lower aspect ratio and smaller size of the texture elements at the upper end of the stimulus to the fact that the surface must be slanted.

## PRIOR KNOWLEDGE AS AN ADDITIONAL CUE

As has been illustrated in other chapters, two cues about the same property can be combined to obtain a more reliable estimate. For example, as described in Chapter 1 of this book, Ernst and Banks (2002) found that humans combine visual and haptic information about the size of a virtually presented bar in a way consistent with linear cue integration. Prior knowledge about the likely sizes of the object whose size is under consideration can serve as yet another cue that, multiplied by the likelihood functions of the other cues, further reduces the variance of the final estimate, as illustrated in Figure 9.4.

There are also situations in which prior knowledge helps to disambiguate which of two alternative interpretations of a stimulus is more likely. For example, the Necker cube (shown in Fig. 9.5A) can be interpreted in two ways, and each interpretation fits equally well with the

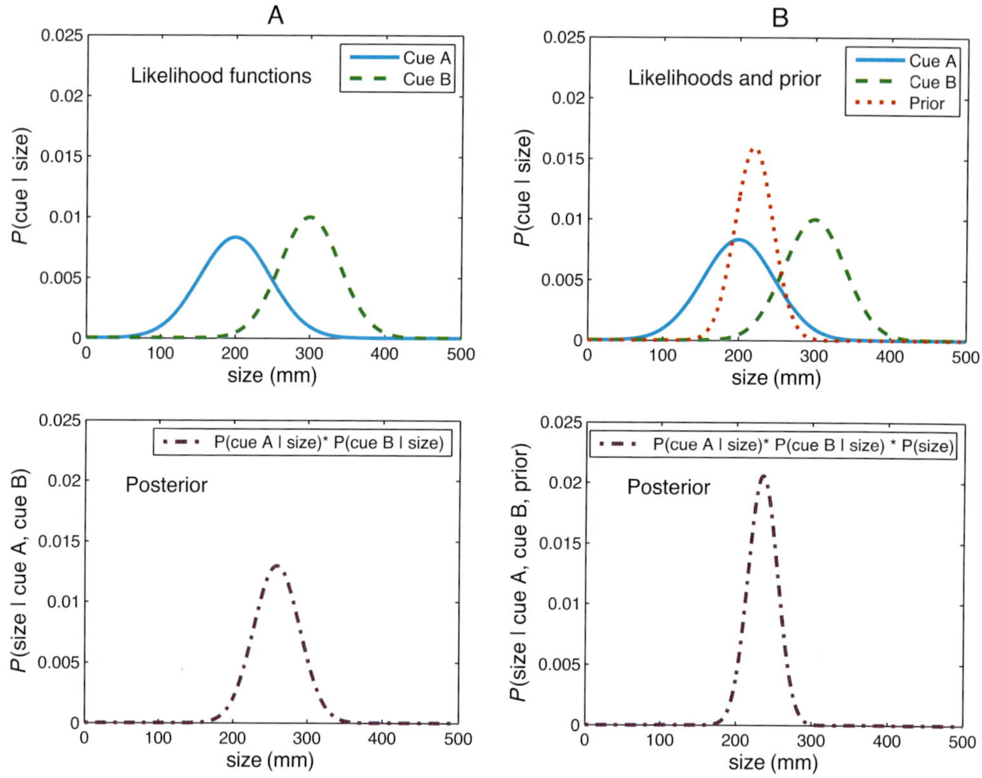


**Figure 9.4** The prior as an additional cue. During cue integration, the likelihood functions for different cues (solid blue line and dashed green line) are multiplied to obtain a posterior (dash-dotted purple line) with lower variance (left column—the lower panel shows the posterior assuming a flat prior on size which has no influence on the shape of the resulting posterior). Prior knowledge (red dotted line) can come in as a third cue to further reduce the variance of the posterior (right column).

sensory information. In this case, the likelihood function is bimodal, with two equally high modes (Fig. 9.5B, solid blue line). Multiplying it with a Gaussian prior (Fig. 9.5B, dashed red line) whose peak is closer to one of the two modes will result in a posterior with a clear global maximum, which will be close to that mode of the likelihood function that was supported by the prior (Fig. 9.5C).

## MULTIPLE CANDIDATE PRIORS AND DIFFERENT WORLD MODELS

In many cases, there are multiple, qualitatively different candidate priors that could be used to disambiguate sensory information. Each of these competing priors (termed so by Yuille and Bülthoff, 1996) would lead to a different interpretation of the stimulus. As mentioned earlier, humans tend to assume that textures are regular, for example, that texture elements are distributed evenly across a surface, are symmetric, or even isotropic. However, this regularity assumption does not always hold, and thus, an alternative prior to use when interpreting the image of a textured surface is that the texture might be random. Since an observer does not generally know a priori which prior constraint holds, it does not seem to be wise to randomly pick one and drop the other, because that means risking picking the wrong prior and arriving at an incorrect stimulus interpretation. Instead, the priors that drive perception are mixtures of the competing candidate priors, as will be described next.

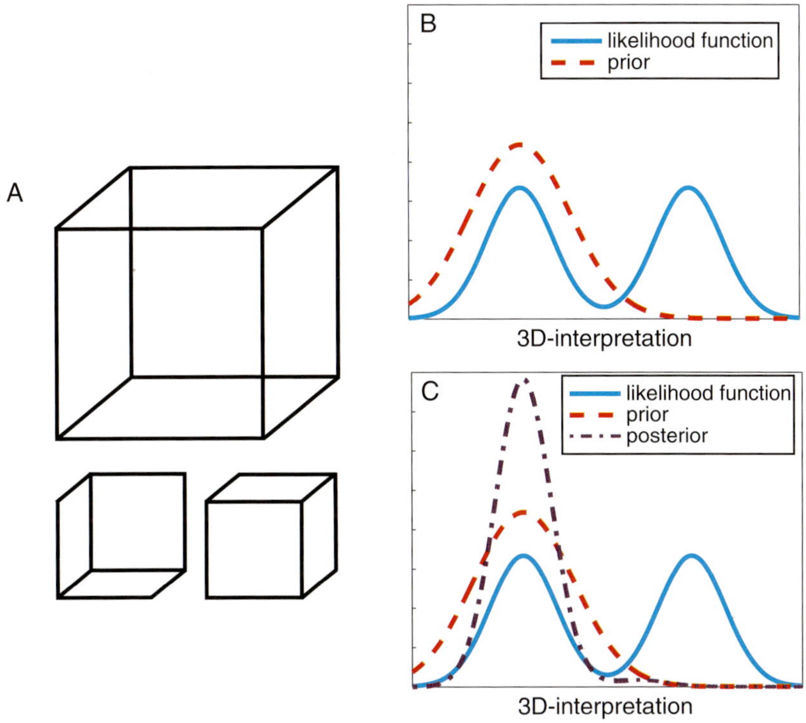


**Figure 9.5** A prior disambiguates a bimodal likelihood function. (A) The Necker cube can be interpreted in two ways (small cubes below). Each of the two interpretations is equally likely, so that the likelihood function (solid blue line) is bimodal (B). A prior, here indicated by the dashed red line, can help to disambiguate which of the two interpretations the observer should rely on, because it pulls the posterior (dash-dotted purple line) toward the mode of the likelihood function that is closer to the peak of the prior (C).

## Mixture Models

Consider the elliptical stimulus shown in Figure 9.6A. Based on the experience that many of the ellipses we see every day are circles viewed from angles that make them appear elliptical (e.g., coins, buttons, hockey pucks, wheels, iris, and pupil), we might assume that it represents a slanted circle; alternatively, it might indeed represent an ellipse. Given the first assumption, the prior on the true aspect ratio of the depicted object is a delta function at 1, because by definition the aspect ratio of a circle is 1. Given the second assumption, the prior on aspect ratio is very broad, because ellipses can come with many different aspect ratios including, but not limited to, 1. In other words, there are two categorically different priors on the true aspect ratio.

Knill (2003, 2007a) proposed to model the prior on true aspect ratio $\alpha$ in the world as a mixture of two qualitatively different priors on aspect ratio, a circle prior $P_{\text{circle}}(\alpha)$ that simply assumes that all ellipses in the world are circles (and thus is modeled by a delta function, which has the value zero everywhere except in a single place where its value is infinitely large, $\alpha = 1$), and an ellipse prior $P_{\text{ellipse}}(\alpha)$ that assumes that ellipses in the world can theoretically have any aspect ratio, but that aspect ratios close to 1 are still the most likely (this was modeled as a log-Gaussian to make sure that the function would be equal for $\alpha$ and $1/\alpha$ so as to be invariant to rotations of the ellipse). The mixture prior on true aspect ratio $\alpha$ thus is described by

$$P(\alpha) = \pi_{\text{circle}} P_{\text{circle}}(\alpha) + \pi_{\text{ellipse}} P_{\text{ellipse}}(\alpha). \quad (9.2)$$

The higher the observer's belief in the circle model, the higher the weight $\pi_{\text{circle}}$ assigned to

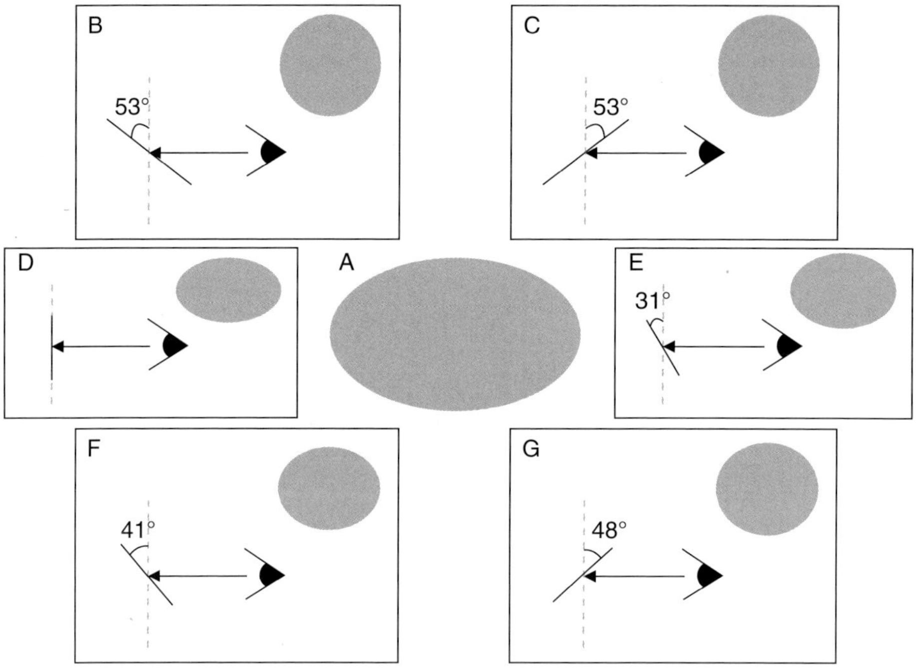


**Figure 9.6** Alternative interpretations of an elliptical stimulus. The ellipse shown in (A) could be interpreted in any of the ways shown around it, and in infinitely many other ways, depending on which prior assumptions are made. Only if the true aspect ratio of the stimulus is assumed can the slant be inferred from the aspect ratio seen in the image.

it in the mixture, and the lower the weight $\pi_{\text{ellipse}}$ assigned to the random-ellipse model. Because the models are mutually exclusive, $\pi_{\text{ellipse}} = 1 - \pi_{\text{circle}}$.

If we assume that the ellipse is slanted about its major axis, and if its true aspect ratio $\alpha$ is known or assumed, its slant $S$ can be inferred from the aspect ratio $A$ in the image, as follows from the cosine law of foreshortening, which states that

$$A = \alpha \cos(S). \tag{9.3}$$

(Note that the foreshortening cue to slant is ambiguous: The image aspect ratio is the same, whether the top or the bottom of the figure is slanted away from the viewer. For simplicity, we will ignore this fact in the following discussion, assuming that other cues can easily disambiguate the sign of slant.) In the case of a circle prior, the assumed $\alpha$ equals 1 so that $S$ can directly be inferred from $A$. In the case of the ellipse prior, there are multiple values of $\alpha$, each of which would lead to a different estimate of $S$, so that inferring $S$ from $A$ requires marginalizing across all these possible $\alpha$ (marginalizing over $\alpha$ is the same as averaging the likelihood functions computed for all possible values of $\alpha$ weighted by the prior probability distribution for $\alpha$). Because the prior on aspect ratio is a mixture of priors, the likelihood function that expresses the probability of observing a certain aspect ratio $A$ in the image given different slants $S$ is a mixture, too. To obtain the likelihood function $P(A|S)$, we extend Eq. 9.3 to account for the fact that a subject's estimate of the image aspect ratio $A$ is corrupted by perceptual noise:

$$A = \alpha \cos(S) + noise_A. \tag{9.4}$$

We assume that the perceptual noise is normally distributed around a mean of 0, with a standard deviation $\sigma_\alpha$. Thus, for a given slant $S$ and true aspect ratio $\alpha$, the likelihood function is

$$P(A|S,\alpha)=\frac{1}{\sqrt{2\pi}\,\sigma_A}\exp\left[\frac{-(A-\alpha\cos(S))^2}{2\sigma_A^2}\right], \tag{9.5}$$

which is simply a bell-shaped probability distribution with standard deviation $\sigma_\alpha$, peaked at $S = \cos^{-1}(A)$. To obtain $P(A|S)$ for a certain $A$ and $S$, we have to compute $P(A|S, \alpha)$ for each possible $\alpha$, and then integrate over all $\alpha$ to get $P(A|S)$.

The first component of the mixture is the likelihood function $P_{\text{circle}}(A|S)$. In the case of the circle prior $\alpha$ is always 1, so that we can use Eq. 9.5 and compute $P_{\text{circle}}(A|S)$ as

$$P_{\text{circle}}(A|S)=\frac{1}{\sqrt{2\pi}\,\sigma_A}\exp\left[\frac{-(A-\cos(S))^2}{2\sigma_A^2}\right]. \tag{9.6}$$

To obtain $P_{\text{ellipse}}(A|S)$, we have to integrate over $\alpha$ (which can range from 0 to $\infty$),

$$P_{\text{ellipse}}(A|S) = \int_0^\infty \frac{1}{\sqrt{2\pi}\,\sigma_A} \times \exp\left[\frac{-(A-\alpha\cos(S))^2}{2\sigma_A^2}\right] P_{\text{ellipse}}(\alpha)\, d\alpha. \tag{9.7}$$

Note that, as each assumed $\alpha$ will lead to a distribution with a peak at a different slant $S$, $P_{\text{ellipse}}(A|S)$ will be broadly distributed over slants, whereas $P_{\text{circle}}(A|S)$ is nicely peaked at the slant suggested by the seen aspect ratio $A$ if the true aspect ratio $\alpha$ is 1. The two likelihood functions are shown in Figures 9.7A and 9.7B.

To obtain the mixture likelihood function $P(A|S)$, the two component likelihood functions are combined in a weighted sum

$$P(A|S)=\pi_{\text{circle}}P_{\text{circle}}(A|S)+\pi_{\text{ellipse}}P_{\text{ellipse}}(A|S), \tag{9.8}$$

where the weight $\pi_{\text{circle}}$ represents the observer's prior belief that a figure is a circle, and the weight $\pi_{\text{ellipse}}$ represents the observer's belief that a figure was randomly drawn from an ensemble of ellipses, and the likelihood functions are defined as in Eqs. 9.6 and 9.7. The resulting mixture model likelihood function (Fig. 9.7C) has a peak at the slant at which the seen aspect ratio $A$ is most likely to be observed if the object is a circle, but in contrast to the likelihood function for a circle prior $P_{\text{circle}}(A|S)$ it has broader tails (Fig. 9.7D).

Knill (2003, 2007a) showed that using mixture models for priors can successfully model robust and nonlinear cue-integration behavior that was similar to observed human data. Further testing the mixture model framework, Knill (2007a, 2007b) found that when judging the three-dimensional orientation of elliptical stimuli, subjects learned to rely less on the observed aspect ratio as a cue to depth if they were confronted with stimuli whose aspect ratio was unambiguously different from 1. The intuitive explanation is that experiencing elliptical stimuli violates the constrained prior assumption that most elliptical stimuli are in fact circles. As a consequence, the belief in the circle assumption is lowered, and the aspect ratio, whose reliability as a cue to slant critically depends on this prior assumption, is effectively used less compared to other cues to slant (such as stereoscopic disparities) whose reliability does not depend on the circle assumption. If, on the other hand, subjects experience many perfectly isotropic circles, the circle assumption is confirmed and the aspect ratio cue is relied upon more strongly. This was also confirmed experimentally.

### Mixture Models and Robust Cue Integration

The particular shape of the mixture-model likelihood function gives rise to a form of robust cue-integration behavior that cannot be modeled if the cue likelihood functions are all Gaussian, namely, cue reweighting or, in extreme cases, cue vetoing. If there were just two Gaussian likelihood functions, $P_{\text{circle}}(A|S)$ and $P(\text{disp}|S)$, multiplication of the two likelihood functions would always result in a posterior that is also a Gaussian and peaked between the two

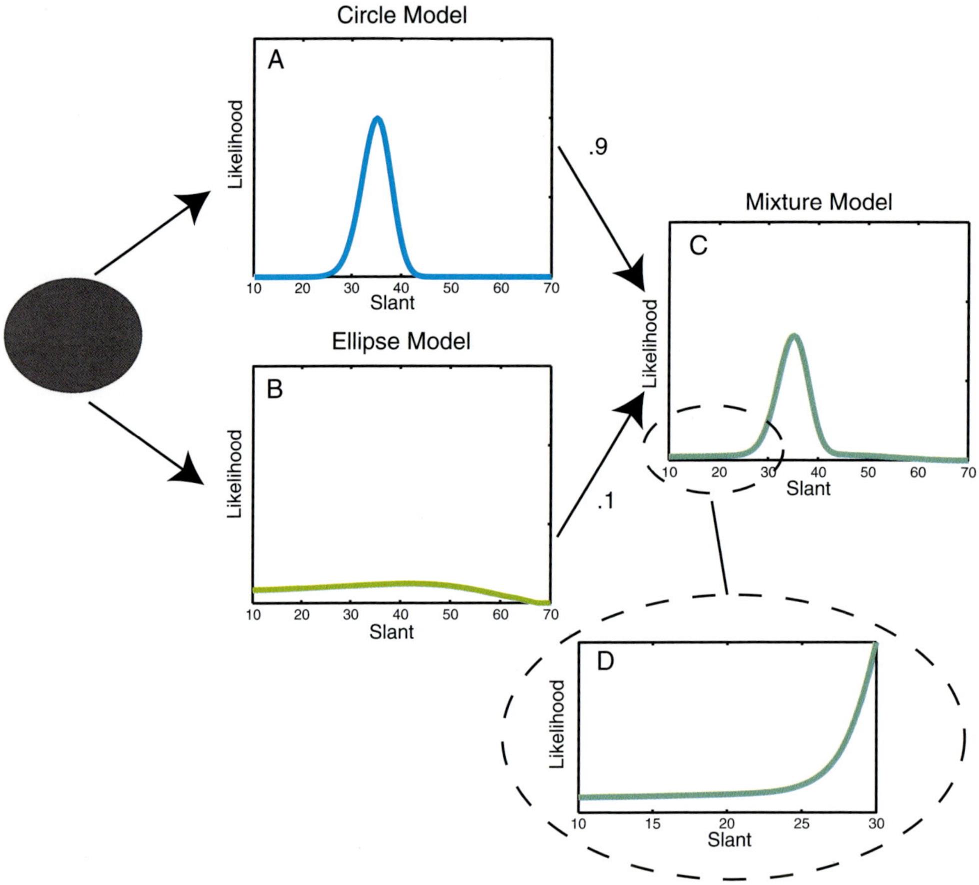


**Figure 9.7** Two likelihood functions for the same cue, obtained assuming two different generative models, are combined into a mixture cue likelihood function. (A) Shape-cue likelihood function assuming that the viewed ellipse is a circle. (B) Shape-cue likelihood function assuming that the viewed ellipse could be an ellipse with any aspect ratio. (C) Mixture likelihood function obtained by building a weighted average of (A) and (B). (D) Note that the resulting mixture has broad tails. (Adapted with permission from Knill, 2007a, Fig. 2.)

likelihood functions. This would also be the case if there were a huge cue conflict and the peaks of the two Gaussians were far apart. The resulting slant estimate (a linear weighted sum of the slants suggested by the two cues) would then be very different from the slants suggested by either cue. However, such a large cue conflict is very unlikely to occur just due to the variability of the two single-cue estimates. It thus indicates that a different generative model should be applied to interpret at least one of the cues. Mixture models take into account that there are multiple possible generative models for a cue (for example, the observed aspect ratio $A$ of an ellipse could arise from a slanted circle but also from a slanted ellipse with an aspect ratio different from 1), which allows for "normal" cue integration as well as down-weighting or vetoing one cue in case of large conflicts. If the slant-from-disparity and the slant-from-$A$ cues roughly agree, the peak of the posterior will fall in between the peaks of the likelihood functions, and the outcome of the cue integration process will look much like weighted averaging (Fig. 9.8A). Effectively, the circle model has been chosen. If the cues disagree strongly, the broad tails of the mixture likelihood

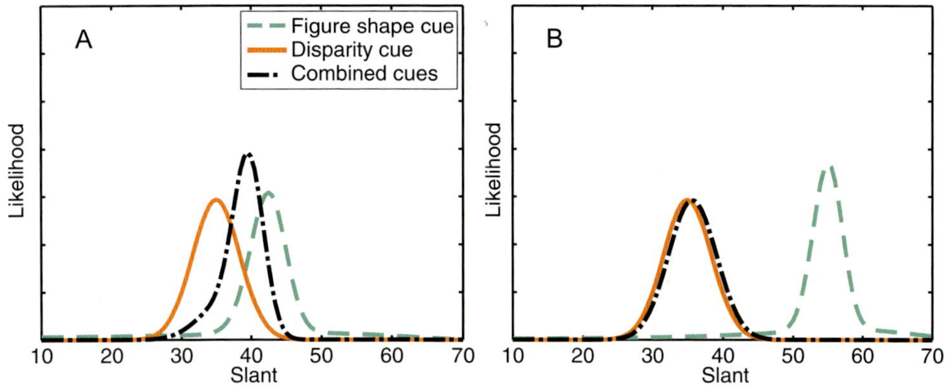


**Figure 9.8** Integration of a mixture likelihood function with broad tails with a Gaussian likelihood function. (A) If the cues (solid orange and dashed turquoise line) roughly agree, the resulting posterior is in between the two cue likelihood function peaks, just as it would be if both cue likelihood functions were Gaussians. (B) If the cues are strongly discrepant, the one with the broad tails (a mixture likelihood function as illustrated in Fig. 9.7) is effectively vetoed. (Adapted with permission from Knill, 2007a, Fig. 3, panels A and C.)

function allow the other cue to maintain its influence on the posterior, whereas the peak of the mixture likelihood function associated with the *A* cue will be suppressed because the likelihood function of the other cue has values close to zero at its location (Fig. 9.8B). Effectively, the circle model has been rejected, and the perceptual impression will be that of a slanted ellipse, not a slanted circle. This way, the integration process becomes robust to outliers and effectively selects between competing prior models. Knill (2007a) showed that the apparent weights that subjects give the foreshortening cue relative to disparity cues changes with the size of cue conflicts in a manner consistent with a Bayesian estimator using a mixed prior on figure shapes.

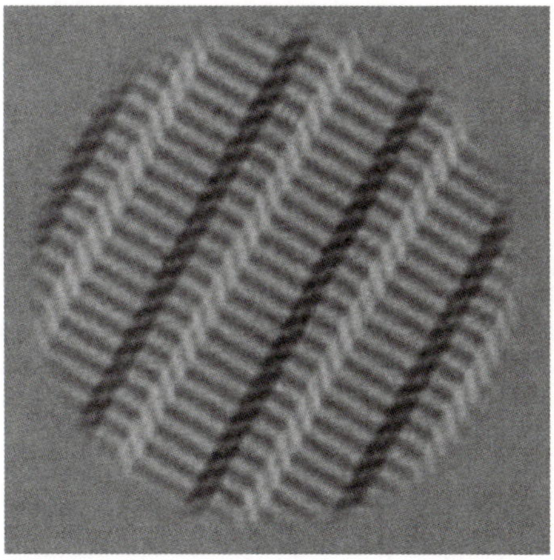

**Figure 9.9** A bistable stimulus. This stimulus (reprinted with permission from Mamassian & Landy, 2001, Fig. 3C), can be viewed as having the broad ridges bulging toward the viewer if one assumes that the light comes from above left and thus the left sides of the wide ridges are in the light, while the right sides are in the shadow. Alternatively, it can be viewed as having the narrow ridges bulging, but this interpretation is inconsistent with the light-from-left-above prior, because in that case the right sides of the ridges are in the light, and the left sides are in the shadow.

### Interactions of Priors

In the aforementioned examples, two different candidate priors competed for interpreting the same cue. However, often the information provided by the individual cues relies on separate, independent priors. In some cases, the stimulus interpretations consistent with the priors can disagree. For example, the stimulus in Figure 9.9 can be interpreted using two different cues to shape: shading and image contours. The shading cue requires a prior assumption about the location of the light source, and it has been shown that observers tend to interpret stimuli assuming that the light source is located above and slightly to the left (Mamassian & Goutcher, 2001; Sun & Perona, 1998). Assuming a light-from-above prior and interpreting the stimulus using the shading cue, the wide ridges seem to bulge, and the narrow ones recede. On the other hand, the image contours are also a cue to shape, provided prior assumptions about the orientation of the surface relative to the viewer are made. Usually, we interpret image contours assuming that our viewpoint is located above the object (Mamassian & Landy, 1998). Given that assumption, the lines on the stimulus give the impression that the narrow ridges are bulging and the broad ones recede. In a fully Bayesian mode, the interpretation of such a stimulus depends on the relative "strength" of the priors; for example, on the spread of the assumed prior probability distribution of light source directions (a broad prior on light source direction is equivalent to a weak prior). Mamassian and Landy (2001) demonstrated how prior assumptions on light source direction, viewpoint on a surface, and surface contours interact to determine subjects' percepts of shaded, contoured surfaces. Their demonstrations showed that the relative influence of different priors on subjects' percepts depended on the contrast of the associated cues; if shading contrast was high and contour contrast low, the light-source prior influenced subjects' judgments more and the viewpoint prior influenced them less. Fitting subjects' shape judgments to a model in which priors were given weights that could depend on stimulus contrast, they found that the resulting weights on the priors varied with stimulus contrast. The authors argued that priors are weighted in the same way cues are weighted in the classical cue-integration model, namely, according to their relative reliability (where reliability is defined as the inverse of the variance of the distribution). This approach to modeling multiple different priors is what the authors themselves call "non-Bayesian heresy," because the variance of the prior probability distribution is modeled to depend on the stimulus, whereas in a strict Bayesian sense the prior should be independent of the data. Whether a properly Bayesian model could account for their data remains to be seen.

### Causal Models

In a similar vein, Körding et al. (2007) use a mixture prior (termed "causal inference model"—see also Chapters 2 and 13) to model the observer's prior belief on whether two sensory cues share a common cause. In their study, subjects saw and/or heard a brief visual and/or auditory stimulus that could come from different locations. They then had to report the location of the auditory stimulus and, in a second experiment, whether the stimuli had a common cause. Because visual localization estimates have a much lower variance than auditory ones, subjects' location judgments for the auditory stimulus were shifted toward the location indicated by the visual stimulus when the two were perceived as coming from the same source. Interestingly, if the stimuli came from moderately different locations and subjects perceived them as having a common cause, the influence of the visual stimulus was less than would be expected by full integration, and it decreased with increasing distance between the two signals. This indicates that even though the "common cause" decision is binary, the integration still depends on what the exact probability of a common cause is assumed to be. In terms of the mixture model approach mentioned earlier, the amount of integration is determined by the relative weight given to the "common cause" and the "no common cause" assumption. Subjects appear to compute the average interpretation across the two models, weighted by the relative likelihood given the sensory data (model averaging), rather than picking the most likely model and using it to interpret the data (model selection).

While conceptually different, the causal model of Körding et al. (2007) acts similarly to a model that assumes some prior "coupling" between different physical variables that give rise to a pair of sensory signals. Ernst (2007) and Roach, Heron, and McGraw (2006) have proposed models that treat sensory signals in different modalities as coming from distinct physical causes (variables) that are probabilistically related to each other through what they refer to as a "coupling" prior. We will illustrate the relationship between the two approaches using the example of auditory-visual localization. Assuming that auditory and visual signals $A$ and $V$ come from distinct physical sources with positions $x_A$ and $x_V$, we can write the posterior density function for $x_A$ and $x_V$ as

$$P(x_A, x_V|A,V) = \frac{P(A,V|x_A, x_V)P(x_A, x_V)}{P(A,V)}, \tag{9.9}$$

where $P(x_A, x_V)$ is the prior density function on the physical locations of the auditory and visual sources, respectively. Ernst (2007) assumes a prior density function that looks like a Gaussian ridge in $x_A$, $x_V$ space; that is,

$$P(x_A, x_V) = Ke^{-(x_A - x_V)^2/2\sigma^2}, \tag{9.10}$$

where $K$ is just a normalizing constant. While this is technically an improper prior (its integral is infinite), one can define bounds on the positions $x_A$, $x_V$ that make it proper. Roach et al. (2006) use a similar prior that is a mixture of a uniform distribution over possible position $x_A$, $x_V$ and a prior like Ernst's,

$$P(x_A, x_V) = \pi\frac{1}{M} + (1 - \pi)Ke^{-(x_A - x_V)^2/2\sigma^2}, \tag{9.11}$$

where $\pi$ is the mixture proportion and $M$ is the area of the region of possible positions. While Roach et al. (2006) did not write the prior in the model in quite this form, we have done so here to bring out the relationship between the resulting model and the causal model. The causal model effectively assumes the same prior as Eq. 9.11. As implemented by Körding et al. (2007), the model effectively had a coupling prior as in Eq. 9.11, taken to the limit of $\sigma \to 0$, since the two-source model had a uniform prior on positions and the single source model assumed that $x_A = x_V$.

While the causal model can be thought of as imposing a coupling prior that is a mixture of different priors associated with each possible causal model, it has a few advantages over using coupling priors to fit data. First, it ties the prior to a particular generative model in the world. This allows one to use knowledge of how the world works to derive, at the least, families of coupling priors that are normative for our environment. Second, it explicitly models the estimation of a causal model. This is arguably an important perceptual function in and of itself. For example, there are likely situations in which it is important to an organism to decide whether sounds and sights emanate from a common source or from different sources. Explicitly constructing causal models allows one to model this function. Finally, as we will discuss further, the causal-modeling approach suggests a natural way to look at learning or at least adds an important dimension to the learning problem.

### Priors: Innate or Acquired?

At this point, there does not seem to be much agreement regarding the question of whether priors are innate. For example, there is a heated and ongoing debate about whether humans are born with the knowledge about a universal grammar (for a discussion in favor of universal grammar, see Chomsky, 1965; for one against it, see Everett, 2005), a set of rules about how language is organized. There is some evidence that the light-from-above prior mentioned earlier might indeed be innate: Hershberger (1970) found that chickens who were raised in an environment where the light came from below nevertheless behaved as though light was coming from above. In the domain of face recognition, it has been argued that face preferences in newborns reflect some innate basic knowledge about the structure of faces (see, for example, Mondloch et al., 1999 and Turati, 2004, for the other side).

The priors observed in the setting of lab experiments mostly match the statistics of natural environments. For example, Geisler, Perry, Super, and Gallogly (2001) developed a Bayesian framework for how contour grouping mechanisms link local edge elements into global contours. For that purpose, they examined the statistical properties of contours in natural images, which presumably drove the evolution of those contour-detecting mechanisms. The idea behind this approach is that the more likely two edge elements with certain relative position (distance between their centers), orientation, contrast, and so forth co-occur in the environment, the more likely it is that they belong to the same contour. Using these edge co-occurrence statistics, Geisler et al.'s (2001) model predicted human contour-detection performance well.

### Priors Can Be Modified through Experience

Some studies have investigated how experience can modify prior assumptions. For example, Adams, Graf, and Ernst (2004) found that the light-from-above prior (one of the priors that determine the likelihood function of a cue, in this case, the shape from shading cue) can be changed (over the course of a 90 min training session) by repeated haptic feedback about the object shape. For example, a subject who initially perceived 70% of the stimuli that were lightest at the 10 o'clock position as bumps and then felt them as dents during training afterward perceived a higher proportion of them as dents. (The prior on light source direction was estimated from the proportions of stimuli perceived as concave for light edges at each clock position.) The change in prior also transferred to a different task where subjects had to indicate which of two sides of an oriented object appeared lighter.

Other studies have demonstrated that subjects can learn experimentally imposed priors. In a study by Tassinari, Hudson, and Landy (2006), subjects were instructed to point at a target whose location was indicated by dots drawn from a distribution centered at the target location (they were told to imagine that the target was a coin flipped into a fountain and the dots were bubbles ascending roughly where the coin fell). In addition to the dots, they also had information about the prior on target location (they were told that the person throwing the coin aimed at the center of the fountain, and they saw in a training session how the actual target locations distributed around screen center). Consistent with optimal Bayesian integration of sensory evidence and prior information—here, the prior serves as an additional cue—subjects relied more strongly on the prior when there were fewer dots providing sensory information about the actual target location.

In a similar study, Körding and Wolpert (2004) had human subjects perform pointing movements toward a visually presented target. Subjects only received visual feedback about the position of their finger halfway through the movement, and this feedback was displaced by an amount randomly drawn from a Gaussian distribution centered at 1 cm to the right. The reliability of this feedback was manipulated (it was given in form of either only one dot, or in form of a Gaussian-distributed cloud of dots with low or high standard deviation, or visual feedback was withheld altogether). Results were in line with the interpretation that in the course of the experiment subjects learned a prior on the sideward displacement (a Gaussian centered at 1 cm), and that—just as they should according to the Bayesian framework—they relied more strongly on the prior as a second cue to finger location when the visual feedback given on a trial was less reliable. An alternative explanation for Körding and Wolpert's results would be that subjects simply adapted to the 1 cm sideward displacement in the sense that they recalibrated the mapping between their visual and sensorimotor estimate of where their finger was at a given point in time and combined their kinesthetic estimate of finger position with the visually specified position in an optimal way—giving more weight to the visual signal as the reliability of that signal increased. However, a second experiment demonstrated that subjects were able to learn a bimodal prior, which cannot be explained in terms of this kind of adaptation. Learning the bimodal prior took subjects significantly longer than learning (or adapting to) the Gaussian displacement. Nevertheless, the second experiment clearly demonstrated that subjects acquired knowledge about the displacement over the course of the experiment and used this knowledge in a way consistent with the Bayesian framework.

In a similar study, Körding, Ku, and Wolpert (2004) had subjects counter a force pulse that was applied to their moving finger and whose amplitude they could infer from a force pulse given earlier in the same trial (sensory information) and from the distribution of force pulses experienced over previous trials (the prior again serving as an additional cue). The results showed that subjects could learn and take into account Gaussian priors with large and small standard deviations. Moreover, subjects who had learned a narrow prior started to rely less on prior knowledge when they were exposed to a new, broader prior. Interestingly, subjects who learned a wide prior first did not rely more on the prior when the prior was changed to have a narrow standard deviation. A similar effect was found by Miyazaki, Nozaki, and Nakajima (2005) in a coincidence-timing task. In this study, subjects were instructed to press a button at the time an LED lit up. To predict when the LED would light up, subjects had two cues: sensory information (the time interval between two previous LED onsets) and prior information (the distribution of time intervals experienced in previous trials). In contrast to Körding et al.'s (2004) results, here, subjects learned to adapt their prior from wide to narrow and from narrow to wide distributions. However, the learning took much longer for the wide-to-narrow change. A possible interpretation for why changes from narrow to wide priors should be learned faster than changes from wide to narrow is that for changes from narrow to wide, subjects suddenly start experiencing cases that are extremely unlikely under the narrow prior; thus, there is positive evidence that the prior needs to be changed. On the other hand, subjects who have learned a broad prior would have to realize that the tails are suddenly underrepresented, and the absence of something is probably less salient than the unexpected presence of something. This intuitive explanation is well in line with the modeling results of DeWeese and Zador (1998), who found that an optimal Bayesian variance estimator displays qualitatively identical behavior, detecting an increase in variance faster than a decrease.

As mentioned earlier, a study by Knill (2007b) demonstrated that after experiencing lots of nonisotropic stimuli, subjects learn to rely less on the prior assumption that objects are isotropic and consequently rely less on monocular cues for whose interpretation this assumption has to be made.

### Flexible and Adaptive Use of Priors

We have now seen evidence that priors reflect environmental statistics and can be modified through experience. Given that different environments can have very different statistics, and that we rapidly move between different environments, it seems inefficient to modify a single prior every time we enter a new environment. For example, human-made environments tend to be more regular (have more right angles, more perfectly homogeneous textures, perfect symmetry and isotropy) than natural environments. Similarly, different object categories often warrant different priors. For example, coins are most likely circular, whereas buttons and brooches also come in different qualitative shapes. As we interact with different objects and move between environments, it would be useful to have separate priors for different environments and object classes, and to adapt them selectively and independently when there is a change in the relevant scene statistics.

Indeed, we recently found experimental evidence for selective adaptation of priors for different object classes (Seydell, Knill, & Trommershäuser, 2010). In all experiments, subjects indicated the perceived slant of a planar figure presented stereoscopically by adjusting a probe so that it was perpendicular to it. The two major cues to slant were the gradient of stereoscopic disparities across the surface and the aspect ratio of the figure. As pointed out earlier, the latter, monocular cue to slant is only useful if assumptions about the true aspect ratio are made—in particular, if it is assumed that the true aspect ratio is 1. Building upon the experiments performed by Knill (2007b), we presented test stimuli in which the slants suggested by the two cues disagreed by 5° randomly interleaved with a large number of training stimuli that could either be slanted surfaces with an aspect ratio of 1 or slanted surfaces with random aspect ratios. We inferred how strongly subjects relied on both cues by fitting their slant judgments for the test stimuli as a weighted sum of the slants suggested by the two slightly conflicting cues.

In a first experiment, our stimuli came from two different object classes defined by their qualitative shape, namely, of ellipses and diamonds. In the first two out of five experimental sessions, we presented only isotropic (we will use the term *isotropic* referring to circles and square diamonds, even though the latter strictly speaking are not isotropic) training stimuli and found that for both shapes, subjects' slant judgments for the test stimuli indicated that subjects relied about equally on the aspect ratio and on stereoscopic disparities as cues to slant. In the following three sessions, we randomized the aspect ratios for the training stimuli of one shape category while keeping the training stimuli of the other shape category isotropic. Consistent with our predictions, subjects who were shown random diamonds and isotropic ellipses learned to rely less on the aspect-ratio cue for diamond test stimuli while relying as strongly on the aspect-ratio cue for ellipse test stimuli as before. The inverse pattern was observed with subjects who were shown random ellipses and isotropic diamonds. This indicates that subjects selectively lowered their belief in isotropy for the object class whose members repeatedly violated the isotropy assumption.

In a second experiment, where we used red circles and purple random ellipses instead of ellipses and diamonds, subjects did not selectively lower their reliance on the aspect ratio cue for purple stimuli. Instead, they generally relied less on the aspect ratio cue once the purple random ellipses were introduced. Even if subjects were explicitly told and reported to be aware that the red stimuli were always perfect circles whereas the purple stimuli could have various aspect ratios, there was no selective adaptation for the two colors. Subjects generalized their learning across colors. This indicates that adapting priors through experience happens implicitly and independent of explicit knowledge, but perhaps more important, that category-contingent learning is not universal. Subjects seem to adapt quickly to some statistical contingencies, but not others; perhaps this is because the brain has prior knowledge of some contingencies but not others.

## SUMMARY

In this chapter, we pointed out the importance of prior knowledge in cue integration and reported studies demonstrating the influence of prior assumptions on human perception and actions. Priors represent knowledge or assumptions that are made independently of the currently available data.

The role of priors in cue integration is threefold: First, prior knowledge can serve as an additional cue, such as when the true size of an apple is inferred from visual information, haptic information, and stored information obtained via prior experience with apples. Second, prior assumptions are often needed to determine the information content of sensory cues. A classical example for this is making inferences about a three-dimensional world from two-dimensional monocular information. Shading, perspective distortion of texture elements, texture density, and many other monocular sources of image information are only useful cues to three-dimensional shape because of certain statistical regularities in the environment. The visual system's ability to use the cues depends on knowledge of these regularities. Third, it has been proposed that priors determine how humans structure and use information. For example, priors on different generative models for cues can determine whether and how the two cues are integrated. Often, priors reflect environmental statistics, which is consistent with the assumption that they are learned and modified through experience. This hypothesis is supported by experimental data that confirm that priors can be modified through experience and that this modification happens implicitly.

## ACKNOWLEDGMENTS

We wish to thank our two anonymous reviewers for helpful comments on an earlier version of this chapter, and Mike Landy for the multiple runs of careful reading and commenting that eventually led to this final version.

## REFERENCES

Adams, W. J., Graf, E. W., & Ernst, M. O. (2004). Experience can change the light-from-above prior. *Nature Neuroscience, 7,* 1057–1058.

Brainard, D. H., & Freeman, W. T. (1997). Bayesian color constancy. *Journal of the Optical Society of America A, 14,* 1393–1411.

Brainard, D. H., Longère, P., Delahunt, P. B., Freeman, W. T., Kraft, J. M., & Xiao, B. (2006). Bayesian model of human color constancy. *Journal of Vision, 6,* 1267–1281.

Chomsky, N. (1965). *Aspects of the theory of syntax.* Cambridge, MA: MIT Press.

DeWeese, M., & Zador, A. (1998). Asymmetric dynamics in optimal variance adaptation. *Neural Computation, 10,* 1179–1202.

Ernst, M. (2007). Learning to integrate arbitrary signals from vision and touch. *Journal of Vision, 7*(5):7, 1–14.

Ernst, M., & Banks, M. (2002). Humans integrate visual and haptic information in a statistically optimal fashion. *Nature, 415,* 429–433.

Everett, D. (2005). Cultural constraints on grammar and cognition in Pirahã: Another look at the design features of human language. *Current Anthropology, 46,* 621–646.

Geisler, W. S., Perry, J. S., Super, B. J., & Gallogly, D. P. (2001). Edge co-occurrence in natural images predicts contour grouping performance. *Vision Research, 41,* 711–724.

Gregory, R. L. (1973). The confounded eye. In R. L. Gregory & C. E. Gombrich (Eds.), *Illusions in nature and art* (pp. 49–95). London, England: Duckworth.

Gregory, R. L. (1997). Knowledge in perception and illusion. *Philosophical Transactions of the Royal Society of London B, 352,* 1121–1128.

Hershberger, W. (1970). Attached-shadow orientation perceived as depth by chickens reared in an environment illuminated from below. *Journal of Comparative and Physiological Psychology, 73,* 407–411.

Knill, D. C. (2003). Mixture models and the probabilistic structure of depth cues. *Vision Research, 43,* 831–854.

Knill, D. C. (2007a). Robust cue integration: A Bayesian model and evidence from cue-conflict studies with stereoscopic and figure cues to slant. *Journal of Vision, 7*(7):5, 1–24.

Knill, D. C. (2007b). Learning Bayesian priors for depth perception. *Journal of Vision, 7*(8):13, 1–20.

Körding, K. P., Beierholm, U., Ma, W. J., Quartz, S., Tenenbaum, J. B., & Shams, L. (2007). Causal inference in multisensory perception. *PLoS ONE, 2*(9): e943.

Körding, K. P., Ku, S., & Wolpert, D. M. (2004). Bayesian integration in force estimation. *Journal of Neurophysiology, 92,* 3161–3165.

Körding, K. P., & Wolpert, D. M. (2004). Bayesian integration in sensorimotor learning. *Nature, 427,* 244–247.

Mamassian, P., & Goutcher, R. (2001). Prior knowledge on the illumination position. *Cognition, 81,* B1–B9.

Mamassian, P., & Landy, M. S. (1998). Observer biases in the interpretation of line drawings. *Vision Research, 38,* 2817–2832.

Mamassian, P., & Landy, M. S. (2001). Interaction of visual prior constraints. *Vision Research, 41,* 2653–2668.

Miyazaki, M., Nozaki, D., & Nakajima, Y. (2005). Testing Bayesian models of coincidence timing. *Journal of Neurophysiology, 94,* 395–399.

Mondloch, C. J., Lewis, T. L., Budreau, D. R., Maurer, D., Dannemiller, J. L., Stephens, B. R., & Kleiner-Gathercoal, K. A. (1999). Face perception during early infancy. *Psychological Science, 10,* 419–122.

Roach, N. W., Heron, J., & McGraw, P. V. (2006). Resolving multisensory conflict: A strategy for balancing the costs and benefits of audio-visual integration. *Proceedings of the Royal Society B, 273,* 2159–2168.

Seydell, A., Knill, D. C., & Trommershäuser, J. (2010). Adapting internal statistical models for interpreting visual cues to depth. *Journal of Vision, 10*(4):1, 1–27.

Stone, L., & Thompson, P. (1992). Human speed perception is contrast dependent. *Vision Research, 32,* 1535–1549.

Sun, J., & Perona, P. (1998). Where is the sun? *Nature Neuroscience, 1,* 183–184.

Tassinari, H., Hudson, T. E., & Landy, M. S. (2006). Combining priors and noisy visual cues in a rapid pointing task. *The Journal of Neuroscience, 26,* 10154–10163.

Turati, C. (2004). Why faces are not special to newborns: An alternative account of the face preference. *Current Directions in Psychological Science, 13,* 5–8.

Von Helmholtz, H. (1867). *Handbuch der physiologischen Optik.* Leipzig, Germany: Voss.

Weiss, Y., Simoncelli, E. P., & Adelson, E. H. (2002). Motion illusions as optimal percepts. *Nature Neuroscience, 5*, 598–604.

Yuille, A. L., & Bülthoff, H. H. (1996). Bayesian decision theory and psychophysics. In D. C. Knill & W. Richards (Eds.), *Perception as Bayesian inference* (pp. 123–161). Cambridge, England: Cambridge University Press.

Zhang, J., Thiele, G. F., & Rowe, R. N. (1995). Gala apple fruit size distribution. *New Zealand Journal of Crop and Horticultural Science, 23*, 85–88.

# CHAPTER 10

## Multisensory Integration and Calibration in Adults and in Children

*David Burr, Paola Binda, and Monica Gori*

Perception can be greatly enhanced by integration of multiple sources of information, both within the senses and between them. Over the past few years, many studies have shown that our nervous system can combine and integrate information from different senses, such as vision, space, and touch (see, e.g., Chapter 1). Although most recent work on multisensory interactions has concentrated on sensory *integration,* an equally important, but somewhat neglected, issue is cross-sensory *calibration.* As George Berkeley (1709) famously asserted 300 years ago, vision has no direct access to physical attributes such as distance, solidarity, or "bigness," and these attributes become tangible only after they have been associated with touch: that is, they need to be *calibrated.*

This chapter discusses recent experiments from our laboratory that study cross-sensory integration and calibration. We first describe a clear example of sensory integration of visual and auditory signals (the "ventriloquist effect") under conditions where audiovisual conflict is introduced artificially and when it is introduced by more natural means, for example, saccadic eye movements. Our results build on many others to show that audiovisual spatial and temporal information is integrated in an optimal manner, where optimality is defined as maximizing precision (Chapter 1). However, young children do not show optimal integration (of visual and haptic information); before 8 years of age, one or the other sense prevails: touch for size, and vision for orientation discrimination. We suggest that the sensory domination may reflect *cross-modal calibration* of vision and touch. Touch does not always calibrate vision (as Berkeley asserted), but the more *robust,* and hence more *accurate* (rather than more *precise*) calibrates the other: touch for size, but vision for orientation. This hypothesis is supported by measurements of haptic discrimination in nonsighted children. Haptic orientation thresholds were greatly impaired compared with age-matched controls, whereas haptic size thresholds were at least as good, and often better. We suggest that the impairment in haptic orientation discrimination results from disruption of cross-modal calibration.

### THE VENTRILOQUIST EFFECT

Ventriloquism is the ancient art of making one's voice appear to come from elsewhere, exploited by the Greek and Roman oracles, and possibly earlier. We regularly experience the effect when watching television and movies, where the voices seem to emanate from the actors' lips rather than from the actual sound source. Originally, ventriloquism was explained by performers *projecting* sound to their puppets by special techniques, and many still believe this (Connor, 2000). Of course, modern physics tells us that it is impossible to "project sound"; it has no option but to emanate from its actual source. More recently, many have suggested that ventriloquism is a perceptual phenomenon, with vision *capturing* sound because of its inherent superiority (Mateeff, Hohnsbein, & Noack, 1985; Pick, Warren, & Hay, 1969; Warren, Welch, & McCarthy, 1981). The spatial displacement of apparent sound sources by vision has since become known as the "ventriloquist effect." Ventriloquists go to great lengths not to move their own lips, and to move their puppets' lips in rough synchrony with the voice. It is assumed that the visual movement of the lips "captures" the sound, so it appears to arise from the wrong source (see Chapters 2 and 13).

But why should vision "capture" sound? Why should vision set the "gold standard" when sight and sound are in discord? The answer is suggested by Eq. 1.1 of Chapter 1: Assuming that cues from the various modalities are statistically independent and roughly Gaussian, the optimal way to combine information is to perform a weighted average, with the weights proportional to the *reliability* of the signal, where reliability is the inverse of the variance of the underlying noise distribution. So if auditory spatial localization were far worse than visual spatial localization, we would expect vision to dominate.

Alais and Burr (2004) tested this idea empirically, under normal conditions and under conditions where visual localization was severely impaired. To estimate the theoretical weights that should be applied, they first measured visual and auditory localization performance in various conditions of image degradation (following Ernst & Banks, 2002). They then measured localization for audiovisual stimuli in "conflict" (different spatial positions, but close enough to be perceived as fused). The results were clear. When visual localization is good, with relatively sharply defined targets, vision does indeed dominate and "capture" sound. However, for severely blurred visual stimuli (that are poorly localized), the reverse holds: Sound captures vision. For moderately blurred stimuli, neither sense dominates; the perceived position lies midway between the sound and flash. The precision of bimodal localization is usually better than either the visual or the auditory unimodal presentation. Thus, the results are not well explained by one sense "capturing" the other, but by a simple model of optimal combination of visual and auditory information.

The results are illustrated in Figure 10.1. Panel A shows sample results for one observer, who was asked to report which of two presentations seemed to be displaced to the right of the other. Both stimuli were audiovisual, comprising a brief click presented together with a visual blob. In one presentation, the *probe*, the click and blob were presented to the same position that varied horizontally over the screen. In the other presentation (randomly first or second), the *conflict stimulus*, the visual stimulus was displaced $\Delta^\circ$ rightward and the sound $\Delta^\circ$ leftward (for the example of Fig. 10.1A $\Delta = 5^\circ$). The abscissa shows the distance of the probe from the center of the conflict stimulus (average of visual and auditory position). When the visual stimuli were small, hence well localizable in space, vision dominated and the psychometric functions were centered around the position of the visual standard, $+5^\circ$ (orange curve). However, when the blobs were heavily blurred, the center of the psychometric function (the "point of subject equality" or PSE) was much closer to the auditory standard, at $-3^\circ$ (pink curve). And for the intermediate blur, the PSE was close to 0, halfway between the auditory and visual standards (dark red curve).

We tested whether the results can be predicted quantitatively by the *ideal-integration* model outlined in Chapter 1. In separate experiments we measured the ability of subjects to localize auditory and visual stimuli presented on their own. The standard deviations ($\sigma$) of those psychometric functions gave estimates of the expected precision or *reliability* ($r$) of the three visual and one auditory stimuli ($r = \sigma^{-2}$), from which we could calculate the relative weights for the audiovisual stimuli (from Eq. 1.2 of Chapter 1). Eq. 1.1 of Chapter 1 then gives the predicted PSEs for the three levels of visual blur, for the various conflicts measured. These are shown on the abscissa of Figure 10.1B, with the measured PSEs shown on the ordinate. Note that for all three observers (different figure shapes) and blur levels (different colors), the measured values followed closely the predictions ($R^2 = 0.87$).

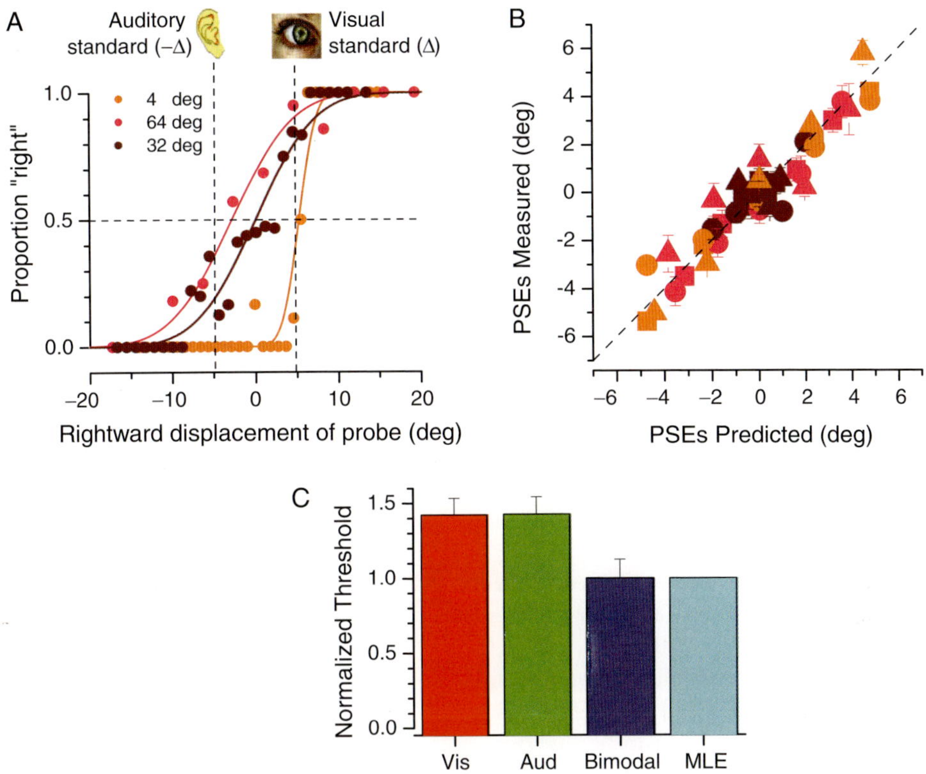


**Figure 10.1** The "ventriloquist" effect (Alais & Burr, 2004). (A) Example psychometric functions for one observer (LM), for one audiovisual conflict ($\Delta = 5°$), for three different levels of blur (see legend). The icons show the positions of the visual and the auditory standard. (B) Results of all observers (different symbols), for five different levels of conflict $\Delta$: color-coding for visual blur as for (A). Measured PSEs (medians of psychometric functions like those of Fig. 10.1A) are plotted against the predictions from the unimodal threshold measurements (Eq. 1.2 of Chapter 1). The points differ little from the dashed diagonal equality line, with $R^2 = 0.87$. Error bars on individual data points obtained by bootstrap (Efron & Tibshirani, 1994). (C) Average normalized thresholds (geometric means after normalizing with MLE predicted thresholds) for five observers, with error bars representing $\pm$ 1 SE of the mean, for discrimination of visual (32° stimuli: red bars), auditory (green), or bimodal (blue). Bimodal data are virtually identical to the MLE predictions (cyan). (Readapted with permission from Alais & Burr, 2004.)

While these results support strongly the ideal-integrator model, they do not provide conclusive proof of integration. Other strategies, like multiplexing (trial-by-trial switching between cues) could produce these types of results (although it would be unlikely to produce them so precisely). The strong proof of integration, perhaps the *signature* of integration, is the improvement of performance observed for multimodal discriminations, because the reliabilities ($\sigma_i^{-2}$) should sum (Eq. 1.3 of Chapter 1). In practice, the maximum-likelihood model does not predict a large improvement in precision for only two modalities: at most $\sqrt{2}$ when the thresholds $\sigma_i$ are similar, and far less when they differ (with the lower one dominating). Figure 10.1C shows average thresholds for the clicks and 32° blobs (similar to each other), together with the measured and predicted audiovisual thresholds. Clearly, the bimodal performance was much better than either unimodal performance, and very close to the theoretical predictions.

Thus, we conclude that the ventriloquist effect is a specific example of near-optimal combination of visual and auditory spatial cues, where each cue is weighted by an inverse estimate of noisiness, rather than one modality capturing the other. As visual localization is usually far superior to auditory localization, vision normally dominates, apparently "capturing" the sound source and giving rise to the classic ventriloquist effect. However, if the visual estimate is corrupted sufficiently by blurring the visual target over a large region of space, the visual estimate can become worse than the auditory one, and optimal localization correctly predicts that sound will effectively capture sight. Note, however, that in order for audition to dominate, vision needed to be blurred nearly to levels of legal blindness!

These results are broadly consistent with other reports of integration of sensory information (Alais & Burr, 2004; Battaglia, Jacobs, & Aslin, 2003; Clark & Yuille, 1990; Ernst & Banks, 2002; Ghahramani, 1995). In this study, for auditory localization to be superior to vision, the visual targets needed to be blurred extensively, over approximately 60°, enough to blur most scenes beyond recognition. However, the location of the audio stimulus was defined by only one cue (interaural timing difference), so auditory localization was only about one-sixth as accurate as normal hearing (Mills, 1958; Perrott & Saberi, 1990). If the effect were to generalize to natural hearing conditions, then 10° blurring would probably be sufficient. This is still a gross visual distortion, explaining why the reverse ventriloquist effect is not often noticed for spatial events. There are cases, however, when it does become relevant, not so much for blurred as for ambiguous stimuli, such as when a teacher tries to locate the pupil talking in a large class.

In the next section, we examine the ventriloquist effect in more natural situations, where vision is degraded not artificially by blurring, but by natural visual processes that occur during saccades. Under natural conditions, eye movements can be initiated by either visual or auditory stimuli and therefore constitute a useful model system to study visual and auditory localization.

## AUDIOVISUAL INTEGRATION AT THE TIME OF SACCADES

Saccades are rapid eye movements made frequently (2–3 times a second) to reposition our gaze across the visual field. While this is a clearly important strategy for extending the resolution of the fovea over the entire visual scene, it also poses serious challenges to the stability and continuity of visual perception; every time we make a saccade, visual images shift rapidly on the retina, generating spurious motion and displacement signals.

The visual system is believed to face these challenges by predictively compensating the consequences of eye movements. Before a saccade, a copy of the oculomotor signal (a "corollary discharge") is sent to visual areas, where it updates spatial representations according to the future postsaccadic gaze position (Fendrich & Corballis, 2001; Wurtz, 2008) and may help in suppressing the perception of spurious motion signals (Burr, Holt, Johnstone, & Ross, 1982; Diamond, Ross, & Morrone, 2000). While this compensation is effective in most conditions, it can lead to perceptual distortions under some conditions, such as when stimuli are briefly flashed just before or during the saccade. These stimuli are grossly mislocalized, systematically displaced in the direction of the endpoint of the saccade (saccadic target) by as much as half the amplitude of the saccade (up to 10° for a 20° saccade; Matin & Pearce, 1965; Morrone, Ross, & Burr, 1997). Because saccadic eye movements are unlikely to affect other modalities (such as audition) that rely on sensors that remain stable during gaze shifts, we took advantage of the saccade-induced selective disruption of visual perception to probe the integration of visual and acoustic information under more natural viewing conditions.

### Spatial Ventriloquism during Saccades

In this section we describe how spatial information from vision and audition seems to be combined in a weighted fashion, following the maximum-likelihood model of ideal cue integration. We measured accuracy and precision of localization for visual, auditory, and audiovisual stimuli briefly presented at the time of saccades (Binda, Bruno, Burr, & Morrone, 2007). Subjects sat before a wide hemispheric screen (covering nearly the whole visual field), where visual stimuli (2° blue blobs flashed for one monitor frame, i.e., 15 ms) were front projected. Auditory stimuli (10 ms bursts of white noise) were played through one of 10 speakers mounted behind the screen. On each trial two stimuli were presented sequentially: a probe, displayed always at the same location, and a test, whose position was variable. In separate sessions, the stimuli were either unimodal (visual or auditory) or bimodal (a flash and a sound displayed to the same location). Subjects reported whether the test (displayed about the time of a saccade) was to the left or right of the probe (two-interval forced-choice alignment task). For each condition and stimulus type we measured a psychometric function, plotting the proportion of "test-seen-right-of-probe" responses against the difference in test and probe position. The median of the curves (PSE) estimates the bias of perceived test location (PSE $< 0^\circ$ implies that the test is mislocalized rightward, in the direction of the saccade). The standard deviation $\sigma$ of the cumulative Gaussian fit gives the threshold or precision of localization.

The uppermost panels of Figure 10.2 compare the localization of unimodal visual (A) or auditory stimuli (B) presented perisaccadically (less than 25 ms before the saccadic onset) and during steady fixation. While auditory localization remains virtually identical in the two conditions, visual localization is dramatically affected by saccades. Not only is there a systematic tendency to perceive the perisaccadic test as mislocalized in the saccade direction (PSE $\ll 0^\circ$) but also the precision of localization is about 10 times lower than in fixation conditions. During fixation, vision is far more precise than audition and both modalities are accurate. Perisaccadically, visual precision is lowered to be similar to that of auditory localization and becomes biased. As audition remains accurate, the two modalities provide conflicting cues to the location of a (physically congruent) bimodal test stimulus. The localization of such a bimodal perisaccadic test stimulus is shown in Figure 10.2C (blue curve; for comparison, visual and auditory perisaccadic curves are replotted in red and green, respectively). The bimodal PSE is intermediate between the two unimodal PSEs, implying that the two modalities are given approximately the same weight. The bimodal curve is slightly steeper than both unimodal curves, meaning that localization is more precise for the bimodal stimulus than for either of its unimodal components. Both these effects are consistent with an optimal (MLE) combination strategy of visual and auditory cues.

Since the exact time of saccadic onset was variable across trials, we were able to measure localization at various delays from the saccade. Figure 10.3 (top and middle panels) shows the time courses of visual, auditory, and bimodal localization, plotting bias and threshold values against the test presentation time (values referring to the steady fixation condition are reported as dashed lines). Visual stimuli (red) were systematically mislocalized when they were presented less than $\sim$ 50 ms before the saccade or during the first $\sim$ 30 ms of its execution, the largest errors occurring at saccadic onset. The change of localization precision follows similar dynamics: In the perisaccadic interval, visual localization thresholds become similar or higher than auditory thresholds. The time courses of bias and threshold for auditory localization (green) are nearly flat, because saccades do not affect them. This also implies that saccades did not impair localization performance in a general way, but rather specifically affected visual representations. The shape of bimodal time courses (blue) is similar to that of visual time courses, but the magnitude of variation is reduced. There is a bias for perisaccadic stimuli, peaking at about the time of saccadic onset. Localization errors, however, are about half the size of those observed for pure visual stimuli. Like visual thresholds, bimodal thresholds increased perisaccadically relative to the steady-fixation condition, but they always remain lower than either unimodal threshold. Based on the visual and auditory time courses, the bimodal time courses of both localization bias and threshold are well predicted by the MLE-integration model (cyan lines show the predicted

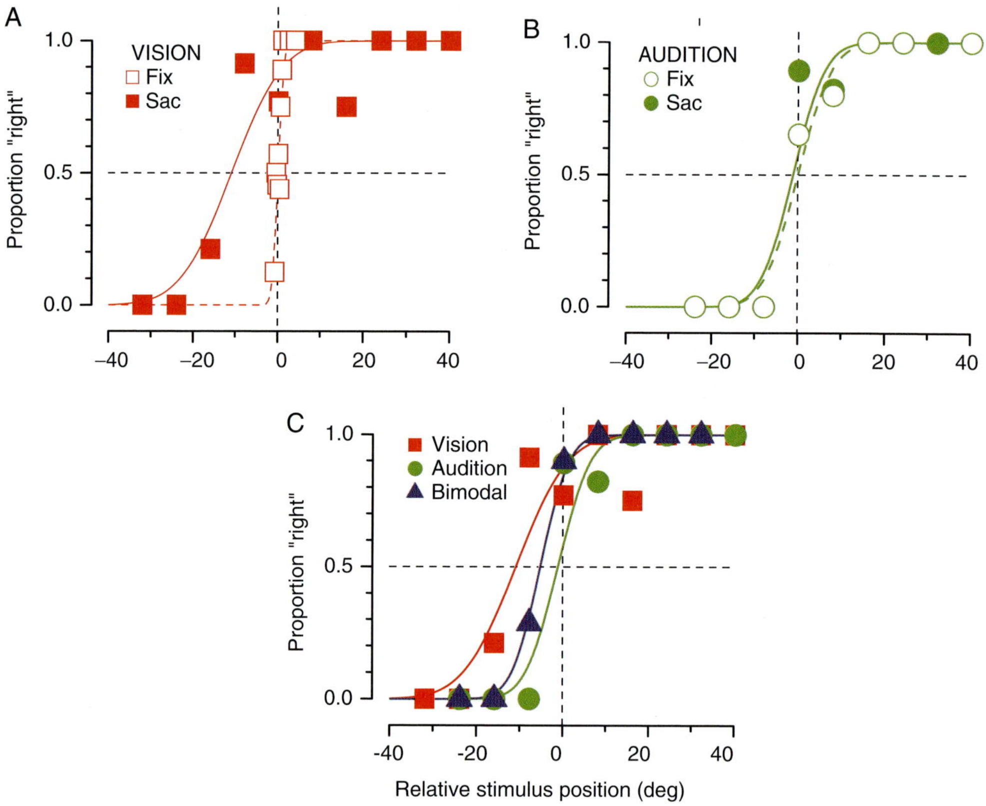


**Figure 10.2** Visual, auditory, and bimodal localization measured during steady fixation and perisaccadically. Subjects compared the locations of two successive audiovisual presentations (SOA = 600 ms), a probe stimulus (fixed position) and a test (variable horizontal location). Stimuli were either visual blobs (displayed on a wide hemispheric screen) or a tone played to one of 10 speakers mounted behind the screen; or they were bimodal, comprising both blob and tone. (A) The proportion of "test-rightward" responses as a function of distance between test and probe for one typical subject. Stimuli were visual blobs presented while subjects maintained steady fixation (hollow symbols) or less than 25 ms before the onset of a saccade. (B) Same as (A), except for auditory tones. (C) Psychometric function for bimodal audiovisual stimuli 25 ms before the onset of a saccade (blue symbols), plotted together with the corresponding visual and auditory unimodal results (replotted from A and B). (Readapted with permission from Binda et al., 2007.)

time courses). Predictions for the localization bias fall very close to the observed data; the predicted precision is most often within ± 1 SE of that observed, and most of the deviations from the model are actually in the direction of greater rather than less improvement. The lower panels of Figure 10.3 plot the variations of visual and auditory integration weights (Eq. 1.2 of Chapter 1) across the time course. The visual weight (red) is progressively reduced as the test presentation approaches the saccadic onset, with the auditory weight (green) increasing commensurately.

In summary, during steady fixation the perceived location of bimodal audiovisual stimuli is usually captured by the visual component. Saccades interfere with this phenomenon, decreasing the extent to which visual cues determine bimodal localization. The distortions induced by saccades on visual space perception are therefore partially rescued when spatial information from another modality (e.g., audition) is provided.

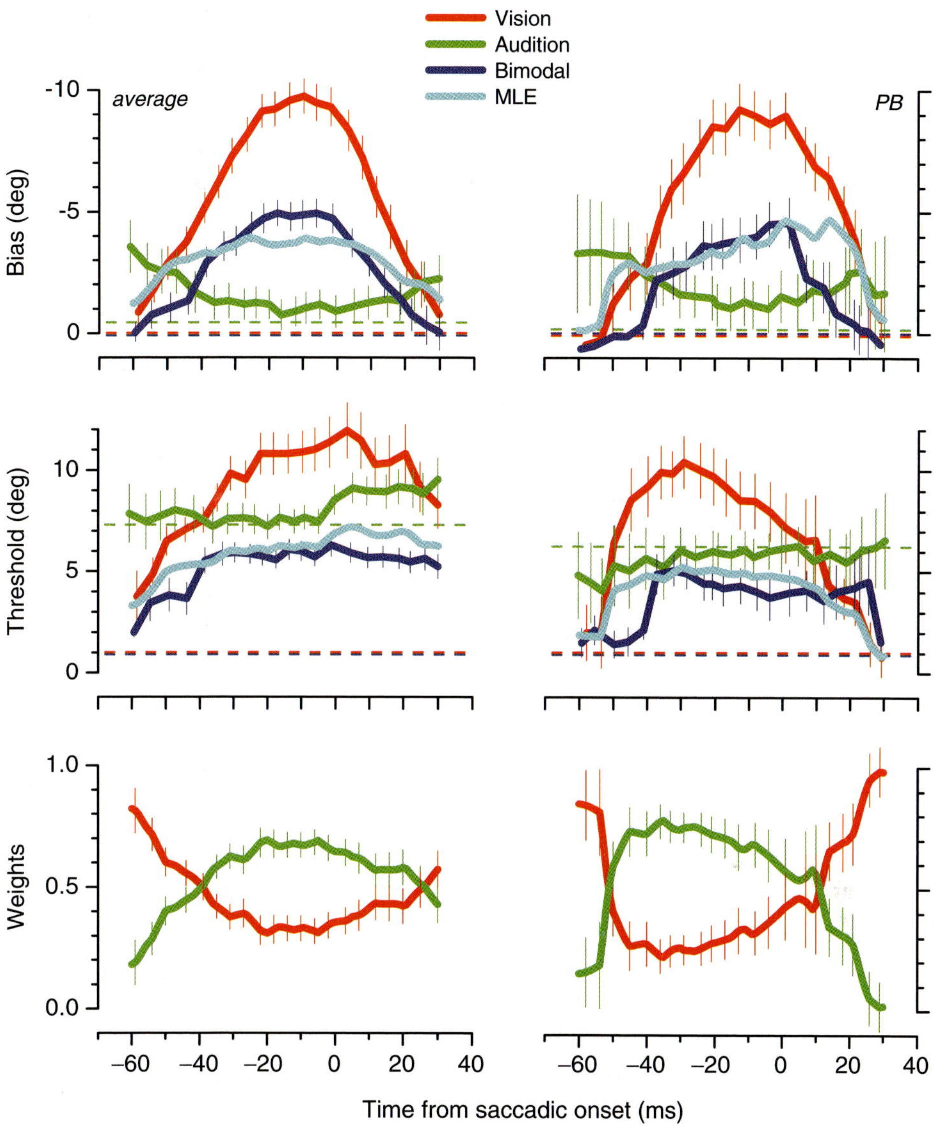


**Figure 10.3** Unimodal and bimodal localization measured at various delays from the start of a saccade. For each stimulus type (visual, auditory, and bimodal), a psychometric function was fitted on a subset of trials, selected by a temporal window of 50 ms width that was iteratively displaced by 5 ms. The resulting bias and threshold values are plotted against the average presentation time of each window. The leftmost panels report averages across PSE and threshold values estimated in three subjects; the behavior of one individual subject is shown in the rightmost panels. Visual and auditory integration weights (calculated from Eq. 1.3 of Chapter 1) are reported in the bottom panels. Error bars were computed with a Monte Carlo simulation where the visual reliability was iteratively reestimated by resampling (with replacement) the visual-only data, whereas the auditory reliability was assigned the value of the average auditory localization precision across the time course. (Readapted with permission from Binda et al., 2007.)

Importantly, the localization of perisaccadic bimodal stimuli presented at various delays from a saccade can be quantitatively predicted by assuming an optimal (MLE) integration of auditory and visual cues, with the accuracy and precision of visual signals changing dynamically. This has two major implications.

First, it suggests that perisaccadic visual signals are already distorted when they are integrated with other sensory cues. They must be biased and imprecise (as suggested by unimodal visual data) when combined with auditory information, or the bimodal localization could not be predicted from the visual and auditory time courses. Saccade-induced distortions of visual space should therefore occur before integration with multisensory spatial cues. Visual signals are initially encoded in a retinotopic frame of reference, where represented positions shift each time the eyes move. For visual perception to remain stable across eye movements, retinotopic representations need to be converted into gaze-invariant (e.g., craniotopic) maps. Such a transformation can be performed by taking into account the position of the eyes (e.g., relative to the head). We propose that, in the case of rapid gaze shifts, eye position information fails in accuracy and precision, resulting in the observed systematic localization errors and in the decrease of localization precision (Binda et al., 2007). Audition, on the other hand, encodes stimuli in craniotopic coordinates, so the spatial cues from the two modalities need to be converted into a common format before integration. A convenient format is craniotopic, which is stable across eye movements. Inaccurate and imprecise eye-position signals will ultimately lead to a distorted representation of those visual signals that constitute the input to the process of multisensory integration. Denève, Latham, and Pouget (2001) demonstrated that a class of neural networks is able both to optimally integrate multisensory signals and to convert each signal into a new reference frame. In principle, such a network is able to simulate our findings in both the unimodal and the bimodal conditions, assuming that the output of the network is required to be craniotopic in all cases, and that the eye-position input is inaccurate and imprecise. A detailed model of how this could occur is presented in Binda et al. (2007).

A second important implication of multisensory integration being near-optimal during saccades is that visual signals must be reweighted dynamically, following the variations of visual precision. At the time of saccades, the neural representations of visual space undergo a rapid and continuous transformation. The coordinates of visual receptive fields in many visual areas transiently change due to the eye-position signal (Duhamel, Colby, & Goldberg, 1992; Sommer & Wurtz, 2006); this transient "remapping" of visual receptive fields is a plausible substrate for the mislocalization of flashed stimuli observed behaviorally (Ross, Morrone, Goldberg, & Burr, 2001). Meanwhile, represented locations become progressively scattered, either because of an enlargement of receptive fields (at the single cell level: Kubischik, 2002) or due to changes at the level of the population code (Krekelberg, Kubischik, Hoffmann, & Bremmer, 2003), and this may result in the observed decrease of localization precision. For visual signals to be optimally weighted in the integration with other sensory cues, the mean and the variance of stimuli position in these rapidly changing maps needs to be estimated instantaneously, that is, without averaging information across time (see Ma, Beck, & Pouget, 2008 and Chapter 21 for a physiologically plausible implementation).[1]

Thus, our results suggest that an instantaneous estimate of visual precision is the optimal strategy for the localization of briefly presented stimuli, whose representation is transiently disrupted by an internal signal (the eye-position signal, which we suggest is responsible for both the dynamic coordinate shift and the transient scattering of represented locations; see Binda

[1]When suggesting that visual weights are updated dynamically, we do not mean that the process of sensory reweighting does not take time. Our results imply that, for each trial, visual precision is reestimated. They also imply that the estimate is based on an instantaneous picture of visual representations because these continually change in the perisaccadic interval. However, the estimation process itself may not be instantaneous. In principle, it could take all the time separating the stimulus presentation from the subject's response.

et al., 2007 for more details). An interesting open question is whether such a strategy would be optimal in contexts other than brief perisaccadic stimulation. When stimuli remain continuously visible, for example, the averaging of information across time could be a preferable solution under the reasonable assumption that the variance associated with the position (or with the size, the form, etc.) of an object remains constant. This assumption may fail when the internal status of the perceptual system changes, as it does during saccades.

### Perceived Timing of Audiovisual Stimuli during Saccades

While vision may be envisaged as an inherently spatial modality, with stimuli represented in a spatial format from the first processing stages (the retina), audition is best suited to process temporal information, as temporal intervals are explicitly encoded as early in the auditory pathway as the cochlea. Given these structural constraints, we may expect vision to be more precise spatially than audition (as we have shown), but audition should be temporally more precise than vision. Indeed, there is good evidence that this is the case, as shown by the phenomena of "auditory driving" (Berger, Martelli, & Pelli, 2003; Gebhard & Mowbray, 1959; Shams, Kamitani, & Shimojo, 2000; Shipley, 1964) and "temporal ventriloquism" (Aschersleben & Bertelson, 2003; Bertelson & Aschersleben, 2003; Burr, Banks, & Morrone, 2009; Hartcher-O'Brien & Alais, 2007; Morein-Zamir, Soto-Faraco, & Kingstone, 2003).

Following similar logic to that of the previous section, we asked whether saccades may interfere with this phenomenon, affecting the relative importance of visual and auditory temporal information (Binda, Morrone, & Burr, 2010; Morrone, Binda, & Burr, 2008). Binda et al. (2010) measured the relative integration weights of visual and auditory temporal cues using a multisensory time-bisection task (similar to that of Burr et al., 2009). We asked subjects to compare the timing of a bimodal-conflicting test stimulus to two temporal markers. The test stimulus was a green vertical bar flashed at the center of the screen together with a 10 ms noise burst, presented before or after the flash (but perceived as a single bimodal event). The two markers (separated by 800 ms) were identical to the test, except that the visual and auditory components were synchronous (see inset in Fig. 10.4). Observers reported whether the test stimulus seemed temporally closer to the first or the second marker (two-alternative forced-choice bisection task). The asynchrony between the auditory and visual components of the test was manipulated in a similar way to the spatial manipulation described previously. The time of presentation of the flash was advanced by $\Delta$ ms and that of the tone delayed by $\Delta$ ms, with $\Delta$ equal to $\pm 25$ ms or $+5$ ms (yielding sound-flash separations of $\pm 50$ ms and $+10$ ms). For each $\Delta$ we measured a psychometric curve, plotting the proportion of "closer to the first marker" responses against the test presentation time (defined as the average presentation time of its auditory and visual components) relative to the two markers. The median of the curves (point of subjective bisection, or PSB) estimates the perceived time of the test stimulus (PSB $> 0$ ms implies that the test was systematically perceived as delayed).

PSB values are reported in Figure 10.4A as a function of $\Delta$. Data points are adequately fitted by a linear function with positive slope (slope of the linear fit across PSBs for all subjects: 0.66 $\pm$ 0.08, implying an auditory weight[2] of 0.83 $\pm$ 0.04). This implies that the perceived timing of the flash changed depending on the asynchrony between its visual and auditory component, and it was determined for the most part ($\sim$ 80%) by the timing of the sound. Thus, in steady-fixation conditions, auditory temporal information is given a stronger weight than visual information and sounds partially capture the perceived timing of bimodal audiovisual stimuli—the temporal-ventriloquism effect. Note that, since we did not measure subjects' performance with unimodal stimuli, we cannot test whether the observed auditory temporal ventriloquism

[2] Auditory weights ($w_a$) can be derived from the slope of the regression line ($\rho$) following the equation: $w_a = 0.5\rho + 0.5$.

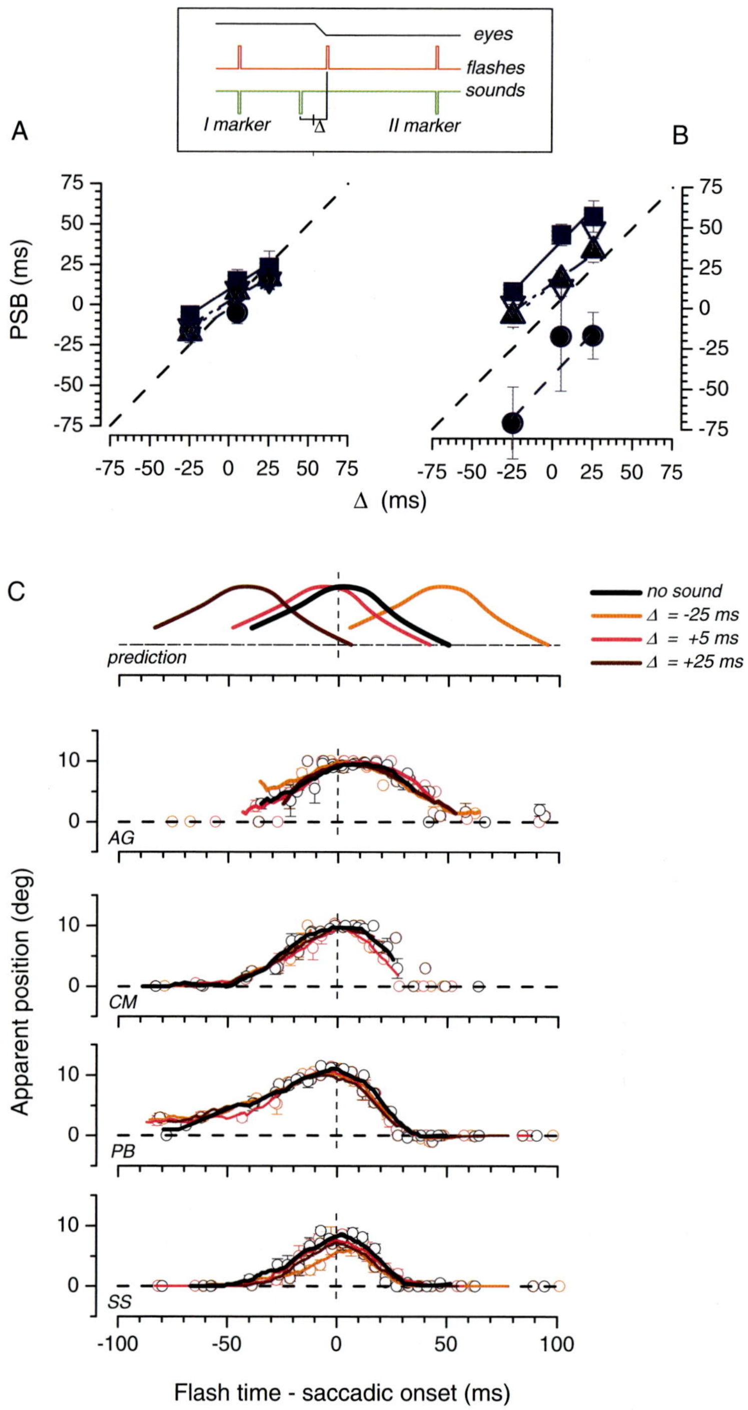


**Figure 10.4** Perceived timing and location for temporally conflicting audiovisual stimuli. (A and B) Results from the temporal bisection task (the inset shows the timing of auditory and visual presentations) in fixation

*Caption continued on next page*

**Figure 10.4** *Continued* conditions (A) and for perisaccadic test stimuli (B). The points of subjective bisection (PSB) are plotted against Δ (the asynchrony between the visual and the auditory components of the test stimulus). Error bars report SE as estimated with a bootstrap resampling at 1000 repetitions (Efron & Tibshirani, 1994). PSB values (different symbols refer to the four tested subjects) were adequately fit by a linear function with high positive slope (dark blue lines), implying that perceived timing of the bimodal test stimulus was mainly determined by the timing of the auditory component. (C) Perceived location of the test stimulus as a function of the time of flash presentation relative to saccadic onset (error bars report bootstrap estimates of SE of the between subjects mean). The upper panel illustrates the predictions from the temporal ventriloquism data if saccadic mislocalization were affected by the sound-induced bias of perceived timing. The lower panels show data from the four tested subjects (hollow symbols: average perceived location in 5 ms time bins; continuous curves: running average of perceived location, computed by taking the average perceived stimulus location within a square temporal window 25 ms wide, sliding along the timings of stimulus presentation by steps of 1 ms). (Readapted with permission from Binda et al., in press.)

is consistent with an optimal integration of information.

We repeated the experiment in a condition where subjects executed a 20° rightward saccade within ±25 ms from the time of the test presentation. In this condition, PSBs were also directly proportional to Δ (see Fig. 10.4B); the linear regression of the PSBs from all subjects estimated a constant of proportionality higher than in fixation conditions (0.89 ± 0.12 implying an auditory weight of 0.95 ± 0.06; averages were computed after weighting each data point by its squared error). The difference in weights in the saccadic and fixation condition was statistically significant ($p < 0.05$).[3] Note that the intercepts of the linear fits also changed with saccades, with a statistically significant average difference between the perisaccadic and fixation data of 18 ms ($p < 0.001$, bootstrap sign test on pooled data). This implies that, for all flash-sound separations, the audiovisual stimulus is perceived as delayed when it is presented at the time of a saccade (in three out of four subjects). This is qualitatively consistent with another study from our lab (Binda, Cicchini, Burr, & Morrone, 2009) showing that saccades cause a delay in the perceived time of the flash. The delay reported in that study (for purely visual stimuli) was 50–100 ms, while here it is ~20 ms. Given the strong auditory temporal capture, the reduced delay is to be expected. In fact, we would have expected an even weaker effect.

These results show that the temporal-ventriloquism effect is also observed at the time of saccades and is even stronger than in steady fixation conditions. This is the opposite of what we observed in the spatial domain, where the magnitude of the spatial-ventriloquism effect is strongly reduced during saccades. In principle, optimal cue combination is able to explain this difference (though we cannot make a quantitative prediction, since we did not measure unimodal performance). During steady fixation, visual spatial cues are more precise and hence dominate auditory spatial cues (Alais & Burr, 2004), but saccades reduce the precision of visual spatial information and consequently reduce its relative weight (see previous section and Binda et al., 2007). In the temporal domain, visual cues are weighted less than auditory cues even during normal fixation, resulting in the temporal-ventriloquism effect (Burr et al., 2009; Morein-Zamir et al., 2003). Given an optimal integration rule, if saccades have an effect on visual temporal information (most plausibly, reducing its precision), it would leave audition as dominant and even increase the dominance, as we observed.

These findings clearly show that the perceived timing of a perisaccadic audiovisual event will depend mainly on the presentation time of

[3]For significance testing, the data from the four subjects were aligned by subtracting the intercept of each regression line and then pooled; the slope of the linear regression for saccade and fixation were compared with a bootstrap sign test.

the auditory stimulus. Will this also affect the dynamics of the perisaccadic mislocalization for brief audiovisual stimuli? Given the sharply defined dynamics of perisaccadic mislocalization (see Fig. 10.3, red lines or blue lines), only flashes presented near saccadic onset should be mislocalized; those presented 50 ms before or afterward are not. So if we assume that space and time are not processed independently (see Binda et al., 2009), leading or trailing sounds should shift the audiovisual event forward or backward substantially in perceived time (given the auditory weight of 0.95, a sound leading a flash by 50 ms should result in a backward shift of perceived flash time of some 47 ms), changing completely the pattern of its mislocalization.

To test this prediction, we asked subjects to report the location of a green vertical bar (flashed at the center of the screen) relative to a previously learned ruler while they made a 20° rightward saccade. The flashed bar was preceded or followed by a brief noise burst, with the same temporal offsets used for the stimulus in the previous experiment. As before, subjects were asked to consider the stimulus as an audiovisual event, but they had to locate it in space rather than time. Figure 10.4C plots the perceived location of the stimulus as a function of the time of flash presentation relative to the saccadic onset for the various conditions (color-coded, see figure caption). The uppermost panel shows the shift predicted by auditory capture. The curves are splines of the average of all data in the unimodal vision condition, shifted by the amount predicted by auditory capture (the audiovisual offset times the auditory weight). The data (lower panels, one for each subject) are clearly inconsistent with the predictions, because all time courses are strikingly similar. For each subject and audiovisual delay, we quantified the amount the sound shifted the curve by sliding it along the time axis to find the point where it coincided best with the no-sound condition (yielding the lowest mean-squared residual). The shift values are very small. We regressed them against the audiovisual delay and found an average linear dependency of $-0.004 \pm 0.016$ ms, which is not statistically different from 0. Note that not only the temporal dynamics of mislocalization but also its magnitude are comparable across conditions; concurrent sounds did not reduce the perisaccadic localization errors. This was probably because in this setup the sounds provided no reliable spatial cues, because they were diffused by a speaker placed above the monitor screen.

We conclude that, while a spatially informative auditory presentation reduces the magnitude of perisaccadic mislocalization (Binda et al., 2007), a temporally informative sound does not alter its dynamics. This is consistent with the hypothesis that the perisaccadic mislocalization of visual signals takes place prior to the integration of visual spatial cues with information from the other modalities: The perceived timing of visual stimuli is altered by sounds, but multisensory integration operates on representations that have already been spatially distorted, following the characteristic dynamics of perisaccadic phenomena.

## Conclusion

We have described a series of experiments studying integration of audiovisual spatial or temporal information during saccades by taking advantage of the selective disruption of eye movements on localization of visual stimuli briefly flashed just before or during a saccade. The results show that the perisaccadic distortions of visual space are greatly reduced when auditory spatial information is provided. Thus, while during steady fixation spatial vision dominates our perception of space (leading to the ventriloquist effect), perisaccadically other sensory modalities become dominant. This can be predicted by assuming an optimal strategy of cue combination (Chapter 1) because, during saccades, visual localization is far less precise than during fixation. Visual signals are therefore dynamically reweighted in the perisaccadic interval, following the rapid variations of localization precision. Our findings also suggest that saccades interfere with visual spatial representations prior to their combination with other sensory cues—biased and imprecise visual spatial signals are provided as input to the multisensory-integration mechanism. A similar conclusion can be drawn from the results of the other two experiments that investigated the combination of visual and auditory temporal cues. Both during fixation and at the time of saccades, audition dominates over vision in determining our perception of time (the temporal-ventriloquism effect). Thus, the perceived time of perisaccadic audiovisual events is determined primarily by the tone. However, the temporal dynamics of their spatial mislocalization is determined exclusively by the timing of the visual stimulus. This suggests that visual stimuli have already undergone perisaccadic mislocalization before they are integrated with auditory cues.

The cues provided from the various modalities are initially encoded in different frames of reference. For them to be combined, they need to be remapped into a common frame of reference. We suggest that saccades interfere with this remapping process because, during rapid "saccadic" gaze shifts, sensory representations cannot be fed with an accurate and precise representation of eye position.

## DEVELOPMENT OF MULTIMODAL INTEGRATION

Mammalian sensory systems are not mature at birth, but they become increasingly refined as the animal develops. In humans, some properties, like visual contrast sensitivity, acuity, and binocular vision, reach near-adult levels within a year of life (Atkinson, 1984), as do some basic tactile tasks (Streri, 2003), while other attributes, like form (Kovács, Kozma, Fehér, & Benedek, 1999), motion perception (Ellemberg et al., 2003), and visual or haptic recognition of a 3D object (Rentschler, Jüttner, Osman, Müller, & Caelli, 2004), continue to develop until 8–14 years of age. There is also a difference in the developmental rate of different sensory systems, with touch developing first, followed by the vestibular, chemical, and auditory senses (all beginning to function prior to birth), and finally vision (Gottlieb, 1971). Some anatomical aspects (such as myelinization of the optic nerve and visual-cortex development) continue to mature through to school age. Cross-sensory integration could also pose particular challenges for maturing sensory systems that have a constant need for *recalibration* to take into account growing limbs, eye length, interocular distances, and so forth.

Several studies show that young children, and even infants, possess a variety of multisensory abilities (see Lewkowicz, 2000, for review). For example, 3-month-old children can match faces with voices on the basis of their synchrony (Bahrick, 2001), and 4-month-old babies can match visual and auditory motion (Lewkowicz, 1992). One recent psychophysical study (Neil, Chee-Ruiter, Scheier, Lewkowicz, & Shimojo, 2006) has shown that integration of visual and auditory orienting responses develops late in humans, after the unimodal orienting responses are well established. These results are also in accord with physiological studies in cats and monkeys that show that, while in adult animals many neurons in the deep layers of superior colliculus show strong integration of multimodal information (Stein, Meredith, & Wallace, 1993), in young animals integration-enhanced response develops later, after the unimodal visual and auditory properties are completely mature (Stein, Labos, & Kruger, 1973; Wallace & Stein, 2001).

However, very few studies to date have investigated cross-sensory integration of spatial attributes, and none has applied the MLE approach of Chapter 1 to examine whether the integration is statistically optimal. We therefore investigated the combination of visual and tactile signals in young children (Gori, Del Viva, Sandini, & Burr, 2008). The results were conclusive, but surprising. Young children do not integrate haptic and visual information in the way that adults do, but one sense completely dominates the other, even though in the conditions of our experiment it was the least precise. That is to say, it is a *loser-take-all* situation. Furthermore, the dominant sense depended on the task: For size judgments touch dominated, and for orientation judgments vision dominated.

The size-discrimination task (top left icon of Fig. 10.5) was a low-technology, child-friendly adaptation of Ernst and Banks' (2002) technique (similar to that used by Helbig & Ernst, 2007),

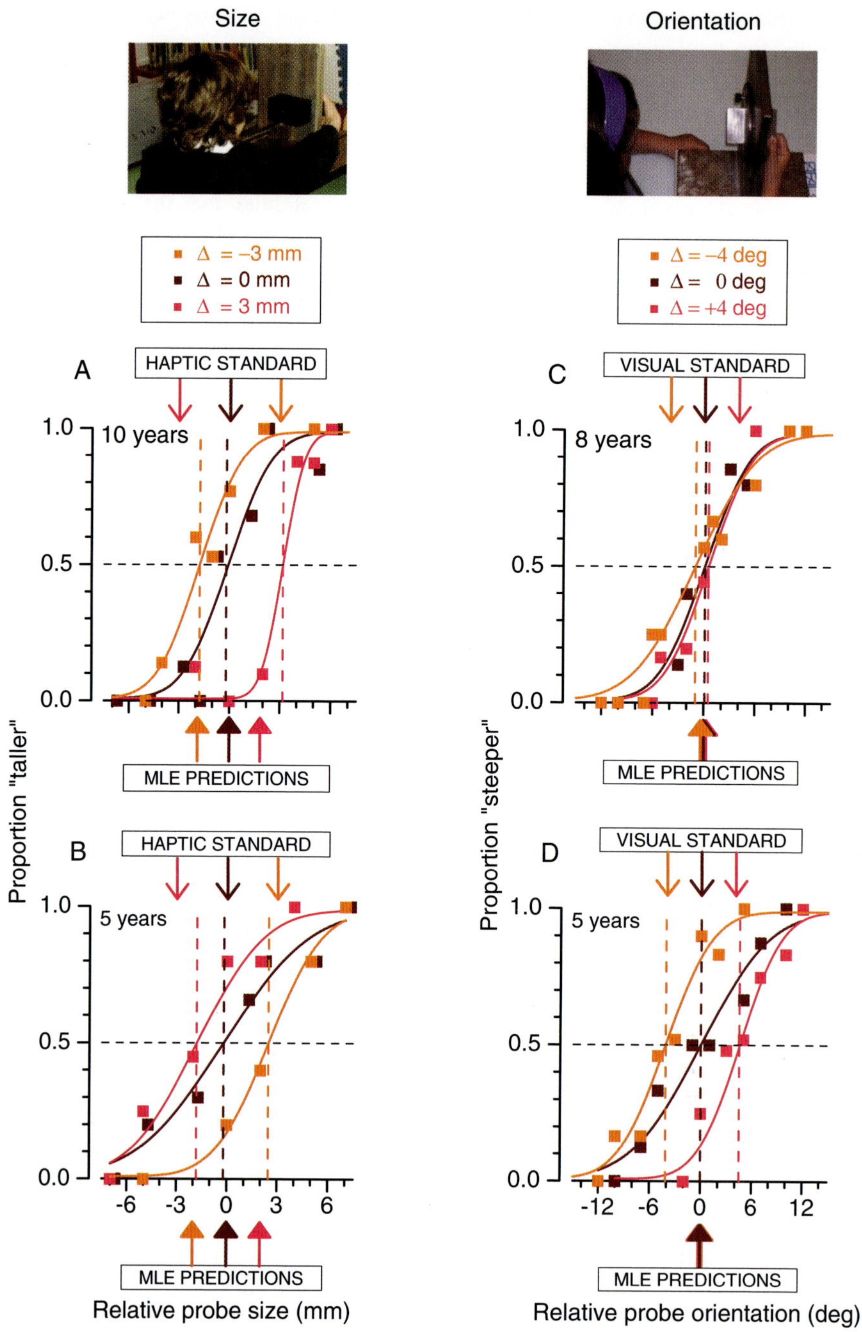


**Figure 10.5** Example psychometric functions for discrimination tasks in four children, with various degrees of cross-modal conflict. (A and B) Size discrimination: SB age 10.2 (A); DV age 5.5 (B); (C and D) Orientation discrimination: AR age 8.7 (C); GF age 5.7 (D). The lower color-coded arrows show the MLE predictions, calculated from threshold measurements (Eq. 1.2, Chapter 1). The upper color-coded arrows indicate the size of the haptic standard (A and B) or the orientation of visual standard (C and D). PSEs for the various curves are shown by dashed colored vertical lines. The older children generally follow the adult pattern, while the 5-year-olds were dominated by haptic information for the size task and visual information for the orientation task. (Readapted with permission from Gori et al., 2008.)

where visual and haptic information were placed in conflict with each other to investigate which dominates perception under various degrees of visual degradation. The stimuli were physical blocks of variable height (48 to 62 mm, in 1 mm increments) displayed in front of an occluding screen for visual judgments, behind the screen for haptic judgments, or both in front and behind for the bimodal judgments. The visual and haptic objects were close enough to each other for multimodal integration to occur (Gepshtein, Burge, Ernst, & Banks, 2005).

All trials used a two-alternative, forced-choice task where the subject judged whether a *standard* block seemed taller or shorter than a *probe* of variable height. For the single-modality trials, one stimulus (randomly first or second) was the *standard*, always 55 mm high, the other was the *probe*, of variable height. The proportion of trials where the probe was judged taller than the standard was computed for each probe height, yielding psychometric functions. The crucial condition was the dual-modality condition, where visual and haptic sizes of the standard were in conflict: The visual block was $55+\Delta$ mm and the haptic block was $55 - \Delta$ mm ($\Delta = 0$ or $\pm 3$ mm). The probe comprised congruent visual and haptic stimuli of variable height (48–62 mm). Despite the visuohaptic conflict of the standard, the blocks appeared as one single stimulus to all adults and children tested.

We validated this technique with adults to demonstrate that optimal cross-modal integration occurs under these conditions. Visual stimuli were blurred by a translucent screen positioned at variable distances from the stimulus, producing results very similar to those obtained by Ernst and Banks (2002): Perceived size of visual-haptic stimuli followed closely the maximum-likelihood estimate (MLE) predictions for all levels of visual blur and, most important, the thresholds for dual-modality presentation were lower than either visual or haptic thresholds.

We then proceeded to measure haptic, visual, and bimodal visuohaptic size discrimination in 5- to 10-year-old children (in conditions with no visual blur). Figures 10.5A and 10.5B show sample psychometric functions for the dual-modality measurements in two children. The pattern of results for the 10-year-old children (Fig. 10.5A) was very much like those for the adult, where negative values of $\Delta$ caused the curves to shift leftward and positive values caused them to shift rightward. That is to say the curves followed the visual standard, suggesting that visual information was dominating the match, as the MLE model suggests it should because the visual thresholds were lower than the haptic thresholds. This is consistent with the MLE model (indicated by color-coded arrows below the abscissae): The visual judgment was more precise and should therefore dominate. For the 5-year-old children (Fig. 10.5B), however, the results were dramatically different. The psychometric functions for the dual-modality presentation shifted in the direction opposite to that of the 10-year-old children, following the bias of the haptic stimulus. The predictions (color-coded arrows under abscissa) are similar for both the 5- and 10-year-olds. For both children visual thresholds were much lower than haptic thresholds, so the visual stimuli should dominate, but for the 5-year-olds the reverse holds, with the haptic standard dominating the match.

Figure 10.6A reports PSEs for all children in each age group for the three conflict conditions, plotted as a function of the MLE predictions from single-modality discrimination thresholds. If the MLE prediction held, the data should fall along the black dotted equality line (like Fig. 10.1B for the ventriloquist effect). For adults this was so. However, at 5 years of age the story was quite different. For the size discriminations, not only do the measured PSEs not follow the MLE predictions, they varied inversely with $\Delta$ (following the haptic standard), lining up almost orthogonal to the equality line. The data for the 6-year-olds similarly do not follow the prediction, but there is a tendency for the data to be more scattered rather than ordered orthogonal to the prediction line. By 8 years of age the data begin to follow the prediction, and by 10 years they fall along it similar to the adult pattern of results.

To ascertain whether the haptic dominance was a general phenomenon, or specific to size

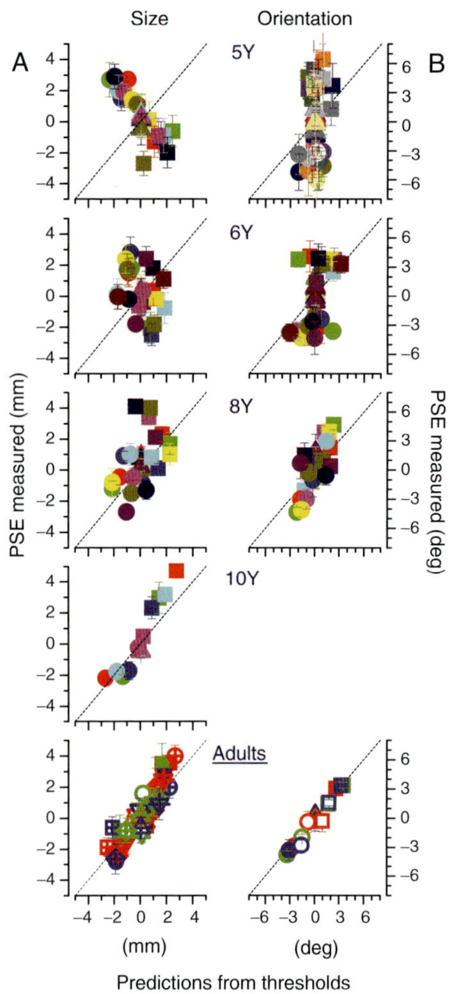


**Figure 10.6** Summary data showing PSEs for all subjects for all conflict conditions, plotted against the predictions, for size (A) and orientation (B) discriminations. Different colors refer to different subjects within each age group and different symbol shapes to the level of cross-sensory conflict (Δ): squares, 3 mm or 4°; circles, –3 mm or –4°; upright triangles, 0; diamonds, 2 mm; inverted triangles, –2 mm. Closed symbols refer to the no-blur condition for the size judgments, and vertical orientation judgments; open symbols to modest blur or oblique orientations; cross in symbols to heavy blur (screen at 39 cm). For both size and orientation discriminations, the predictions are far from the measured results for children younger than 8. Error bars on individual data points obtained by bootstrap (Efron & Tibshirani, 1994). (Readapted with permission from Gori et al., 2008.)

judgments, we repeated the series of experiments with another spatial task: orientation discrimination, a very basic visual task which could in principle be computed by neural hardware of primary visual cortex (Hubel & Wiesel, 1968). The procedure was similar to the size-discrimination task, using a simple, low-technology technique (top right icon of Fig. 10.5). Subjects were required to discriminate which bar of a dual presentation (standard and probe) was rotated more counterclockwise. Rather than blurring the bar, visual discrimination was made more difficult by using an oblique rather than vertical standard, the so-called *oblique effect*, that also occurs in children but does not seem to affect haptic judgments (Appelle, 1972).

As with the size discriminations, we first measured thresholds in each separate modality, then visuohaptically, by varying degrees of conflict ($\Delta = 0$ or $\pm 4°$), with visual standards rotated clockwise by $+\Delta^{\circ}$ and the haptic standards by $-\Delta^{\circ}$. Figures 10.5C and 10.5D show sample psychometric functions for the dual-modality measurements for an 8- and 5-year-old child. As with the size judgments, the pattern of results for the 8-year-old was very much like those for the adult, with the functions of the three different conflicts (Fig. 10.5C) falling very much together, as predicted from the single-modality thresholds by the MLE model (arrows under abscissae). Again, however, the pattern of results for the 5-year-old was quite different (Fig. 10.5D). Although the MLE model predicts similar curves for the three conflict conditions, the psychometric functions followed very closely the visual standards (indicated by the arrows above the graphs), the exact opposite pattern to that observed for size discrimination.

Figure 10.6B plots measured against predicted PSEs for all children in each age group for the three conflict conditions. At 5 years of age, the predictions bore no relation to the measured PSEs, (nearly proportional to $+\Delta$) following the visual stimulus. The data for the 6-year-old children begin to become more scattered but still do not follow predictions. By 8 years of age, the data begin to follow the prediction reasonably well, approaching the adult results where measured PSEs follow well the MLE predictions.

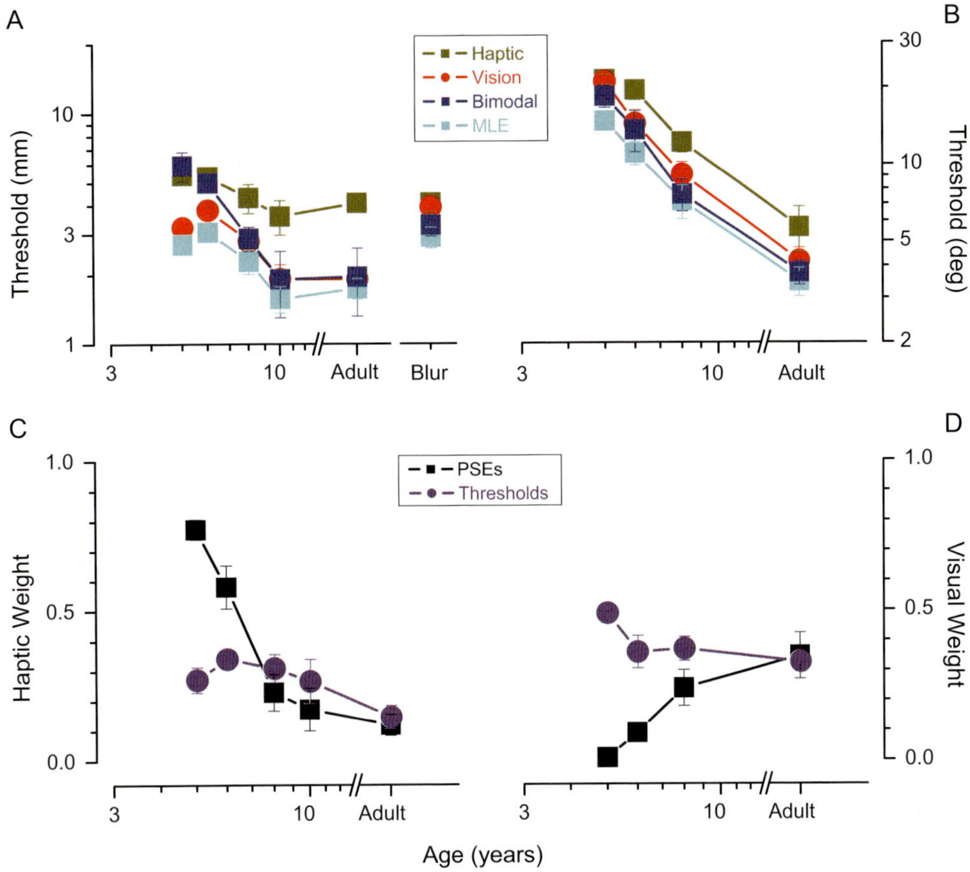


**Figure 10.7** (A and B) Geometric averages of thresholds for haptic (dark yellow), visual (red), and visuohaptic (blue) size and orientation discrimination, together with the average MLE predictions (cyan), as a function of age. The predictions were calculated individually for each subject, then averaged. The tick labeled "blur" shows thresholds for visual stimuli blurred by a translucent screen 19 cm from the blocks. (C and D) Haptic and visual weights for the size and orientation discrimination, derived from thresholds via the MLE model or from PSE values. Weights were calculated individually for each subject, then averaged. After 8–10 years the two estimates converge, suggesting that the system begins to integrate visual and haptic information in a statistically optimal manner. Error bars represent ± 1 SEM. (Readapted with permission from Gori et al., 2008.)

Figures 10.7A and 10.7B show how the thresholds vary with age for the various conditions. For both tasks, visual and haptic thresholds decreased steadily with age up until 10 years (orientation more so than size). The light-blue symbols show the thresholds predicted from the MLE model (Eq. 1.3, Chapter 1). For the adults, the predicted improvement was close to the best single-modality threshold, and indeed the dual-modality thresholds were never worse than the best single-modality threshold. A quite different pattern was observed for the 5-year-old children. For the size discrimination, the dual-modality thresholds were as high as the haptic thresholds, not only much higher than the MLE predictions, but twice the best single-modality (visual) thresholds. This result shows not only that integration is not optimal; it is not even a close approximation, like "winner take all." Indeed, it shows a "*loser* take all" strategy. This reinforces the PSE data in showing that these young children do not integrate cross-modally in a way that benefits perceptual discrimination.

Figures 10.7C and 10.7D tell a similar story, plotting the development of theoretical and observed visual and haptic weights. Violet symbols show the theoretical MLE-predicted weights, and the black symbols indicate the actual weights that were applied for the judgments (calculated from the PSE vs. conflict functions). For both size and orientation judgments, the theoretical haptic weights were fairly constant over age, 0.2–0.3 for size and 0.3–0.4 for orientation. However, the haptic weights necessary to predict the 5-year-old PSE size data are 0.6–0.8, far greater than the prediction, implying that these young children give considerably more weight to touch for size judgments than is optimal. Similarly, the haptic weights necessary to predict the orientation judgments are around 0, far less than the prediction, suggesting that these children base orientation judgments almost entirely on visual information. In neither case does anything like optimal cue combination occur.

Another recent study reinforces our evidence that children under the age of 8 can take advantage of information from only one sense at a time, with optimal multisensory integration developing in middle childhood. Nardini, Jones, Bedford, and Braddick (2008) studied the use of multiple spatial cues for short-range navigation in children and adults. They provided subjects with two cues to navigation: visual landmarks and self-motion. While adults were able to take advantage and integrate both cues, increasing the precision of their navigation when both sources of information were available, children of 4–5 or 7–8 years showed no improvement in precision in the bimodal condition. In the bimodal condition, adults weighted each spatial cue with its reliability (Eq. 1.2, Chapter 1) as we have seen in many other examples in this book. But young children failed completely to integrate cues, alternating between them from trial to trial. These results suggest that the development of the two individual spatial representations occurs before they are integrated within a common unique reference frame. Taken together with our study, it would seem to be a general conclusion that optimal multisensory integration of spatial information only occurs after 8 years of age.

## CROSS-SENSORY CALIBRATION

Our experiments described previously show that before 8 years of age children do not integrate information between senses, but one sense will dominate. Which sense dominates depends on the situation: For size judgments, touch dominates; for orientation, vision dominates. Given the overwhelming body of evidence for optimal integration in adults, the result was not expected, and it suggests that multisensory interaction in infants is fundamentally different from that in adults. How could it differ? Although most recent work on multisensory interactions has concentrated on sensory *fusion* (the efficient combination of information from all the senses), an equally important but somewhat neglected potential role is that of *calibration.* In his famous 300-year-old *Essay towards a new theory of vision,* Bishop George Berkeley (1709) correctly observed that vision has no direct access to attributes such as distance, solidarity, or "bigness." These become tangible only after they have been associated with touch (proposition 45); that is, "touch educates vision," perhaps better expressed as "touch *calibrates* vision." Calibration is probably necessary at all ages, but during the early years of life, when children are effectively "learning to see, reach, and grasp," calibration may be expected to be more important. It is during these years that limbs are growing rapidly and eye length and eye separation are increasing, necessitating constant recalibration between sight and touch. Indeed, many studies suggest that the first 8 years in humans corresponds to the critical period of plasticity for many attributes and properties such as binocular vision (Banks, Aslin, & Letson, 1975) and the acquisition of accent-free language (Doupe & Kuhl, 1999).

So, before 8 years of age, *calibration* may be more important than *integration.* The advantages of fusing sensory information are probably more than offset by those of keeping the evolving system calibrated; and using one system to calibrate another precludes fusion of the two. If we accept Berkeley's ideas that vision must be calibrated by touch, we may explain why size-discrimination thresholds are dominated by touch, even though touch is less precise than vision. But why are orientation thresholds dominated by vision? Perhaps Berkeley was not quite right and touch does not always calibrate vision, but the more robust sense for a particular task is the calibrator. In the same way that the more *precise* and *reliable* sense has the highest weights for sensory fusion, perhaps the more *robust* and *accurate* sense is used for calibration. And the more accurate need not be the more precise. Accuracy is defined in absolute terms, as the distance from physical reality, whereas precision is a relative measure, related to the reliability or repeatability of the results. It is therefore reasonable that, for size, touch will be more accurate, because vision cannot code it directly, but only through a complex calculation of retinal size and estimate of distance. Orientation, on the other hand, is coded directly by primary visual cortex (Hubel & Wiesel, 1968; Tootell et al., 1998) and calculated from touch only indirectly, via complex coordinate transforms.

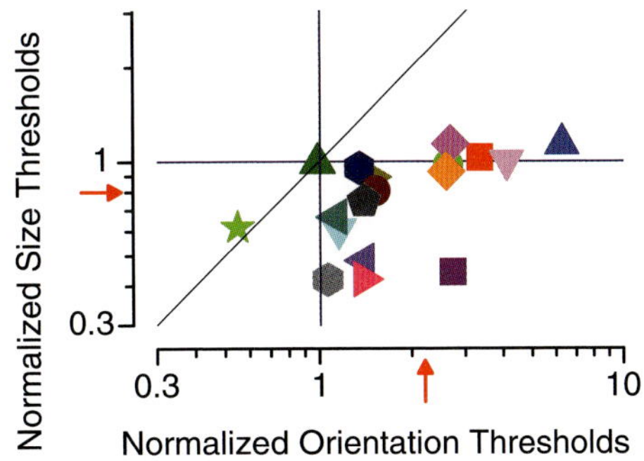


**Figure 10.8** Normalized orientation thresholds plotted against normalized size thresholds. Different colors refer to different subjects. Individual values were normalized by the average threshold in age-matched control (estimated by interpolating the dark yellow curves in Figs. 10.7A and 10.7B for size and orientation, respectively). Most points lie in the lower right quadrant, implying better size and poorer orientation discrimination. The arrows refer to group averages, 2.2 ± 0.3 for orientation and 0.8 ± 0.06 for size. The green star in the lower left quadrant is the acquired low-vision child. (Readapted with permission from Gori et al., 2009.)

## HAPTIC ORIENTATION-DISCRIMINATION IN NONSIGHTED CHILDREN

If the idea of calibration is correct, then early deficits in one sense should impact on the function of other senses that rely on it for calibration. Specifically, haptic impairment should lead to poor visual discrimination of size, and visual impairment to poor haptic discrimination of orientation. We have tested and verified the latter of these predictions (Gori, Sandini, Martinoli, & Burr, 2010). In 17 congenitally visually impaired children (aged 5–19 years), we measured haptic discrimination thresholds for both orientation and size, and we found that orientation, but not size thresholds, were impaired. Figure 10.8 plots size against orientation thresholds, both normalized by age-matched normally sighted children. Orientation discrimination thresholds were all worse than the age-matched controls (> 1), on average twice as high, whereas size discrimination thresholds were generally better than the controls (<1). Interestingly, one child with an acquired visual impairment (star symbol) showed a completely different pattern of results, with no orientation deficit. Although we have only one such subject, we presume that his fine orientation thresholds result from the early visual experience (before 2½ years of age) that may have been sufficient for the visual system to calibrate touch.

The suggestion that specific perceptual tasks may require cross-modal calibration during development could have practical implications, possibly leading to improvements in rehabilitation programs. Where cross-sensory calibration has been compromised, for example, by blindness, it may be possible to train people to use some form of "internal" calibration or to calibrate by another modality such as sound.

## CONCLUSIONS

This chapter has presented several examples of how information from different senses can either be integrated within the human brain to improve perceptual precision or, alternatively, can be used to calibrate other senses with less direct access to physical reality. Spatial information from vision and audition is combined in a linearly weighted fashion, with the weights proportional to the reliability of the signals,[4] both when the signal reliability is degraded artificially, and when it is degraded "naturally" during saccadic eye movements. The weights seem to be updated dynamically, on the fly, taking into account the momentary precision of the visual localization that varies predictably with time from a saccade. The audiovisual combination appears to occur after the saccade has influenced perceived position.

On the other hand, the developmental study showed that young children do not integrate visual and haptic information, but one sense dominates over the other: touch for size discrimination and vision for orientation discrimination. We suggest that the lack of integration in young children reflects cross-sensory calibration, which necessarily precludes integration. The study showing that congenitally blind children have poor haptic orientation-discrimination thresholds, but good haptic size-discrimination thresholds compared with age-matched controls, provides strong support for the calibration hypothesis. We suggest that the poor orientation thresholds in congenitally but not acquired blind children reflect disruption to early cross-modal visual calibration.

## ACKNOWLEDGMENTS

This research was supported by the Italian Ministry of Universities and Research and by EC projects "MEMORY" (FP6-NEST) and "STANIB" (FP7 ERC). The authors would like to thank all the members of the Pisa Vision Lab for fruitful discussions about the work presented here.

[4]But see also Chapters 2 and 13 demonstrating nonlinear combination of auditory and visual signals.

## REFERENCES

Alais, D., & Burr, C. D. (2004). The ventriloquist effect results from near-optimal bimodal integration. *Current Biology, 14*, 257–262.

Appelle, S. (1972). Perception and discrimination as a function of stimulus orientation: The "oblique effect" in man and animals. *Psychological Bulletin, 78*, 266–278.

Aschersleben, G., & Bertelson, P. (2003). Temporal ventriloquism: Crossmodal interaction on the time dimension. 2. Evidence from sensorimotor synchronization. *International Journal of Psychophysiology, 50*, 157–163.

Atkinson, J. (1984). Human visual development over the first 6 months of life. A review and a hypothesis. *Human Neurobiology, 3*, 61–74.

Bahrick, L. E. (2001). Increasing specificity in perceptual development: Infants' detection of nested levels of multimodal stimulation. *Journal of Experimental Child Psychology, 79*, 253–270.

Banks, M. S., Aslin, R. N., & Letson, R. D. (1975). Sensitive period for the development of human binocular vision. *Science, 190*, 675–677.

Battaglia, P. W., Jacobs, R. A., & Aslin, R. N. (2003). Bayesian integration of visual and auditory signals for spatial localization. *Journal of the Optical Society of America A: Optics, Image Science, and Vision, 20*, 1391–1397.

Berger, T. D., Martelli, M., & Pelli, D. G. (2003). Flicker flutter: Is an illusory event as good as the real thing? *Journal of Vision, 3*, 406–412.

Berkeley, G. (1709). *An essay towards a new theory of vision.* Indianapolis, IN: Bobbs-Merrill.

Bertelson, P., & Aschersleben, G. (2003). Temporal ventriloquism: Crossmodal interaction on the time dimension. 1. Evidence from auditory-visual temporal order judgment. *International Journal of Psychophysiology, 50*, 147–155.

Binda, P., Bruno, A., Burr, D. C., & Morrone, M. C. (2007). Fusion of visual and auditory stimuli during saccades: A Bayesian explanation for perisaccadic distortions. *Journal of Neuroscience, 27*, 8525–8532.

Binda, P., Cicchini, G. M., Burr, D. C., & Morrone, M. C. (2009). Spatiotemporal distortions of visual perception at the time of saccades. *Journal of Neuroscience, 29*, 13147–13157.

Binda, P., Morrone, M. C., & Burr, C. D. (2010). Temporal auditory capture does not affect the time-course of saccadic mislocalization of visual stimuli. *Journal of Vision, 10*(2):7, 1–13.

Burr, D., Banks, M. S., & Morrone, M. C. (2009). Auditory dominance over vision in the perception of interval duration. *Experimental Brain Research, 198*, 49–57.

Burr, D. C., Holt, J., Johnstone, J. R., & Ross, J. (1982). Selective depression of motion sensitivity during saccades. *Journal of Physiology, 333*, 1–15.

Clark, J. J., & Yuille, A. L. (1990). *Data fusion for sensory information processing systems.* Boston, MA: Kluwer.

Connor, S. (2000). *Dumbstruck: A cultural history of ventriloquism.* Oxford, England: Oxford University Press.

Denève, S., Latham, P. E., & Pouget, A. (2001). Efficient computation and cue integration with noisy population codes. *Nature Neuroscience, 4*, 826–831.

Diamond, M. R., Ross, J., & Morrone, M. C. (2000). Extraretinal control of saccadic suppression. *Journal of Neuroscience, 20*, 3449–3455.

Doupe, A. J., & Kuhl, P. K. (1999). Birdsong and human speech: Common themes and mechanisms. *Annual Review of Neuroscience, 22*, 567–631.

Duhamel, J. R., Colby, C. L., & Goldberg, M. E. (1992). The updating of the representation of visual space in parietal cortex by intended eye movements. *Science, 255*, 90–92.

Efron, B., & Tibshirani, R. (1994). An introduction to the bootstrap. *Monographs on Statistics and Applied Probability* (Vol. 57). New York, NY: Chapman & Hall.

Ellemberg D., Lewis, T. L., Meghji, K. S., Maurer, D., Guillemot, J. P., & Lepore, F. (2003). Comparison of sensitivity to first- and second-order local motion in 5-year-olds and adults. *Spatial Vision, 16*, 419–428.

Ernst, M., & Banks, M. (2002). Humans integrate visual and haptic information in a statistically optimal fashion. *Nature, 415*, 429–433.

Fendrich, R., & Corballis, P. M. (2001). The temporal cross-capture of audition and vision. *Perception and Psychophysics, 63*, 719–725.

Gebhard, J. W., & Mowbray, G. H. (1959). On discriminating the rate of visual flicker and auditory flutter. *American Journal of Experimental Psychology, 72*, 521–528.

Gepshtein, S., Burge, J., Ernst, M. O., & Banks, M. S. (2005). The combination of vision and touch depends on spatial proximity. *Journal of Vision, 5*, 1013–1023.

Ghahramani, Z. (1995). *Computation and psychophysics of sensorimotor integration.* Doctoral dissertation, Department of Brain and Cognitive Sciences, Massachusetts Institute of Technology, Cambrige, MA.

Gori, M., Del Viva, M., Sandini, G., & Burr, D. C. (2008). Young children do not integrate visual and haptic form information. *Current Biology, 18*, 694–698.

Gori, M., Sandini, G., Martinoli, C., & Burr, D. C. (2010). Poor haptic orientation discrimination in non-sighted children may reflect disruption of crosssensory calibration. *Current Biology, 20*(3), 223–225.

Gottlieb, G. (1971). *Development of species identification in birds: An inquiry into the prenatal determinants of perception.* Chicago, IL: University of Chicago Press.

Hartcher-O'Brien, J., & Alais, D. (2007, July). *Temporal ventriloquism: Perceptual shifts forwards and backwards in time predicted by the maximum likelihood model.* Paper presented at the 8th Annual Meeting of the International Multisensory Research Forum, University of Sydney, Australia.

Helbig, H. B., & Ernst, M. O. (2007). Optimal integration of shape information from vision and touch. *Experimental Brain Research, 179*, 595–606.

Hubel, D. H., & Wiesel, T. N. (1968). Receptive fields and functional architecture of monkey striate cortex. *Journal of Physiology (London), 195*, 215–243.

Kovács, I., Kozma, P., Fehér, A., Benedek, G. (1999). Late maturation of visual spatial integration in humans. *Proceedings of the National Academy of Sciences USA, 96*, 12204–12209.

Krekelberg, B., Kubischik, M., Hoffmann, K. P., & Bremmer, F. (2003). Neural correlates of visual localization and perisaccadic mislocalization. *Neuron, 37*, 537–545.

Kubischik, M. (2002). Dynamic spatial representations during saccades in the macaque parietal cortex. Bochum, Germany: Ruhr-Universitaet Bochum.

Lewkowicz, D. J. (1992). Infants' responsiveness to the auditory and visual attributes of a sounding/moving stimulus. *Perception and Psychophysics, 52*, 519–528.

Lewkowicz, D. J. (2000). The development of intersensory temporal perception: An epigenetic systems/limitations view. *Psychological Bulletin, 126*, 281–308.

Ma, W. J., Beck, J. M., & Pouget, A. (2008). Spiking networks for Bayesian inference and choice. *Current Opinion in Neurobiology, 18*, 217–222.

Mateeff, S., Hohnsbein, J., & Noack, T. (1985). Dynamic visual capture: Apparent auditory motion induced by a moving visual target. *Perception, 14*, 721–727.

Matin, L., & Pearce, D. G. (1965). Visual perception of direction for stimuli flashed during voluntary saccadic eye movements. *Science, 148*, 1485–1488.

Mills, A. (1958). On the minimum audible angle. *Journal of the Acoustical Society of America, 30*, 237–246.

Morein-Zamir, S., Soto-Faraco, S., & Kingstone, A. (2003). Auditory capture of vision: Examining temporal ventriloquism. *Brain Research Cognitive Brain Research, 17*, 154–163.

Morrone, M. C., Binda, P., & Burr, D. C. (2008). Spatiotopic selectivity for location of events in space and time. *Journal of Vision, 8*(6): 819.

Morrone, M. C., Ross, J., & Burr, D. C. (1997). Apparent position of visual targets during real and simulated saccadic eye movements. *Journal of Neuroscience, 17*, 7941–7953.

Nardini, M., Jones, P., Bedford, R., & Braddick, O. (2008). Development of cue integration in human navigation. *Current Biology, 18*, 689–693.

Neil, P. A., Chee-Ruiter, C., Scheier, C., Lewkowicz, D. J., & Shimojo, S. (2006). Development of multisensory spatial integration and perception in humans. *Developmental Science, 9*, 454–464.

Perrott, D., & Saberi, K. (1990). Minimum audible angle thresholds for sources varying in both elevation and azimuth. *Journal of the Acoustical Society of America, 87*, 1728–1731.

Pick, H. L., Warren, D. H., & Hay, J. C. (1969). Sensory conflict in judgements of spatial direction. *Perception and Psychophysics, 6*, 203–205.

Rentschler, I., Jüttner, M., Osman, E., Müller, A., Caelli, T., (2004). Development of configural 3D object recognition. *Behavioral Brain Research, 149*, 107–111.

Ross, J., Morrone, M. C., Goldberg, M. E., & Burr, D. C. (2001). Changes in visual perception at the time of saccades. *Trends in Neurosciences, 24*, 113–121.

Shams, L., Kamitani, Y., & Shimojo, S. (2000). Illusions. What you see is what you hear. *Nature, 408*, 788.

Shipley, T. (1964). Auditory flutter-driving of visual flicker. *Science, 145*, 1328–1330.

Sommer, M. A., & Wurtz, R. H. (2006). Influence of the thalamus on spatial visual processing in frontal cortex. *Nature, 444*, 374–377.

Stein, B. E., Labos, E., & Kruger, L. (1973). Sequence of changes in properties of neurons of superior colliculus of the kitten during maturation. *Journal of Neurophysiology, 36*, 667–679.

Stein, B. E., Meredith, M. A., & Wallace, M. T. (1993). The visually responsive neuron and beyond: Multisensory integration in cat and monkey. *Progress in Brain Research, 95*, 79–90.

Streri, A. (2003). Cross-modal recognition of shape from hand to eyes in human newborns. *Somatosensory and Motor Research, 20*, 13–18.

Tootell R. B., Hadjikhani, N. K., Vanduffel, W., Liu, A. K., Mendola, J. D., Sereno, M. I., & Dale, A. M. (1998). Functional analysis of primary visual cortex (V1) in humans. *Proceedings of the National Academy of Sciences USA, 95*, 811–817.

Wallace, M. T., & Stein, B. E. (2001). Sensory and multisensory responses in the newborn monkey superior colliculus. *Journal of Neuroscience, 21*, 8886–8894.

Warren, D. H., Welch, R. B., & McCarthy, T. J. (1981). The role of visual-auditory "compellingness" in the ventriloquism effect: Implications for transitivity among the spatial senses. *Perception and Psychophysics, 30*, 557–564.

Wurtz, R. H. (2008). Neuronal mechanisms of visual stability. *Vision Research, 48*, 2070–2089.

# CHAPTER 11

# The Statistical Relationship between Depth, Visual Cues, and Human Perception

*Martin S. Banks, Johannes Burge, and Robert T. Held*

## INTRODUCTION

Estimating the three-dimensional (3D) structure of the environment is a hard problem because the third dimension, depth, is not directly available in the retinal images. This "inverse optics problem" has been a core area of study in vision science for centuries (Berkeley, 1709; von Helmholtz, 1867). The traditional approach to studying 3D perception defines "cues" as identifiable sources of depth information that could in principle provide useful information. This approach can be summarized with a depth-cue taxonomy, a categorization of potential cues and the sort of depth information they provide (Palmer, 1999). The categorization is usually based on a geometric analysis of the relationship between scene properties and the retinal images they produce.

The relationship between the values of depth cues and the 3D structure of the viewed scene is always uncertain, and the uncertainty has two general causes. The first is noise in the measurements by the visual system. For example, the estimation of depth from disparity is uncertain because of errors internal to the visual system in measuring retinal disparity (Cormack, Landers, & Ramakrishnan, 1997) and eye position (Backus, Banks, van Ee, & Crowell, 1999). The second cause is the uncertain relationship between the properties of the external environment and retinal images. For example, the estimation of depth from aerial perspective is uncertain because the current properties of the atmosphere and the illumination and reflectance properties of the object affect the contrast, saturation, and hue of the retinal image (Fry, Bridgeman, & Ellerbrock, 1949). It is unclear how to incorporate those uncertainties in the classical geometric model of depth perception.

This classical approach is being replaced with one based on statistics: Bayesian inference. This approach gracefully incorporates both uncertainty due to internal noise and uncertainty due to external properties that are unknown to the observer. Here, we use the Bayesian framework to explore the information content of some underappreciated sources of depth information: the shape of the contour dividing two image regions and the pattern of blur across the retinal image. The work on contour shape and blur is described in greater detail, respectively, in Burge, Fowlkes, and Banks (2010) and Held, Cooper, O'Brien, and Banks (2010). Contour shape and blur do not directly signal depth, so if they were presented in isolation, the viewer could not use them to determine the 3D structure of the stimulus. However, when these information sources are presented in the context of other information that is normally present in natural viewing of real scenes, their potential usefulness becomes apparent.

Before beginning, we need to define some terms that have been used inconsistently in the literature. "Depth" has been used to describe various aspects of distance. In some cases, it refers to absolute distance, in others it refers to ratios of distances, and in yet others, it refers to ordering in distance. In our discussion, we require quite specific definitions so that we can discuss depth information precisely. Accordingly, we will define four types of distance measurement: *(1)* "absolute distance" refers to distance from the eye to a point in the scene, and the units are distance units such as meters; *(2)* "distance ratio" is the ratio of the absolute distances to two points in the scene and is unitless; *(3)* "distance separation" is the absolute distance to one point minus the absolute distance to another, and its units are distance units such as meters; *(4)* "distance order" is the ordering of points in the scene according to their increasing absolute distance and is unitless. "Depth" will be used as a superordinate term for all four measurements. "Metric depth" will be any measure that is expressed in units of distance, referring to either absolute distance or distance separation. "Nonmetric depth" will be the other categories of distance ratio and distance ordering. We will use these definitions to describe more precisely the information provided by various depth cues.

## CAN FIGURE-GROUND CUES PROVIDE METRIC DEPTH?

To estimate depth as accurately and precisely as possible, all relevant information should be used. Experimental evidence suggests that the visual system combines information from multiple metric-depth cues in a statistically optimal fashion (Hillis, Watt, Landy, & Banks, 2004; Knill & Saunders, 2003). However, it is unclear how information from ordinal and metric cues should be combined (Landy, Maloney, Johnston, & Young, 1995). Distance-ordering information constrains only the sign of depth between pairs of surfaces, so the ordering cue is either consistent with the metric cue and provides no additional numerical information, or the cues are inconsistent and it is not obvious how to resolve the conflict. And yet the shape of an occluder's silhouette affects the depth perceived from disparity; that is, the imaged shape of the occluding object changes the amount of depth that is perceived between the occluder and the background (Bertamini, Martinovic, & Wuerger, 2008; Burge et al., 2010; Burge, Peterson, & Palmer, 2005). Perhaps we can understand this counterintuitive result by considering the depth information potentially provided by the involved depth cues; in particular, it may be productive to consider the statistical relationship between each cue and its associated distribution of depths in the natural environment (Brunswik & Kamiya, 1953; Hoiem, Efros, & Hebert, 2005; Saxena, Chung, & Ng, 2005).

We know that metric depth can be estimated from disparity, provided that the viewer also has estimates of viewing distance and azimuth that can be obtained from extraretinal, eye-position signals and vertical disparity (Backus et al., 1999; Gårding, Porrill, Mayhew, & Frisby, 1995). Uncertainty arises due to noise in measuring the disparities (Cormack et al., 1997) and extraretinal signals (Backus et al., 1999). Can metric depth be estimated from occlusion? More specifically, can the properties of the contour at an occlusion provide metric depth information? At face value, the answer would seem to be negative because there is no *a priori* geometric reason that contour shape provides any metric depth information. This point is illustrated in Figure 11.1, which shows that various arrangements of contour shape and surface ordering in depth could produce the same contour in the retinal image. However, the convexity of an image region (e.g., the convexity of a silhouette) may be statistically correlated with depth in natural viewing. If this were the case, convexity could impart information about metric depth and the visual system could exploit it.

### Natural-scene Analysis

To evaluate the hypothesis that image-region shape provides metric depth information, we investigated the relationship between convexity and distance separation in natural scenes. Again, distance separation is defined as the difference

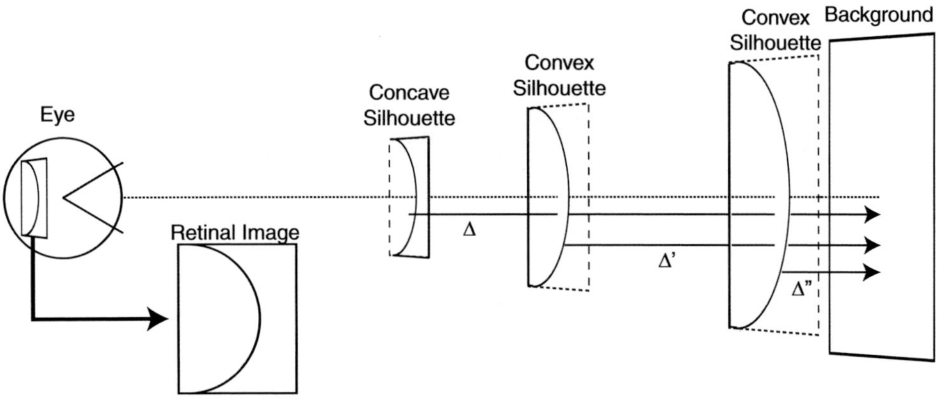


**Figure 11.1** The geometric information in occlusion. The same retinal image is generated by different combinations of the contour shape of the boundary of the occluding surface and the distance ordering of the occluding and occluded surfaces. Thus, there is no geometric constraint to indicate that the shape of the occluding contour is related to metric depth.

in viewing distance for two points along a line of sight. We examined the figure-ground cue of convexity because it can be readily measured in images of natural scenes (Fowlkes, Martin, & Malik, 2007) and because it is known to affect figure-ground assignment (Kanizsa & Gerbino, 1976; Metzger, 1953). We measured the joint statistics of convexity and distance separation in a collection of indoor and outdoor scenes by analyzing a collection of luminance and range images (Potetz & Lee, 2003; Yang & Purves, 2003). Figure 11.2A is an example of a luminance image and Figure 11.2B is the corresponding range image.

Contours in the images were hand-selected by naive participants using the procedure of Fowlkes et al. (2007) (Figs. 11.2C and 11.2D). We then computed the convexity of the local image regions on either side of the contour. Our measure of convexity is described in the figure caption. Figure 11.2E shows convexity along each selected contour in the expanded region from Figure 11.2A. Finally, we examined the frequency of different distance separations as a function of region convexity.

Figure 11.3A shows the distribution of convexities for the contours we analyzed. Figure 11.3B shows the statistical relationship between convexity and distance separation, where separation is the difference in the viewing distances of the two surfaces on opposite sides of a contour. This plot shows that metric depth information is provided by the two-dimensional (2D) shape of image regions, a striking result given the lack of a geometric relationship. The most likely distance separation is zero because many contours correspond to rapid changes in surface orientation or changes in reflectance due to surface markings. Nonetheless, distance separation is clearly dependent on convexity. For all positive separations, a region is always more likely to be near than far if its bounding contour makes it convex. Put another way, if the contour is convex, the distance between the occluding and the occluded surface is likely to be larger than if the contour is concave. To our knowledge, this is the first evidence that a depth cue with no known geometric relationship to depth—the figure-ground cue of convexity—is statistically correlated with metric depth. The effect is small, but consistent. Presumably, the cause of the statistical relationship is that objects are mostly convex.

We further examined these statistical relationships for conditions that are similar to the ones used in our experiment. The disparity-specified separations in the experiments were not large, so we focused the scene analysis on separations of 0–2 m. We also focused on image regions whose convexities were nearly equal

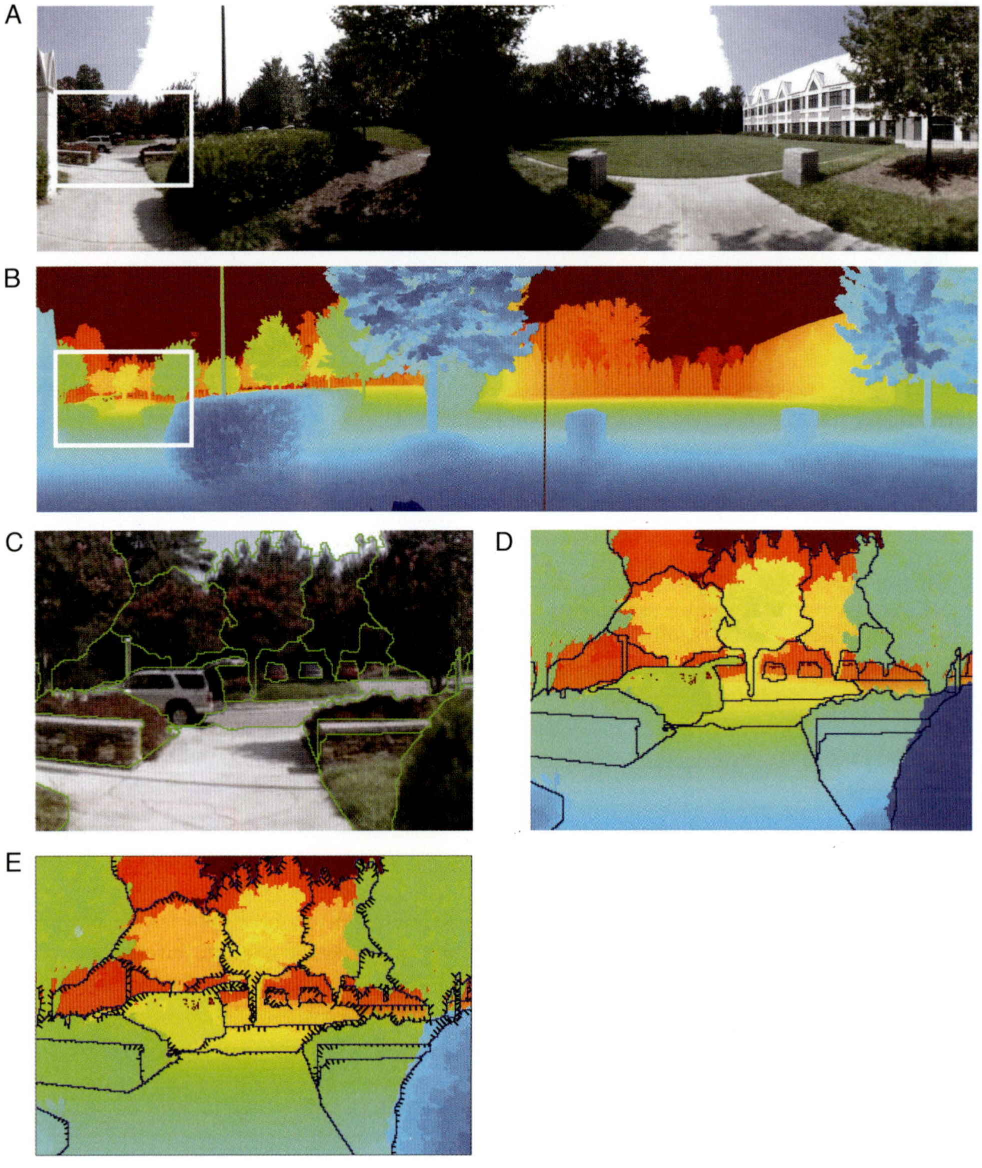


**Figure 11.2** Luminance and range images. (A) An example luminance image. (B) Corresponding range image. Blue indicates nearer distances, yellow intermediate distances, and red farther distances. (C) Close-up of the luminance image with a representative hand segmentation overlaid. (D) Close-up of the associated range image with the same segmentation overlaid. (E) The same image as (D), but with convexity flags added. Flags point toward the image region that was classified as more convex. Longer flags correspond to larger convexity values. For each point along a selected contour, we computed the convexity of the local image regions on either side of the contour using the technique of Fowlkes et al. (2007). A circular analysis window of fixed radius (2.16°, 15 pixels) was centered at each point along a selected contour. We sampled pairs of points inside both regions and recorded the fraction of pairs for which a line segment connecting them lay completely within the region. Convexity, $c$, is the log ratio of the two fractions.

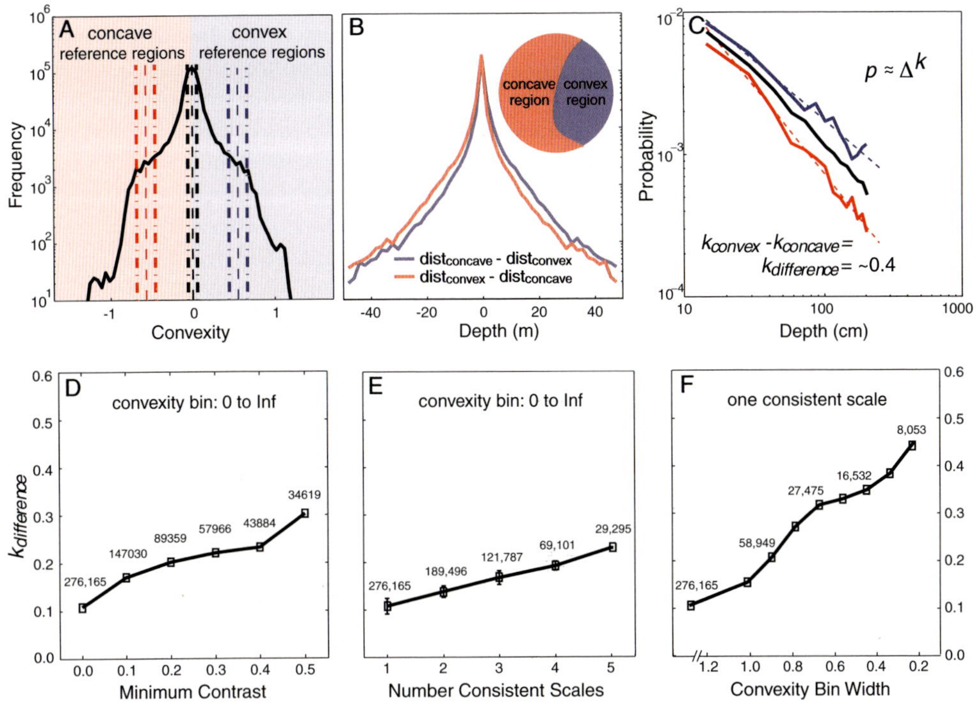


**Figure 11.3** Natural-scene statistics computed from ~450,000 sampled contour points. (A) Frequency of different convexities. A circular analysis window was centered at each point along a selected contour. One of the two regions inside the window was arbitrarily chosen as the *reference region*. Positive values indicate that the reference region was more convex than the other region (light blue shading); negative values indicate that the reference region was more concave (pink shading). (B) Joint statistics of convexity and distance separation. Frequency of occurrence plotted as a function of separation for all convex (light blue) and concave (pink) reference regions. When the reference region is nearer ("figure"), separations are positive. When the reference region is farther ("ground"), separations are negative. The two curves are mirror images because every curved contour has a convex region on one side and a concave region on the other. (C) Joint statistics of convexity and distance separation for 0–2 m and for convexities similar to those in the psychophysical experiments. The means of the bins defined by the dashed vertical lines in (A) are similar to the convexities of the three stimulus types in the psychophysical experiments: convex (blue), concave (red), and straight-contoured (black). The straight bin has approximately 10 times more samples than the convex and concave bins, so the black curve is smoother. Dotted lines are power-law fits to the data. Except for separations of ~0, the data are well fit by a power law. The difference between the convex and concave power-law exponents, $k_{difference} = k_{convex} - k_{concave}$, is approximately 0.4. (D) $k_{difference}$ as a function of the minimum contrast that was analyzed. As the minimum contrast increases, the analyzed contours have greater contrast on average. $k_{difference}$ increases monotonically as the minimum contrast becomes greater. (E) Change in $k_{difference}$ as a function of the number of spatial scales for which the sign of region convexity is consistent (i.e., contours that are more and more circular). $k_{difference}$ increases monotonically as the number of scales for which convexity is consistent increases. These data are discussed later in the chapter. (F) Change in $k_{difference}$ as a function of the narrowness of the convexity bins. $k_{difference}$ is always positive and increases monotonically as the bins become increasingly narrow. These data are also discussed later on.

(e.g., straight contours) or were quite different (defined in Fig. 11.3A). The distributions conditioned on these three convexities for 0–2 m separations are shown in Figure 11.3C. The distributions are well described by power laws (linear on log-log plots) for all separations except ~0. We will take advantage of the power-law property and henceforth describe distributions by the difference in the exponents $k$ of the best-fitting functions: $k_{difference} = k_{convex} - k_{concave}$.

## Psychophysical Experiments on Convexity and Depth

We conducted two experiments. Two experienced and visually normal observers participated in the first experiment and seven in the second. All were naive to the experimental hypotheses. The stimuli were two adjacent equal-area regions textured with random dots that were separated by a curved or a straight luminance contour (Fig. 11.4). One region was black with white dots, and the other was white with black dots. Disparity specified that one region was in front of the other. There were three kinds of stimuli: consistent, inconsistent, and neutral. In consistent stimuli, the disparity-specified near region was made convex by the contour (Fig. 11.4A). In neutral stimuli, the contour was a vertical line (Fig. 11.4B). In inconsistent stimuli, the disparity-specified near region was concave (Fig. 11.4C). In the two-interval procedure, there were five conditions: consistent versus consistent (i.e., two consistent stimuli were presented on a trial), neutral versus neutral, inconsistent versus inconsistent, consistent versus neutral, and inconsistent versus neutral.

Two stimuli were presented sequentially on each trial: a standard and comparison. Observers indicated the stimulus in which they perceived more separation in depth between the two regions. The disparity of the standard was fixed at one of eight values: 2.5–20 arcmin in 2.5-arcmin steps. These disparities corresponded to simulated separations of ~12–157 cm at the viewing distance of 325 cm. We used this rather long distance to reduce the reliability of disparity and thereby increase the probability of observing an effect of convexity. An adaptive staircase adjusted the disparity of the comparison relative to the standard disparity.

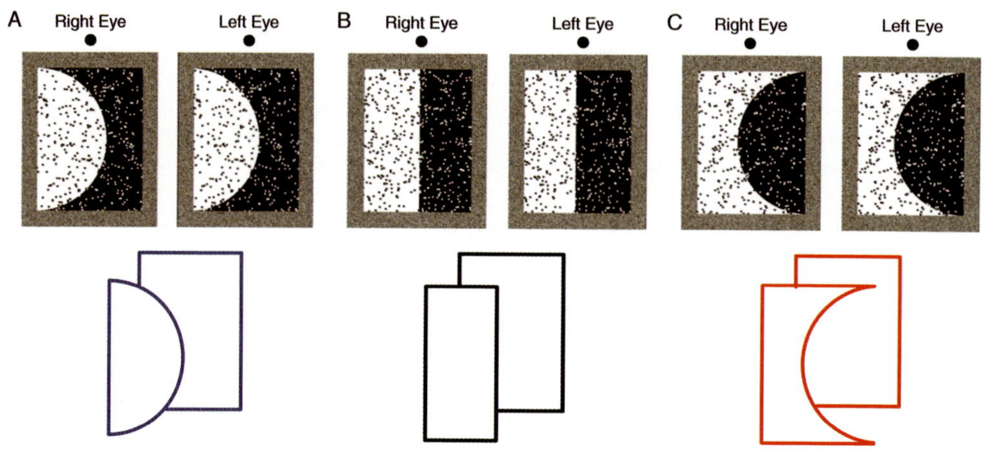


**Figure 11.4** Examples of the experimental stimuli. The upper row contains stereograms that can be cross-fused to reveal two regions at different distances. The lower row depicts the disparity-specified depth for each stimulus type. (A) Consistent stimulus: Disparity and convexity both indicate that the white region is nearer than the black region. (B) Neutral stimulus: Disparity specifies that the white region is nearer, while convexity does not indicate which region is nearer. (C) Inconsistent stimulus: Disparity specifies that the white region is nearer and convexity suggests that it is farther. A reader who examines the stereograms closely might perceive a difference in distance separation between the different stimuli, but as our data show, the perceptual effect is small.

Only the disparity of the far region changed, so observers could not base judgments on the depth separation between the frame and the near region. Observers indicated the interval that contained the greater apparent separation in depth between the near and far regions. No feedback was provided.

Figure 11.5 illustrates the expected influence of contour shape on depth judgments. The upper row depicts the probability distributions associated with consistent stimuli (Fig. 11.4A) in which convexity and disparity both indicate that one side is nearer. The posterior distribution, given by the product of the distributions in the left panel, is shifted slightly toward less depth than specified by disparity. The lower row depicts the probability distributions associated with inconsistent stimuli (Fig. 11.4C). The product of the two distributions in the left panel is now shifted toward less depth than occurs with consistent stimuli. Therefore, the observer should perceive less depth with inconsistent stimuli (concave occluders) than with consistent stimuli (convex occluders) when the disparity-specified depth is the same.

We assume that the influence of convexity on depth percepts will be based on the variance of depth from convexity relative to the variance of depth from disparity (Ernst & Banks, 2002; Knill & Saunders, 2003). Therefore, the influence of convexity on perceived separation in depth should increase with increasing disparity because the variance of depth from disparity increases as the disparity increases; specifically, discrimination thresholds increase in proportion to disparity (Blakemore, 1970; McKee, Levi, & Bowne, 1990; Morgan, Watamanuik, & McKee, 2000). As a result, the difference in the posteriors on the right side of Figure 11.5 should increase as disparity increases, that is, the influence of convexity on depth judgments should increase as the disparity in the stimulus increases.

The results are shown in Figure 11.6. The PSE changes in the two panels of Figure 11.6A show that, to produce the same perceived separation, consistent stimuli required less disparity than

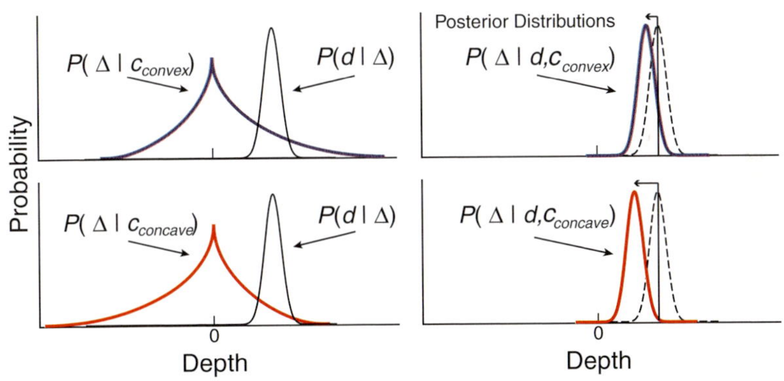


**Figure 11.5** Predicted depth percepts for different combinations of convexity and disparity. The stimulus is composed of two regions separated by a contour. The left panels show probability distributions associated with convexity and disparity expressed over distance separation. The abscissa is the depth between the regions on the two sides of the contour. Positive numbers indicate that the putative figural region is closer than the opposing ground region. The blue and red curves are schematics representing the probability distributions derived from the natural-scene statistics (Fig. 11.3) for convex and concave reference regions, respectively. The black curves represent the distribution over depths derived from an intrinsically noisy disparity signal that specifies that the assigned region is nearer than the opposing region; although the distribution is solid in the left panel and dashed in the right, the two are the same distribution. The right panels show the posterior distributions (solid curves) and the disparity likelihood functions (dashed curves) for the same two situations. The posterior distributions are shifted relative to the disparity likelihood functions by different amounts depending on the convexity-depth probability distribution.

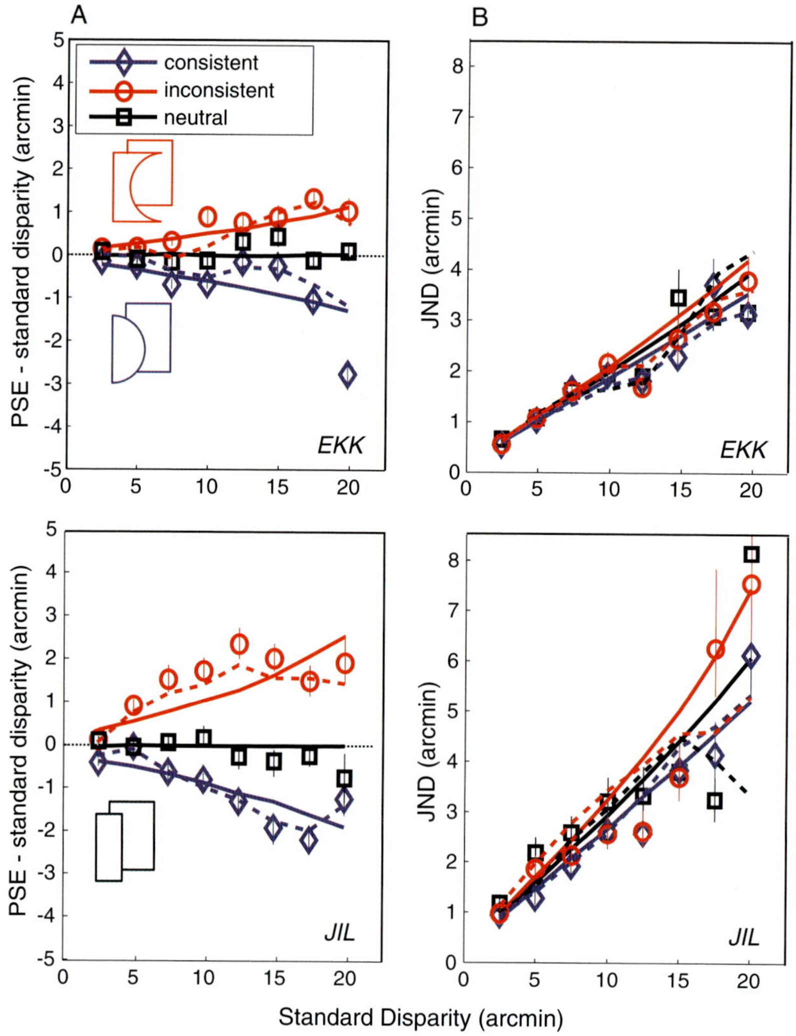


**Figure 11.6** Experimental results. Upper and lower rows show data from observers EKK and JIL, respectively. (A) Points of subjective equality (PSEs) plotted against the disparity of the standard. The ordinates are the disparity of the comparison stimulus minus the disparity of the standard stimulus at the PSE. The abscissas are the disparity of the standard stimulus. Data points are the mean of the cumulative Gaussian that best fit the psychometric data in each condition. Blue indicates the neutral-consistent stimulus pairing, red the neutral-inconsistent pairing, and black the neutral-neutral pairing. Error bars are bootstrapped 95% confidence intervals (Wichmann & Hill, 2001). Dotted lines represent predictions of a nonparametric model. Solid lines represent the predictions of a power-law model. If convexity did not affect perceived separation in depth, the data would lie on a horizontal line through zero. (B) Just-noticeable differences (JNDs) plotted against disparity of the standard. This is the disparity difference that was required for observers to respond that the comparison stimulus had greater depth than the standard 84% of the time. The three sets of data are for neutral versus neutral (black), consistent versus consistent (blue), and inconsistent versus inconsistent (red). Symbols represent the standard deviation of the best-fitting cumulative Gaussian for each condition. Error bars are 95% confidence intervals. Dotted and solid lines are again the predictions of nonparametric and power-law models, respectively.

neutral stimuli and inconsistent stimuli required more. For example, at a standard disparity of 15 arcmin, EKK and JIL needed 1.1 and 3.9 arcmin less disparity, respectively, in consistent than in inconsistent stimuli to perceive the same separation. This effect is consistent with observers using the relationship between contour convexity and distance separation in judging the separation of the near and far regions in our stimuli. Notice that the effect of contour shape increased systematically with increasing disparity. This is expected because of the decreases in the reliability of depth from disparity with increasing disparity, which allows an increasing influence of contour shape. The results thus suggest that contour shape provides metric depth information to human observers.

Figure 11.6B shows that just-noticeable differences (JNDs) rose systematically with increasing disparity, as expected, but that they did not vary significantly across consistent versus consistent, inconsistent versus inconsistent, and neutral versus neutral conditions. Convexity had a larger influence in the observer (JIL) with higher discrimination thresholds, the expected result if both observers had internalized the same natural-scene statistics for convexity and depth.

To test for the generality of these results, we conducted a shorter experiment on more observers. The stimuli and procedure were the same as in the first experiment with a few exceptions. Instead of convex, concave, and straight contours, there were only convex and concave contours. Instead of five stimulus conditions, there were four: consistent-consistent, inconsistent-inconsistent, consistent-inconsistent, and inconsistent-consistent. The standard stimulus had only one value: 15 arcmin.

The results are shown in Figure 11.7. Figure 11.7A shows that the seven observers exhibited the same pattern of results as the observers in the first experiment; Figure 11.7B shows the data averaged across observers.

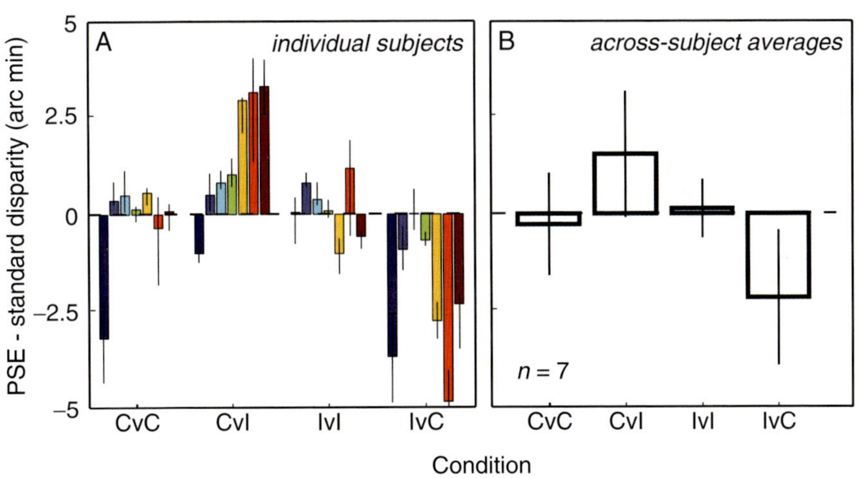


**Figure 11.7** Results from the second experiment. (A) Points of subjective equality (PSEs) from individual observers. Four stimulus pairings were presented: consistent-consistent (CvC), consistent-inconsistent (CvI), inconsistent-inconsistent (IvI), and inconsistent-consistent (IvC). The first member of each pair is the standard stimulus; the second is the comparison. PSE minus standard disparity is plotted for each observer: the disparity increment of the comparison stimulus, relative to the standard disparity, that on average yielded the same apparent separation in depth as the standard stimulus. Error bars are bootstrapped 95% confidence intervals (Wichmann & Hill, 2001). The dashed horizontal lines through zero represent the expected data if region convexity did not affect perceived separation. (B) PSEs averaged across observers minus the standard disparity for the four pairings. To perceive separation as the same, observers needed more disparity in inconsistent comparison stimuli than in consistent standard stimuli. The reverse was true for consistent comparisons and inconsistent standards. Error bars represent one standard deviation of the group mean.

On average, consistent stimuli required about 2.1 arcmin less disparity than inconsistent stimuli to produce the same apparent separation in depth.

Recently, Gillam, Anderson, and Rizwi (2009) reported a failure to observe an effect of the consistency between contour convexity and the disparity-specified distance separation, a finding that disagrees with that of Burge et al. (2005, 2010) and Bertamini et al. (2008). They, however, presented their stimuli at a viewing distance of 85 cm where disparity is a much more reliable signal than at the 325 cm viewing distance of our experiments. We collected data at the two distances and found that the convexity effect was significantly greater at the longer distance.

## Modeling the Psychophysical Experiments on Convexity and Depth

The results from the psychophysical experiments are qualitatively consistent with the expected behavior of an ideal observer who has incorporated the natural-scene statistics associated with region convexity and metric depth. Specifically, the results show that convexity has an effect on the perceived distance separation between two image regions. But are these results quantitatively consistent with incorporation of the natural-scene statistics? To answer this, we fit the observers' responses with a probabilistic model of depth estimation to determine the probability distributions that provided the best quantitative account of those responses. In doing this, we modeled the computation of the depth percept as a probabilistic process. Assuming conditional independence, Bayes' rule states:

$$P(\Delta|d, c) = \frac{P(d|\Delta)P(c|\Delta)P(\Delta)}{P(d, c)}. \quad (11.1)$$

That is, the posterior probability of a particular distance separation, $\Delta$, given a measurement of disparity, $d$, across a contour bounding an image region with convexity $c$, is equal to the product of the likelihood of the disparity measurement for a particular depth, $P(d|\Delta)$, the likelihood of the convexity measurement for a particular depth, $P(c|\Delta)$, and the prior distribution of depths, $P(\Delta)$, divided by a normalizing constant, $P(d, c)$, for all such contours. We can use the product rule, which states that $P(c, \Delta) = P(c|\Delta)P(\Delta)$, to combine the latter two terms in the numerator into the joint probability of $c$ and $\Delta$: $P(\Delta|d, c) = P(d|\Delta)P(c, \Delta)/P(d, c)$. Next, we use the fact that $P(c, \Delta) = P(\Delta, c)$ and regroup again using the product rule. Rearranging yields:

$$P(\Delta|d, c) = \left(\frac{1}{P(d, c)/P(c)}\right)P(d|\Delta)P(\Delta|c), \quad (11.2)$$

where $1/\left(P(d, c)/P(c)\right)$ is a normalizing constant, $P(d|\Delta)$ is the disparity likelihood, and $P(\Delta|c)$ is the convexity-depth distribution, which is the distribution we measured in the natural-scene, luminance-range images. The depth prior, $P(\Delta)$, has been absorbed by $P(\Delta|c)$.

It is convenient to express these probability distributions using common units. Fortunately, a deterministic relationship between distance separation and disparity is given by the equation:

$$d = f(\Delta) = 2\left(\tan^{-1}(I/2z_0) - \tan^{-1}(I/2(z_0 + \Delta))\right), \quad (11.3)$$

where $z_0$ is the fixation distance and $I$ is the interocular separation (Howard & Rogers, 2002). Solving for $\Delta$ allows us to map disparity signals into distance separations.

In this model, the convexity and disparity of an image region both affect the expected perceived depth. This is illustrated schematically in Figure 11.5, which shows probability distributions associated with image-region convexity and disparity (left) and the posterior distributions generated from the products of those distributions (right). The disparity signal indicates that the region on one side of the contour is nearer than the region on the other side. If the region is bounded by a contour that makes it convex (upper left), the convexity-depth distribution is skewed toward larger depths than when the region is concave (lower left). As a consequence, the estimated depth will be greater in the convex (upper right) than in the concave case (lower right). Said another way, when region convexity and disparity are consistent with one another (i.e., both indicate that the same region is nearer than the other), perceived depth should be greater than when they are inconsistent.

Assuming that the convexity-depth distribution is locally linear on a log-linear plot when depth is plotted as disparity (i.e., assuming that locally, in the neighborhood of $\Delta = f^{-1}(d)$, $\log P(\Delta|c) \approx m_d(c, d)f(\Delta) + b(c, d)$, we can approximate the posterior in disparity as Gaussian:

$$P(\Delta|d, c) \propto \exp\left[-\frac{(f(\Delta) - d)^2}{2\sigma^2(d)} + m_d(c, d)f(\Delta) + b(c, d)\right]. \quad (11.4)$$

That is, although $P(\Delta|d, c)$ itself is not Gaussian, when stated as a function of disparity, it takes a Gaussian form with mean disparity $d + m_d(c, d)\sigma^2(d)$ and standard deviation $\sigma(d)$; $m_d(c, d)$ is local slope in the convexity-depth distribution mapped into disparity, and $b(c, d)$ is absorbed into a scaling factor that ensures the posterior distribution integrates to 1. We modeled the process that generated the psychophysical data by computing posterior distributions for the standard and comparison stimuli on each trial. We used signal-detection theory to model the discrimination and generate psychometric functions. The psychometric functions were the cumulative probability that the comparison stimulus was perceived as having more distance separation than the standard stimulus:

$$P\left(\hat{\Delta}_{comp} > \hat{\Delta}_{std}\right) = \int_0^{\infty} P\left(\hat{\Delta}_{comp}|d_{comp}, c_{comp}\right) \times \int_0^{\hat{\Delta}_{comp}} P\left(\hat{\Delta}_{std}|d_{std}, c_{std}\right). \quad (11.5)$$

With the Gaussian approximation to the posterior in hand, the psychometric functions can be computed in closed form as a function of the parameters.

We first examined how the disparity-likelihood distributions we estimated from the psychophysical data compared with previous findings in the literature (McKee et al., 1990). The agreement was good. This is important because it shows that our analysis recovered reasonable values for the disparity distributions, and it supports our assumption that disparity and convexity provide conditionally independent depth estimates.

Figure 11.8A shows the convexity-depth distributions estimated from data in the first experiment. In this case, we used a nonparametric model, which makes very few assumptions about the shapes of the distributions and has 26 free parameters. The estimated distributions are similar in many respects to the convexity-depth distributions recovered from the natural-scene statistics (Fig. 11.3): *(1)* the distributions are skewed such that large distance separations are more probable across contours that bound convex regions than straight-contoured or concave regions; *(2)* all three distributions have much heavier tails than Gaussians; *(3)* the estimated convexity-depth distributions are roughly linear in a log-log plot, which means that they are similar to power laws. Figure 11.8B shows the distributions that were recovered from the psychophysical data when we fit them using a power-law model. By fitting only the power-law exponents, the number of free parameters was reduced from 26 to 5 (two for disparity and three for convexity-depth distributions).

We assessed the goodness of fit between the data and the nonparametric and power-law models. We computed the squared error for a coin-flipping model with no degrees of freedom and a psychometric-fitting model with 80 degrees of freedom. The nonparametric ($df$=26) and power-law ($df$=5) models provided nearly as good a fit to the data as the psychometric-fitting model and significantly better fits than the coin-flipping model. Because the power-law model provided nearly as good a fit to the data as the nonparametric model, we conclude that power laws are excellent descriptions of the internal convexity-depth distributions.

While the convexity-depth distributions estimated from the psychophysical experiment and natural-scene measurements were similar in many ways, they did differ in one interesting

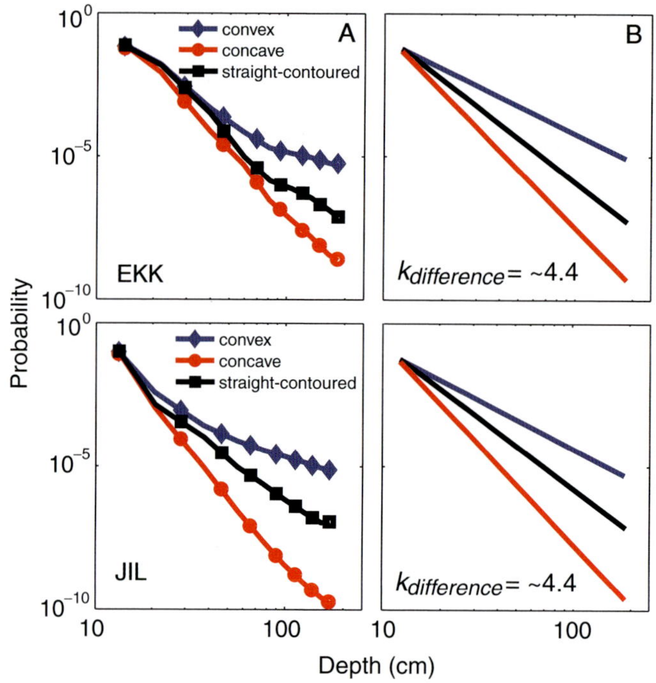


**Figure 11.8** Convexity-depth distributions estimated from the first experiment. Blue represents the distribution for convex reference regions, red the distribution for concave reference regions, and black the distribution for straight-contoured reference regions. (A) Convexity-depth distributions recovered from fitting the psychometric data with the nonparametric model. The distributions are approximately linear in these log-log plots, suggesting that they were well described by a power law. (B) Convexity-depth distributions that were recovered by refitting the psychometric data with the power-law model. Note the similarity to the nonparametric distributions in (A). One free parameter, one local slope of the straight-contoured distribution, had to be set to uniquely determine these fits. The differences between the estimated distributions were unaffected by the value of that parameter because it was the differences in the slopes that mattered. The standard errors for the best-fitting parameters were estimated by redoing the fitting procedure 30 times with bootstrapped sets of psychometric data. The standard errors were small, so if they were plotted they would generally not be visible in this figure.

respect: The effect of convexity was much larger in the psychophysically estimated distributions; $k_{difference}$, the difference between the exponents of the best-fitting power laws from the experiment was ~4.4, whereas $k_{difference}$ from the natural statistics was 0.1 to 0.5, depending on which set of contours was included (Fig. 11.3).

There is a plausible explanation for this discrepancy. The contours presented in the psychophysical experiments were different from the great majority of contours analyzed in the natural scenes. In the experiments, the contours were high contrast, and the regions they bounded were circular, so they had consistent convexity across scale (e.g., the silhouette of a basketball). In the natural-scene dataset, many contours were low contrast, and the regions they bounded were convex at some spatial scales and concave at others (e.g., the silhouette of a tree). To examine the possibility that the discrepancy was due to the use in the psychophysical experiment of high-contrast contours with consistent convexity, we recomputed the natural-scene statistics and focused our analysis, to the best degree possible, on contours with those properties. Figures 11.3D, 11.3E, and 11.3F show the convexity-depth distributions for natural-scene contours after selection with more or less restrictive criteria. When the contours included in the natural-scene analysis are most similar to those in the psychophysical experiments (i.e., high-contrast edges, consistent classification as convex or concave across scale, a narrow range of convexities), $k_{difference}$ becomes more similar to the value recovered from the psychophysical experiments. Thus, conditioning on additional visual features that restrict the contours under consideration to contours similar to the experimental stimuli, yields natural-scene distributions that are quantitatively more similar to the distributions recovered from the psychophysics. Unfortunately, we cannot further refine the selection of contours from the database on other visual features because doing so yields too few samples to calculate meaningful statistics. As more natural-scene data become available, one could pursue this further.

To summarize the first part of this chapter, we found, in an analysis of natural-scene statistics, that convexity provides information about depth in natural scenes. The convexity of an image region can, therefore, provide information about the probability of different distance separations across the contour bounding that region. We constructed a probabilistic model of how that information would be used to maximize the accuracy of depth estimates. In psychophysical experiments, we showed that convexity affects perceived distance separation in a manner consistent with such a model. Our work thus establishes the ecological validity of the figure-ground cue of convexity and its usefulness to the human viewers. And it exemplifies the utility of the Bayesian framework for representing the use of such a cue in perceiving the 3D structure of the environment.

We now turn to the next depth cue that we analyzed in the probabilistic framework: image blur.

## BLUR AS A CUE TO METRIC DEPTH

### Background

Our subjective impression of the visual world is that everything is in focus. This impression is reinforced by the common practice in photography and cinematography of creating images that are in focus everywhere (i.e., images with infinite depth of focus). Our subjective impression, however, is quite incorrect because, with the exception of the image on the fovea, most parts of the retinal image are significantly blurred. Here, we explore how blur affects depth perception.

Previous research on blur as a depth cue has produced mixed results. For instance, Mather and Smith (2000) found that blur had little effect on perceived depth when it was presented with binocular disparity. They manipulated blur independently of disparity and measured the perceived distance separation between the two regions. Blur only had an effect when it was greatly exaggerated and therefore specified a much larger separation than disparity. Watt, Akeley, Ernst, and Banks (2005) found no effect of blur on the perceived slant of disparity-specified planes (although they did find an effect with perspective-defined planes viewed monocularly). Other investigators have stated that blur has no discernible effect on depth percepts when reliable cues like structure from motion are available (e.g., Caudek & Proffitt, 1993; Hogervorst & Eagle, 1998, 2000).

There are, however, convincing demonstrations that blur can provide distance-ordering information. Consider two adjoining regions, one with a blurred texture and one with a sharp texture. When the border between the regions is blurred, it appears to belong to the region with blurred texture, and people perceive that region as nearer and as occluding a sharply textured background. When the border is sharp, it seems to belong to the sharply textured region, and people tend to see that region as nearer (Marshall, Burbeck, Ariely, Rolland, & Martin, 1996; Mather, 1996, 1997; Mather & Smith, 2002; O'Shea, Govan, & Sekuler, 1997; Palmer & Brooks, 2008). From these results and others, vision scientists have concluded that blur is at best a weak depth cue. Mather and Smith (2002), for example, stated that blur acts as "a relatively coarse, qualitative depth cue" (p. 1211).

Despite the widely held view that blur is a weak depth cue, there is also evidence that it can affect the perception of metric distance and size. For example, cinematographers make miniature models appear much larger by reducing the camera's aperture, thereby reducing the blur variation throughout the scene (Fielding, 1985). The opposite effect is created by the striking photographic manipulation known as the tilt-shift effect: A full-size scene is made to look much smaller by adding blur with either a special camera or postprocessing software (Flickr, 2009; Laforet, 2007). In photography, the apparent enlarging associated with reduced blur and the miniaturization associated with added blur are called depth-of-field effects (Kingslake, 1992). The images in Figure 11.9 demonstrate miniaturization. The upper-left image is a photograph of an urban scene taken with a small aperture. The upper-right image has been rendered using a blur pattern consistent with a shorter focal distance and, therefore, with a smaller scene; the added blur makes it look like a scale model. The panels in the lower row demonstrate an approximate technique for manipulating apparent size. The left image is a photograph taken with a small aperture. In the right image, a vertical blur gradient has been applied (i.e., pixels were blurred according to their position in the image rather than their distances) and this causes the scene to look much smaller. These and related demonstrations show that blur can have a profound effect on perceived size, which is presumably caused by an effect on perceived absolute distance.

These examples, combined with the literature cited earlier, present a mixed picture of whether blur is a useful cue to depth. To resolve the conflict, we turn to blur's optical origins and examine how it could, in principle, be used to estimate distance.

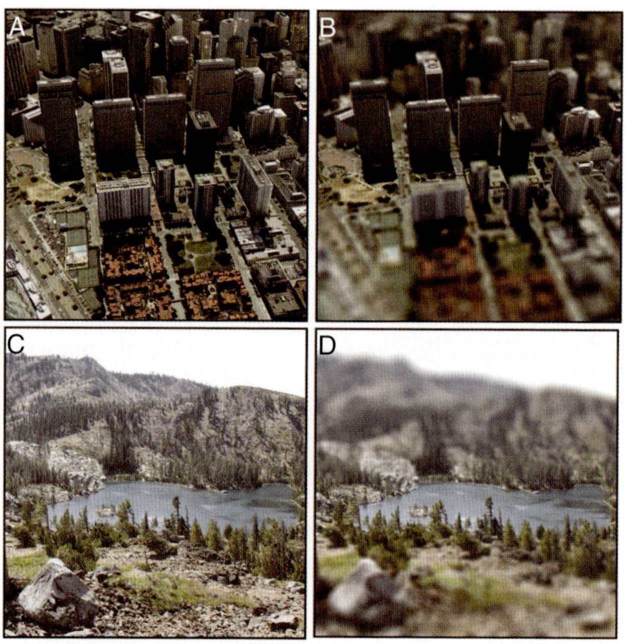


**Figure 11.9** Blur and perceived size and distance. Top two images: Rendering with a shallow depth of field makes a scene appear miniature. The left image is rendered with a pinhole aperture; the right is rendered with a virtual 60 m aperture. Bottom two images: achieving the same effect with a blur gradient whose orientation is the same as the distance gradient. The left image is a photograph with a small aperture, while the right has a blur gradient applied in Photoshop. See http://www.tiltshiftphotography.net/ for convincing images. (Original city images and data from GoogleEarth are copyright Terrametrics, SanBorn, and Google. Lake image copyright 2009, Casey Held.)

### Probabilistic Modeling of Blur as a Distance Cue

In an ideal lens with focal length $f$, the light rays emanating from a point at some near distance $z$ in front of the lens will be focused to another point on the opposite side of the lens at distance $s$, where the relationship between these distances is given by the thin-lens equation:

$$1/s + 1/z = 1/f. \tag{11.6}$$

If the image plane is at distance $s_0$ behind the lens, then light emanating from features at distance $z_0 = 1/(1/f - 1/s_0)$ will be focused on the image plane (Fig. 11.10). The plane at distance $z_0$ is the focal plane, so $z_0$ is the focal distance of the imaging device. Objects at other distances will be out of focus, and hence will generate blurred images on the image plane. We can express the amount of blur by the diameter $b$ of the blur circle for an object at distance $z_1$,

$$b = \frac{As_0}{z_0}\left|1 - \frac{z_0}{z_1}\right|, \tag{11.7}$$

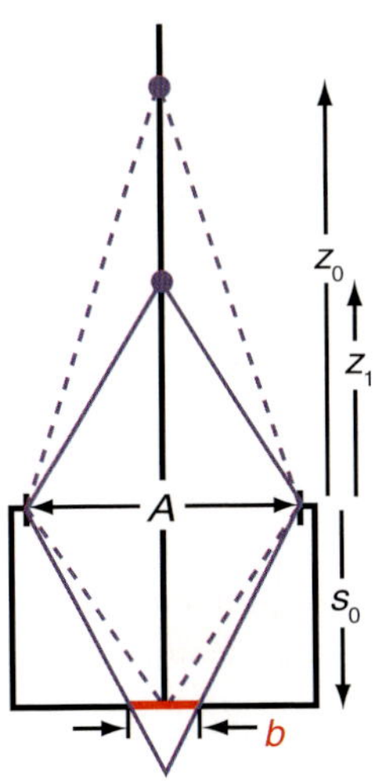


**Figure 11.10** Optics and formation of blurred images. The box represents a camera with aperture diameter $A$. The camera lens forms an image in the film plane at the back of the box. Two objects at distances $z_0$ and $z_1$ are presented with the camera focused at $z_0$, so $z_1$ creates a blurred image with width $b$.

where $A$ is the diameter of the aperture. It is convenient to substitute $r$ for the distance ratio $z_1/z_0$, yielding:

$$b = \frac{As_0}{z_0}\left|1 - \frac{1}{r}\right|. \tag{11.8}$$

Real imaging devices, like the eye, have imperfect optics and more than one refracting element, so Eq. 11.8 is not strictly correct. Later in this chapter, we describe those effects and show that they do not affect our analysis.

If an object is blurred, is it possible to recover its distance from the viewer? To answer this, we examine the implications of Eq. 11.8. Now the aperture $A$ is the diameter of a human pupil, $z_0$ is the distance to which the eye is focused, and $r$ is the distance ratio $(z_1/z_0)$. Figure 11.11 shows the probability of measuring a given amount of blur, given values of $z_0$ and $r$, assuming $A$ is 4.6 mm (±1 mm; Spring & Stiles, 1948). For each blur magnitude, infinite combinations of $z_0$ and $r$ are possible. The distributions for large and small blur differ; large blur diameters are consistent with a range of short focal distances, and small blur diameters are consistent with a range of long distances. Nonetheless, one cannot estimate focal distance or distance ratio from one observation of blur or from a set of such observations. How then does the change in perceived size and distance in Figure 11.9 occur?

The images in Figure 11.9 contain other pictorial cues that specify the distance ratios among objects in the scene. Such cues are scale ambiguous, with the possible exception of familiar size, so they cannot directly signal the absolute distance to objects. Here, we will focus on perspective cues (e.g., linear perspective, texture gradient, relative size) that are commonplace in natural scenes. We can determine absolute distance from the combination of blur and perspective. To do this, we again employ Bayes' rule. Assuming conditional independence,

$$P(z_0, r|b, p) = \frac{P(b|z_0, r)P(p|z_0, r)P(z_0, r)}{P(b, p)}, \tag{11.9}$$

where $p$ is the perspective information, $b$ is the blur-circle diameter, $r$ is the distance ratio,

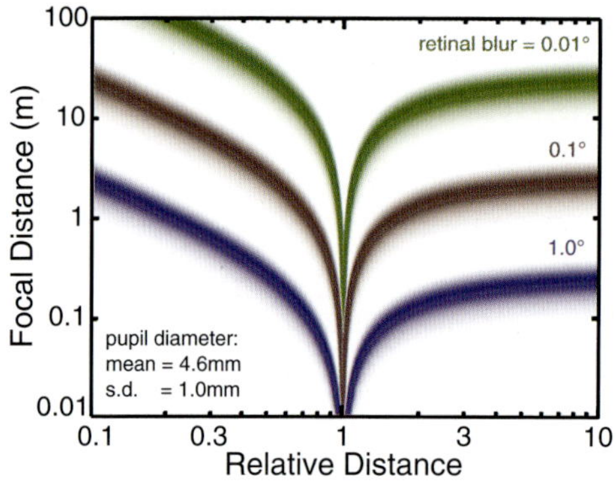


**Figure 11.11** Focal distance as a function of retinal-image blur and relative distance. Relative distance is the ratio of the distance to an object and the distance to the focal plane. The three colored curves represent different amounts of image blur expressed as the diameter of the blur circle, *b*. The variance in the distribution was determined by assuming that pupil diameter is Gaussian distributed with a mean of 4.6 mm and standard deviation of 1 mm (Spring & Stiles 1948). We assume the observer has no knowledge of current pupil diameter. For a given amount of blur, it is impossible to recover the original focal distance without knowledge of the relative distance. Note that as the relative distance approaches 1, the object moves closer to the focal plane. There is a singularity at a relative distance of 1, because the object is by definition completely in focus.

and $z_0$ is the absolute distance to which the eye is focused. By regrouping the terms in a similar fashion to our derivations for the convexity cue, we obtain:

$$P(z_0, r|b, p) = \left(\frac{1}{P(b, p)/P(p)}\right) P(b|z_0, r)P(z_0, r|p). \quad (11.10)$$

As with the combination of convexity and disparity, it would be more useful to have the distributions expressed over common units so that the posterior can be obtained via pointwise multiplication. Here, we would like to have both terms on the right expressed over the absolute distance and distance ratios, $z_0$ and $r$, respectively. Fortunately, just as there is a deterministic relationship between distance separation and disparity, there is a deterministic relationship between focal distance and distance ratio, and retinal blur due to defocus. This relationship, given by Eq. 11.8, can be inverted to map blur back into a focal distance and distance ratio:

$$z_0, r = f^{-1}(b). \quad (11.11)$$

The distributions in Figure 11.11 show the possible values for $z_0$ and $r$, given retinal blur, $b$.

Figure 11.12 illustrates the estimation of depth from blur and perspective. Figure 11.12A is the distribution of absolute distances and distance ratios given the observed blur. Figure 11.12B is the distribution of distances given the observed perspective, and Figure 11.12C is the combined estimate based on both cues. Notice that the absolute distance and distance ratio are now reasonably well specified by the image data. We use the distribution in Figure 11.12C to make depth estimates.

Figure 11.12 illustrates the Bayesian model for estimating distance from blur. We made some simplifying assumptions, all of which can be avoided as we learn more.

First, we assumed that the visual system's capacity to estimate depth from blur is limited only by the optics of retinal-image formation. Of course, the visual system must measure the blur from the images and this measurement is subject to error (Georgeson, May, Freeman, & Hesse, 2007; Mather & Smith, 2002; Walsh & Charman, 1988). If we included this observation, the blur distributions in Figures 11.11 and 11.12A would have larger variance than the ones shown. This would decrease the precision of estimation, but it should not affect the accuracy. The measurement of blur has been investigated in the computer- and biological-vision literatures (Farid & Simoncelli, 1998; Georgeson et al., 2007; Mather & Smith, 2000; Pentland, 1987). Naturally, the interpretation of a blur measurement depends on the contents of the scene because the same blur can be observed at the retina when a sharp edge in the world is viewed with inaccurate focus and when a blurred edge (e.g., a shadow border) is viewed with accurate focus.

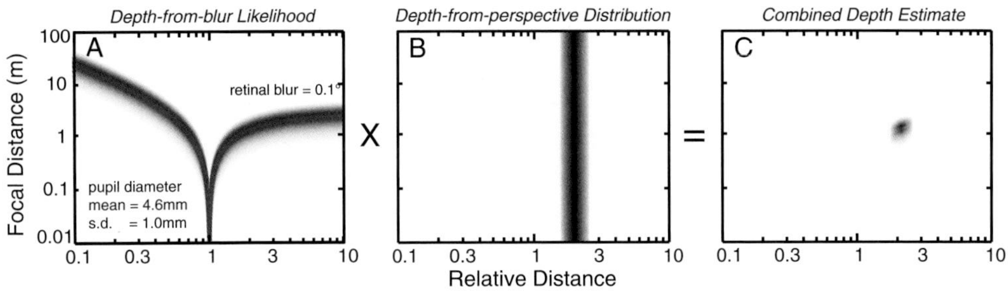


**Figure 11.12** Bayesian model of blur as an absolute cue to distance. (A) The probability distribution $P(z_0, r|b)$, where $b$ is the observed image blur diameter (in this case, 0.1°), $z_0$ is the focal distance, and $r$ is the ratio of distance ($z_1/z_0$; object/focal). One cannot estimate the absolute or relative distance to points in the scene from observations of their blur. (B) The probability distribution $P(z_0, r|p)$, where $p$ is the observed perspective. Perspective specifies the relative but not the absolute distance: It is scale ambiguous. (C) The product of the distributions in (A) and (B). From this posterior distribution, the absolute and relative distances of points in the scene can be estimated.

Second, we assumed a representative variance for the measurement of perspective, but this would certainly vary significantly across different types of images. The measurement of perspective has also been extensively investigated in computer and biological vision (Brillaut-O'Mahony, 1991; Coughlan & Yuille, 2003; Knill, 1998; Okatani & Deguchi, 2007). The ability to infer distance ratios from perspective depends, of course, on the scene contents. If the scene consists of homogenous, rectilinear structures, like the urban scenes in Figure 11.9, the variance of $P(z_0, r|p)$ would be small and distance ratios could be estimated accurately. If the scene is devoid of such structures, the variance of the distribution would be larger and ratio estimation more prone to error. As you can see from Figure 11.12, high variance in the perspective distribution can compromise the ability to estimate absolute distance from the two cues. We predict, therefore, that altering perceived size by manipulating blur will be more effective in scenes that contain rich perspective than in scenes with weak perspective.

Third, we assumed that the other pictorial cues provide distance-ratio information only. In fact, the images also contain the cue of familiar size, which conveys some absolute distance information. We could have incorporated this into the theory by modifying the perspective distribution in Figure 11.12B. The distribution would become a 2D Gaussian with different variances horizontally and vertically. We chose not to add this feature in order to keep the presentation simple, and because we have little idea of what the relative horizontal and vertical variances would be. It is interesting to note, however, that including familiar size might help explain anecdotal observations that the miniaturization effect is hard to obtain in some images.

Fourth, we represented the eye's optics with an ideal lens, free of aberrations. Image formation by real human eyes is affected by diffraction due to the pupil, at least for pupil diameters of 2–3 mm or smaller, and is also affected by a host of higher-order aberrations, including coma and spherical aberration at larger pupil diameters (Wilson, Decker, & Roorda, 2002). Incorporating diffraction and higher-order aberrations into our calculations in Figure 11.12A would yield greater retinal-image blur than shown for distances at or very close to the focal distance: The trough in the blur distribution would be deeper; the rest of the distribution would be unaffected. As a consequence, the ability to estimate absolute distance would be unaffected by incorporating diffraction and higher-order aberrations as long as a sufficiently large range of distance ratios was available in the stimulus.

Fifth, we assumed for the purposes of the experiment and modeling described in the following text, that the eye's optics are fixed when subjects view photographs. Of course, the optical power of the eye varies continually due to accommodation (adjustments of the shape of the crystalline lens), and the muscle command sent to the muscles controlling the shape of the lens is a cue to distance, albeit a highly variable and weak one (Fisher & Ciuffreda, 1988; Mon-Williams & Tresilian, 1999; Wallach & Norris, 1963). In viewing real scenes, accommodation turns blur into a dynamic cue that may allow the visual system to glean more distance information than we have assumed. The inclusion of accommodation into our modeling would have had little effect on our interpretation of the demonstration in Figure 11.9 or our psychophysical experiment because the stimuli are photographs, so the changes in the retinal image as the eye accommodated did not mimic the changes that occur in real scenes. Inclusion of accommodation would, however, definitely affect the use of blur in real scenes. We intend to pursue the use of dynamic blur and accommodation using volumetric displays that yield a reasonable approximation to the relationship in real scenes (e.g., Akeley, Watt, Girshick, & Banks, 2004; Love et al., 2009).

### Predictions of the Model

The model predicts that the visual system estimates absolute distance by finding the focal distance that is most consistent with the blur and perspective in a given image. If the blur and perspective are consistent with one another, accurate and precise distance estimates can be obtained. If they are inconsistent, the estimates will be generally less accurate and precise. We examined these predictions by considering images with three types of blur: *(1)* blur that is completely consistent with the distance ratios in a scene, *(2)* blur that is mostly correlated with the distances, and *(3)* blur that is uncorrelated with the distances. Fourteen scenes from GoogleEarth were used. Seven had a large amount of depth variation (skyscrapers) and seven had little depth variation (one- to three-story buildings). The camera was placed 500 m above the ground and oriented down 35° from earth-horizontal. The average distance from the camera to the buildings in the center of each scene was 785 m.

We used a standard depth-of-field rendering approach (Haeberli & Akeley, 1990) to create blur consistent with different scales of the GoogleEarth locales. We captured several images of the same locale from positions on a jittered grid covering a circular aperture. We translated each image to ensure that objects in the center of the scene were aligned from one image to another, and then averaged the images. The diameters of the simulated camera apertures were 60.0, 38.3, 24.5, 15.6, and 10.0 m. The unusually large apertures were needed to produce blur consistent with what a human eye with a 4.6 mm pupil would receive when focused at 0.06, 0.09, 0.15, 0.23, and 0.36 m, respectively. Figures 11.13B and 11.13C show example images with simulated 24.5 and 60 m apertures.

If the object is a plane, the distances in the image will form a gradient that runs along a line in the image. The pattern of blur is also a gradient that runs in the same direction (McCloskey & Langer, 2009). If we added the appropriate sign to the blur (i.e., removed the absolute value in Eq. 11.8), the blur gradient is also linear (i.e., $b$ is proportional to height in the image). Larger gradients are associated with greater slant between the object and image planes. The GoogleEarth scenes, particularly the ones with low depth variation, are approximately planes with the distance gradient running from bottom to top in the image. Thus, to create the second blur condition, we applied a linear blur gradient (apart from the sign) running in the same direction in the image as the distance gradient. This choice was motivated, in part, by the fact that most of the miniaturized images available online were created by applying linear blur gradients in postprocessing (Flickr, 2009). To create the third blur condition, we applied a horizontal blur gradient to images in which the distance gradient was vertical. Thus, the blur gradient was orthogonal to the distance gradient and, therefore, the blur was not highly correlated with distance in the scene.

Each row or column of pixels (for vertical or horizontal gradients, respectively) was assigned

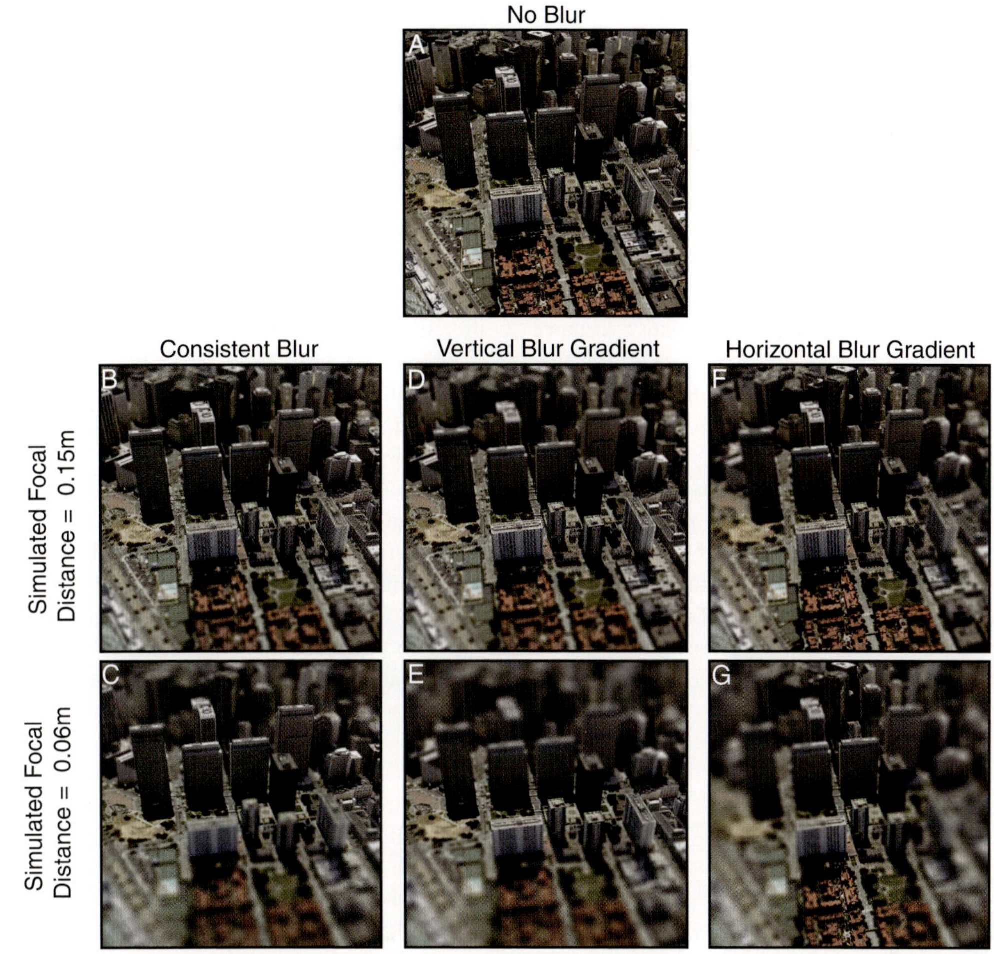


**Figure 11.13** Four types of blur used in the analysis and experiment: (A) no blur, (B and C) consistent blur, (D and E) linear vertical blur gradient, and (F and G) linear horizontal blur gradient. Simulated focal distances of 0.15 m (B, D, and F) and 0.06 m (C, E , and G) are shown. In approximating the blur produced by a short focal length, the consistent-blur condition produces the most accurate blur, followed by the vertical gradient, the horizontal gradient, and the no-blur condition. (Original city images and data from GoogleEarth are copyright Terrametrics, SanBorn, and Google.)

a blur magnitude based on its position along the gradient. Each row or column was then blurred independently using a cylindrical blur kernel of the appropriate diameter. Finally, all of the blurred pixels were recombined to create the final image. The maximum amounts of blur in the horizontal and vertical gradients were assigned to the average blur magnitudes along the top and bottom of the consistent-blur images. Thus, the histograms of blur magnitude were roughly equal across the three types of blur manipulation. Figures 11.13D–11.13G are examples of the resulting images.

We examined how the three types of blur manipulation might affect estimates of focal distance. We know that the blur in the consistent condition is completely consistent with focal distance and distance ratios, so we focused the analysis on the vertical- and horizontal-blur-gradient conditions. We first selected pixels in image regions containing contrast by employing the Canny edge detector (Canny, 1986).

The detector's parameters were set such that it found the subjectively most salient edges. We later verified that the choice of parameters did not affect the model's predictions. We then took the distance ratios $r$ in the scene from the video card's z-buffer while running GoogleEarth. These recovered distances constitute the depth map. If we implemented the Bayesian model in Eq. 11.10, there would, of course, be additional uncertainty due to the estimation of blur from images and the estimation of relative distance from perspective in the images. For the two incorrect blur conditions, the blur for each pixel was determined by the applied gradients. We assumed $A = 4.6$ mm and $s_0 = 17$ mm. We also assumed that observers use perspective to estimate $r$ correctly for each pixel relative to the pixels in the best-focused region. Having determined $b$ and $r$ from the images, and knowing $s_0$ and $A$, we used Eq. 11.8 to solve for $z_0$. All of the estimates were combined to produce a marginal distribution of estimated focal distances. The median of the distribution could be used to estimate absolute distance

Figure 11.14A shows the focal-distance estimates based on the blur and distance-ratio data from the consistent-blur image in Figure 11.13C. Because the blur was rendered correctly for the distance ratios, all of the estimates indicate the intended focal distance of 0.06 m. Therefore, the marginal distribution of estimates has zero variance and the final estimate is accurate and precise.

Figure 11.14B plots the blur/distance-ratio data from the vertical-blur image in Figure 11.13E. The focal-distance estimates now vary widely, though the majority lies close to the intended value of 0.06 m. Thus, vertical blur gradients should influence estimates of focal distance, but in a less compelling and consistent fashion than consistent blur does. It is not shown here, but scenes with larger depth variation produced marginal distributions with higher variance. This makes sense because the

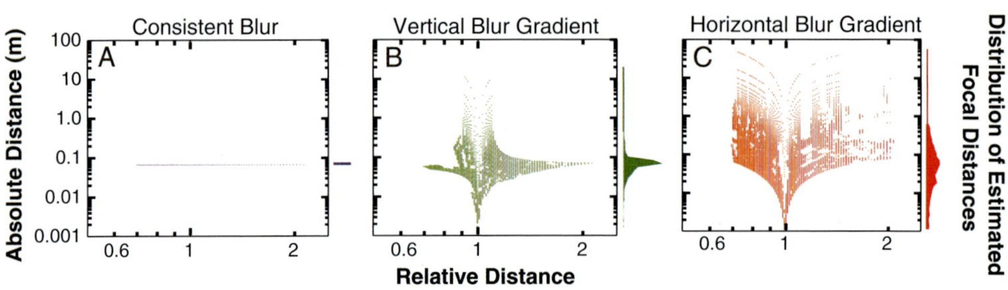


**Figure 11.14** The relationship between focal distance, blur, and perspective for images with consistent blur, vertical blur gradients, and horizontal blur gradients. Intended focal distance was 0.06 m. The left panel shows the relationship for the consistent-blur images in which the blur was completely consistent with focal distance and the distance ratio in various parts of the image. The middle and right panels show the relationship for the vertical and horizontal blur gradients. To construct these panels, we first extracted the distance ratio $r$ from the z-buffer of the video card (that is, not by using an algorithm to estimate $r$ from the image). We extracted $b$ from the blur gradients applied to the images. We then calculated $z_0$ from Eq. 11.8 using the known values of $b$, $r$, and $A$ (4.6 mm for the human eye). Each point in each panel represents a pair of $z_0$ and $r$ for a small region in the corresponding image. All of the focal distance estimates can be accumulated to form a marginal distribution of estimates (shown on the right of each panel). One could estimate $z_0$ from the median of the marginal distribution. The data from consistent-blur rendering yield a marginal distribution of zero variance because all estimates are the same. Though the vertical blur gradient incorrectly blurs several pixels, it is well correlated with the depths in the scene, so it too produces a marginal distribution with low variance. The blur applied by the horizontal gradient is mostly uncorrelated with depth, resulting in a marginal distribution with large variance and therefore the least reliable estimate.

vertical blur gradient is a closer approximation to consistent blur as the scene becomes more planar.

Figure 11.14C plots the blur/relative-distance data from the horizontal-blur image in Figure 11.13G. In horizontal gradient images, the blur is mostly uncorrelated with the relative depths in the scene, so focal-distance estimates are scattered. Although the median of the marginal distribution is similar to the ones obtained with consistent blur and the vertical gradient, the variance of the distribution is much greater. The analysis, therefore, suggests that the horizontal gradient will have the smallest influence of the three blur types on perceived distance.

## Psychophysical Experiment on Estimating Absolute Distance from Blur

We next compared human judgments of perceived distance to our model's predictions. We used the same blur-rendering techniques to generate stimuli for the psychophysical experiment: consistent blur, vertical blur gradient, and horizontal blur gradient. An additional stimulus was created by rendering each scene with no blur. The stimuli were generated from the same 14 GoogleEarth scenes on which we conducted the analysis in Figure 11.14.

The seven subjects were unaware of the experimental hypotheses. They were positioned with a chin rest 45 cm from a CRT and viewed the stimuli monocularly. Each stimulus was displayed for 3 seconds. Subjects were told to look around the scene in each image to get an impression of its distance and scale. After each stimulus presentation, subjects entered an estimate of the distance from a marked building in the center of the scene to the camera that produced the image. There were 224 unique stimuli, and each stimulus was presented seven times in random order for a total of 1568 trials.

Figure 11.15 shows the results averaged across subjects. The left and right panels show the data for the low- and high-depth-variation images, respectively. The abscissas represent simulated focal distance (the focal distance used to generate the blur in the consistent-blur condition); the values for the vertical and horizontal blur gradients are those that yielded the same maximum blur magnitudes as in the consistent-blur condition. The ordinates represent the average reported distance to the marked object in the center of the scene, divided by the average reported distance for the no-blur control condition. Lower values mean that the scene was seen as closer and therefore presumably smaller.

All subjects exhibited a statistically significant effect of blur magnitude (three-way, repeated-measures ANOVA, $p < 0.00001$), indicating that

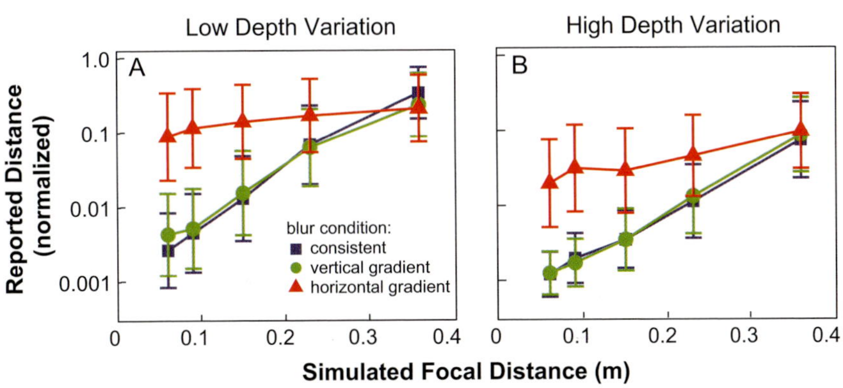


**Figure 11.15** Results of the psychophysical experiment averaged across all seven subjects. (A) and (B), respectively, show the data when the images had low and high depth variation. The type of blur manipulation is indicated by the colors and shapes of the data points. Blue squares indicate consistent blur, green circles indicate vertical blur gradient, and red triangles indicate horizontal blur gradient. Error bars represent standard errors.

the marked object appeared smaller when the blur was large. The effect of magnitude was much larger in the consistent-blur and vertical-blur-gradient conditions than in the horizontal-gradient condition, so there was a significant effect of blur type ($p < 0.00001$). There was a tendency for the high-depth-variation scenes to be seen as closer, but for blur magnitude to have a larger effect for the low-depth-variation scenes ($p = 0.18$, n.s.).

The results show that perceived absolute distance is influenced by the pattern and magnitude of blur just as the model predicts. Consistent blur and vertical-gradient blur yield systematic and predictable variations in perceived distance. Horizontal-gradient blur yields a much less systematic variation in perceived distance. Thus, two cues—blur and perspective—that by themselves do not convey absolute distance information can be used in combination to make reliable estimates of absolute distance and size.

## DISCUSSION

### Reconsidering Blur as a Depth Cue

As we mentioned earlier, previous work on humans' ability to extract depth from blur has concluded that blur is at best a coarse, qualitative cue providing no more than ordinal depth information. Can the probabilistic model presented here explain why previous work revealed no quantitative effect of blur?

Some investigators have looked for an effect of blur when disparity was present. Mather and Smith (2000) found no effect of blur in a distance-separation task except when blur specified a much larger separation than disparity, and even then the effect was quite small. Watt et al. (2005) found no effect of blur in a slant-estimation task when disparity was present. To reexamine these studies, it is useful to note that disparity and blur share a fundamental underlying geometry. Disparity is the difference in image positions created by the differing vantage points of the two eyes. Defocus blur is caused by the difference in image positions created by the differing vantage points of different parts of the pupil. In other words, they both allow an estimation of depth from triangulation. We can formalize this similarity by rewriting Eq. 11.8, which relates the diameter of the blur circle in the image to the viewing situation. Replacing the aperture $A$ with the interocular distance $I$, we obtain:

$$d = \frac{Is_0}{z_0}\left(1 - \frac{1}{r}\right), \tag{11.12}$$

where $d$ is the horizontal disparity. By combining the above equation with Eq. 11.8, we obtain:

$$\frac{b}{|d|} = \frac{A}{I}, \tag{11.13}$$

which means the blur and horizontal disparity are affected by the same viewing parameters (e.g., viewing distance, need for scaling), but that disparities are generally much larger than blur circles because $A/I$ is $\sim 1/12$ for most viewing situations. If we incorporate the signals required for disparity scaling and correction in the mapping function, we can represent the disparity likelihood function as $P(d|z_0, r)$, where $d$ is disparity (Backus et al., 1999; Gårding et al., 1995). In the format of Figure 11.12, disparity and eye-position signals together specify both distance ratio and absolute distance. Numerous psychophysical experiments have shown that very small depths can be discerned from disparity (Blakemore, 1970); much smaller than can be discriminated from changes in blur (Walsh & Charman, 1988). For this reason, the variance of the depth-from-disparity distribution is generally small, so the product distribution is affected very little by the blur. The theory, therefore, predicts little, if any, effect from blur when the depth step is specified by disparity, and this is consistent with the experimental observations of Mather and Smith (2000) and Watt et al. (2005). This does not mean of course that blur is not used as a depth cue; it just means that the disparity estimate is often so low in variance that it dominates in those viewing conditions. One would have to make the disparity signal much noisier to test for an effect from blur. It is interesting in this regard to note that disparity-discrimination thresholds worsen much more rapidly in front of and behind fixation (Blakemore, 1970) than blur-discrimination thresholds do (Walsh & Charman, 1988). Because of the difference in how discrimination thresholds worsen away from fixation, blur might well be a more reliable depth signal than disparity for points in front of and behind where one is looking.

Other investigators have examined the use of blur in distance ordering. When the stimulus consists of two textured regions with a neutral border between them, the depth between the regions is not specified. However, when the texture in one region is blurrier than the texture in the other, the blur of the border determines perceived distance ordering (Marshall et al., 1996; Mather, 1996; Palmer & Brooks, 2008). The border appears to belong to the region whose texture has similar blur, and that region is then seen as figure while the other region is seen as ground. We can represent this relationship between border and region blur with a probability distribution. The distribution would have zero probability for all distance ratios less than 1 and nonzero probability for all distance ratios greater than 1 (or the opposite, depending on whether the interregion border is blurred or sharp). The product of that distribution and the distribution derived from region blur (Fig. 11.12A) then reduces to one of the two wings of the blur function; this specifies the distance ordering, which is consistent with the previous observations (Marshall et al., 1996; Mather, 1996; Palmer & Brooks, 2008).

We conclude that previous claims that blur is a weak depth cue providing only coarse ordinal information are incorrect. When the depth information contained in blur is represented in the Bayesian framework, we can see that it provides useful information about metric depth when combined with information from nonmetric depth cues like perspective.

## Reconsidering Figure-Ground Cues as Information about Metric Depth

The role of figure-ground cues in biological and machine vision has been extensively investigated (Bertamini et al., 2008; Burge et al., 2005, 2010; Driver & Baylis, 1996; Fowlkes et al., 2007; Palmer, 1999; Peterson, Harvey, & Weidenbacher, 1991; Rubin, 1921; Vecera, Vogel, & Woodman, 2002), but no comprehensive theory of how figure-ground cues affect contour assignment and depth perception has emerged. We suggest that such a theory could be based on the statistics associated with viewing natural scenes. We showed here how this theory works for the figure-ground cue of convexity. Many other figure-ground cues could affect metric depth percepts. Consider, for example, the figure-ground cue of lower region. In images containing two regions separated by a neutral contour, the lower region tends to be seen as figure (Vecera et al., 2002). The ground plane is present in most views of natural scenes, so positions low in the visual field are likely to be nearer to the viewer than positions high in the field (Huang, Lee, & Mumford, 2000; Potetz & Lee, 2003; Yang & Purves, 2003). When we analyzed the natural-scene statistics, we observed that the asymmetry in the probability distribution of depth conditioned on elevation is greater than the asymmetry in the distribution conditioned on convexity. If the visual system has incorporated the statistics associated with lower region, we would therefore expect generally larger perceptual effects from lower region than from convexity. Psychophysical experiments confirm this expectation: lower region and convexity determine figural assignment ~70% and ~60% of the time, respectively (Peterson & Skow, 2008; Vecera et al., 2002). Lower region is also a better predictor than convexity of depth-ordering judgments in images of natural scenes (Fowlkes et al., 2007).

Other figure-ground cues—size, symmetry, familiarity, contrast, and brightness—should be amenable to the same sort of analysis.

Two motion-in-depth phenomena are consistent with our claim that figure-ground cues provide metric depth information. First, a monocularly viewed sequence of stacking disks generates a vivid sense of movement toward the viewer (Engel, Remus, & Sainath, 2006). By the traditional taxonomy, the depth cues in this stimulus provide only distance-ordering information: T-junctions (Palmer, 1999) and the figure-ground cues of surroundedness and small area (Rubin, 1921). When the stacking sequence ceases, an after-effect of movement away from the viewer occurs (Engel et al., 2006). Second, a monocularly viewed moving disk that occludes a background of vertical bars when translating leftward, and is occluded by the bars when moving rightward, is perceived as moving elliptically in depth; it also elicits vergence eye movements consistent with an elliptical path (Ringach, 1996). If cues to occlusion only provided distance-ordering information, it would be difficult to understand these motion-in-depth percepts and the induced vergence eye movements. However, if occlusion cues provide metric information, as proposed here, the percepts and accompanying eye movements are readily understood.

In addition to the figure-ground cues, many depth cues such as aerial perspective (Fry et al., 1949; Troscianko, Montagnon, Le Clerc, Malbert, & Chanteau, 1991) and shading (Koenderink & van Doorn, 1992) are regarded as nonmetric because, from the cue value alone, one cannot uniquely determine depths in the scene. This view stems from considering only the geometric relationship between retinal-image features associated with the cue and depth; with these cues, there is no deterministic relationship between relevant image features and depth in the scene. We propose instead that the visual system uses the information in those cues probabilistically, much as it uses convexity. From this, it follows that all depth cues have the potential to affect metric depth estimates as long as there is a nonuniform statistical relationship between the cue value and depth in the environment.

Consider, for example, contrast, saturation, and brightness. O'Shea, Govan, and Sekuler (1994) showed that the relative contrast of two adjoining regions affects perceived distance ordering: the region with higher contrast is typically perceived as nearer than the low-contrast region. Egusa (1983) and Troscianko et al. (1991) showed that desaturated images appear farther than saturated images. The retinal-image contrast and saturation associated with a given object are affected by increasing atmospheric attenuation across distance in natural scenes (Fry et al., 1949). Thus, these two perceptual effects are undoubtedly due to the viewer incorporating statistics relating contrast, saturation, and absolute distance. Brightness affects perceived distance ordering as well (Egusa, 1983): brighter regions are seen as nearer than darker ones. This effect is also understandable from natural-scene statistics because dark regions tend to be farther from the viewer than bright regions (Potetz & Lee, 2003).

We argue that all depth cues should be conceptualized in a probabilistic framework. Such an approach has recently been explored in computer vision where machine-learning techniques were used to combine statistical information about depth and surface orientation provided by a diverse set of image features (Hoiem et al., 2005; Saxena et al., 2005). Some of these features were similar to known monocular depth cues; others were not. From the information contained in a large collection of these features, the algorithms were able to generate reasonably accurate estimates of 3D scene layout. These results show that useful metric information is available from image features that have traditionally been considered nonmetric depth cues. Interestingly, the results also show that useful depth information is available from image features that have not yet been identified as depth cues.

Our results and the aforementioned computer-vision results indicate that the conventional, geometry-based taxonomy that classifies depth cues according to the type of distance information they provide is unnecessary. By capitalizing on the statistical relationship between images and the environment to which our visual systems have been exposed, the probabilistic approach used here will yield a richer understanding of how we perceive 3D layout.

### Experimental Verification of Bayesian Models

Many observations in the perception literature are compatible with the Bayesian framework. These include the observations that the variances of different sources of sensory information are taken into account in essentially optimal fashion when multiple sources are available (e.g., Alais & Burr, 2004; Ernst & Banks, 2002; Knill & Saunders, 2003). They also include observations that prior information affects perception (Mamassian & Goucher, 2001; Weiss, Simoncelli, & Adelson, 2002). However, from the standpoint of theory testing, there is something missing here.

A key idea in the Bayesian characterization of perceptual processing is that perceptual systems have internalized the statistical properties of the natural environment and the noises involved in sensory measurement, and that the systems use those properties efficiently to make optimal inferences. But on closer examination, previous work has not demonstrated that perceptual systems do in fact make optimal inferences. An example helps explain this point.

Many perceptual effects cannot be explained from *a priori* geometric constraints alone. For example, perceived speed decreases when the contrast of the moving stimulus is reduced (Stocker & Simoncelli, 2006; Weiss et al., 2002). This effect can be understood in the Bayesian framework if we assume that the visual system has a prior for slow motion. If such a prior exists, we would expect lower contrast objects to be perceived as slower than higher contrast objects: With lower contrast, the variance of sensory measurement increases and the prior would have greater influence, pulling perceived speed toward zero. Using this observation, Stocker and Simoncelli (2006) estimated the prior for speed from psychophysical data. Their analysis yielded a prior for speed that was peaked at zero and had longer tails than a Gaussian distribution. Although the estimated prior is consistent with a variety of phenomena in motion perception (Weiss et al., 2002), there is no evidence that the estimated prior actually corresponds to the state of the natural environment. To determine whether it does would require knowledge of what the speed prior for the natural environment is, so that one could compare the estimated prior to "ground truth." Thus, it cannot be argued from that analysis alone that the visual system has internalized statistical properties of the environment accurately.

The figure-ground work described here attempts to close this gap by measuring the statistics from natural scenes and seeing whether observers have internalized those same statistics. We showed that people behave as though they use an asymmetric convexity-depth distribution when making depth judgments in the presence of a region-bounding contour. The distribution they appear to be using is like the distribution for natural scenes in that it is well fit by power laws with different exponents for positive and negative distance separations. Our experiment thus demonstrated the ecological validity of convexity as a cue to metric depth and explained its usefulness to the visual system. But we too did not close the aforementioned gap because the distributions we estimated from the psychophysical data were not quantitatively the same as the distributions we measured from natural scenes. Thus, with the possible exceptions of findings in contour grouping (Elder & Goldberg, 2002; Geisler, Perry, Super, & Gallogly, 2001; Ren & Malik, 2002) and figure-ground assignment (Fowlkes et al., 2007), the field still awaits evidence that the internalized statistics really do match the statistics of natural scenes.

### Natural-Scene Statistics and Depth Perception

The importance of natural-scene statistics in perceptual tasks was first articulated by Brunswik (Brunswik & Kamiya, 1953), who argued that Gestalt cues could and should be ecologically validated. The role of natural-scene statistics has since been investigated in relation to several perceptual tasks: contour grouping (Elder & Goldberg, 2002; Geisler et al., 2001; Ren & Malik, 2002), figure-ground assignment (Fowlkes et al., 2007), and length estimation (Howe & Purves, 2002). It is useful to distinguish this work from a much larger literature on how the statistics of natural images relate to neural coding. Current thinking in natural-image work is that processing in early visual pathways evolved to code and transmit information about retinal images as efficiently as possible (Barlow, 1961; Simoncelli & Olshausen, 2001). To determine the encoding efficiency, one needs to know the statistics of the image properties to be encoded, so recent work has focused on measuring natural-image statistics and determining whether visual cortical neurons are constructed to exploit those statistics (Olshausen & Field, 1996; Vinje & Gallant, 2000). It is unclear, however, that efficient encoding is the primary task of early visual processing.

To make strong claims about the role of natural statistics in perception, it is important to study tasks that are known to be critical for the biological system under study. By knowing that the task is critical, one can determine that a failure to exploit the task-relevant statistics is due to suboptimal performance in a necessary task, rather than to a mistaken hypothesis about what the system was designed to do. Surely one of the most important perceptual tasks is to estimate the 3D layout of the environment because such estimation is required for guidance of visuomotor behavior in that environment (Geisler, 2008). For this reason, we chose to focus our work on the task of estimating 3D layout. We found in the analysis of convexity that people have, in fact, incorporated depth information contained in natural-scene statistics. We found in the analysis of blur that people have, in fact, incorporated depth information contained in how retinal images are formed.

## REFERENCES


Akeley, K., Watt, S. J., Girshick, A. R., & Banks, M. S. (2004). A stereo display prototype with multiple focal distances. *ACM Transactions in Graphics, 23*, 804–813.

Alais D., & Burr, D. (2004). The ventriloquist effect results from near-optimal cross-modal integration. *Current Biology, 14*, 257–262.

Backus, B. T., Banks, M. S., van Ee, R., & Crowell, J. A. (1999). Horizontal and vertical disparity, eye position, and stereoscopic slant perception. *Vision Research, 39*, 1143–1170.

Barlow, H. B. (1961). Possible principles underlying the transformation of sensory messages. In W. A. Rosenblith (Ed.), *Sensory communication* (pp. 217–234). Cambridge, MA: MIT Press.

Berkeley, G. (1709). *An essay toward a new theory of vision.* Dublin, Ireland: Pepyat.

Bertamini, M., Martinovic, J., & Wuerger, S. M. (2008). Integration of ordinal and metric cues in depth processing. *Journal of Vision, 8*(2):10, 1–12.

Blakemore, C. (1970). The range and scope of binocular depth discrimination in man. *Journal of Physiology, 211*, 599–622.

Brillaut-O'Mahony, B. (1991). New method for vanishing point detection. *CVGIP: Image Understanding, 54*, 289–300.

Brunswik, E., & Kamiya, J. (1953). Ecological cue validity of "proximity" and of other gestalt factors. *American Journal of Psychology, 66*, 20–32.

Burge, J., Fowlkes, C. C., & Banks, M. S. (2010). Natural-scene statistics predict the influence of the figure-ground cue of convexity on human depth. *Journal of Neuroscience, 30*, 7269–7280.

Burge, J., Peterson, M. A., & Palmer, S.E. (2005). Ordinal configural cues combine with metric disparity in depth perception. *Journal of Vision, 5*, 534–542.

Canny, J. F. (1986). A computational approach to edge detection. *IEEE Transactions Pattern Analysis and Machine Intelligence, 8*, 679–698.

Caudek, C., & Proffitt, D. R. (1993). Depth perception in motion parallax and stereokinesis. *Journal of Experimental Psychology: Human Perception and Performance, 19*, 32–47.

Cormack, L. K., Landers, D. D., & Ramakrishnan, S. (1997). Element density and the efficiency of binocular matching. *Journal of Optical Society of America A, 14*, 723–730.

Coughlan, J. M., & Yuille, A. L. (2003). Manhattan world: Orientation and outlier detection by Bayesian inference. *Neural Computation, 15*, 1063–1088.

Driver, J., & Baylis, G. (1996). Edge-assignment and figure-ground organization in short term visual matching. *Cognitive Psychology, 31*, 248–306.

Egusa, H. (1983). Effects of brightness, hue, and saturation on perceived depth between adjacent regions in the visual field. *Perception, 12*, 167–175.

Elder, J. H., & Goldberg, R. M. (2002). Ecological statistics of Gestalt laws for the perceptual organization of contours. *Journal of Vision, 2*, 324–353.

Engel, S. A., Remus, D. A., & Sainath, R. (2006). Motion from occlusion. *Journal of Vision, 6*, 649–652.

Ernst, M. O., & Banks, M. S. (2002). Humans integrate visual and haptic information in a statistically optimal fashion. *Nature, 415*, 429–433.

Farid, H., & Simoncelli, E. P. (1998). Range estimation by optical differentiation. *Journal of the Optical Society of America A, 15*, 1777–1786.

Fielding, R. (1985). *Special effects cinematography.* Oxford, England: Focal Press.

Fisher, S. K., & Ciuffreda, K. J. (1988). Accommodation and apparent distance. *Perception, 17*, 609–621.

Flickr. (2009). Flickr group: Tilt shift miniaturization fakes. Retrieved from http://www.flickr.com/groups/59319377@N00

Fowlkes, C. C., Martin, D. R., & Malik, J. (2007). Local figure/ground cues are valid for natural images. *Journal of Vision, 7*(8):2, 1–9.

Fry, G. A., Bridgeman, C. S., & Ellerbrock, V. J. (1949). The effects of atmospheric scattering on binocular depth perception. *American Journal of Optometry and Archives of American Academy of Optometry, 26*, 9–15.

Gårding, J., Porrill, J., Mayhew, J. E. W., & Frisby, J. P. (1995). Stereopsis, vertical disparity and relief transformations. *Vision Research, 35*, 703–722.

Geisler, W. S. (2008). Visual perception and the statistical properties of natural scenes. *Annual Review of Psychology, 59*, 10.1–10.26.

Geisler, W. S., Perry, J. S., Super, B. J., & Gallogly, D. P. (2001). Edge co-occurrence in natural images predicts contour grouping performance. *Vision Research, 41*, 711–724.

Georgeson, M. A., May, K. A., Freeman, T. C. A., & Hesse, G. S. (2007). From filters to features: Scale-space analysis of edge and blur coding in human vision. *Journal of Vision, 7*(13):7, 1–21.

Gillam, B. J., Anderson, B. L., & Rizwi, F. (2009). Failure of facial configural cues to alter metric stereoscopic depth. *Journal of Vision, 9*(1):3, 1–5.

Haeberli, P., & Akeley, K. (1990). The accumulation buffer: Hardware support for high-quality rendering. *ACM SIGGRAPH Computer Graphics, 24*, 309–318.

Held, R. T., Cooper, E. A., O'Brien, J. F., & Banks, M. S. (2010). Using blur to affect perceived distance and size. *ACM Transactions on Graphics, 29*(2), Article 19, 1–16.

Hillis, J. M., Watt, S. J., Landy, M. S., & Banks, M. S. (2004). Slant from texture and disparity cues: Optimal cue combination. *Journal of Vision, 4*, 967–992.

Hogervorst, M. A., & Eagle, R. A. (1998). Biases in three-dimensional structure-from-motion arise from noise in early the visual system. *Proceedings of the Royal Society of London B, 265*, 1587–1593.

Hogervorst, M. A., & Eagle, R. A. (2000). The role of perspective effects and accelerations in perceived three-dimensional structure-from-motion. *Journal of Experimental Psychology: Human Perception and Performance, 26*, 934–955.

Hoiem, D., Efros, A. A., & Hebert, M. (2005). Geometric context from a single image. *Proceedings of the IEEE International Conference on Computer Vision*, 1–8, 654–661.

Howard, I. P., & Rogers, B. J. (2002). *Seeing in depth, Vol. 2. Depth perception.* Toronto, Canada: I. Porteous.

Howe, C. Q., & Purves, D. (2002). Range image statistics can explain the anomalous perception of length. *Proceedings of the National Academy of Sciences USA, 99*, 13184–13188.

Huang, J., Lee, A. B., & Mumford, D. (2000). Statistics of range images. *Proceedings of the IEEE Conference on Computational Vision and Pattern Recognition, 1*, 324–331.

Kanizsa, G., & Gerbino, W. (1976). Convexity and symmetry in figure-ground organization. In M. Henle (Ed.), *Vision and artifact* (pp. 25–32). New York, NY: Springer.

Kingslake, R. (1992). *Optics in photography.* Bellingham, WA: SPIE Optical Engineering Press.

Knill, D. C. (1998). Discrimination of planar surface slant from texture: Human and ideal observers compared. *Vision Research, 38*, 1683–1711.

Knill, D. C., & Saunders, J.A. (2003). Do humans optimally integrate stereo and texture information to slant? *Vision Research, 43*, 2539–2558.

Koenderink, J. J., & van Doorn, A. J. (1992). Surface shape and curvatures scales. *Image and Vision Computing, 10*, 557–565.

Laforet, V. (2007, May 31). A really big show. *New York Times.*

Landy, M. S., Maloney, L. T., Johnston, E. B., & Young, M. (1995). Measurement and modeling of depth cue combination: In defense of weak fusion. *Vision Research, 35*, 389–412.

Love, G. D., Hoffman, D. M., Hands, P. J. W., Gao, J., Kirby, A. K., & Banks, M. S. (2009). High-speed switchable lens enables the development of a volumetric stereoscopic display. *Optics Express, 17*, 15716–15725.

Mamassian, P., & Goucher, R. (2001). Prior knowledge on the illumination position. *Cognition, 81*, B1–B9.

Marshall, J., Burbeck, C., Ariely, D., Rolland, J., & Martin, K. (1996). Occlusion edge blur: A cue to relative visual depth. *Journal of the Optical Society of America A, 13*, 681–688.

Mather, G. (1996). Image blur as a pictorial depth cue. *Proceedings of the Royal Society of London B: Biological Sciences, 263*, 169–172.

Mather, G. (1997). The use of image blur as a depth cue. *Perception, 26*, 1147–1158.

Mather, G., & Smith, D. R. R. (2000). Depth cue integration: Stereopsis and image blur. *Vision Research, 40*, 3501–3506.

Mather, G., & Smith, D. R. R. (2002). Blur discrimination and its relationship to blur-mediated depth perception. *Perception, 31*, 1211–1219.

McCloskey, S., & Langer, M. (2009, June). Planar orientation from blur gradients in a single image. *Proceedings of the IEEE Conference on Computer Vision and Pattern Recognition*, 2318–2325.

McKee, S. P., Levi, D. M., & Bowne, S. F. (1990). The imprecision of stereopsis. *Vision Research, 30*, 1763–1779.

Metzger, F. (1953). *Gesetze des Sehens.* Frankfurt-am-Main, Germany: Waldemar Kramer.

Mon-Williams, M., & Tresilian, J. R. (1999). Ordinal depth information from accommodation? *Ergonomics, 43*, 391–404.

Morgan, M. J., Watamanuik, S. N. J., & McKee, S. P. (2000). The use of an implicit standard for measuring discrimination thresholds. *Vision Research, 40*, 2341–2349.

Okatani, T., & Deguchi, K. (2007). Estimating scale of a scene from a single image based on defocus blur and scene geometry. *Computer Vision and Pattern Recognition*, 1–8.

Olshausen, B., & Field, D. (1996). Emergence of simple-cell receptive field properties by learning a sparse code for natural images. *Nature, 381*, 607–609.

O'Shea, R. P., Blackburn, S., & Ono, H. (1994). Contrast as a depth cue. *Vision Research, 34*, 1595–1604.

O'Shea, R. P., Govan, D. G., & Sekuler, R. (1997). Blur and contrast as pictorial depth cues. *Perception, 26*, 599–612.

Palmer, S. E. (1999). *Vision science: Photons to phenomenology.* Cambridge, MA: MIT Press.

Palmer, S. E., & Brooks, J. L. (2008). Edge-region grouping in figure-ground organization and depth perception. *Journal of Experimental Psychology: Human Perception and Performance, 24*, 1353–1371.

Pentland, A. P. (1987). A new sense for depth of field. *IEEE Transactions on Pattern Analysis and Machine, 9*, 523–531.

Peterson, M. A., Harvey, E. H., & Weidenbacher, H. L. (1991). Shape recognition contributions to figure-ground organization: Which route counts? *Journal of Experimental Psychology: Human Perception and Performance, 17*, 1075–1089.

Peterson, M. A., & Skow, E. (2008). Inhibitory competition between shape properties in figure-ground perception. *Journal of Experimental Psychology, 32*, 251–267.

Potetz, B., & Lee, T. S. (2003). Statistical correlations between 2D images and 3D structures in natural scenes. *Journal of Optical Society of America A, 20*, 1292–1303.

Ren, X., & Malik, J. (2002). A probabilistic multi-scale model for contour completion based on image statistics. *Proceedings of the 7th ECCV, Vol. 1*, 312–327. New York, NY: Springer.

Ringach, D. L. (1996). Binocular eye movements caused by the perception of three-dimensional structure from motion. Doctoral dissertation New York University, New York, NY.

Rubin, E. (1921). *Visuell Wahrgenommene Figuren.* Kobenhaven, Germany: Glydenalske Boghandel.

Saxena, A., Chung, S. H., & Ng, A. Y. (2005). Learning depth from single monocular images. In Y. Weiss, B. Schölkopf, & J. Platt (Eds.), *Advances in neural information processing systems 18* (pp. 1161–1168). Cambridge, MA: MIT Press.

Simoncelli, E. P., & Olshausen, B. A. (2001). Natural image statistics and neural representation. *Annual Review of Neuroscience, 24*, 1193–1216.

Spring, K., & Stiles, W. S. (1948). Variation of pupil size with change in the angle at which the light stimulus strikes the retina. *British Journal of Ophthalmology, 32*, 340–346.

Stocker, A. A., & Simoncelli, E. P. (2006). Noise characteristics and prior expectations in human visual speed perception. *Nature Neuroscience, 9*, 578–585.

Troscianko, T., Montagnon, R., Le Clerc, J., Malbert, E., & Chanteau, P. (1991). The role of color as a monocular depth cue. *Vision Research, 31,* 1923–1930.

Vecera, S. P., Vogel, E. K. & Woodman, G. F. (2002). Lower region: A new cue for figure-ground assignment. *Journal of Experimental Psychology, 131,* 194–205.

Vinje, W. E., & Gallant, J. L. (2000). Sparse coding and decorrelation in primary visual cortex during natural vision. *Science, 287,* 1273–1276.

von Helmholtz, H. (1867). *Handbuch der Physiologischen Optik.* Leipzig, Germany: Leopold Voss.

Wallach, H., & Norris, C. M. (1963). Accommodation as a distance cue. *American Journal of Psychology, 76,* 659–664.

Walsh, G., & Charman, W. N. (1988). Visual sensitivity to temporal change in focus and its relevance to the accommodation response. *Vision Research, 28,* 1207–1221.

Watt, S. J., Akeley, K., Ernst, M. O., & Banks, M. S. (2005). Focus cues affect perceived depth. *Journal of Vision, 5,* 834–862.

Weiss, Y., Simoncelli, E. P., & Adelson, E. H. (2002). Motion illusions as optimal percepts. *Nature Neuroscience, 5,* 598–604.

Wichmann, F. A., & Hill, N. J. (2001). The psychometric function: II. Bootstrap-based confidence intervals and sampling. *Perception and Psychophysics, 63,* 1314–1329.

Wilson, B. J., Decker, K. E., & Roorda, A. (2002). Monochromatic aberrations provide an odd-error cue to focus direction. *Journal of the Optical Society of America A, 19,* 833–839.

Yang, Z., & Purves, D. (2003). A statistical explanation of visual space. *Nature Neuroscience, 6,* 632–640.

# CHAPTER 12

# Multisensory Perception: From Integration to Remapping

*Marc O. Ernst and Massimiliano Di Luca*

## INTRODUCTION

The brain receives information about the environment from all the sensory modalities, including vision, touch, and audition. To interact efficiently with the environment, this information must eventually converge to form a reliable and accurate multimodal percept. This process is often complicated by the existence of noise at every level of signal processing, which makes the sensory information derived from the world unreliable and inaccurate. We define *reliability* as the inverse variance of the probability distribution that describes the information a sensory signal contributes to the perceptual estimation process. In contrast, *accuracy* is defined as the probability with which the sensory signal truly represents the magnitude of the real-world physical property that it reflects. In other words, it is inversely related to the probability of a sensory signal being biased with respect to the world property. There are several ways in which the nervous system may minimize the negative consequences of noise in terms of reliability and accuracy. Two key strategies are to combine redundant sensory estimates and to use prior knowledge. There is behavioral evidence that the human nervous system employs both of these strategies to reduce the adverse effects of noise and thus to improve perceptual estimates.

In this chapter, we elaborate further on how these strategies may be used by the nervous system to obtain the best possible estimates from noisy signals. We first describe how weighted averaging can increase the reliability of sensory estimates, which is the benefit of multisensory integration. Then, we point out that integration can also come at a cost of introducing inaccuracy in the sensory estimates. This shows that there is a need to balance the benefits and costs of integration. This is done using the Bayesian approach, with a joint likelihood function representing the reliability of the sensory estimates (e.g., $\hat{S}_V$ and $\hat{S}_H$, for visual and haptic sensory estimates) and a joint prior probability distribution providing the co-occurrence statistics of sensory signals $p(S_V, S_H)$, that is, the prior probability of jointly encountering an ensemble of sensory signals derived from the world. This framework naturally leads to a continuum of integration between fusion and segregation. We further show how this framework can be used to model the breakdown of integration by having the joint prior conditioned on multisensory discordance (i.e., a separation of the sensory signals in time, space, or some other measure of similarity). If the multisensory signals differ constantly over a period of time, because they may be consistently inaccurate, recalibration of the multisensory estimates will be the result. The rate of recalibration can be described using a Kalman-filter model, which can also be derived from the Bayesian approach. We conclude by proposing how integration and recalibration can be jointly described under this common approach.

## MULTISENSORY INTEGRATION

For estimating a specific environmental property, such as the size of an object in the world $S_W$, there are often multiple sources of sensory information available. For example, an object's size can be estimated by sight and touch (haptics), $S_V$ and $S_H$. Typical models of sensory integration assume unbiased (accurate) sensory signals (i.e., $S_V = S_H$) with normally distributed noise sources that are independent, a situation in which sensory integration is beneficial (see Chapter 1; Landy, Maloney, Johnston, & Young, 1995). For the estimation of an object's size from vision and touch, the assumption of independent noise sources is likely to be true since most of the neuronal processing for sensory signals, that is, their transmission from sensory transducers to the brain, is largely independent. As was introduced in Chapter 1, Figure 12.1 illustrates the optimal mechanism of sensory combination given these assumptions and given that the goal is to compute a minimum-variance estimate. This can be considered the standard model of sensory integration. The likelihood functions represent two independent estimates of size, the visual size estimate $\hat{S}_V$ and the haptic size estimate $\hat{S}_H$, based on sensory measurements $(z_V, z_H)$ that are corrupted by noise (with standard deviations $\sigma_V$ and $\sigma_H$). The integrated multisensory estimate $\hat{S}_{VH}$ is a weighted average of the individual sensory estimates with weights $w_V$ and $w_H$ that sum up to unity (Cochran, 1937):

$$\hat{S}_{VH} = w_V \hat{S}_V + w_H \hat{S}_H, \text{ where } w_V + w_H = 1. \quad (12.1)$$

To achieve optimal performance, the chosen weights need to be proportional to the reliability $r$, which is defined as the inverse of the signal variance:

$$w_j = \frac{r_j}{\sum_i r_i}, \text{ with } r_i = \frac{1}{\sigma_i^2}. \quad (12.2)$$

The indices $i$ and $j$ refer to the sensory modalities $(V, H)$. The modality that provides more reliable information in a given situation is given a higher weight, and so has a greater influence on the final percept. In the example shown in Figure 12.1, visual information about the size of the object is four times more reliable than the haptic information. Therefore, the combined estimate (the weighted sum) is "closer" to the visual estimate than the haptic one (in the present example the visual weight is 0.8 according to Eq. 12.2). In another circumstance where the haptic modality might provide a more reliable estimate, the situation would be reversed.

Given this weighting scheme, the benefit of integration is that the variance of the combined estimate from vision and touch is less than that of either of the individual estimates that are fed into the averaging process. Therefore, the combined estimate arising from integration of multiple sources of independent information shows greater reliability and diminished effects of noise. Mathematically, this is expressed by the combined reliability $r$ being the sum of the individual reliabilities:

$$r = \sum_i r_i. \quad (12.3)$$

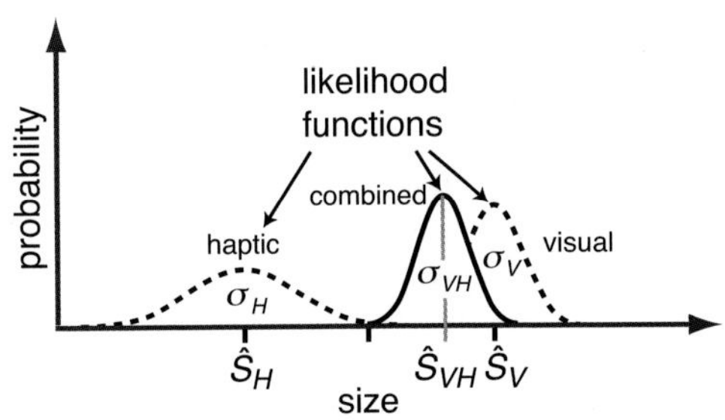


**Figure 12.1** Schematic representation of the likelihood functions of the individual visual and haptic size estimates $\hat{S}_V$ and $\hat{S}_H$ and of the combined visual-haptic size estimate $\hat{S}_{VH}$, which is a weighted average according to Eq. 12.1. The variance associated with the visual-haptic distribution is less than either of the two individual estimates (Eq. 12.3). (Adapted from Ernst & Banks, 2002.)

Given that all estimates are unbiased, this integration scheme can be considered statistically optimal, since it provides the lowest possible variance of its combined estimate. Thus, this form of sensory combination is the best way to reduce uncertainty given the assumptions that all estimates are accurate and contain Gaussian-distributed, independent noise (Chapter 1). Even if the noise distributions of the individual signals displayed a correlation, averaging of sensory information would still be advantageous and the combined estimate would still be more reliable than each individual estimate alone (Oruç, Maloney, & Landy, 2003).

Several studies have tested this integration scheme empirically (e.g., Gharahmani, Wolpert, & Jordan, 1997; van Beers, Sittig, & Denier van der Gon, 1998, 1999). In 2002, Ernst and Banks showed that humans integrate visual and haptic information in such a statistically optimal fashion. It has further been demonstrated that this finding of optimality also holds across and within other sensory modalities, for example, vision and audition (e.g., Alais & Burr, 2004; Hillis, Watt, Landy, & Banks, 2004; Knill & Saunders, 2003; Landy & Kojima, 2001). Thus, weighted averaging of sensory information appears to be a general strategy employed by the perceptual system to decrease the detrimental effects of noise.

If redundant sources of sensory information are absent or if the noises of these sources are perfectly correlated, averaging different estimates is not an option to reduce noise. However, because the world is structured quite regularly, the nervous system can use prior knowledge about such statistical regularities to reduce the uncertainty and ambiguity in neuronal signals. Prior knowledge can also be formalized as a probability distribution in a manner similar to that for sensory signals corrupted by noise. For example, let us consider the distribution of velocities for all objects. While some objects in our environment do move around occasionally, from a purely statistical point of view, on average most objects are likely to remain stationary at most times, that is, the velocity of an object is most likely to be zero. Thus, a reasonable probability distribution describing the velocity of all objects is centered at zero with some variance (Stocker & Simoncelli, 2006; Weiss, Simoncelli, & Adelson 2002). This prior knowledge can be combined with unreliable sensory evidence in order to minimize the uncertainty in the final velocity estimate. If all the probability distributions are Gaussian, using Bayes' rule it is possible to derive that the combined posterior estimate (the maximum a posteriori or MAP estimate) is a weighted average as well; however, now it is a weighted average between the prior and the likelihood function, that is, the sensory evidence:

$$\hat{S}_{MAP} = w_{likelihood}\hat{S}_{likelihood} + w_{prior}\hat{S}_{prior}. \quad (12.4)$$

The reliability of the MAP estimate then is given by:

$$r_{MAP} = r_{likelihood} + r_{prior}. \quad (12.5)$$

The principles of weighted averaging and the use of prior knowledge can be combined and placed into a larger mathematical framework of optimal statistical estimation and decision theory, known as Bayesian decision theory (Chapter 1; Mamassian, Landy, & Maloney, 2002). This approach is illustrated in Figure 12.2 in the context of the action-perception loop. Psychophysical experiments have confirmed that at least some aspects of human perception and action that deal with noise and uncertainty can be described well using this Bayesian framework (e.g., Adams, Graf, & Ernst, 2004; Kersten, Mamassian, & Yuille, 2004; Körding & Wolpert, 2004; Stocker & Simoncelli, 2006).

## THE COST OF INTEGRATION

While weighted averaging of sensory measurements or use of prior knowledge has the benefit of reducing noise and uncertainty in perceptual estimates, it also incurs a potential cost. The cost is the introduction of potential biases into perception. Biases can occur, for example, when the sensory estimates ($\hat{S}_V$ and $\hat{S}_H$) as defined by the likelihood functions and thus sensory signals ($S_V$ and $S_H$) do not accurately represent the physical stimuli ($S_{W_V}$ and $S_{W_H}$). Accuracy of

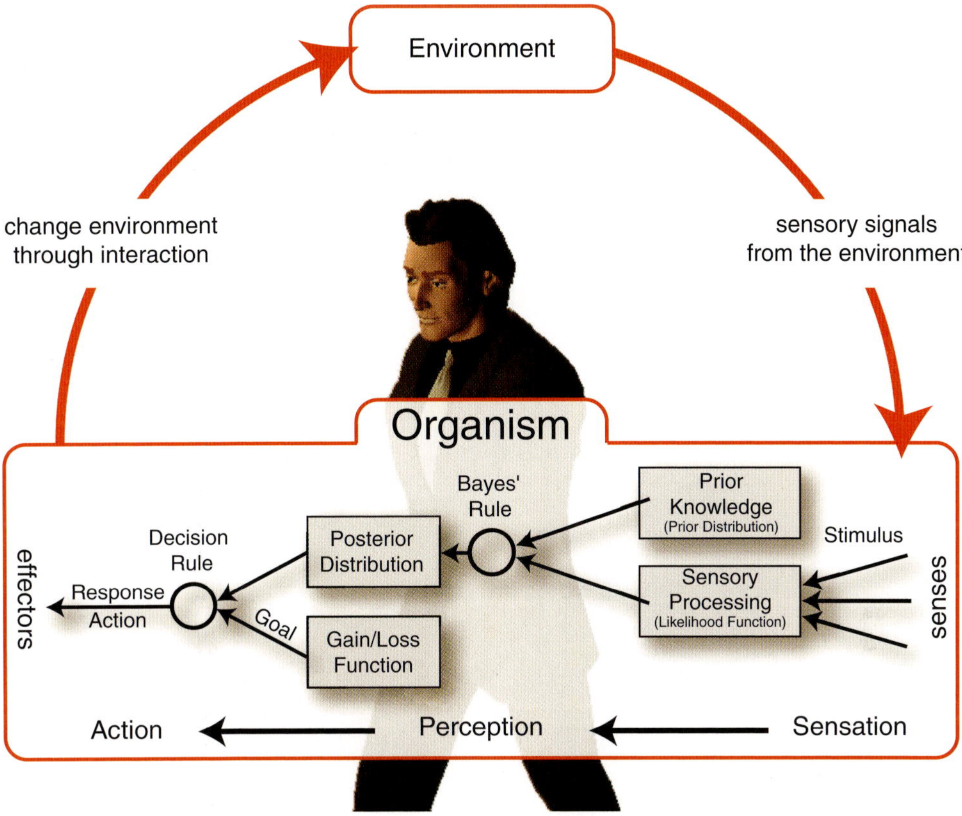


**Figure 12.2** The action/perception-loop schematically illustrates the processing of information according to Bayesian decision theory. Multiple sensory signals are averaged during sensory processing and then combined with prior knowledge, to derive the most reliable, unbiased estimate (posterior) that can be used in a task that has a goal as defined by a gain or loss function. (Adapted from Ernst & Bülthoff, 2004.)

the sensory estimates was one of the assumptions made in the previous section for deriving the optimal integration scheme (Chapter 1). However, if the estimates are no longer accurate due to external or internal influences on the signals, the potential cost of biases has to be considered.[1] Examples of sources of inaccuracies in signals may be muscle fatigue, variance in grip posture, or wearing gloves. Additionally there might be glasses that distort the visual image and so affect visual position estimates, or effects of temperature or humidity that affect sound propagation and thus affect auditory estimates, to name just a few. Figure 12.3A illustrates some examples of processes that might affect the accuracy of visual-haptic size estimates. The top panel shows sensory signals ($S_V$ and $S_H$) that are accurate with respect to the world property $S_W$ (so $S_W = S_{W_V} = S_{W_H} = S_V = S_H$) to be estimated (i.e., the size of the object at a specific position), followed by three examples of $S_V$ and $S_H$ signals that are inaccurate and contain an additional bias $B$ (i.e., $S_V = S_{W_V} + B_V$ and $S_H = S_{W_H} + B_H$). For now we assume that the signals are derived from the same location, so the visual and haptic sizes to be estimated are identical: $S_W = S_{W_V} = S_{W_H}$.

If the sensory signals $S_V$ and $S_H$, and hence the sensory estimates derived from these signals,

[1]Throughout the paper we are only considering additive biases, although the general scheme can be extended to other forms of biases, for example, multiplicative biases.

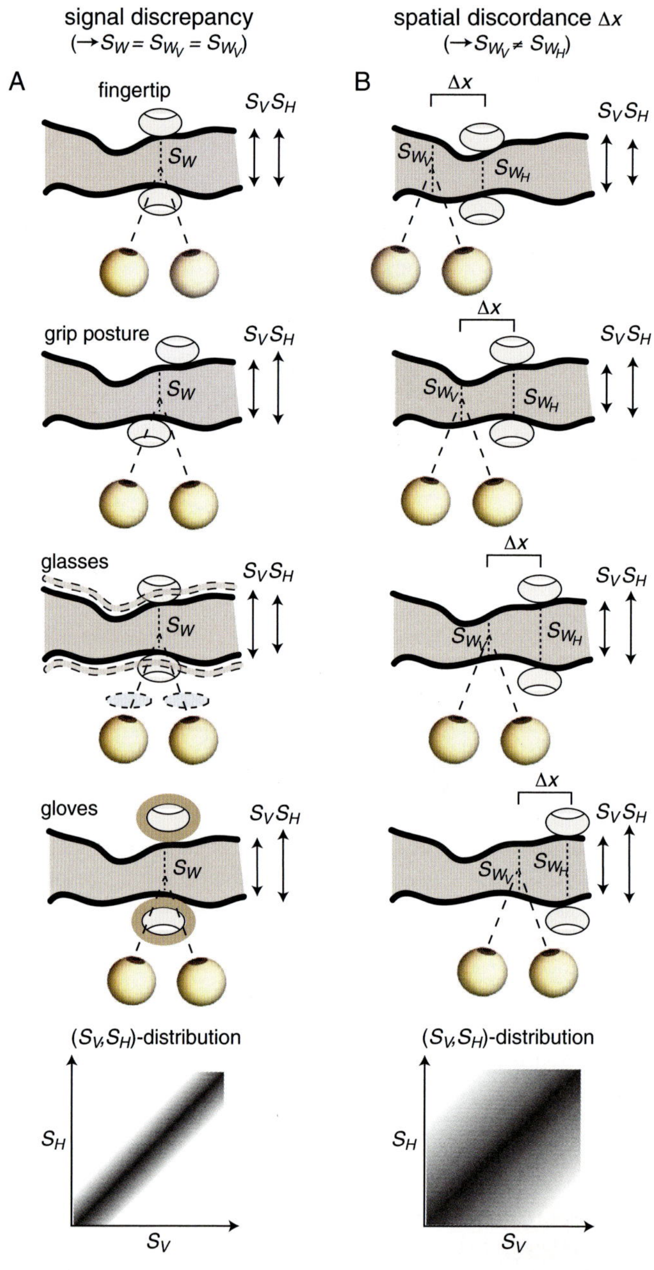


**Figure 12.3** (A) Visual and haptic size signals $S_V$ and $S_H$ measured near the same location on an object at which the true size is $S_W$. In this case visual and haptic sizes are identical ($S_{W_V} = S_{W_H}$). The sensory signals can be corrupted by various disturbances, which affect their accuracy, such as different grip postures, glasses, or gloves. (B) Visual and haptic size signals $S_V$ and $S_H$ derived from locations on an object in close proximity (offset horizontally by $\Delta x$). In this case visual and haptic sizes may differ slightly ($S_{W_V} \neq S_{W_H}$). Thus, the visual and haptic size signals will also differ slightly due to variations in the shape of the object. However, in general there will still be a correlation between the $S_V$ and $S_H$ signals as the object's size varies smoothly. Most probably this correlation will decrease with increasing $\Delta x$. In both cases, the lower panel labeled ($S_V$, $S_H$)–distribution provides the co-occurrence statistics of the signal values $S_V$ and $S_H$ that build the basis for the prior used for multisensory integration.

$\hat{S}_V$ and $\hat{S}_H$,[2] are inaccurate, that is, if they are biased by $B = (B_V, B_H)$ with respect to the world property $S_W$ or with respect to each other (sensory discrepancy $D = S_V - S_H = (S_W + B_V) - (S_W + B_H)$), their respective values need not necessarily agree even when they are derived from the same location ($S_W = S_{W_V} = S_{W_H}$). In such a case, weighted averaging of the estimates derived from these biased signals will inevitably also bias the combined estimate. To avoid the cost of biased estimates, the perceptual system must be able to infer how accurate the signals are. *This is a difficult problem that cannot be determined directly from the sensory estimates, because these estimates do not carry information about their own accuracy.* Reliability, on the other hand, which is the inverse variance associated with the estimates, can be directly assessed from sensory measurements. Furthermore, the mere existence of a discrepancy between sensory estimates $\hat{D} = \hat{S}_V - \hat{S}_H$ does not reveal whether some of the estimates are inaccurate, because even when they are accurate, the presence of noise in the estimation process will cause the respective peaks of their likelihood functions to disagree slightly (as illustrated in Fig. 12.1). We will discuss later in the chapter how persistently biased estimates may be avoided through the process of recalibration.

A problem regarding potential biases also exists while using prior knowledge to reduce perceptual uncertainty. If the prior probability distribution does not *accurately* describe the statistics of the current environment and if the mean of the prior distribution differs from the mean of the sensory measurements, it will introduce a bias in the final perceptual estimates. Evidence for this phenomenon can be found in several perceptual illusions, for instance, the one illustrated in Figure 12.4. Both pictures show footprints in the sand. However, most people see the left image as an indentation in the sand, whereas they see the right image as if it were embossed or raised from the surface. The reason for this counterintuitive perception is the inherently ambiguous nature of the image and the need to make certain prior assumptions in order to interpret it (Rock, 1983). The prior assumption we make in this case is that the light

[2]Variables with a hat always denote noisy sensory estimates, whereas variables without a hat represent world signals from which the sensory estimates are derived.

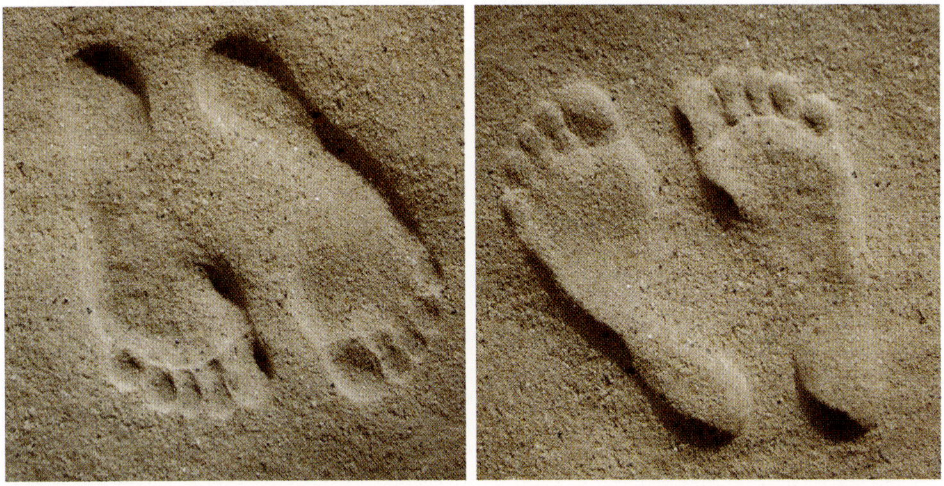

**Figure 12.4** Effect of the light-from-above prior on perception using ambiguous images. The left and right images show footprints in the sand. In the left image the light illuminating the scene is actually coming from above, and the footprint is correctly seen as an indentation. In the right image, which is the left image presented upside down, the light is coming from below. Employing the light-from-above prior in this situation causes the footprint to be seen as embossed or raised from the surface.

source in the image is placed above the surface (Brewster, 1826; Mamassian & Goutcher, 2001). The assumption reflects our common world experience of always having artificial or natural light from above (Dror, Willsky, & Adelson, 2004). In the illustration, this assumption is only correct for the left image. The illusion arises when one views the right image. In the right image the footprints are actually illuminated from below. Thus, making prior assumptions about light from above, that is, using an inappropriate prior for the current situation, forces our perception toward a bias that causes us to see the footprints raised from the surface.

To interact successfully with the environment in order to, say, point to an object, *the goal of the sensorimotor system must be to derive accurate estimates for the motor actions to be performed.* For example, we might wish to interact with the environment by touching one of the toes of the footprints shown in Figure 12.4. Evoking an inappropriate prior will introduce a bias into the inferred depth used for pointing. That is, in the right part of Figure 12.4 we would wrongly point to the illusory perceived embossed toe instead of the actual imprinted toe (Hartung, Schrater, Bülthoff, Kersten, & Franz, 2005). Therefore, biases such as those discussed earlier are undesirable and should be avoided. This, in turn, predicts that multisensory integration must break down with an increase of conflicting information between the multisensory sources. For this reason prior knowledge should be disregarded if it is evident that the sensory information is derived from an environment with statistical regularities that conflict with those represented by the prior probability distributions. There is experimental evidence to back up both these claims, which will be discussed next.

As indicated earlier, there are many perceptual illusions that arise because prior assumptions bias the percept. Another example is the use of prior knowledge about symmetry or isotropy in visual slant perception (Palmer, 1985). When asked for the three-dimensional interpretation of an ellipse, humans consistently see the ellipse as a circle slanted in depth. This perceptual effect is explained using a prior for symmetry which when evoked interprets the ellipse as a circle. This may make sense because, considering the statistics of our world, we are more likely to encounter circles than ellipses. Therefore, under these statistical considerations, for the unlikely event that the ellipse is really an ellipse, this prior will give rise to a biased percept. Knill (2007a) showed that we down-weight such prior knowledge for seeing circles if we are placed in an environment where ellipses or irregular shapes occur more frequently. This is consistent with the idea that we begin to ignore the prior when there is statistical evidence against the symmetry assumption. As a consequence, this strategy saves us from acquiring biases based on false prior assumptions. Along the same lines, Adams et al. (2004) showed that the light-from-above prior (as demonstrated in Fig. 12.4) adapts when observers are put in an environment where the light source is placed predominantly to the left or right, instead of above.

There is also empirical evidence for biases in multisensory perception and for the breakdown of multisensory integration with large discrepancies between the sensory estimates. For example, multisensory integration has been studied experimentally by the deliberate introduction of small discrepancies between sensory signals such that the perceptual consequences of integration are evident in a bias resulting from weighted averaging; a method termed "perturbation analysis" (Young, Landy, & Maloney, 1993). Some notable demonstrations of multisensory biases induced by weighted averaging include shifts in perceived location (Alais & Burr, 2004; Bertelson & Radeau, 1981; Pick, Warren, & Hay, 1969; Welch & Warren, 1980), perceived rate of a rhythmic stimulation (Bresciani, Dammeier, & Ernst 2006, 2008; Bresciani & Ernst, 2007; Bresciani et al., 2005; Gebhard & Mowbray, 1959; Myers, Cotton, & Hilp, 1981; Recanzone, 2003; Shams, Kamitami, & Shimojo, 2002; Shipley, 1964; Welch, DuttonHurt, & Warren, 1986), or perceived size (Ernst & Banks, 2002; Helbig & Ernst, 2007). With larger experimentally induced discrepancies between the perceptual estimates, however, the integration and weighted averaging process breaks down (Knill, 2007b). Integration breaks down even more rapidly if there is additional evidence that the sources of information do not originate from the same object or event. For example, Gepshtein, Burge, Banks, and Ernst (2005) showed that visual and haptic size integration breaks down rapidly if the visual and haptic information do not come from the same location. That is, location information is used in addition to determine whether to integrate the size estimates. Several studies have shown this breakdown of integration with spatial discordance in a similar way (Jack & Thurlow, 1973; Jackson, 1953; Warren & Cleaves, 1971; Witkin, Wapner, Leventhal, 1952; but see also Recanzone, 2003). The breakdown also happens with temporal discrepancies (e.g., Bresciani et al., 2005; Radeau & Bertelson, 1987; Shams et al., 2002; van Wassenhove, Grant, & Poeppel, 2007). This breakdown of integration with increasing discordance in space and time defines the spatial and temporal windows of integration. It is more generally referred to as robustness of integration.

We have now identified two competing goals of the perceptual-motor system: the first goal, discussed in the previous section, was to achieve the most reliable estimates possible; the second goal, discussed in this section, was to avoid inaccuracy of the estimates, that is, to achieve the most accurate estimates. *To maximize the gain from integration, these two competing goals must be best balanced.* For this the precision (reliability) and accuracy of the sensory estimates has to be known to the system. As mentioned earlier, reliability can in principle be determined online from analyzing the estimates. However, there is no direct information in the sensory signals or estimates that would allow one to determine their accuracy. In the following we will therefore concentrate on the question of how the brain determines whether sensory signals and estimates are accurate, whether there is a discrepancy between the sensory estimates, and so whether to integrate. The same question arises for the use of prior knowledge as well and whether it conforms to the statistics of the present environment. To keep matters simple, however, from now on we will concentrate on the first question.

## BALANCING BENEFITS AND COSTS

Whether to integrate different multisensory estimates depends on the presence of an actual difference $D$ between the multiple sensory signals. The perceptual system, however, does not have direct access to the sensory signals but only to the estimates derived from these signals. Thus, to estimate what constitutes an actual difference $D$ between the signals is a question that is itself shrouded in uncertainty because of the noise in the estimation process. That is, when we make estimates $\hat{D}$ of sensory discrepancies, we are unable to do so reliably because of the noise in such estimates (see Wallace et al., 2004). For this reason, it is practically impossible to determine an absolute threshold for whether to integrate. Every time a discrepancy is detected between two estimates, the perceptual system must determine (either implicitly or explicitly) the reason for such a discrepancy. If the discrepancy $\hat{D}$ arises from random noise in the processing of the neuronal signals, the discrepancy changes randomly from trial to trial. In this case, by integrating the two estimates, the perceptual system could average out the influence of such noise as shown in the beginning of this chapter. However, if the discrepancy in the estimates $\hat{D}$ were due to a systematic difference $D$ between the signals, then the best strategy would require the perceptual system to not integrate the multisensory information. This may occur, for example, in a scenario where the sensory signals to be combined show some inaccuracy (in form of an additive bias $B$) with respect to the world (i.e., $S_V = S_{W_V} + B_V$ or $S_H = S_{W_H} + B_H$), or with respect to one another (i.e., $D = S_V - S_H$). Figure 12.3A illustrates this with a few examples showing how the sensory signals ($S_V$ and $S_H$) may become inaccurate with respect to the world property $S_W = (S_{W_V}, S_{W_H})$ to be estimated. As a consequence, determining the reason for the discrepancies in the sensory estimates is a credit-assignment problem with two possibilities: The reason for the discrepancy could either be a difference between the signals or a random perturbation as a result of noise, where both possibilities are uncertain. Since both possibilities are plausible and have associated uncertainty, the optimal strategy would be to use them both and weight each according to its relative certainty. We call this optimal because it balances the benefit of multisensory integration while minimizing the potential costs associated with it. This intuitive concept forms the basis of a model that we discuss further in the next section.

## MODELING FUSION, PARTIAL FUSION, AND SEGREGATION

To summarize, no matter how small it may be, a discrepancy *always* exists between perceptual estimates derived from different signals ($\hat{D} = \hat{S}_V - \hat{S}_H$). Such discrepancies could either be caused by random noise in the estimates (with standard deviations $\sigma_V$ and $\sigma_H$), which is unavoidable and always present, or it could be caused by a systematic difference $D$ in magnitude between the sensory signals. To make the best possible use of such discrepant information, the brain must use different and antithetical strategies for random noise and systematic difference. Information should be fused if the discrepancy was caused by random noise in the estimates, and it should be segregated if the discrepancy was caused by an actual difference in the signals. Interestingly, the very determination of the source of the discrepancy, random or systematic, is itself uncertain and difficult to estimate and so the reason for any discrepancy can only be determined with uncertainty. Thus, the best solution to model such a process is to use a fully probabilistic approach.

While our nervous system is capable of processing many complex signals and sources at once, we try to keep matters simple here by considering a discrepancy between only two estimates, each of which represents a property $S_W = (S_{W_V}, S_{W_H})$ specified by sensory signals $S = (S_V, S_H)$. Thus, it is reasonable to think of the integration process in a 2D space (Fig. 12.5), although the problem can be extended easily to higher dimensions. We now continue with the example we used earlier (Eq. 12.1) in which visual and haptic estimates are combined to determine the size of an object $S_W = (S_{W_V}, S_{W_H})$ with $S_{W_V} = S_{W_H}$. Let $S = (S_V, S_H)$ be the sensory signals derived from the world $S_W = (S_{W_V}, S_{W_H})$, which may be biased ($B = (B_V, B_H)$; Fig. 12.3) with respect to some world property or with respect to one another, and let $z = (z_V, z_H)$ be the sensory measurements derived from $S$. Both the visual and haptic measurements are corrupted by independent Gaussian noise with variance $\sigma_i^2$, so $z_i = S_i + \varepsilon_i$ with $i$ referring to the individual sensory modality $(V, H)$[3]. With these assumptions, the joint likelihood function takes the form of a Gaussian density function:

$$p(z|S) = N(\hat{S}, \Sigma_z)$$

$$\text{with } \Sigma_z = \begin{pmatrix} \sigma_V^2 & 0 \\ 0 & \sigma_H^2 \end{pmatrix}, \qquad (12.6)$$

which is a bivariate normal distribution with mean $\hat{S} = (\hat{S}_V, \hat{S}_H) = (z_V, z_H)$ (i.e., the maximum-likelihood estimates of the sensory signals equal the noisy measurements) and covariance matrix $\Sigma_z$ (left column in Fig. 12.5).

The likelihood function represents the sensory measurements on a given trial. The goal of this task will be the estimation of a property of the world, such as $S_W$, while taking into account both sensory imprecision (due to random noise) and inaccuracy (additive bias). In the rest of this chapter, we will develop a Bayesian model of this process that proceeds in two steps. In the first stage, discussed in this section and the next, we describe how the observer can use Bayes' rule to calculate a posterior distribution of the sensory signals given the noisy measurements, $P(S_V, S_H | z_V, z_H)$, and MAP estimates of those sensory signals, $\hat{S}^{MAP}$, that take into account prior knowledge of the correlations between the signals, $p(S_V, S_H)$. In subsequent sections, we describe how the observer can use prior knowledge of the likely inaccuracy in each modality $(B_V, B_H)$ along with current estimates of the discrepancy between

[3]As previously, we assume the visual and haptic estimates are normally distributed and statistically independent. Oruç et al. (2003) and Ernst (2005) describe an analysis of how such a system behaves in case the estimates are not independent and how this may give rise to negative weights.

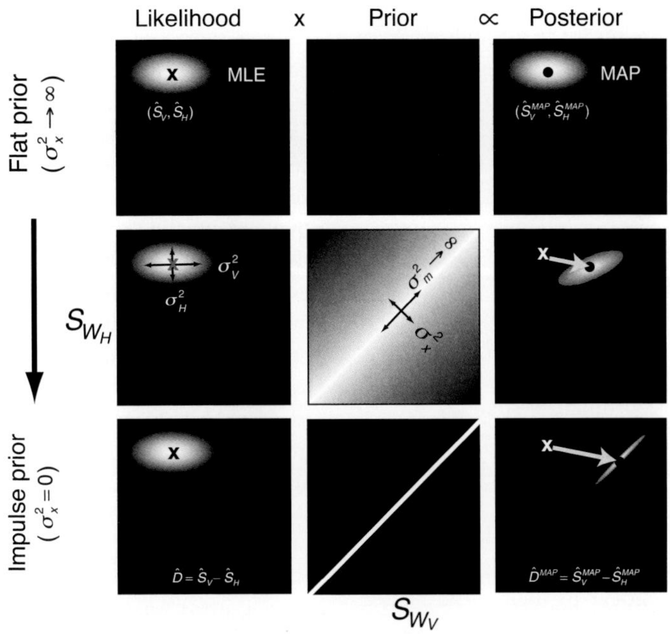


**Figure 12.5** The combination of visual and haptic measurements with different prior distributions. (Left column) Likelihood functions resulting from noise with standard deviation $\sigma_V$ twice as large as $\sigma_H$; x indicates the maximum-likelihood estimate (MLE) of the sensory signals $\hat{S} = (\hat{S}_V, \hat{S}_H)$. (Middle column) Prior distributions with variance $\sigma_m^2 \rightarrow \infty$, but different variances $\sigma_x^2$. Top: flat prior $\sigma_x^2 \rightarrow \infty$; middle: intermediate prior $0 < \sigma_x^2 < \infty$; bottom: impulse prior $\sigma_x^2 = 0$. (Right) Posterior distributions, which are the normalized product of the likelihood and prior distributions. A dot indicates the maximum a posteriori (MAP) estimate $\hat{S}^{MAP} = (\hat{S}_V^{MAP}, \hat{S}_H^{MAP})$. Arrows correspond to bias in the MAP estimate relative to the MLE estimate. The orientation of the arrows indicates the weighting of the $\hat{S}_V$ and $\hat{S}_H$ estimates. The length of the arrow indicates the degree of fusion. (Adapted with permission from Ernst, 2007. Copyright ARVO.)

sensory signals ($\hat{D}^{MAP} = \hat{S}_V^{MAP} - \hat{S}_H^{MAP}$) after integration occurred to solve iteratively the credit-assignment problem: What portion of $\hat{D}^{MAP}$ should be attributed to the bias $B_i$ or the world property $S_{W_i}$ of each modality? The solution of this problem will allow the observer to remap each modality, as a means of providing the best possible (low bias and low uncertainty) estimate of $S_W$.

To begin, we assume that the system has acquired a priori knowledge about the probability of jointly encountering a combination of sensory signals encoded in the prior $p(S_V, S_H)$. Some examples of visual and haptic signals to size $(S_V, S_H)$ that might be encountered in conjunction when trying to estimate the world property $S_W$ are provided in Figure 12.3. The lower row in Figure 12.3 shows what such a distribution of jointly encountered signals might look like. Figure 12.3A shows cases where the signals are derived from the same location for which we can assume that $S_{W_V} = S_{W_H}$. All these examples show signals with varying accuracy ($B_i = S_{W_i} - S_i$). The point here is that the variance in the joint distribution and hence the variance of the prior learned from these signals is affected by the variability in accuracy of the two signals. Figure 12.3B illustrates a similar example of co-occurrence of visual and haptic signals, but here these signals are derived from slightly disparate locations $\Delta x$ for which in general $S_{W_V} \neq S_{W_H}$. We return to this example in a later section of this chapter when we discuss the link between integration and remapping.

Assuming for now that all the joint distributions are Gaussians, a prior that fulfills what we have discussed thus far can be defined as:

$$p(S)=p(S_V, S_H)=N(n,\Pi)$$
$$\text{with} \quad \Pi=R^T\begin{pmatrix} \sigma_m^2 \to \infty & 0 \\ 0 & \sigma_x^2 \end{pmatrix}R, \quad (12.7)$$

which is a bivariate normal distribution with mean $n = (0, 0)$ and covariance matrix $\Pi$. $\sigma_m^2$ and $\sigma_x^2$ are the variances of the prior along its principal axes and $R$ is an orthogonal matrix that rotates the coordinate system by 45° so that the prior is aligned with the diagonal where $S_V = S_H$ (Fig. 12.5, middle column). We choose the variance along the positive diagonal to be $\sigma_m^2 \to \infty$, which indicates that the probability of jointly encountering two signals $(S_V, S_H)$ is independent of their mean value.[4] The second variance, $\sigma_x^2$, indicates the spread of the joint distribution, which represents the a priori distribution of possible discrepancies between the signals. Therefore, the probability that the source of any detected discrepancy $\hat{D}$ is not random noise but an actual difference between the signals $D = S_V - S_H$ is a function of the variance $\Pi$ (i.e., $\sigma_x^2$) of this prior. The diagonal with $S_V = S_H$ represents the mapping between the signals since it provides the functional relationship between the two. We can therefore also refer to $\sigma_x^2$ as the *mapping uncertainty*. Furthermore, this distribution also provides a measure of redundancy between the two signals; the smaller the variance $\sigma_x^2$, the more redundant the signals are with respect to one another.

Figure 12.5 illustrates three examples of the model described earlier for prior distributions with different $\sigma_x^2$ (middle column) ranging from very large (top row) to near zero (bottom row). A prior probability with $\sigma_x^2 \to \infty$ corresponds to a state in which any possible combination of $S_V$ and $S_H$ signals contains roughly an equal a priori probability of occurrence. Such a prior is often referred to as a "flat prior." In this extreme case of $\sigma_x^2 \to \infty$, there is no mapping between the sensory signals or estimates derived from them and thus the discrepancy between the estimates is ill defined. Theoretically, however, one might argue that the accuracy of the signals with respect to this ill-defined mapping approaches zero. This has also been referred to as signals that are invalid (with respect to the property defined by the mapping). Such a situation is an example of signals $S_V$ and $S_H$ that do not carry redundant information. Thus, as an example we could take any set of nonrelated signals, such as the luminance and the stiffness of an object, which are highly unlikely to carry any redundant information (Ernst, 2007) and can co-occur in any possible combination.

A prior probability with $\sigma_x^2 = 0$, on the other hand, corresponds to a state in which signals occur only for the condition $S_V = S_H$. Such a prior relates to signals that are always perfectly accurate (with respect to the property of interest). In this situation the prior probability of encountering an actual difference $D$ between the signals is zero. Thus, in this situation the sensory signals are completely redundant. While such a scenario would be purely theoretical because there is always some variance present, indirect empirical evidence that humans use very tight priors was provided by Hillis, Ernst, Banks, and Landy (2002), who found close to mandatory fusion of disparity and texture estimates to slant (see later discussion).

An intermediate value of $\sigma_x^2$ corresponds to a state in which the probability distribution indicates some uncertainty with respect to the possible co-occurrence of signal values $S_V$ and $S_H$. Such a prior relates to signals that display some inaccuracy with respect to the mapping and thus there exists a nonzero probability of encountering various differences $D$ between the signals. The signals in this situation are thus only *partially* redundant (with respect to one another). Since this prior refers to the probability of co-occurrence of certain signals, that is, it represents the prior probability of jointly encountering an ensemble of sensory estimates, in earlier work this prior $p(S_V, S_H)$ has also been referred to as the "coupling prior" (Bresciani et al., 2006; Ernst, 2005, 2007). Realistically, all

[4]Thus, $n$ could have any value with $S_V = S_H$. We arbitrarily choose $n = (0, 0)$.

cases of multisensory integration, such as size estimation from vision and touch, fall into this category (Ernst, 2005; Hillis et al., 2002). This is because there is always some probability that the signals are inaccurate due to external or internal factors, such as muscle fatigue, optical distortion, or other environmental or bodily influences (Fig. 12.3A).

Using Bayes' rule (see Chapter 1), the joint likelihood function obtained from the sensory signals is combined with prior knowledge about the co-occurrence statistics of these signals. This gives rise to a final estimate of the sensory signals $\hat{S}^{MAP} = (\hat{S}_V^{MAP}, \hat{S}_H^{MAP})$ based on the posterior distribution $p(S_V, S_H|z_V, z_H) \propto p(z_V, z_H|S_V, S_H)p(S_V, S_H)$, which balances the benefit of reduced variance with the cost of a potential bias in the estimate (Fig. 12.5, right column). Note that this step does not yet provide an estimate of the world property $S_W = (S_{W_V}, S_{W_H})$ or the biases $B = (B_V, B_H)$. How we estimate $S_W$ and $B$ will be discussed in the later section, "From Integration to Remapping." However, from the MAP estimate of the sensory signals we can derive the best estimate of the current discrepancy $D$ between the signals, which is $\hat{D}^{MAP} = \hat{S}_V^{MAP} - \hat{S}_H^{MAP}$.

The posterior estimate $\hat{S}^{MAP}$ is shifted with respect to the likelihood $\hat{S}$. This shift is highlighted by the arrow in Figure 12.5, right column. The length of the arrow indicates the strength of the integration, whereas the direction of the arrow indicates the weighting of the sensory estimates. In the following we will more closely investigate this shift (captured by the two parameters of the arrow) for the three values of $\sigma_x^2$.

If the prior is flat ($\sigma_x^2 \rightarrow \infty$; Fig. 12.5, top row), the posterior becomes identical to the likelihood function, which implies that the multisensory estimates are not integrated but kept independent, that is, they are segregated (no shift). Since the signals are independent, any form of integration in this case would only introduce a bias into the final estimates. Given this situation, there can also be no benefit from integration in the form of reduced variance because the signals do not carry redundant information.

In contrast, a prior with $\sigma_x^2 = 0$ gives rise to a posterior that results in complete fusion (Fig. 12.5, bottom row). As can be observed from the figure, such an impulse prior denotes the existence of only those signals for which $S_V = S_H$. Thus, in the case of fusion, the maximum a posteriori (MAP) estimate $\hat{S}^{MAP}$ coincides with the prior $p(S_V, S_H)$. The direction $\alpha$ in which the estimate is shifted is solely determined by $\sigma_V^2$ and $\sigma_H^2$ of the likelihood function (Bresciani et al., 2006):

$$\alpha = \arctan\left(\frac{\sigma_H^2}{\sigma_V^2}\right). \tag{12.8}$$

In this particular case, the MAP estimate maximally benefits from fusion by acquiring the smallest possible variance in the combined estimate. The prior with $\sigma_x^2 = 0$ applies to a situation with entirely accurate and perfectly redundant signals. Thus, whatever detected discrepancy exists must be a consequence of measurement noise. This case where $\sigma_x^2 = 0$ is identical to the previously discussed *standard model* of cue integration, which also assumed unbiased (accurate) signals and estimates derived from the same world property (see section on "Multisensory Integration" in this chapter and Chapter 1).

For cases where $0 < \sigma_x^2 < \infty$, the MAP estimate $\hat{S}^{MAP} = (\hat{S}_V^{MAP}, \hat{S}_H^{MAP})$ is situated midway between the maximum-likelihood estimates $(\hat{S}_V, \hat{S}_H)$ and the diagonal (Fig. 12.5, middle row). In other words, the result here lies between the "no fusion" case and "complete fusion" case, and thus we refer to it as "partial fusion." The strength of integration is indicated by the length $L$ of the arrow, which has been normalized to the size of the conflict and can be described as a weighting function between the likelihood and the prior in the direction of $\alpha$ (the direction of bias $\alpha$ can be determined from Eq. 12.8):

$$L = \frac{\sigma_{likelihood}^2(\alpha)}{\sigma_{likelihood}^2(\alpha) + \sigma_{prior}^2(\alpha)}. \tag{12.9}$$

Any measured discrepancy $\hat{D} = \hat{S}_V - \hat{S}_H$ is the result of both measurement noise ($\sigma_V$ and $\sigma_H$) and an actual discrepancy ($D = S_V - S_H$) due to bias $B$ (inaccuracy in $S_V$ and/or $S_H$, assuming $S_{W_V} = S_{W_H}$). Combining the likelihood with the prior, resulting in this weighting function (Eq. 12.9), provides the best balance between reliability and accuracy of the estimates of the sensory signals (in the MAP sense). The overall variance of the final estimate resulting from partial integration of the sensory signals lies in between that resulting from pure segregation and complete integration (Fig. 12.5, right column). It must be noted, however, that the final estimate can only profit from the integration process to the extent to which the signals are redundant. Thus, this weighting scheme constitutes the best balance between the costs of introducing a bias in the estimates and benefits of reducing their variances. The remaining difference in the MAP estimates $\hat{D}^{MAP} = \hat{S}_V^{MAP} - \hat{S}_H^{MAP}$ corresponds to the best current estimate of the actual discrepancy $D$ between the sensory signals. The predictions of this model, both regarding bias and variance, have been confirmed by an experimental study of the perceived quantity of visual and haptic events (Bresciani et al., 2006).

This theoretical framework can also explain how we can learn to integrate over an artificially enforced, statistical relationship between two arbitrary signals (Ernst, 2007). In this study, participants were trained by presenting previously unrelated aspects of a stimulus, for example, the luminance and the stiffness of an object, in correlation for some time. Participants learned this correlation; they began to exhibit integration of the two aspects of the stimulus which were previously unrelated. This was interpreted as the learning of a new prior probability that certain combinations of the two stimulus aspects—luminance and stiffness—are likely to co-occur. Once such a relationship is learned, the newly acquired prior knowledge can be used to integrate the estimates and therefore observers can benefit from a reduction in estimation noise. Thus, during the experiment, the participants switched their behavior from treating the estimates as completely independent to a more intermediate perception of the estimates exhibiting "partial fusion."

## BREAKDOWN OF INTEGRATION

It is important to note that in the model described in the previous section, the extent of the discrepancy between the maximum-likelihood estimates $\hat{D} = \hat{S}_V - \hat{S}_H$ does not influence the integration process (i.e., whether estimates are integrated or segregated). The weighting between the estimates, that is, the weighting between the likelihood and the prior, as well as the direction of shift $\alpha$, are all independent of the extent of the discrepancy given the assumptions of this model. Thus, this model so far does not capture the breakdown of integration. This is because the shape of the prior and the shape of the likelihood are both assumed to be Gaussian. The problem arises at larger conflicts between signals where, in order to behave robustly, integration should break down. Roach, Heron, and McGraw (2006) suggested relaxing the Gaussian assumption to account for this possibility. In particular, they introduced "heavy tails" to the Gaussian distribution of the prior. This transforms the prior in a very sensible way: Close to the diagonal the prior by and large keeps its Gaussian shape with a reasonable variance. Far from the diagonal the prior does not approach zero probability as a Gaussian would, but maintains a nonzero probability. In essence Roach et al. (2006) suggest a linear combination of a flat coupling prior that is used for modeling segregation (Fig. 12.5, upper row) and a coupling prior that is used for modeling partial fusion or fusion. As a result, the system continues to behave as it did without the long tails when the discrepancies are reasonably small, since the central Gaussian part of the prior plays the dominant role. For larger discrepancies, however, this prior ensures that the process converges toward segregation, because of the increased influence of the flat part of the prior.

This model can further be extended to *orthogonal dimensions* to include, for example, spatial and temporal discordance as well.[5]

[5] We call a conflict along the dimension to be estimated (e.g., size) discrepancy, whereas when we refer to a conflict in an orthogonal dimension (e.g., space or time) we call this discordance.

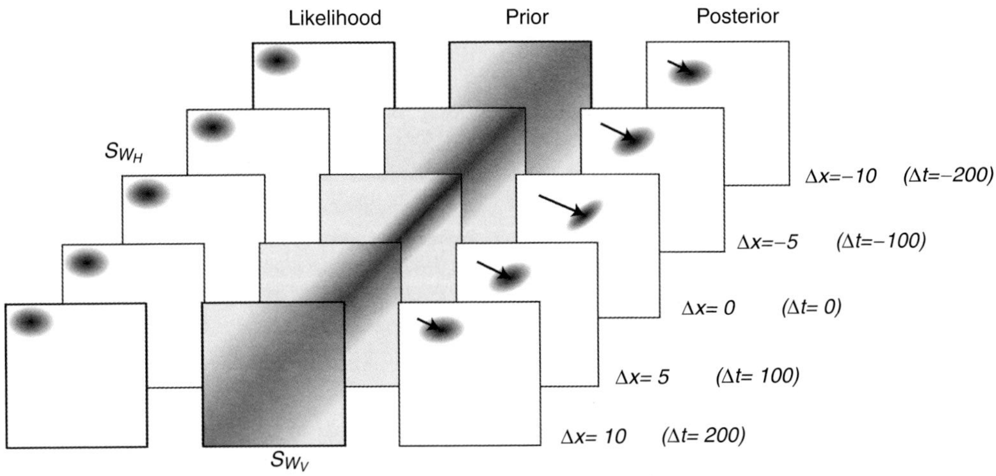


**Figure 12.6** Schematic illustration demonstrating robust estimation, that is, the breakdown of integration. The coupling prior is assumed to be of Gaussian shape with heavy tails (Roach et al., 2006). The variance of the Gaussian increases with increasing spatial or temporal discordance between the two signals, reflecting a lower correlation between the signals (Fig. 12.3B). Thus, with small discrepancies between the $S_V$ and $S_H$ signals, the weight of the prior decreases with temporal asynchrony and spatial disparity and so the effect of integration disappears. With large spatial inconsistencies or temporal asynchronies the two signals can then be perceived independently of one another as the correlation tends to disappear and the coupling prior becomes flat. (Adapted with permission from Ernst, 2007. Copyright ARVO.)

The conceptual basis of the model is illustrated in Figure 12.3B. We assume that under most circumstances, objects and the environment tend to change in their properties over space and time in a smooth, continuous way rather than a discontinuous and chaotic manner. Thus, despite the spatial or temporal discordance, generally there will still be a correlation between the multisensory signals. This correlation implies that despite some spatial and temporal discordance there is still redundancy in the multisensory signals. This redundancy should be used by the brain to improve its estimates. An example of a distribution of spatially discordant $S_V$ and $S_H$ size signals is indicated in the lower panel of Figure 12.3B. With increasing spatial discordance $\Delta x$, this correlation becomes weaker and weaker until finally the co-occurrence statistics of signals derived from vision and touch will result in a flat distribution. This change in the co-occurrence statistics with increasing spatial or temporal discordance is illustrated in Figure 12.6. The left column shows a likelihood function, which is identical for all five situations depicted since the sensory measurements are assumed to be identical in all cases. The effect of spatial and temporal discordance is reflected in the prior. For $\Delta x = 0$ $(\Delta t = 0)$ such a prior would resemble a central Gaussian with intermediate variance (analogous to Fig. 12.5, middle row), which also has heavy tails to account for the integration breakdown with increasing disparity in the size estimates (the flat tails are indicated by the gray background in the prior). With increasing spatial or temporal discordance ($\Delta x \neq 0$ or $\Delta t \neq 0$), the variance of the central part of the prior increases. This is because the prior probability of encountering combinations of $S_V$ and $S_H$ signals, for which the discrepancy $D = S_V - S_H$ is large, increases with the discordance in space or time ($\Delta x$ or $\Delta t$). As a consequence, as the discordance in space or time increases, the influence that the Gaussian part of the prior exerts on the likelihood function decreases. This process is represented by the arrows in Figure 12.6 (right column). This phenomenon corresponds to a breakdown of the integration process across space and time, which upon experimentation manifests itself as the spatial and temporal windows of integration.

The exact shape of the prior distribution reflects the co-occurrence statistics of the sensory signal values $S_V$ and $S_H$. This in turn determines the point at which the integration falloff occurs and therefore also determines the dimensions of the temporal or spatial window of integration. It is likely that all these priors have flat tails, because even at large discrepancies there will always be some remaining probability of encountering outliers in the co-occurrence statistics. The tails enable the independent treatment of signals at large inconsistencies. In principle, it should be possible to reconstruct the observers' embodiment of such a prior from experiments that measure the spatial and temporal integration windows. This could be achieved, for example, by extending the methods introduced by Stocker and Simoncelli (2006) to this two-dimensional estimation problem.

Recently, a few other approaches have been proposed to model this elusive aspect of the robustness or breakdown of integration. Some of these methods have also been described in this book (Chapters 2 and 13). We will discuss two of the more prominent proposals in this direction, both of which closely resemble the proposal presented here. The first proposes that the likelihood function is a mixture of Gaussians (Knill, 2007b) to explain the breakdown of integration, whereas the second approach formalizes the concept of causal inference to achieve the same purpose (Körding et al., 2007). Both approaches model the transition from fusion to segregation successfully; however, they both relate to special cases and specific scenarios for which they might be considered optimal.

The mixture-of-Gaussians approach by Knill (2007b) refers to a specific scenario in which a texture signal to slant is modeled by a likelihood function, which is composed of a central Gaussian with heavy tails. This proposal resembles what we have discussed earlier in this chapter, except that the heavy tails are added to the probability distributions of one of the sensory estimates and not to a coupling prior. The primary argument in this theory is that in order for texture to be a useful signal, we must make some prior assumptions about the isotropy of the texture that, in statistical considerations, could possibly fail in some cases. This argument provides a suitable justification for the use of heavy tails. The argument, however, is specific to the texture signal and can therefore not be easily extended to other within- or cross-modal sensory signals.

The second proposal attempts to formalize the concept of causal inference to model why integration breaks down with highly discrepant information (Körding et al., 2007). The proposal has the same intuitive basis that we have been referring to from time to time, that is, segregation at large discrepancies, integration when there is no apparent discrepancy. This model, however, concentrates on the causal attribution aspects of combining different signals. Two signals could either have one common cause, if they are generated by the same object/event, or they may have different causes when generated by different objects/events. In the former case, the signals should be integrated, and in the latter case they should be kept apart. The model takes into account a prior probability $p_{common}$ of whether a common source or separate sources exist for a given set of multisensory signals. $p_{common} = 1$ corresponds to perfect knowledge that there is a common source and thus complete fusion. As discussed previously, complete fusion can be described by a coupling prior corresponding to an impulse prior with $\sigma_x^2 = 0$. $p_{common} = 0$ corresponds to complete knowledge that there are two independent sources and thus complete segregation. Complete segregation was previously described by a flat coupling prior with $\sigma_x^2 \to \infty$. Whenever two sensory signals are detected, in general there will be some probability $p_{common}$ of a common cause and some probability $1 - p_{common}$ of independent causes. This probability depends on many factors such as, for example, temporal delays, visual experience, context, and many more (Körding et al., 2007), so it is not easy to predict. In any case, however, it will lead to a weighted combination of the two priors for complete fusion and segregation, and will thus in essence be analogous to a coupling prior, which has the form of an impulse prior with flat, heavy tails (Körding et al., 2007, supplement). In this sense, the causal-inference model is a special case of the model described earlier. It does not allow for variance in the prior describing the common cause (i.e., the impulse prior), because just like the standard model of integration (see Chapter 1), the causal-inference model is based on the assumption that all sensory signals with a common cause are perfectly correlated and accurate (i.e., the sensory estimates are assumed to be unbiased). Because it does not consider a weaker correlation between the co-occurring signals (i.e., the situation illustrated in Fig. 12.3B) and because it does not take into account the (in)accuracy of the signals (i.e., the situation in Fig. 12.3A), the causal-inference model does not optimally balance the benefits and costs of multisensory integration, that is, reduced variance and potential biases, respectively.

## REMAPPING

As discussed earlier, multisensory integration breaks down with increasing discrepancy between the estimates. However, if the discrepancy is systematic and persists over several measurements, we adapt to such a discrepancy and doing so brings the conflicting sensory maps (or sensorimotor maps) back into correspondence. This process of adaptation is therefore also referred to as remapping or recalibration. In this section, we review optimal linear models of remapping in the context of a visuomotor task. In the next section, we apply this model to the problem of combining visual and haptic size signals while simultaneously determining the best remapping of each.

There are many examples of such sensory and sensorimotor adaptation processes (e.g., Adams, Banks, & van Ee, 2001; Bedford, 1993; Frissen, Vroomen, & de Gelder, 2003; Pick et al., 1969; Welch, 1978; Welch & Warren, 1980, 1986). The most classic examples of this phenomenon are the experiments on prism shifts first studied by Hermann von Helmholtz (1867). In these experiments observers were asked to point to a visual target in "open loop" using fast pointing movements. Here, the use of open loop refers to the absence of online feedback to control the movement. The visual feedback can only be procured at the end of the pointing movement upon observing the location where the finger landed. Let this position of the estimated location of the feedback signal be $\hat{S}_F$ and the estimated target location be $\hat{S}_L$. After each trial of such open loop pointing, an error in pointing response can be detected that corresponds to the difference between the feedback- and target-position estimates: $\hat{D} = \hat{S}_F - \hat{S}_L$. It is this error that adaptation seeks to minimize.

A typical visuomotor adaptation experiment consists of three phases: a baseline, in which the accuracy of pointing performance is assessed (Fig. 12.7, trial $<60$). Once the baseline is established, observers receive spectacles fitted with prisms that shift the visual world by some constant amount (e.g., 10°). Once observers wear the prism-fitted spectacles, they exhibit an initial error in their pointing response, which is equivalent to the extent of the prism shift. After only a few pointing movements, however, observers begin to correct for the error induced by the prism and eventually "adapt" to this change (Fig. 12.7, $60 \leq$ trial $\leq 110$). After adaptation has been achieved, the removal of these prism glasses results in recalibration back to baseline (Fig. 12.7, trial $>110$).

An interesting aspect of this phenomenon is the rate at which people adapt to these changes. This rate varies enormously depending on the experimental condition. For instance, the rate of adaptation strongly depends on the nature of the conflicting signals provided to the observer. In visuomotor tasks, like pointing to targets, usually the first few trials after wearing prism-spectacles are sufficient for reaching an almost constant minimization of the error, that is, reaching an asymptote for the newly introduced change. In contrast, adaptation purely within the visual domain, for instance, for texture and binocular disparity signals, has been known to take up to several days until adaptation saturates and a constant minimization of the error has been achieved (Adams et al., 2001). Four

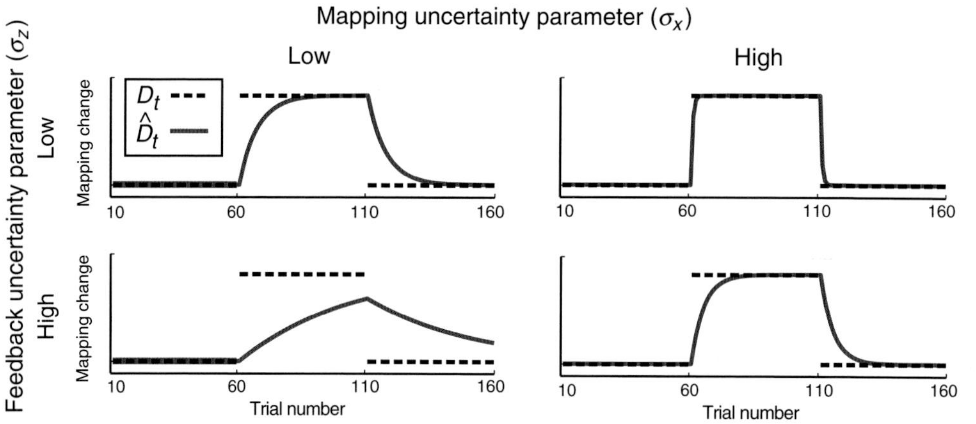


**Figure 12.7** Kalman-filter responses to step changes. The dashed black lines in each panel represent the relationship between the position of the reach endpoint and the position of the visual feedback. This relationship is the visuomotor mapping. As in our experiments, there are three phases: prestep (trials 1–60), step (61–110), and poststep (111–160). A first step change in the mapping occurs at the end of the prestep phase; the initial mapping is then restored after the step phase. The blue curves represent the visuomotor mapping estimates $\hat{D}_{t+}^{MAP}$ over time. The upper and lower rows show models of the estimates when the measurement uncertainty $\sigma_z^2$ is small and large, respectively. An increase in $\sigma_z^2$ causes a decrease in adaptation rate. The left and right columns show responses when the mapping uncertainty $\sigma_x^2$ is small and large, respectively. An increase in $\sigma_x^2$ causes an increase in adaptation rate; the effect is larger when $\sigma_z^2$ is large. (Adapted with permission from Burge et al., 2008. Copyright ARVO.)

examples of adaptation profiles with different rate parameters are provided in Figure 12.7. Even though adaptation has been actively researched for over a 100 years, the search for a computational framework for it only began in recent times with models that tried to describe the process underlying remapping (e.g., Baddley, Ingram, & Miall, 2003; Burge, Ernst, & Banks, 2008; Gharahmani et al., 1997).

In 2008, we investigated how the statistics of the environment and the system together influence the rate of adaptation in visuomotor tasks (Burge et al., 2008). The problem can be formulated in a manner almost analogous to that faced in integration. When a conflict $\hat{D}_t = \hat{S}_{F,t} - \hat{S}_{L,t}$ is detected on a given trial $t$, which in this case would be the difference between the estimated feedback and target positions, the perceptual system must ask itself, what is the source of this conflict.[6] Upon consideration, we find that the answer is twofold: The conflict could be caused by an actual discrepancy between the sensory (or the sensorimotor) maps $D_t$. Alternatively, it could merely be due to measurement noise $\sigma_z^2$ when acquiring the sensory estimates $\hat{D}_t$. If this latter is indeed the case and the discrepancy is caused solely by measurement noise, there would be a new random discrepancy from trial to trial, which would best be ignored by the system. In other words, the system should not attempt to adapt to this randomly fluctuating change in discrepancy caused by measurement noise because to do so would actually make things worse. In sharp contrast, if the discrepancy instead arose due to an actual mismatch in the sensorimotor maps $D_t$, it would cause a systematic and sustained discrepancy over trials. Because the occurrence of this discrepancy is persistent and systematic, it would be appropriate for the system to adapt to it.

Analogous to what has been discussed for integration, also for remapping the estimates of both types of error, random versus systematic, contain uncertainty. That is, on a given trial the

[6] In the earlier example, we would define $\hat{D}_t = \hat{S}_{V,t} - \hat{S}_{H,t}$.

system can only determine the discrepancy with some uncertainty. The measure of uncertainty for random errors is the variance $\sigma_z^2$ of the measurement $z$. As noted in the previous sections on integration, detecting a systematic error presents more challenge for the system. This is because such an error cannot be determined from one trial observation alone. We must accumulate prior knowledge about the error signal over several observations and use this information to successfully identify a systematic error. Those data, however, also contain uncertainty: the uncertainty $\sigma_x^2$ associated with the mapping.

Since it is likely that visuomotor tasks contain both systematic and random errors, the nervous system must be able to weight the error estimates flexibly based on their relative uncertainties to solve this credit-assignment problem and to create an optimal estimate of the current mapping. We now turn to a computational framework that formalizes these arguments.

Let us consider that the purpose of the system is primarily to obtain the best possible estimate of the visuomotor mapping in order to remain accurate. The best estimate of the current systematic discrepancy on a given trial, $\hat{D}_{t+}^{MAP}$ (the MAP estimate derived from the posterior), is a weighted average of the conflict currently measured, $\hat{D}_t = \hat{S}_{F,t} - \hat{S}_{L,t}$ (the MLE estimate), and the prediction based on past history, $\hat{D}_{t-}$ (derived from the prior):

$$\begin{aligned}\hat{D}_{t+}^{MAP} &= w_x\hat{D}_{t-} + w_z\hat{D}_t \\ &= \hat{D}_{t-} + K(\hat{D}_t - \hat{D}_{t-}).\end{aligned} \quad (12.10)$$

The value $K$ is a proportion of the error signal by which the visuomotor mapping is adjusted. In the framework we propose further, we refer to this proportion as the Kalman gain. The "+" on the index indicates that this conflict estimate is used in the next trial to update the mapping; the "−" on the index indicates that this prior information is derived from previous trials, whereas no modifier on the index indicates that it is the measurement derived on the current trial. In an optimal scenario, the weights would be inversely proportional to the relative uncertainties associated with error estimates based on measurements and prior knowledge:

$$w_x = \frac{\sigma_z^2}{\sigma_z^2 + \sigma_x^2} \quad \text{and} \quad w_z = \frac{\sigma_x^2}{\sigma_z^2 + \sigma_x^2}. \quad (12.11)$$

From Eqs. 12.10 and 12.11, we obtain

$$K = \frac{\sigma_x^2}{\sigma_z^2 + \sigma_x^2}. \quad (12.12)$$

Since $\hat{D}_{t+}^{MAP}$ is the optimal current estimate of the systematic error that determines the discrepancy, recalibration in any given trial should occur based on this combined estimate.

Adaptation is an iterative process where every trial $t$ results in an updated combined estimate of the current error signal, which is used for updating the prior in the next step, thereby enabling the efficient tracking of the changes that occur in the mapping. Many experiments show that the brain can adapt under quite complex conditions. For the sake of simplicity, however, here we consider a linear system, which has achieved steady state. Under these assumptions, and following our arguments for Bayesian optimality, the Kalman filter presents an optimal solution to these modeling efforts (for the derivation, refer to Burge et al., 2008). In doing so, we treat the performance of a visuomotor task as a control system in which the error signal is adjusted by the proportion $K$, which represents the Kalman gain of such a system.

Figure 12.7 shows the response of a Kalman-filter model to step changes in the mapping. Such a step change is analogous to introducing a prism and later removing it. As the filter adjusts the visuomotor mapping, the error between target and reach position decreases exponentially with time. In other words, human subjects compensate for the error on a trial-by-trial basis to achieve exponentially a constant asymptote at which they have minimized their error. Therefore, we use the exponent $\lambda$ to express the adaptation rate, which is a function of $K$:

$$\lambda = -\log(1 - K). \quad (12.13)$$

From this equation, we find that the model predicts faster adaptation rates for higher gains and low adaptation rates for lower gains. The measurement uncertainty $\sigma_z^2$ and the mapping uncertainty $\sigma_x^2$ affect the Kalman gain and thus the adaptation rate in contrasting ways (Eq. 12.12). These opposing effects are illustrated in Figure 12.7. With an increase in measurement uncertainty $\sigma_z^2$, the adaptation rate slows down, whereas with an increase in mapping uncertainty $\sigma_x^2$, adaptation becomes faster.

These predictions have been tested empirically by systematically varying the measurement noise using various blur conditions on the visual feedback signals, thus making them less reliable to estimate (Burge et al., 2008). They found that observers did indeed adapt more slowly with an increase in the blur of the feedback stimuli. When they introduced a perturbation into the mapping on a trial-by-trial basis instead of blurring the feedback signal, however, they found that a random but statistically stationary error in the feedback did not elicit any change in the rate of adaptation. That trial-by-trial variation did not affect the rate of recalibration suggests that the measurement noise may be estimated online in any given trial, but not over trials.

In a second experiment Burge et al. (2008) perturbed the mapping from trial to trial with time-correlated noise in a random-walk fashion. To put it simply, in each trial a new random variable drawn from a Gaussian distribution was added to the previous mapping. If correctly learned, this manipulation affects the mapping uncertainty as the mapping is constantly changing in a time-correlated fashion. Consistent with the predictions of the optimal adaptor, the results showed an increased adaptation rate for an increase in the variance of the random-walk distribution. In conclusion, it seems that to a first approximation (e.g., assuming stationary statistics) the Kalman-filter model is a good predictor of human adaptation performance.

## FROM INTEGRATION TO REMAPPING

In this section we apply the Bayesian (Kalman-filter) model of remapping to the visual-haptic size-estimation task and combine it with the partial-integration model from earlier in this chapter. This is illustrated in Figure 12.8. We assume there is a sequence of trials at times $t$ in which the observer has sensory estimates $\hat{S}_{V,t}$ and $\hat{S}_{H,t}$, and tries to estimate $S_W = (S_{W_V}, S_{W_H})$. For simplicity, we assume the perceptual situation to be constant throughout the trials, so that $S_W$, $S_i$, and $B_i$ are all independent of $t$. Furthermore, for now we assume that $S_{W_V} = S_{W_H}$, which implies that we are estimating the identical world property by vision and touch. The initial situation for estimating $S_W$ is that there may exist an unknown additive bias $B = (B_V, B_H)$ in the visual and haptic signals $S = (S_V, S_H) = (S_{W_V} + B_V, S_{W_H} + B_H)$ leading to a discrepancy $D = S_V - S_H$ between the sensory signals. At first, we do not know these biases, so at time step $t = 0$, before any measurement is performed, the initial bias estimate is $\hat{B}_0 = 0$, the initial prediction for the discrepancy is $\hat{D}_{t^-=0} = 0$, and the initial coupling prior $p_0(S_V, S_H) = p(S_{V,0}, S_{H,0})$ is unbiased, that is, it is centered on the diagonal $S_V = S_H$. For every time step $t = 1,2,3,\ldots$, the observer begins by deriving the maximum-likelihood estimate $\hat{S}_t = (\hat{S}_{V,t}, \hat{S}_{H,t})$ of the current signals $S_t = (S_{V,t}, S_{H,t})$. These MLE estimates contain a discrepancy $\hat{D}_t = \hat{S}_{V,t} - \hat{S}_{H,t}$. In the leftmost column of Figure 12.8 this is indicated by the red Gaussian blobs being off the diagonal (equivalent to Fig. 12.5, left column).[7] The variance of the likelihood function $\Sigma_z$ indicates the measurement uncertainty. Next, to solve the credit-assignment problem of whether this discrepancy $\hat{D}_t$ is caused by noise $\Sigma_z$ or an actual difference $D$ between the signals, the Bayesian integration scheme is applied, combining the maximum-likelihood estimate with prior knowledge about the joint distribution of $S_{V,t}$ and $S_{H,t}$, that is, the mapping between the signals. That is, the column labeled "prior" in Figure 12.8 shows an example of an intermediate "coupling prior" with variance $\sigma_x^2$. This variance

[7] For illustrative purposes we assume that at every trial the same noise value $\varepsilon$ is added to the measurement $z_{i,t} = S_{i,t} + \varepsilon_{i,t}$ so the likelihood function is identical in each row of Figure 12.8.

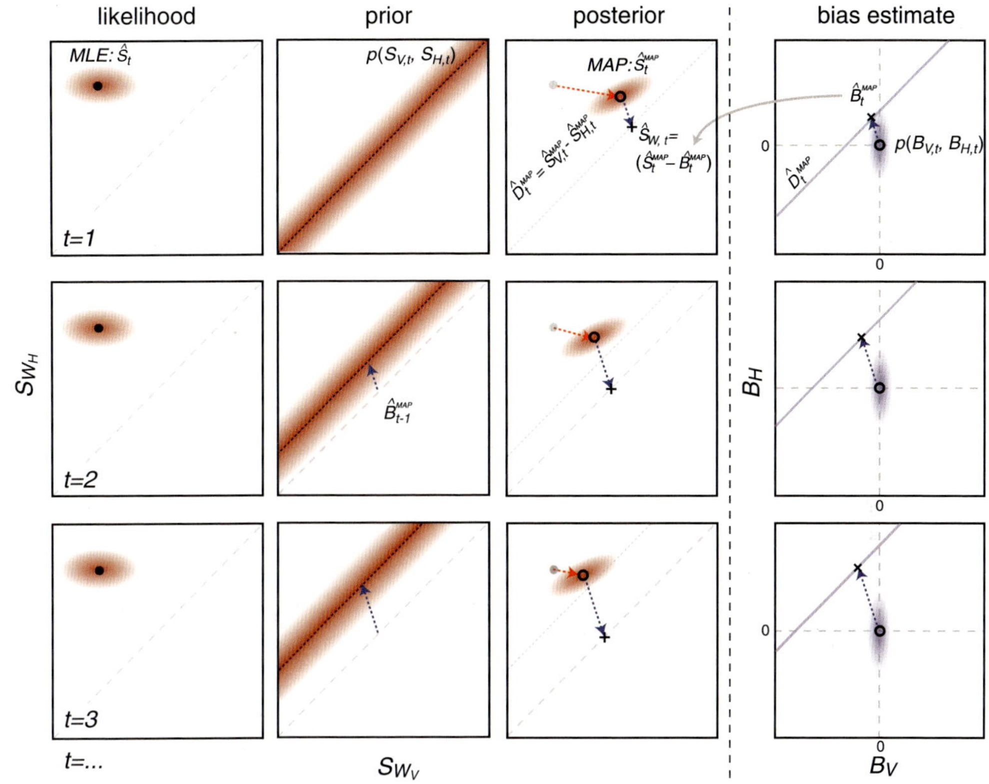


**Figure 12.8** Illustration of the link between integration and remapping of visual and haptic size estimates. The leftmost column illustrates the maximum-likelihood estimates $\hat{S}_t = (\hat{S}_{V,t}, \hat{S}_{H,t})$ indicated by a dot with the corresponding measurement noise $\Sigma_z$ indicated by the red Gaussian blob. The column labeled "prior" gives a coupling prior $p(S_{V,t}, S_{H,t}) = p_0(S_{V,t} - \hat{B}^{MAP}_{V,t-1}, S_{H,t} - \hat{B}^{MAP}_{H,t-1})$ with corresponding mapping uncertainty $\sigma_x^2$ indicated by the red shaded area. The column labeled "posterior" shows the maximum a posteriori (MAP) estimate, indicated by the o, together with its variance. The MAP estimate is the result of the Bayes' product between likelihood and prior. The amount of integration and the weighting of the signals are given by the length and the orientation of the red arrow, respectively, just as in Figure 12.5. The estimate of discrepancy resulting from the MAP estimate is given by $\hat{D}^{MAP}_{t+} = \hat{S}^{MAP}_{V,t} - \hat{S}^{MAP}_{H,t}$. To determine the part of $\hat{D}^{MAP}_{t+}$ that can be attributed to a visual or haptic bias is again an ambiguous problem. This new credit-assignment problem is solved in the rightmost column labeled "bias estimate." Here the ambiguous $\hat{D}^{MAP}_{t+}$ estimate is represented by the diagonal line. Additionally, there is prior information $p(B_V, B_H)$ about potential biases occurring in the visual and haptic modality, which is indicated by the blue Gaussian blob. The discrepancy estimate combined with the bias prior according to Bayes' rule results in the current bias estimate $\hat{B}^{MAP}_t$. This resulting bias estimate is used for shifting the coupling prior in the next time step. The estimate $\hat{B}^{MAP}_t$ is indicated by x and the blue arrow. The size estimate of the object is the combination of the MAP and the bias estimate according to $\hat{S}_{W,t} = \hat{S}^{MAP}_t - \hat{B}^{MAP}_t = (\hat{S}^{MAP}_{V,t} - \hat{B}^{MAP}_{V,t}, \hat{S}^{MAP}_{H,t} - \hat{B}^{MAP}_{H,t})$. This is indicated by the sum of the red and blue arrow in the "posterior" column. Each row provides a new time step in the remapping process. Repeating the same estimation over several trials $t$, the bias estimate $\hat{B}^{MAP}_t$, as indicated by the blue arrow, is exponentially increasing so that in the end the system reaches the calibrated steady state.

corresponds to the mapping uncertainty. Applying Bayes' rule $p(S_{V,t}, S_{H,t}|z_{V,t}, z_{H,t}) \propto p(z_{V,t}, z_{H,t}|S_{V,t}, S_{H,t})p(S_{V,t}, S_{H,t})$ results in the optimal current estimates of the sensory signals $\hat{S}_t^{MAP} = (\hat{S}_{V,t}^{MAP}, \hat{S}_{H,t}^{MAP})$, thereby maximally reducing the variance in the sensory estimates while at the same time providing the best possible estimate of the current discrepancy $\hat{D}_{t+}^{MAP} = \hat{S}_{H,t}^{MAP} - \hat{S}_{H,t}^{MAP}$ at time step $t$. Thus, the MAP estimate of the discrepancy $\hat{D}_{t+}^{MAP}$ is smaller than $\hat{D}_t$ to the extent that the two sensory signals are coupled. The result of combining likelihood with prior knowledge using Bayes' rule is illustrated in Figure 12.8 in the column labeled "posterior." The result of integration corresponds to Eq. 12.10: $\hat{D}_{t+}^{MAP} = w_x\hat{D}_{t-} + w_z\hat{D}_t = \hat{D}_{t-} + K(\hat{D}_t - \hat{D}_{t-})$. This integration process, illustrated by the red distributions and the red arrow, is identical to what was shown in Figure 12.5. The MAP estimate $\hat{S}_t^{MAP} = (\hat{S}_{V,t}^{MAP}, \hat{S}_{H,t}^{MAP})$ at each time step is the best current estimate of the size signals available. The best current discrepancy estimate between the size signals corresponds to $\hat{D}_{t+}^{MAP} = \hat{S}_{V,t}^{MAP} - \hat{S}_{H,t}^{MAP}$.

Note, up to now we have no estimate of bias $\hat{B}_t$ and no estimate of visual and haptic object size $S_W = (S_{W_V}, S_{W_H})$. What we do have is the discrepancy estimate $\hat{D}_{t+}^{MAP}$, but to what extent the visual and haptic biases contribute to this discrepancy

$$\begin{aligned}\hat{D}_{t+}^{MAP} &= (S_{W_V} + \hat{B}_{V,t}^{MAP}) - (S_{W_H} + \hat{B}_{H,t}^{MAP}) \\ &= \hat{B}_{V,t}^{MAP} - \hat{B}_{H,t}^{MAP}, \qquad (12.14)\end{aligned}$$

given that we are assuming $S_{W_V} = S_{W_H}$, is still unknown. This ambiguity in the discrepancy estimate after integration is indicated by the blue diagonal line in the rightmost column of Figure 12.8. It illustrates that there is an infinite combination of visual and haptic biases that are consistent with $\hat{D}_{t+}^{MAP}$. For now, we assume that we know for sure that the visual and haptic sizes are identical ($S_{W_V} = S_{W_H}$), so the discrepancy estimate given by the blue line contains no noise, that is, is not blurry. The attribution of visual and haptic bias to the discrepancy estimate is a second credit-assignment problem, and in order to solve it we need additional prior knowledge.

In the following we will discuss how to best resolve this new credit-assignment problem. Gharahmani and colleagues (1997) proposed that the discrepancy in the sensory estimates should be resolved in proportion to their variances ($\sigma_V^2, \sigma_H^2$), that is, more credit should be given to a signal with higher variance. However, since the variance of an estimate does not necessarily determine the probability of it containing a bias (i.e., its contribution to the discrepancy), this might lead to a suboptimal strategy. A better way to resolve the credit assignment problem resulting from the "bias ambiguity" may be to use prior knowledge about the probability of the signals being biased $p(B_V, B_H)$. We call this the "bias prior." We need to use prior knowledge because there is no direct information in the sensory signals about whether they are accurate or biased. For example, if the estimates derived from the haptic modality have often been biased in the past, it is more likely that the haptic modality provides the biased signal also in the current situation. This prior knowledge encoding the probability of a bias in a sensory signal is indicated by the blue Gaussian blob in the rightmost column of Figure 12.8. The variance of this prior distribution determines the probability of the signal to be biased. In the example of Figure 12.8, the visual signal is less likely to be biased than the haptic signal. Consequently, in the absence of any other evidence as to what may have caused the discrepancy, the ambiguity in the discrepancy estimate will be resolved once again using Bayes' rule. This time we use Bayes' rule to combine the discrepancy estimate $\hat{D}_{t+}^{MAP}$ with this bias prior $p(B_V, B_H)$. This will result in the current best bias estimate $\hat{B}_t^{MAP} = (\hat{B}_{V,t}^{MAP}, \hat{B}_{H,t}^{MAP})$ indicated by the blue arrow in the rightmost column of Figure 12.8. The proportion $\hat{B}_{V,t}^{MAP}/\hat{B}_{H,t}^{MAP}$ and thus the direction of the blue arrow are solely dependent on the variance of the bias prior $p(B_V, B_H)$. Now that we have a bias estimate we also have an estimate of the visual and haptic size of the object, which was our objective from the start of this chapter. The visual and haptic sizes are given by $\hat{S}_{W,t} = \hat{S}_t^{MAP} - \hat{B}_t^{MAP} = (\hat{S}_{V,t}^{MAP} - \hat{B}_{V,t}^{MAP}, \hat{S}_{H,t}^{MAP} - \hat{B}_{H,t}^{MAP})$ as indicated in Figure 12.8 by the sum of the red and blue arrows in the column labeled "posterior."

With this our estimation problem is solved and at the end of the time step we have the best current estimate of the sensory signals $\hat{S}_t^{MAP}$, the sizes of the objects $\hat{S}_{W,t}$, and the biases $\hat{B}_t^{MAP}$. However, to achieve even more accurate estimates in the future, we have to recalibrate our system based on these bias estimates.

The iterative recalibration process is described next. Each row in Figure 12.8 denotes a new time step $t - 1$. After integration at time step $t - 1$ the perceptual system is left with a bias estimate $\hat{B}_{t-1}^{MAP} = (\hat{B}_{V,t-1}^{MAP}, \hat{B}_{H,t-1}^{MAP})$. It is this bias estimate that is used during recalibration (remapping) to change the mapping at time $t$ defined by the coupling prior. Thus, the coupling prior at time $t$ will be shifted to be consistent with the current estimate of the bias, so that $p(S_{V,t}, S_{H,t}) = p_0(S_{V,t} - \hat{B}_{V,t-1}^{MAP}, S_{H,t} - \hat{B}_{H,t-1}^{MAP})$, indicated by the blue arrow in the "prior" column of Figure 12.8.[8]

This iterative updating process corresponds to the Kalman-filter approach to remapping that we discussed in the last section. As can be seen from Figure 12.8, while the direction of the blue arrow stays constant, the length of the blue arrow continuously increases with every time step, providing an increasingly accurate estimate of the bias $\hat{B}_t^{MAP}$ and the world property $\hat{S}_{W,t}$. Thereby, it is the discrepancy estimate $\hat{D}_{t+}^{MAP}$ that determines the extent to which one must adapt at each time step, and this in turn determines the rate of adaptation. This is consistent with the exponential adaptation response discussed in the previous section (Fig. 12.7 and Eq. 12.13). After several time steps the system eventually reaches steady state. This steady state, however, can only be reached if the bias $B$ is constant over several trials, such as for example when wearing glasses (Fig. 12.3A, third row). In contrast, if the bias $B$ is constantly changing from trial to trial, such as for example when using different grip postures with every size measurement (Fig. 12.3A, second row), recalibration will never saturate and reach steady state.

There is empirical evidence that the bias assignment during recalibration can be situation dependent, indicating the use of different bias priors depending on the exact stimulation condition. This was shown by Di Luca, Machulla, and Ernst (2009) in a recent study on visual-auditory adaptation to temporal asynchrony. For colocated visual-auditory signals, they found that it is the visual estimates that exhibit adaptation. On the other hand, when auditory signals were presented via headphones, they found that participants adapted the auditory estimates. In this study they argue that the manipulation, headphones versus no headphones, alters the probability of the auditory estimate to be biased, which is reflected in a change of the bias prior. They argue that this is because, when presented via headphones, the auditory signal becomes the "odd one out" and is thus more likely biased. The change in bias prior with spatial discrepancy (i.e., with headphones) is similar to the change in the coupling prior with spatial discordance we discussed earlier for modeling the breakdown of integration. With headphones the bias prior will have a larger variance for $B_A$ than for $B_V$, so that with headphones it is predominantly the auditory modality that becomes recalibrated.

So far we have not discussed that the discrepancy estimate $\hat{D}_{t+}^{MAP}$ may contain uncertainty as well. We assumed that we are seeing and touching the object at the same location so that the size of the object is equal in vision and touch $S_{W_V} = S_{W_H}$. In this case any discrepancy detected $\hat{D}_{t+}^{MAP}$ must be the result of a bias so there is no uncertainty in the discrepancy estimate. However, if we consider the situation depicted in Figure 12.3B when we are seeing and touching the object at discrepant locations, $S_{W_V}$ may be different from $S_{W_H}$. This way the discrepancy $\hat{D}_{t+}^{MAP}$ could either result from a bias in one of the sensory signals or from an actual difference in the visual and haptic sizes of the object $(S_{W_V}, S_{W_H})$. If there is such an uncertainty in the discrepancy estimate $\hat{D}_{t+}^{MAP}$, the blue diagonal line representing this discrepancy in Figure 12.8 becomes blurry as well, with the blur representing the

[8]The prior update corresponds to a linear shift. In general, however, also the variance of the prior should be updated. This however, goes beyond the scope of this chapter.

uncertainty. As a result, the Bayes product of the discrepancy estimate with the bias prior will result in a reduced bias estimate $\hat{B}_t^{MAP}$ (compared to the situation when $\hat{D}_{t+}^{MAP}$ was certain). Subtracting this reduced bias estimate $\hat{B}_t^{MAP} = (\hat{B}_{V,t}^{MAP}, \hat{B}_{H,t}^{MAP})$ from the MAP estimate $\hat{S}_t^{MAP} = (\hat{S}_{V,t}^{MAP}, \hat{S}_{H,t}^{MAP})$ will again result in the best current size estimate (Fig. 12.8 sum of red and blue arrow in column labeled "posterior"). However, with the reduced bias estimate, the size estimates for vision and touch will differ: $\hat{S}_{W,t} = \hat{S}_t^{MAP} - \hat{B}_t^{MAP} = (\hat{S}_{V,t}^{MAP} - \hat{B}_{V,t}^{MAP}, \hat{S}_{H,t}^{MAP} - \hat{B}_{H,t}^{MAP})$. Given the situation in Figure 12.3B, this is the optimal estimate of the visual and haptic sizes, their biases, and their signals. As $\hat{B}_t^{MAP}$ becomes smaller with increasing uncertainty in $\hat{D}_{t+}^{MAP}$ the amount of bias recalibration per time step will decrease accordingly.

This brings us to a question that we invoked in the previous section, which we can now answer more comprehensively. This question pertains to why the rate of adaptation varies so much in differing scenarios. The answer is that this is because the rate is a function of both the measurement noise $\Sigma_z$ and the mapping uncertainty $\sigma_x$. A lower measurement noise $\Sigma_z$ causes an increased adaptation rate and so does higher mapping uncertainty $\sigma_x$. Similarly, we have discussed earlier that the extent of integration increases with an increase in measurement noise $\Sigma_z$ and a decrease of mapping uncertainty $\sigma_x$. This dependency between the rate of adaptation and the degree of integration appears to have empirical support. For instance, texture and binocular disparity signals within the visual domain have been shown to be integrated such that they exhibit almost complete fusion (Hillis et al., 2002). This corresponds well to the fact that adaptation of texture and disparity signals can take up to 2 or 3 days (Adams et al., 2001). In contrast, the extent of integration between visual and haptic signals seems significantly far from complete fusion (Ernst, 2005; Hillis et al., 2002), which corresponds to the relatively fast adaptation rate found in the sensorimotor domain and for visual-haptic estimates. From this we may conclude that the mapping uncertainty ($\sigma_x$; the variance of the coupling prior) is very low for the texture and disparity signals in the visual domain and it is comparatively high for sensorimotor and visual-haptic signals. This makes sense because the two visual signals, texture and disparity, originate from the same receptors on the retina, so discrepancies between these two signals are not very likely to occur. The absence of discrepancies means there is no need for adaptation, and thus the estimates can be mandatorily fused. For visual-haptic estimates, however, the situation is different, because there are different receptors responsible for the sensory signals. A discrepancy between the senses is generated, for example, every time we use tools. For example, when we grasp an object using a gripper or a big glove, we have to adjust the mapping between the visual and haptic signals to use these tools in open loop. To adjust quickly to such novel situations, errors in the feedback signals have to be detected, which they could not be if the signals were mandatorily fused. Thus, in the case of visual-haptic estimates the mapping uncertainty $\sigma_x$ is higher than in the case of texture and disparity estimates, leading to a faster adaptation rate and to signals that are not mandatorily fused.

## CONCLUDING REMARKS AND SOME OPEN QUESTIONS

We began this chapter by describing the standard model of integration (see Chapter 1) because it has proven successful in the description of many experimental results. During the course of this chapter, our goal was to argue that the process of integration is more complex than the standard model leads us to believe. The standard model seeks to reduce the noise in perceptual estimates through integration and focuses on what we have earlier referred to as the benefits of integration. However, it assumes perfectly correlated and unbiased (accurate) estimates and therefore disregards the potential cost of integration. The price we pay for such an assumption is that we disregard the fact that the estimates may actually become biased during integration. If we take into account that signals may be inaccurate, by balancing costs and benefits in a probabilistic way as we have suggested here, we achieve a unified framework that can explain the process of integration as well as the process of remapping.

This framework assumes that for both integration and remapping, there exists a precise representation of the probability distributions that represent the measurement process as well as prior knowledge about the mapping between different sensory signals, that is, their co-occurrence statistics, and about the probability of occurrence of a discrepancy between the sensory signals $S_i$ and the world property $S_W$. This includes knowing not only the mean and the variance of the distributions but also the entire shape, because knowledge of the shape of the probability distributions has proven to be crucial, especially in the efforts to model the breakdown of integration. Up to now, however, our knowledge about how these distributions are represented in the human brain is very limited. There are some indications from computational neuroscience that the utilization of such probability distributions may be implemented in a neuronal population code. Pouget, Denève, and Duhamel (2002) demonstrated that processing with such population codes can perform integration and remapping of sensory estimates equally well (see also Chapter 21; Ma, Beck, Latham, & Pouget, 2006; Pouget et al., 2002). There is also some recent evidence from monkey physiology that Bayes-optimal integration of visual and vestibular estimates of perceived direction of motion may be conducted in populations of neurons in area MSTd of the monkey brain (see Chapter 16; Gu, Angelaki, & Deangelis, 2008).

One major problem that we face currently with the Bayesian approach is that the prior distributions, which are used to represent the statistics of the sensory signals derived from the environment, are merely postulated. The reason that they are only postulated is that they are not easily measurable. Future research needs to address how priors can be determined, measured, or manipulated independently. There are several ways to achieve this. One method entails the study of how priors are learned in one context and then to investigate how the learning of these priors is transferred to other situations or tasks. This has successfully been demonstrated by Adams et al. (2004), who adapted the light-from-above prior in one context and demonstrated transfer of the learning effect to another context and task, thereby undoubtedly demonstrating the updating of a priori knowledge. Alternatively, one can indirectly infer the prior by varying the reliability of the signal estimates using a method proposed by Stocker and Simoncelli (2006). Ideally, such an inferred prior distribution should then be compared to the statistics of the environment as measured independently by some physical measurement device. Recently, this approach has been employed by Banks, Burge, and Held (Chapter 11) for the visual perception of depth at an occluding contour. In their experiments, Burge et al. found a good qualitative agreement between the empirically inferred prior and the physically measured statistics of the environment. Future research must strive to demonstrate such correspondence between postulated priors and the statistics of the environment in order to justify the Bayesian approach to human perception.

## ACKNOWLEDGMENTS

We thank Mike Landy for very helpful comments on earlier drafts of this chapter and Devika Narain for outstanding help in the editing process. This work was supported by the EU grant ImmerSence (IST-2006-027141), the EU grant THE (IST-2009-248587), and the HFSP Research Grant (2006) "Mechanisms of associative learning in human perception."

## REFERENCES

Adams, W. J., Banks, M. S., & van Ee, R. (2001). Adaptation to three-dimensional distortions in human vision. *Nature Neuroscience, 4*, 1063–1064.

Adams, W. J., Graf, E. W., & Ernst, M. O. (2004). Experience can change the "light-from-above" prior. *Nature Neuroscience, 7*, 1057–1058.

Alais, D., & Burr, D. (2004). The ventriloquist effect results from near optimal crossmodal integration. *Current Biology, 14*, 257–262.

Baddeley, R. J., Ingram, H. A., & Miall, R. C. (2003). System identification applied to a visuomotor task: Near-optimal human performance in a noisy changing task. *Journal of Neuroscience, 23,* 3066–3075.

Bedford, F. L. (1993). Perceptual learning. In D. Medin (Ed.), *The psychology of learning and motivation* (pp. 1–60). New York, NY: Academic Press.

Bertelson, P., & Radeau, M. (1981). Cross-modal bias and perceptual fusion with auditory–visual discordance. *Perception and Psychophysics, 29,* 578–584.

Bresciani, J-P., Dammeier, F., & Ernst, M. O. (2006). Vision and touch are automatically integrated for the perception of sequences of events. *Journal of Vision, 6,* 554–564.

Bresciani, J-P., Dammeier, F., & Ernst, M. O. (2008). Tri-modal integration of visual, tactile and auditory signals for the perception of sequences of events. *Brain Research Bulletin, 75,* 753–760.

Bresciani, J-P., & Ernst, M. O. (2007). Signal reliability modulates auditory-tactile integration for event counting. *NeuroReport, 18,* 1157–1167.

Bresciani, J-P., Ernst, M. O., Drewing, K., Bouyer, G., Maury, V., & Kheddar, A. (2005). Feeling what you hear: Auditory signals can modulate tactile taps perception. *Experimental Brain Research, 162,* 172–180.

Brewster, D. (1826). On the optical illusion of the conversion of cameos into intaglios and of intaglios into cameos, with an account of other analogous phenomena. *Edinburgh Journal of Science, 4,* 99–108.

Burge, J., Ernst, M. O., & Banks, M. S. (2008). The statistical determinants of adaptation rate in human reaching. *Journal of Vision, 8*(4):20, 1–19.

Cochran, W. G. (1937). Problems arising in the analysis of a series of similar experiments. *Journal of the Royal Statistical Society, 4*(Suppl.), 102–118.

Di Luca, M., Machulla, T-K., & Ernst, M. O. (2009). Recalibration of multisensory simultaneity: Crossmodal transfer coincides with a change in perceptual latency. *Journal of Vision, 9*(12):7, 1–16.

Dror, R., Willsky, A., & Adelson, E. (2004). Statistical characterization of real-world illumination. *Journal of Vision, 4,* 821–837.

Ernst, M. O. (2005). A Bayesian view on multimodal cue integration. In G. Knoblich, I. Thornton, M. Grosjean, & M. Shiffrar (Eds.), *Human body perception from the inside out* (pp.105–131). New York, NY: Oxford University Press.

Ernst, M. O. (2007). Learning to integrate arbitrary signals from vision and touch. *Journal of Vision, 7*(5):7, 1–14.

Ernst, M. O., & Banks, M. S. (2002). Humans integrate visual and haptic information in a statistically optimal fashion. *Nature, 415,* 429–433.

Ernst, M. O., & Bülthoff, H. H. (2004). Merging the senses into a robust percept. *Trends in Cognitive Sciences, 8,* 162–169.

Frissen, I., Vroomen, J., & de Gelder, B. (2003). The aftereffects of ventriloquism: Are they sound-frequency specific? *Acta Psychologica, 113,* 315–327.

Gebhard, J. W., & Mowbray, G. H. (1959). On discriminating the rate of visual flicker and auditory flutter. *The American Journal of Psychology, 72,* 521–529.

Gepshtein, S., Burge, J., Banks, M. S., & Ernst, M. O. (2005). Optimal combination of vision and touch has a limited spatial range. *Journal of Vision, 5,* 1013–1023.

Ghahramani, Z., Wolpert, D. M., & Jordan, M. I. (1997). Computational models of sensorimotor integration. In P. G. Morasso & V. Sanguineti (Eds.), *Self-organization, computational maps and motor control* (pp. 117–147). Amsterdam, Netherlands: Elsevier Press.

Gu, Y., Angelaki, D. E., & Deangelis, G. C. (2008). Neural correlates of multisensory cue integration in macaque MSTd. *Nature Neuroscience, 11,* 1201–1210.

Hartung, B., Schrater, P. R., Bülthoff, H. H., Kersten, D., & Franz, V. H. (2005). Is prior knowledge of object geometry used in visually guided reaching? *Journal of Vision, 5,* 504–514.

Helbig, H. B., & Ernst, M. O. (2007). Optimal integration of shape information from vision and touch. *Experimental Brain Research, 179,* 595–606.

Hillis, J. M., Ernst, M. O., Banks, M. S., & Landy, M. S. (2002). Combining sensory information: mandatory fusion within, but not between, senses. *Science, 298,* 1627–1630.

Hillis, J. M., Watt, S., Landy, M. S., & Banks, M. S. (2004). Slant from texture and disparity cues: Optimal cue combination. *Journal of Vision, 4,* 1–24.

Jack, C. E., Thurlow, W. R. (1973). Effects of degree of visual association and angle of displacement on the "ventriloquism" effect. *Perceptual and Motor Skills, 37,* 967–979.

Jackson, C. V. (1953). Visual factors in auditory localization. *Quarterly Journal of Experimental Psychology, 5*, 52–65.

Kersten D., Mamassian, P., & Yuille, A. (2004). Object perception as Bayesian inference. *Annual Review of Psychology, 44*, 271–304.

Knill, D. C. (2007a). Learning Bayesian priors for depth perception. *Journal of Vision, 7*(8):13, 1–20.

Knill, D. C. (2007b). Robust cue integration: A Bayesian model and evidence from cue-conflict studies with stereoscopic and figure cues to slant. *Journal of Vision, 7*(7):5, 1–24.

Knill, D. C., & Saunders, J. A. (2003). Do humans optimally integrate stereo and texture information for judgments of surface slant? *Vision Research, 43*, 2539–2558.

Körding, K. P., Beierholm, U., Ma, W., Quartz, S., Tenenbaum, J., Shams, L., & Sporns, O. (2007). Causal inference in multisensory perception. *PLoS ONE, 2*, e943.

Körding, K. P., & Wolpert, D. M. (2004). Bayesian integration of sensorimotor learning. *Nature, 427*, 244–247.

Landy, M. S., & Kojima, H. (2001). Ideal cue combination for localizing texture-defined edges. *Journal of the Optical Society of America A, 18*, 2307–2320.

Landy, M. S., Maloney, L. T., Johnston, E. B., & Young, M. J. (1995). Measurement and modeling of depth cue combination: In defense of weak fusion. *Vision Research, 35*, 389–412.

Ma, J. W., Beck, J. M., Latham, P. E., & Pouget A. (2006). Bayesian inference with probabilistic population codes. *Nature Neuroscience, 9*, 1432–1438.

Mamassian, P., & Goutcher, R. (2001). Prior knowledge on the illumination position. *Cognition, 81*, B1–B9.

Mamassian, P., Landy, M., & Maloney, L. T. (2002). Bayesian modelling of visual perception. In P. N. Rao, B. A. Olshausen, & M. S. Lewicki (Eds.), *Probabilistic models of the brain* (pp. 13–60). Cambridge, MA: MIT Press.

Myers, A. K., Cotton, B., & Hilp, H. A. (1981). Matching the rate of concurrent tone bursts and light flashes as a function of flash surround luminance. *Perception and Psychophysics, 30*, 33–38.

Oruç, I., Maloney, T. M., & Landy, M. S. (2003). Weighted linear cue combination with possibly correlated error. *Vision Research, 43*, 2451–2468.

Palmer, S. (1985). The role of symmetry in shape perception. *Acta Psychologica, 59*, 67–90.

Pick, H., Warren, D., & Hay, J. (1969). Sensory conflict in judgments of spatial direction. *Perception and Psychophysics, 6*, 203–205.

Pouget, A., Denève, S., & Duhamel, J. (2002). Opinion: A computational perspective on the neural basis of multisensory spatial representations. *Nature Reviews Neuroscience, 3*, 741–747.

Radeau, M., & Bertelson, P. (1987). Auditory-visual interaction and the timing of inputs. Thomas (1941) revisited. *Psychological Research, 49*, 17–22.

Recanzone, G. H. (2003). Auditory influences on visual temporal rate perception. *Journal of Neurophysiology, 89*, 1078–1093.

Roach, N., Heron, J., & Mcgraw, P. (2006). Resolving multisensory conflict: A strategy for balancing the costs and benefits of audio-visual integration. *Proceedings of the Royal Society of London B: Biological Sciences, 273*, 2159–2168.

Rock, I. (1983). *The logic of perception.* Cambridge, MA: MIT Press.

Shams, L., Kamitani, Y., & Shimojo, S. (2002). Visual illusion induced by sound. *Cognitive Brain Research, 14*, 147–152.

Shipley, T. (1964). Auditory flutter-driving of visual flicker. *Science, 187*, 802.

Stocker, A. A., & Simoncelli, E. P. (2006). Noise characteristics and prior expectations in human visual speed perception. *Nature Neuroscience, 9*, 578–585.

van Beers, R. J., Sittig, A. C., & Denier van der Gon, J. J. (1998). The precision of proprioceptive position sense. *Experimental Brain Research, 122*, 367–377.

van Beers, R. J., Sittig, A. C., & Denier van der Gon, J. J. (1999). Integration of proprioceptive and visual position information: An experimentally supported model. *Journal of Neurophysiology, 81*, 1355–1364.

van Wassenhove, V., Grant, K., & Poeppel, D. (2007). Temporal window of integration in auditory-visual speech perception. *Neuropsychologia, 45*, 598–607.

von Helmholtz, H. (1867). *Handbuch der physiologischen Optic* (Vol. 3). Leipzig, Germany: Leopold Voss.

Wallace, M. T., Roberson, G. E., Hairston, W. D., Stein, B. E., Vaughan, J. W., & Schirillo, J. A. (2004). Unifying multisensory signals across time and space. *Experimental Brain Research, 158*, 252–258.

Warren, D. H., & Cleaves, W. T. (1971). Visual-proprioceptive interaction under large amounts of conflicts. *Journal of Experimental Psychology, 90,* 206–214.

Weiss, Y., Simoncelli, E. P., & Adelson, E. H. (2002). Motion illusions as optimal percepts. *Nature Neuroscience, 5,* 598–604.

Welch, R. B. (1978). *Perceptual modification: Adapting to altered sensory environments.* New York, NY: Academic Press.

Welch, R. B., DuttonHurt, L., & Warren, D. (1986). Contributions of audition and vision to temporal rate. *Perception and Psychophysics, 39,* 294–300.

Welch, R. B., & Warren, D. H. (1980). Immediate perceptual response to intersensory discrepancy. *Psychological Bulletin, 88,* 638–667.

Welch, R. B., & Warren, D. H. (1986). Intersensory interactions. In K. R. Boff, L. Kaufman, & J. P. Thomas (Eds.), *Handbook of perception and human performance* (pp. 25.1–25.36). New York, NY: J. Wiley & Sons.

Witkin, H. A., Wapner, S., & Leventhal, T. J. (1952). Sound localization with conflicting visual and auditory cues. *Journal of Experimental Psychology, 43,* 58–67.

Young, M., Landy, M., & Maloney, L. (1993). A perturbation analysis of depth perception from combinations of texture and motion cues. *Vision Research, 33,* 2685–2696.

# CHAPTER 13

## Humans' Multisensory Perception, from Integration to Segregation, Follows Bayesian Inference

*Ladan Shams and Ulrik Beierholm*

### INTRODUCTION

Humans are almost always surrounded by multiple objects and, therefore, multiple sources of sensory stimulation. At any given instant, the brain is typically engaged in processing sensory stimuli from two or more modalities. To achieve a coherent and valid perception of the physical world, it must determine which of these temporally coincident sensory signals are caused by the same physical source and thus should be integrated into a single percept. However, integration of sensory signals that originate from different objects/events can be detrimental; therefore, it is equally important for the nervous system to determine which signals should be segregated. The signals of different modalities are more likely to be integrated if they are spatially congruent (Spence, Pavani, Maravita, & Holmes, 2004). For example, when in a parking lot, we tend to fuse the sound of a car honk with the image of a car that is spatially closest to the honk. Furthermore, signals are more likely to be integrated if they are structurally congruent. The sound of a TV program is normally integrated with the pictures on the TV screen; however, such integration would not occur if the speakers play the sound from a news program while the video displays a children's show. Thus, the determination of which set of temporally coincident sensory signals are to be bound together and which are to be segregated seems to be based on the degrees of spatial and structural consistency of the signals, which can vary from situation to situation.

In this chapter, we will first discuss experimental findings showing that multisensory perception encompasses a spectrum of phenomena ranging from full integration (or fusion), to partial integration, to complete segregation. Next, we will describe two Bayesian causal-inference models that can account for the entire range of combinations of two or more sensory cues. We will show that one of these models, which is a hierarchical Bayesian model, is a special form of the other one (which is a nonhierarchical model). We will then compare the predictions of these models with human data in multiple experiments and show that Bayesian causal-inference models can account for the human data remarkably well. Finally, we will present a study that investigates the stability of priors in the face of drastic change in sensory conditions.

### RANGE OF INTERACTIONS BETWEEN TWO MODALITIES

We have explored the question of when and how the different sensory signals are integrated using two paradigms, one in which the degree of structural consistency between signals is varied, and one in which the degree of spatial consistency is varied. One paradigm uses the task of temporal numerosity judgment, and the other one uses the task of spatial localization. These two paradigms are complementary in the sense that the temporal numerosity judgment task primarily involves temporal processing, whereas spatial localization is obviously a spatial task. In one case (numerosity judgment) hearing dominates the percept, whereas in the other (spatial localization) vision dominates under natural conditions. Another feature of these paradigms is that in both of them strong interactions occur between modalities under some conditions, leading to well-known illusions: the sound-induced flash illusion (Shams, Kamitani, & Shimojo, 2000) and the ventriloquist effect (Howard & Templeton, 1966).

First, we discuss the human data in these two experimental settings. In the numerosity-judgment experiment (Shams, Ma, & Beierholm, 2005), a variable number of flashes paired with a variable number of beeps (each ranging from zero to four) were presented in each trial and the subject was asked to report both the number of flashes and the number of beeps they perceived at the end of each trial. The center of trains of flashes and beeps were temporally aligned in all trials. Figure 13.1 shows the group data from 10 observers. Strong sound-induced flash illusions can be found in a large fraction of trials in the panels corresponding to 1 flash + 2 beeps and 2 flashes + 1 beep, where a single flash is perceived as two flashes, and where two flashes are perceived as one flash, respectively.

In the spatial localization experiment (Körding et al., 2007), observers were presented in each trial with either a brief visual stimulus in one of five locations (along the horizontal direction in the frontoparallel plane, ranging from $-10°$ to $+10°$ of visual field equally spaced), or a brief sound at one of the same five locations, or both simultaneously. Their task was to report the location of the visual stimulus as well as the location of the sound in each trial by a key press in a forced-choice paradigm. All 35 combinations of these stimuli (except for no flash and no sound) were presented in pseudorandom order. The group data from 19 observers are shown in Figure 13.2. The ventriloquist illusion can be found in several conditions, for example, in V2A3 (i.e., visual stimulus at $-5°$, auditory at $0°$) where the location of sound is captured by vision in a large fraction of trials.

In these illusion trials, in which perception in one modality is completely captured by the other modality or the percepts in two modalities are shifted toward each other and converge, the two modalities are fused. The two modalities are also fused when there is no discrepancy between the stimuli as in conditions along the diagonal in which the auditory and visual pulsations or locations are the same. Inspecting the matrix of joint auditory-visual responses (not shown here) confirms that indeed in these conditions the subjects generally report seeing and hearing the same thing simultaneously. At the other extreme, little or no interaction between the two modalities is found when there is a large discrepancy between the two stimuli, for example, in 1 flash + 4 beeps or 4 flashes + 1 beep conditions (Fig. 13.1) or in V1A5 or V5A1 conditions (Fig. 13.2). More interestingly, there are also many trials in which the two modalities are neither completely fused nor segregated, but partially shifted toward each other. We refer to this phenomenon as "partial integration." It occurs when the discrepancy between the two modalities is moderate. Examples can be found in the 3 flashes + 1 beep condition in which two flashes and one beep are perceived (Figs. 13.1 and 13.3), and in the V3A5 condition where V3 and A4 locations are perceived (Fig. 13.2) in a large fraction of trials. In summary, when the discrepancy between the two modalities is none or small, the two modalities are fused; when the discrepancy is large, the two modalities are segregated; and when the discrepancy is moderate, partial integration can occur (Fig. 13.4A). Small discrepancy can be caused by environmental or neural noise even when the two signals originate from the same object. Therefore, it makes sense for the nervous system to fuse the signals when the discrepancy is minute. Similarly, large discrepancy is often due to the fact that the two signals are not caused by the same object, and therefore it makes sense for the nervous system to segregate them. It is

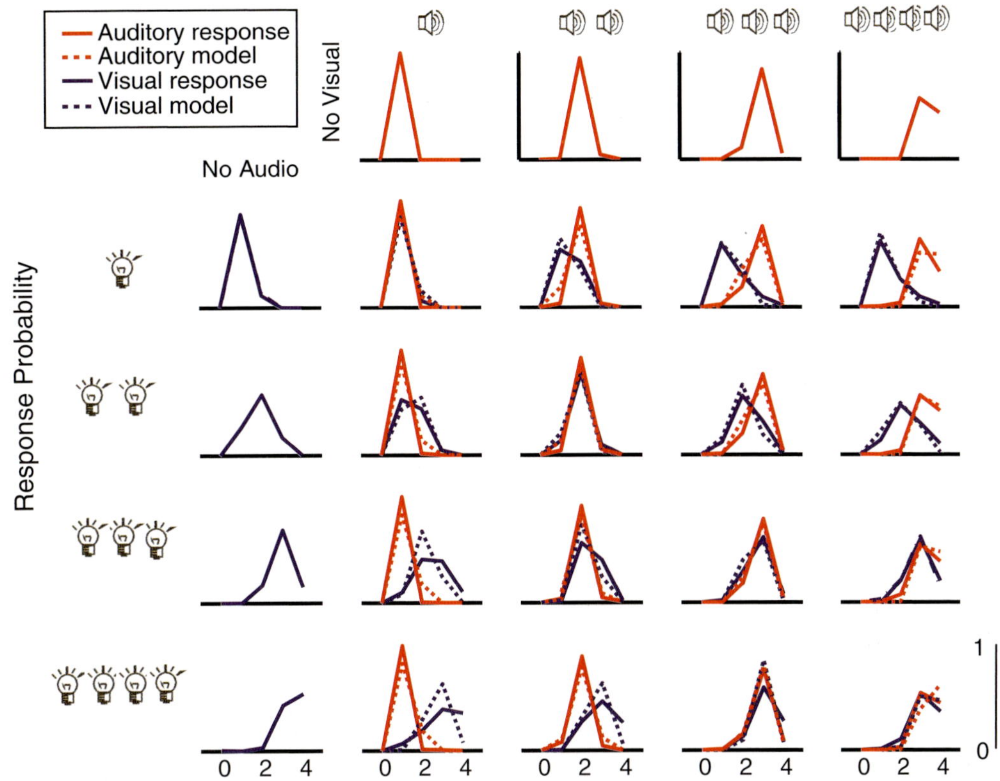


**Figure 13.1** Human observers' response profiles in the temporal-numerosity-judgment task. To facilitate interpretation of the data, instead of presenting a 5x5 matrix of joint posterior probabilities for each condition, only the two one-dimensional projections of the joint response distributions are displayed; that is, in each condition, instead of showing 25 auditory-visual responses, 10 marginalized distributions are shown (5 auditory and 5 visual). The auditory and visual judgments of human observers are plotted in red and blue, respectively. Each panel represents one of the conditions. The first row and first column represent the auditory-alone and visual-alone conditions, respectively. The remaining panels correspond to conditions in which auditory and visual stimuli were presented simultaneously. The horizontal axes represent the response category (with zeros denoting absence of a stimulus and 1–4 representing the number of flashes or beeps). The vertical axes represent the probability of a perceived number of flashes or beeps.

not obvious, however, what the advantage of partial integration is for stimuli of moderate discrepancy. What would be gained by only partially integrating the information from two modalities? The goal of this work is to find computational principles that can explain this entire range of cross-modal interaction.

To examine whether there is a sharp divide between the situations of integration and segregation, we quantified the cross-modal integration in each condition (see Fig. 13.4 caption for details) and plotted the amount of integration as a function of discrepancy between the two modalities. Figures 13.4B and 13.4C show the results of this analysis for the two experiments described earlier. As can be seen, integration between the two modalities degrades smoothly as the discrepancy between the two modalities increases. The model presented later accounts for this graded integration/segregation scheme using one single inference process.

It is not uncommon in daily life to have simultaneous stimulation in more than two sensory modalities. How do cues from three

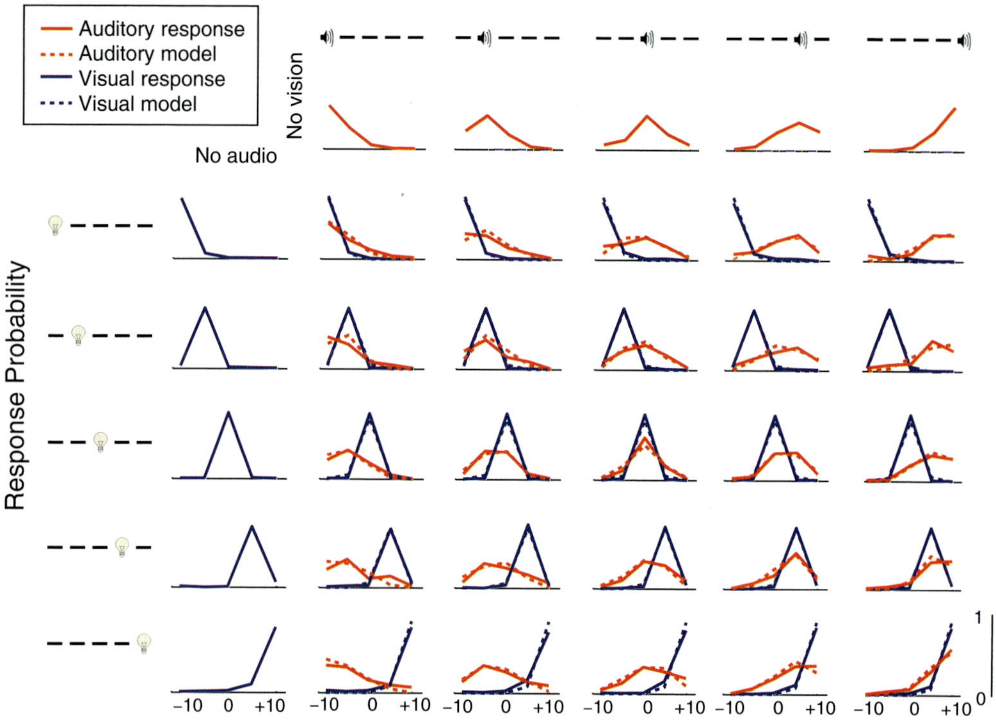


**Figure 13.2** Human data in the spatial-localization experiment. As in Figure 13.1, to facilitate interpretation of the data, marginalized posteriors are shown. The representation of the human data is identical to Figure 13.1, with the exception that the response categories range from –10 to +10 degrees of azimuth.

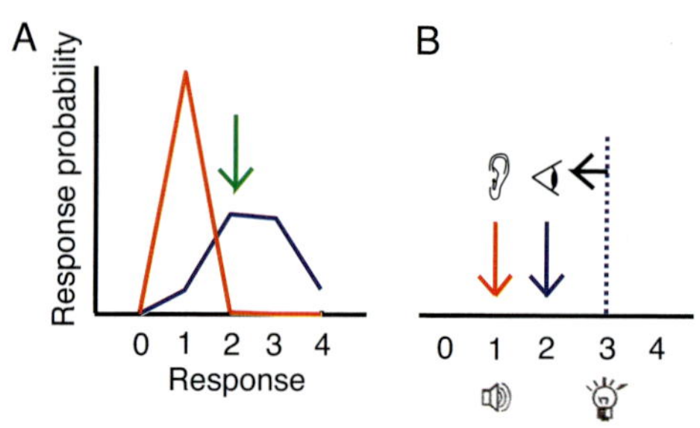


**Figure 13.3** (A) In the temporal-numerosity-judgment task, in the 3 flashes-1 beep condition, one beep and two flashes are perceived in many trials (green arrow). (B) This is an example of partial integration in which the visual percept is shifted toward the auditory percept but only partially.

modalities interact? We tested trisensory cue combination using the numerosity-judgment paradigm where a variable number (ranging from 0 to 2) of flashes, beeps, and taps were presented in each trial and the subjects were asked to judge all three in each trial. Figure 13.5 shows the human data for the various stimulus conditions. This experiment revealed a number of different illusions, both of fusion (when two pulses are perceived as one) and fission (when one pulse is perceived as two) type, across almost all pairs and triplets of modalities. In almost all conditions where there was a discrepancy between the modalities, an illusion was found, showing that these interactions are indeed the rule rather than the exception in human perceptual processing.

## BAYESIAN MODEL OF INTEGRATION AND SEGREGATION

Traditional models of cue combination (Fig. 13.6A) (Alais & Burr, 2004; Bülthoff & Mallot, 1988; Knill, 2003; Landy, Maloney, Johnston, & Young, 1995; Yuille & Bülthoff,

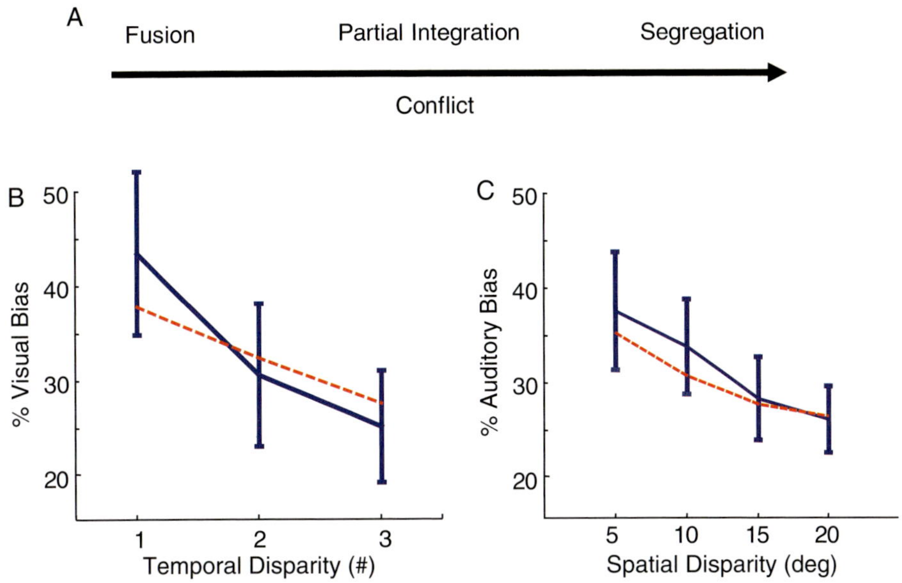


**Figure 13.4** (A) The spectrum of perceptual phenomena as a function of degree of conflict between two modalities. When there is no or small discrepancy between two modalities, the signals tend to be fused. When the discrepancy is moderate, partial integration may occur. When the discrepancy is large, the signals are segregated. (B) Bias (auditory influence on vision) as a function of discrepancy between the two modalities. Bias is here defined as the absolute deviation from veridical, divided by discrepancy. (C) Bias (influence of vision on auditory perception) as a function of spatial disparity between the auditory and visual stimuli.

1996) have been successful in accounting for the fusion phenomenon (e.g., Alais & Burr, 2004; Ernst & Banks, 2002; Ghahramani, Wolpert, & Jordan, 1997; Hillis, Ernst, Banks, & Landy, 2002; van Beers, Sittig, & Denier van der Gon, 1999), but they are unable to account for the segregation and partial-integration range of interactions. As discussed earlier, the full integration only occurs when the discrepancy (spatial, temporal, structural) between the two signals is small. Moderate and large discrepancies result in different percepts in different modalities, which cannot be explained by traditional models.

## Implicit Causal-Inference Model

We developed a Bayesian observer model (see Fig. 13.6B) that does not assume such forced fusion (Shams et al., 2005). Instead, our model assumes a source for each signal; however, the sources are not taken to be statistically independent. Thus, the model allows inference about both cases in which separate entities have caused the sensory signals (segregation) and cases in which sensory signals are caused by one source (integration). The model uses Bayes' rule to make inferences about the causes of the various sensory signals. This framework is very general and can be extended to any number of signals and any combination of modalities (Fig. 13.6C). However, for the purpose of illustration, we first focus on the combination of audition and vision.

We assume that the auditory and visual signals are statistically independent given the auditory and visual causes. This is a common assumption, motivated by the hypothesis that the noise processes that corrupt the signals in the different sensory pathways are independent. The information about the likelihood of sensory signal $x_A$ occurring given an auditory cause $s_A$ is represented by the probability distribution $P(x_A|s_A)$. Similarly, $P(x_V|s_V)$ represents the likelihood of sensory signal $x_V$ given a source $s_V$ in the physical world. The priors $P(s_A, s_V)$ denote the perceptual knowledge of the observer about

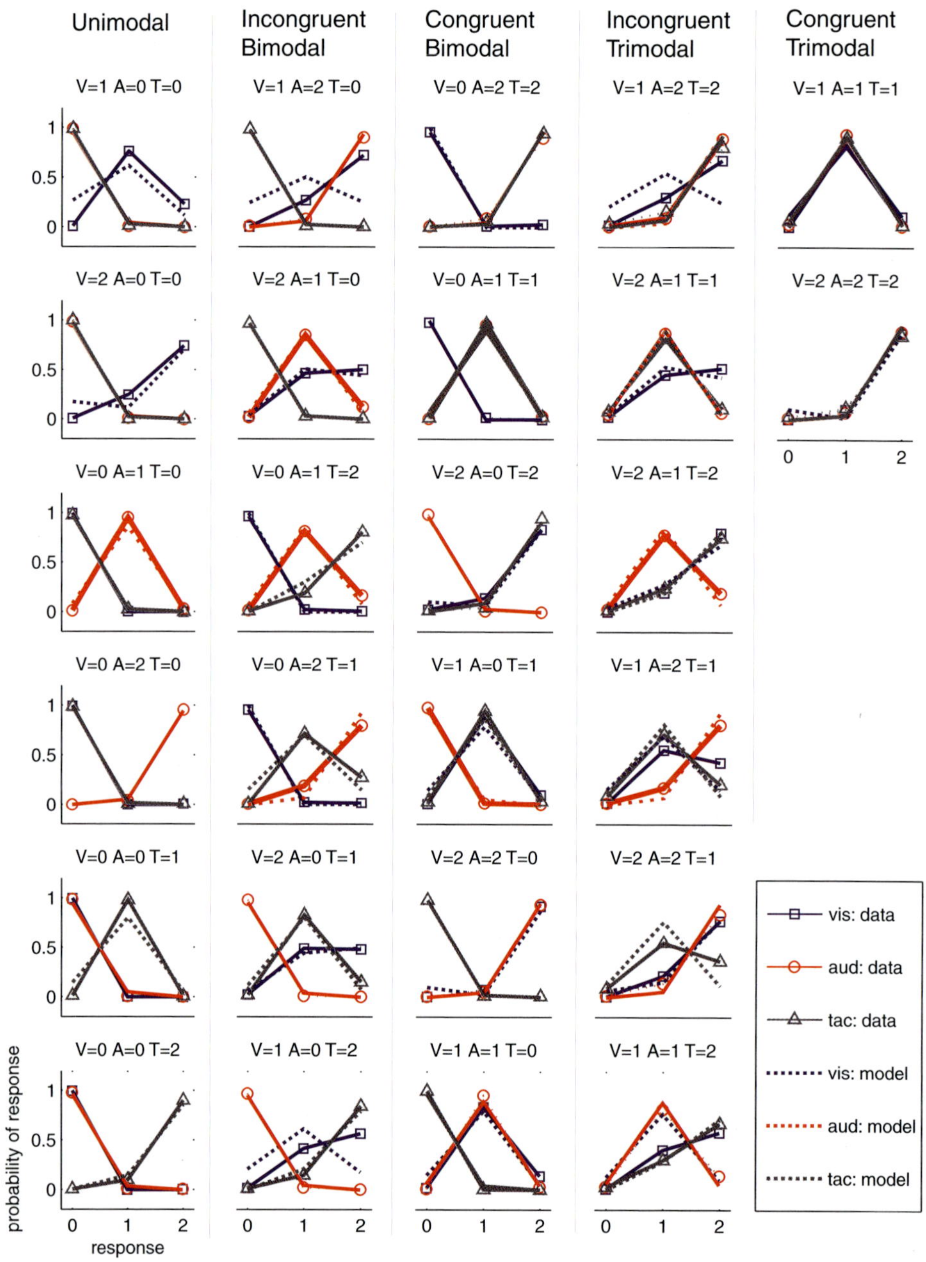


**Figure 13.5** Human data and fits of the Bayesian observer model in the trisensory numerosity-judgment task. Each panel corresponds to one of the stimulus conditions. Blue, red, and black represent visual, auditory, and tactile responses, respectively. Symbols and solid lines represent data and broken lines represent model fits. The horizontal axis is the response category, and the vertical axis is the response probability.

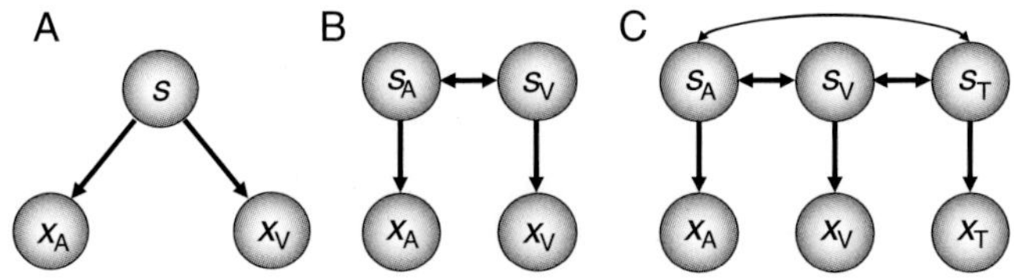


**Figure 13.6** Generative models of different cue-combination models. The graph nodes represent random variables, and arrows denote potential conditionality. The absence of an arrow represents statistical independence between the two variables. (A) This Bayes net represents the traditional model of cue combination, in which the cues are assumed to be caused by one object. (B) This graph represents the model of Shams et al. (2005) in which the two cues may or may not be caused by the same object. The double arrow represents interdependency between the two variables. (C) This graph represents the model of Wozny, Beierholm, and Shams (2008) in which three cues are considered and any one or two or three of them may be caused by the same or distinct sources.

the auditory-visual events in the environment. This prior probability encodes the interaction between the two modalities, and thus it can be referred to as an interaction prior. If the two modalities are independent of each other, the two-dimensional distribution will be factorizable (e.g., like an isotropic Gaussian; Fig. 13.7A). In contrast, if the two modalities are expected to be consistent in all conditions, that is, highly coupled together, then it will have a diagonal form (with all other nondiagonal values equal to zero, Fig. 13.7B). An ideal observer would try to make the best possible estimate of the physical sources $s_A$ and $s_V$, based on the knowledge $P(x_A|s_A)$, $P(x_V|s_V)$ and $P(s_A, s_V)$. These estimates are based on the posterior probabilities $P(s_A, s_V|x_A, x_V)$, which can be calculated using Bayes' rule, and simplified by the assumptions represented by the model structure (Fig. 13.6B), resulting in the following inference rule:

$$P(s_A, s_V|x_A, x_V) = \frac{P(x_A|s_A)P(x_V|s_V)P(s_A, s_V)}{P(x_A, x_V)}. \qquad (13.1)$$

This inference rule simply states that the posterior probability of events $s_A$ and $s_V$ is the normalized product of the single-modality likelihoods and joint prior.

This model can account for the observer's data in both experiments (Beierholm, 2007; Shams et al., 2005). It can also be easily extended to a combination of three modalities. Figure 13.6C shows the extension of the model to auditory-visual-tactile combination (Wozny, Beierholm, & Shams, 2008). We tested this model on the trisensory numerosity-judgment task. We assumed a univariate Gaussian distribution for likelihood functions and a trivariate Gaussian function for the joint prior. The standard deviations of the auditory, tactile, and visual likelihood functions were estimated from unisensory-condition data. It was assumed that the means, variances, and covariances of the multivariate prior distribution were all equal across the three senses; that is, all three means are identical, all three variances are identical, and all three covariances are identical. Thus, the model had only three free parameters, corresponding to the variance, covariance, and mean values of the prior distribution. To produce predictions of the model, we ran Monte Carlo simulations. On each trial, the mean of each likelihood function was assumed to have been sampled from a Gaussian distribution with a mean at the veridical location and a standard deviation equal to that estimated from unisensory data. This results in different posterior distribution on each trial (of the same stimulus condition). We assume the observers minimize the mean squared error of their responses, and thus the optimal estimate is the mean of the posterior distribution (which in this case is equivalent to the maximum, as the posterior is a Gaussian). In this fashion, for each stimulus condition, we obtained a distribution of responses, and this distribution was compared

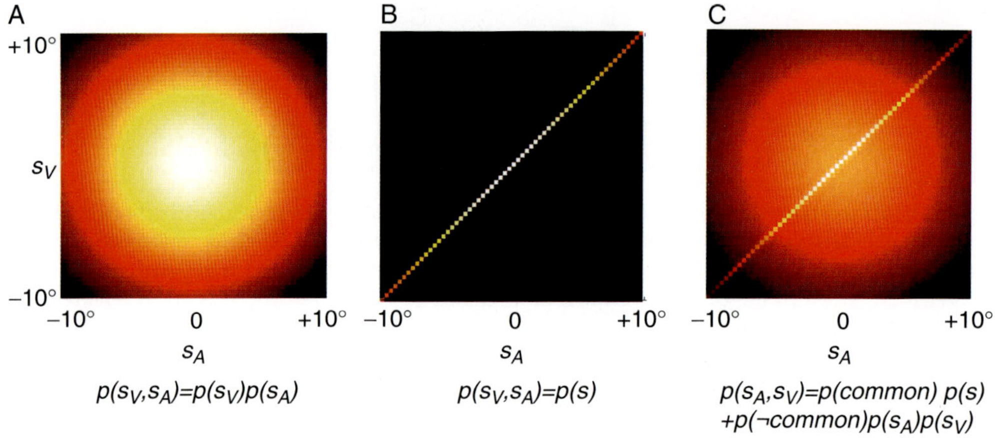


**Figure 13.7** The interaction prior. The horizontal and vertical axes represent auditory and visual sources, respectively. (A) This isotropic Gaussian function is factorizable and indicates that the two sources are independent of each other. (B) This prior indicates that the two sources are always the same and cannot take on different values. (C) This prior is a mixture of the priors shown in (A) and (B). This is the prior distribution for the causal-inference model.

with the response distribution obtained from human observers. As can be seen in Figure 13.5, the model can account for all two-way and three-way interactions. Using only three free parameters, the model can provide a remarkable account ($R^2 = 0.95$) for 676 data points.

## Explicit Causal-Inference Model

While the model just described can account for the entire range of interactions from integration, to partial integration, to segregation, it does not make explicit predictions about the perceived causal structure of the events. To be able to make predictions directly about the causal structure of the stimuli, one needs a hierarchical model in which a variable encodes the choice between different causal structures (Fig. 13.8). Assuming that observers minimize the mean squared error of their responses, this generative model (Fig. 13.8) would result in the following inference. The probability of a common cause is determined using Bayes' rule as follows:

$$p(C=1|x_V,x_A)=\frac{p(x_V,x_A|C=1)\,p(C=1)}{p(x_V,x_A)} \tag{13.2}$$

In other words, the probability of common cause depends on the similarity between the two sensations and the prior belief in a common cause. Notably, the optimal estimate of the two modalities turns out to be a weighted average of two optimal estimates: the optimal estimate corresponding to the independent-causes hypothesis, and the optimal estimate corresponding to the common-cause hypothesis, each weighted according to its respective probability:

$$\hat{s} = p\left(C=1|x_V,x_A\right)\hat{s}_{C=1} + p\left(C=2|x_V,x_A\right)\hat{s}_{C=2}. \tag{13.3}$$

This is a nonlinear combination of the two sensations and results in partial integration.

## Relationship between the Two Models

Although the models shown in Eqs. 13.1 and 13.3 and Figures 13.6B and 13.8 look very different, they are intimately related. The hierarchical model is a special case of the nonhierarchical model. By integrating out the variable $C$, the hierarchical model can be recast as a special form

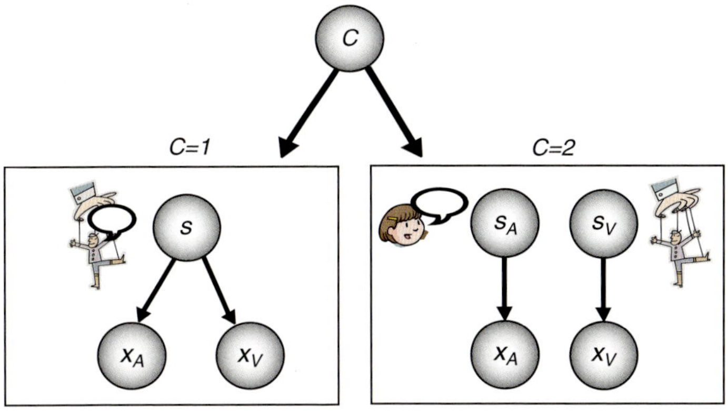


**Figure 13.8** The generative model for the hierarchical causal-inference model.

of the nonhierarchical model:

$$p(s_A, s_V | x_A, x_V) = \frac{p(x_A | s_A)p(x_V | s_V)p(s_A, s_V)}{p(x_A, x_V)}, \quad (13.4)$$

where $p(s_A, s_V) = p(C = 1)p(s) + p(C = 2) p(s_A)p(s_V)$.

This formulation also makes it obvious that the hierarchical causal-inference model is a mixture model, where the joint prior (Fig. 13.7C) is a weighted average of the prior corresponding to a common cause (Fig. 13.7B) and a prior corresponding to independent causes (an isotropic two-dimensional Gaussian, Fig. 13.7A), each weighted by its respective prior probability. Mathematically, this model is equivalent to the mixture model proposed by Knill (2003).

## COMPARISON WITH HUMAN DATA

We compared the hierarchical causal-inference model with human data in the two tasks discussed in this chapter; the spatial-localization task and the temporal-numerosity-judgment task. The prior and likelihoods were all modeled using Gaussian distributions. In the spatial-localization task, the mean of each likelihood function was sampled in each trial from a Gaussian distribution with a mean at the veridical location and a standard deviation that was a free parameter. The mean of the prior over space was at the center, representing a bias for straight-ahead location. As described earlier for the trisensory model, to produce model predictions we ran Monte Carlo simulations. We assume the observers minimize the mean squared error of their responses, and hence the optimal estimate would be the mean of the posterior distribution. In this fashion, for each stimulus condition, we obtained a distribution of responses, and this distribution was compared with the response distribution obtained from human observers. The model had four free parameters: the width of the visual likelihood, the width of the auditory likelihood, the width of the prior over space, and the prior probability of a common cause. These parameters were fitted to the data, and the results are shown in Figure 13.2. As can be seen, the model can account for the data in all conditions well. The model accounts for 97% of the variance in 1225 datapoints, using only four free parameters. The same model can also account for the data reported by Wallace et al. (2004), where the subjects were asked to report their judgment of unity (common cause) (see Chapter 2 for more details).

Other models, including the traditional forced-fusion model, a model that does not integrate the stimuli at all, as well as two recent models that do not assume forced fusion were tested on the same dataset (data shown in Fig. 13.2; Körding et al., 2007) and compared with the causal-inference model. The causal-inference model outperformed all other models (Körding et al., 2007).

The hierarchical causal-inference model was also tested on the numerosity-judgment task. The data and model fits are shown in Figure 13.1. As can be seen, the model also accounts for the data in all conditions well here. Accounting for 567 data points, the model explains 86% of the variance using only four free parameters.

In summary, the causal inference model can account for two complementary tasks, for data from two different laboratories, and outperforms other models. These results taken together suggest that human auditory-visual perception is consistent with Bayesian inference.

## INDEPENDENCE OF PRIORS AND LIKELIHOODS

The findings described in this chapter suggest that humans are Bayes optimal in auditory-visual perceptual tasks given the (fitted) subjective priors. How is this achieved in the brain? The general understanding of Bayesian inference is that priors represent the statistics of the environment, whereas likelihoods correspond to the sensory representations. In other words, it is generally assumed that likelihoods and priors are independent of each other. Does demonstration of Bayes optimality under one condition indicate that the priors and likelihoods are independent? The answer to this question is no. The Bayes optimality in a given task under a certain condition only implies that the performance of the observers is consistent with a Bayesian observer, but it could very well be the case that if we change the likelihoods, for example, by modifying the stimuli, the estimated priors would change and vice versa. Because we can estimate the likelihoods and priors using our model, we can empirically test this question.

Specifically, we asked whether priors are independent of likelihoods, that is, whether a change in likelihoods would cause a change in priors (Beierholm, Quartz, & Shams, 2009). We tried to induce a change in visual likelihoods by altering the parameters of the visual stimuli. Namely, we tested two different visual stimulus contrasts in the same spatial-localization task described earlier. To make sure that any potential learning of the priors within one session did not affect the results of the other session, we tested subjects in these two conditions 1 week apart, so that exposure to the statistics of real scenes would remove the effects of any possible learning within the first session. Therefore, the same observers were run in two sessions (low visual contrast and high visual contrast) using the same task, but with a 1-week interval between the two sessions.

Indeed, comparing the performance in the unisensory visual and auditory conditions between the two sessions, no significant difference was found in the auditory performance, whereas the visual performance was as much as 41% poorer in the low-contrast conditions. The lack of change in the auditory performance is to be expected because the auditory stimuli were not changed between the two sessions. The drastic change in visual performance confirms that the change in the visual stimulus was a substantial change. The model fits to the high-contrast condition were shown in Figure 13.2. The model was also fitted to the low-contrast data and was found to account for the data well ($R^2 = 0.75$).

In summary, we find that the performance of the observers is Bayes optimal in both high-contrast and low-contrast conditions given their subjective priors, and there is a substantial difference between the responses (and hence, the posteriors) in the low-contrast and high-contrast conditions. Therefore, it remains to be tested whether the likelihoods and priors are the same or different between the two sessions. If the priors are the same between the two sessions, then swapping the priors of the two sessions should not cause a change in the goodness of fit to the data. To test this, we used the priors that were estimated from the low-contrast data to predict the high-contrast data, and vice versa. In both cases, the goodness of fit of the model remained mostly unchanged (going from $R^2 = 0.97$ to $R^2 = 0.95$ for the high-contrast data, and from $R^2 = 0.75$ to $R^2 = 0.74$ for the low-contrast data). This finding suggests that the priors are nearly constant between the two sessions.

We also compared the parameters of the likelihoods and prior distributions for the two sessions directly with each other. For the group

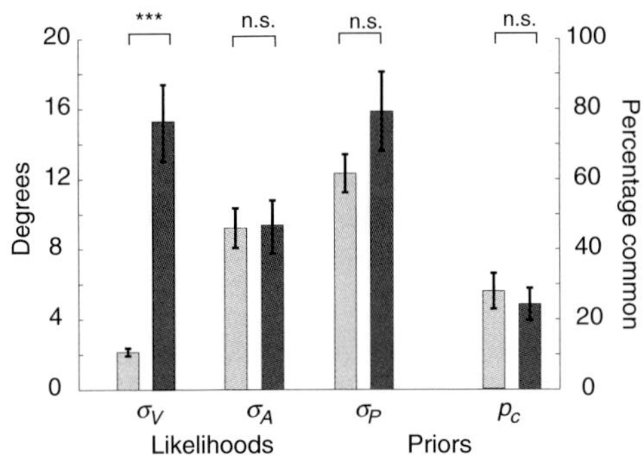


**Figure 13.9** Mean parameter values across observers. Light gray bars represent values for the high-visual-contrast condition, and dark gray bars represent those of low-contrast condition. Error bars denote the standard error of the mean.

data, the variance of the auditory likelihood was highly similar between the two sessions, whereas the variance of the visual likelihood was much larger for the low-contrast session. These results confirm that these parameters are not some arbitrary free parameters fitted to the data, but indeed capture the notion of likelihood functions. The prior parameters, namely the probability of a common cause and the width of the prior over space, were highly similar between the two sessions, suggesting that the priors were not different between the two sessions. To be able to test whether any of the differences between the parameters (albeit very small) are statistically significant, we fitted the model to the individual observers' data and performed paired $t$-tests between the two sessions. The mean and standard errors of the four parameters across observers are shown in Figure 13.9. As can be seen, there is no statistically significant difference for the prior parameters or auditory likelihood between the two conditions. The only parameter that is significantly different ($p < 0.0005$) is the visual noise (i.e., standard deviation of visual likelihood), which is much higher in the low-contrast condition. Therefore, these results indicate that despite a large change in likelihoods, the priors remained the same, suggesting that priors are indeed independent of likelihoods.

## DISCUSSION AND CONCLUSIONS

The results presented here altogether suggest that the brain uses a mechanism similar to Bayesian inference for combining auditory, visual, and tactile signals for deciding whether, to what degree, and how (in which direction) to integrate the signals from two or more modalities. It should also be noted that two important and very different auditory-visual illusions (Howard & Templeton, 1966; Shams et al., 2000) can be viewed as the result of one coherent and statistically optimal computational strategy. We discussed a model that allows for both common cause and independent causes and can account for the entire range of interactions among auditory, visual, and tactile modalities. This model only implicitly performs causal inference. We also presented a special form of this general model, a hierarchical model that explicitly assumes that one of two causal structures gave rise to the stimuli, and it makes explicit predictions about the perceived causal structure of the stimuli. This model is useful for accounting for data on judgments of unity, in experiments where the observers are explicitly probed for this judgment. It is, however, not clear whether under natural conditions, observers do make a commitment to one or another causal structure. Future research can investigate this question empirically. While the hierarchical causal-inference model has the advantage of making direct predictions about perceived causal structure of events, it can become exceedingly complex for situations where three or more sensory signals are present simultaneously, as the number of possible causal structures becomes prohibitively large. For example, for the auditory-visual-tactile task discussed earlier, the nonhierarchical Bayesian model of Eq. 13.1 is substantially simpler than an extension of the hierarchical model of Eq. 13.3 to three modalities would have been.

While several previous studies have shown that human perception is consistent with a Bayesian observer (e.g., Bloj, Kersten, & Hurlbert, 1999; Stocker & Simoncelli, 2006; Weiss, Simoncelli, & Adelson, 2002), the demonstration of Bayes optimality does not indicate that the priors and likelihoods are encoded independently of each other as is the general interpretation of Bayesian inference. We discussed results that provide evidence for the priors being independent of likelihoods. This finding is consistent with the general notion of priors encoding the statistics of the environment and therefore being invariant to the sensory conditions at any given moment.

## REFERENCES


Alais, D., & Burr, D. (2004). The ventriloquist effect results from near-optimal bimodal integration. *Current Biology, 14*, 257–262.

Beierholm, U. R. (2007). Bayesian modeling of sensory cue combinations. Unpublished doctoral dissertation. Pasadena, CA: California Institute of Technology.

Beierholm, U. R., Quartz, S. R., & Shams, L. (2009). Bayesian priors are encoded independently from likelihoods in human multisensory perception. *Journal of Vision, 9*(5):23, 1–9.

Bloj, M. G., Kersten, D., & Hurlbert, A. C. (1999). Perception of three-dimensional shape influences colour perception through mutual illumination. *Nature, 402*, 877–879.

Bülthoff, H. H., & Mallot, H. A. (1988). Integration of depth modules: Stereo and shading. *Journal of Optical Society of America A, 5*, 1749–1758.

Ernst, M. O., & Banks, M. S. (2002). Humans integrate visual and haptic information in a statistically optimal fashion. *Nature, 415*, 429–433.

Ghahramani, Z., Wolpert, D. M., & Jordan, M. I. (1997). Computational models of sensorimotor integration. In P. G. Morasso & V. Sanguineti (Eds.), *Self-organization, computational maps, and motor control* (pp. 117–147). Amsterdam, Netherlands: North-Holland/Elsevier Press.

Hillis, J. M., Ernst, M. O., Banks, M. S., & Landy, M. S. (2002). Combining sensory information: Mandatory fusion within, but not between, senses. *Science, 298*, 1627–1630.

Howard, I. P., & Templeton, W. B. (1966). *Human spatial orientation*. London, England: Wiley.

Knill, D. C. (2003). Mixture models and the probabilistic structure of depth cues. *Vision Research, 43*, 831–854.

Körding, K., Beierholm, U., Ma, W. J., Tenebaum, J. M., Quartz, S., & Shams, L. (2007). Causal inference in multisensory perception. *PLoS ONE, 2*, e943.

Landy, M. S., Maloney, L. T., Johnston, E. B., & Young, M. (1995). Measurement and modeling of depth cue combination: In defense of weak fusion. *Vision Research, 35*, 389–412.

Shams, L., Kamitani, Y., & Shimojo, S. (2000). What you see is what you hear. *Nature, 408*, 788.

Shams, L., Ma, W. J., & Beierholm, U. (2005). Sound-induced flash illusion as an optimal percept. *Neuroreport, 16*, 1923–1927.

Spence, C., Pavani, F., Maravita, A., & Holmes, N. (2004). Multisensory contributions to the 3-D representation of visuotactile peripersonal space in humans: Evidence from the crossmodal congruency task. *Journal of Physiology (Paris), 98*, 171–189.

Stocker, A. A., & Simoncelli, E. P. (2006). Noise characteristics and prior expectations in human visual speed perception. *Nature Neuroscience, 9*, 578–585.

van Beers, R. J., Sittig, A. C., & Denier van der Gon, J. J. (1999). Integration of proprioceptive and visual position information: An experimentally supported model. *Journal of Neurophysiology, 81*, 1355–1364.

Wallace, M. T., Roberson, G. H., Hairston, W. D., Stein, B. E., Vaughan, J. W., & Schirillo, J. A. (2004). Unifying mulitsensory signals across time and space. *Experimental Brain Research, 158*, 252–258.

Weiss, Y., Simoncelli, E., & Adelson, E. H. (2002). Motion illusions as optimal percepts. *Nature Neuroscience, 5*, 508–510.

Wozny, D. R., Beierholm, U. R., & Shams, L. (2008). Human trimodal perception follows optimal statistical inference. *Journal of Vision, 8*(3):24, 1–11.

Yuille, A. L., & Bülthoff, H. H. (1996). Bayesian decision theory and psychophysics. In D. C. Knill, & D. C. Richards (Eds.), *Perception as Bayesian inference* (pp. 123–161). Cambridge, England: Cambridge University Press.

# CHAPTER 14

## Cues and Pseudocues in Texture and Shape Perception

*Michael S. Landy, Yun-Xian Ho, Sascha Serwe, Julia Trommershäuser, and Laurence T. Maloney*

### INTRODUCTION

In estimating properties of the world, we often use multiple sources of information. For example, in estimating the three-dimensional (3D) layout of a scene, there are many sources of information or "cues" available for the estimation of depth and shape (Kaufman, 1974). These include binocular cues (disparity, vergence), motion cues (motion parallax, the kinetic depth effect), pictorial cues (texture, linear perspective, occlusion, etc.), and more. Human observers often combine these cues in a near-optimal fashion so as to maximize the precision of their estimates of scene layout (see Chapter 1, also Landy, Maloney, Johnston, & Young, 1995).

Some cues are acquired after birth. In infancy, the motion and binocular cues appear to develop around 3–4 months of age, with use of the pictorial cues beginning some 3 months later (Kellman & Arterberry, 1998, 2006). The onset of responses to binocular disparity appears to be based on maturation of the required vergence control and cortical architecture (binocular, disparity-tuned cells). On the other hand, it is not known whether the onset of the response to pictorial depth cues is the result of maturation or learning.

If a new depth cue is to be learned, the visual system has to note a correlation between values of that cue and other indicators of the values of the environmental variable being estimated. For example, consider the pattern of texture as a cue to slant. For observers to learn how to use texture, they must associate larger texture gradients (rapid changes in the size and density of texture elements across the image) or larger values of foreshortening (in which circles on the surface appear as eccentric ellipses in the retinal image) with larger values of surface slant. An observer could do so by noting the correlation of these image features with previously learned cues to surface slant such as the gradient of binocular disparities, or by using haptic cues as the observer handles the surface manually.

Backus and colleagues (see Chapter 6; Backus & Haijiang, 2007; Haijiang, Saunders, Stone, & Backus, 2006) investigated the visual system's ability to learn new depth cues. They did so by artificially pairing different values of a new, arbitrary "cue" with depth cues on which the visual system already relies. In their experiment, observers viewed Necker cubes that rotated about a vertical axis (Fig. 14.1). A Necker cube (Necker, 1832) is a picture of a transparent cube in which only the edges are drawn. It is an ambiguous figure; every few seconds the perception of the cube "switches" so that the face that was previously seen as behind is now perceived to be in front, and vice versa. When such a figure is rotated, the perceived direction of rotation reverses along with perceived depth.

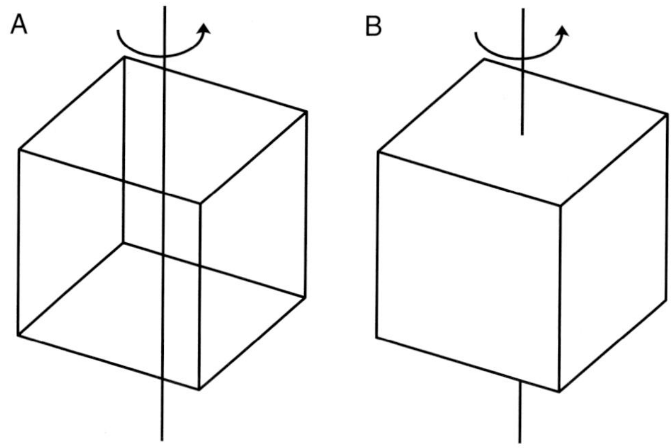


**Figure 14.1** The experiments of Backus and colleagues (Chapter 6; Backus & Haijiang, 2007; Haijiang et al., 2006). (A) In these experiments, observers viewed rotating Necker cubes that spontaneously reverse in perceived depth and rotation direction. (B) In a training session, unambiguous cubes (with occlusion as shown here as well as binocular disparity) were shown, and rotation direction was paired with a new cue (e.g., position in the display). After training, perception of rotation direction of ambiguous stimuli was affected by the value of the newly recruited cue.

In their experiment, the direction of rotation was disambiguated by including disparity and occlusion cues (the cube was now opaque, so the rear face was not visible, and binocular disparities were consistent with the pictorial depth; Fig. 14.1B). In addition, another aspect of the display varied in concert with the rotation direction. For example, if the cube rotated front to the right, it was shown in the upper half of the display. If it rotated front to the left, it was shown in the lower half of the display. After a sequence of such learning trials, the experimenters presented test trials with no disparity or occlusion cues. These displays consisted of standard rotating Necker cubes, which as described previously are normally ambiguous as to rotation direction. However, after learning, the previously irrelevant "cue", that is, the position in the display (upper vs. lower), had a substantial influence on perceived rotation direction. This "cue recruitment" paradigm is analogous to conditioning; however, the conditioning results in an increased frequency of occurrence of a particular percept rather than an overt behavior.

The recruited cues explored by Backus and colleagues are all binary; the cue is either a higher or lower display location, movement in the left or right direction, and so forth. They can be used to disambiguate a rotating cube but cannot, in and of themselves, provide a cue that could be used to quantify depth. The strength of these cues can be measured experimentally, and indeed these cues can trade off against trusted cues such as binocular disparity to determine which of two possible percepts (front rightward vs. front leftward) is obtained (Backus & Haijiang, 2007). However, by themselves they do not provide a continuously valued estimate of depth that combines with other depth cues. Note that binary depth cues such as occlusion can also trade off against continuously valued depth cues (e.g., binocular disparity) in the perception of depth (Burge, Peterson, & Palmer, 2005).

In this chapter, we review several studies that provide evidence that the visual system uses additional cues beyond those traditionally discussed for the estimation of scene properties, including shape, depth, and 3D surface texture. Figure 14.2 shows several example stimuli from one of these studies (Ho, Landy, & Maloney, 2006) in which observers were asked to judge surface roughness. These computer-rendered stereograms depict bumpy, pitted surfaces that include several cues to depth and shape. Figure 14.2B depicts a larger range of depth

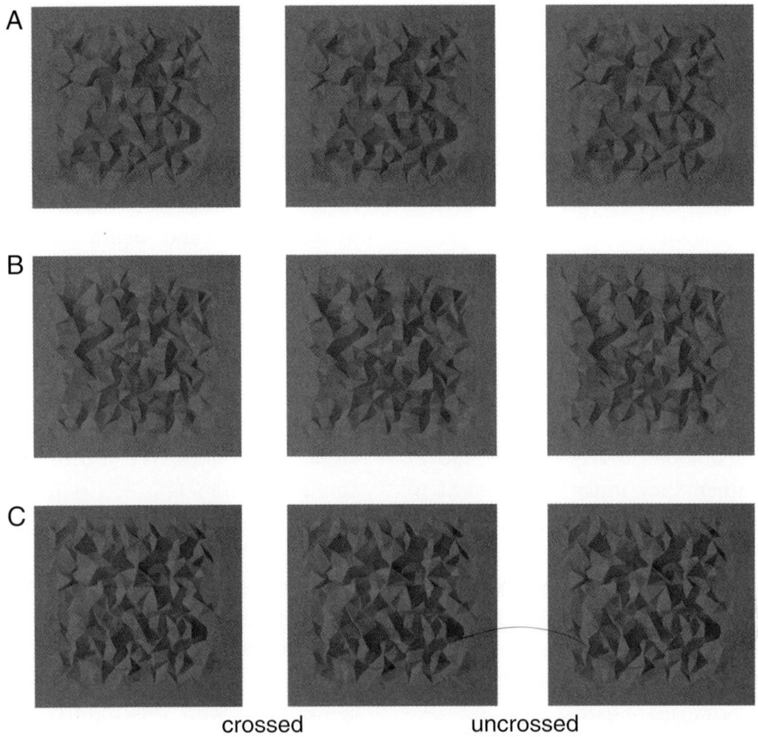


**Figure 14.2** Cast shadows as a pseudocue. (A) This stereogram shows a sample stimulus from the study of Ho and colleagues (Ho et al., 2006). A random bumpy surface was computer-rendered using a combination of ambient illumination and a single point source. (B) If we increase the range of depth in the surface, the amount of the image in cast shadow increases. (C) If, instead of increasing the range of depth, we move the light source to a more glancing angle relative to the surface, the amount of cast shadows also increases. As a result, perceived depth and surface roughness increase as well, even though there was no change of rendered depth as compared to (A). (Reprinted from Ho et al., 2006. Copyright ARVO; used with permission.)

values across the bumps and valleys, and hence appears rougher than Figure 14.2A. Figure 14.2C appears rougher than Figure 14.2A as well, but in this case the parameters used to generate the bumpy surface are identical. Rather, all that has changed is the pattern of illumination. In Figure 14.2C, the point illuminant is located such that the surface is illuminated from a more glancing angle, resulting in more and deeper cast shadows. Relative to Figure 14.2A, both Figures 14.2B and 14.2C have an increase in the amount of visible cast shadow, and both appear to be rougher surfaces than Figure 14.2A.

We refer to the proportion of the surface in cast shadow (and several related image statistics) as a "pseudocue" for the estimation of both surface roughness (in Fig. 14.2) and depth (for an experiment we discuss below). We call this a pseudocue because it is a cue to an object or surface property that confounds changes in that property with changes in irrelevant properties of the surface, object, or viewing environment. The proportion of cast shadow is a pseudocue for surface roughness in the sense that an increase in the variance of depths of textural elements comprising the surface, that is, an increase in roughness, results in an increase in the amount of cast shadow given that all other variables in the scene are constant. But a change in light-source position can also increase the value of this pseudocue, with no concomitant change in physical roughness. This pseudocue would be a valid cue to roughness if all aspects of the scene except for the range of depth values were fixed, including the position of the illuminant, the location of the observer relative to the surface, and the class of surface geometry. However, observers appear to use this pseudocue as though it were a valid tool for estimating surface roughness across varying illumination and viewing conditions, resulting in failures of "roughness constancy."

This definition of *pseudocue* is related to the idea of *cue promotion* described by Landy and colleagues (1995). For example, the raw data for binocular stereopsis are the binocular disparity values for various points in the retinal images. These data do not provide estimates of depth or surface slant in and of themselves; rather, they must be *promoted* to depth estimates after scaling disparities based on additional parameters. These additional parameters describe the viewing geometry and include ocular vergence, version, and torsion. Use of the raw disparity values as a direct indication of depth results in failures of depth constancy with changes of gaze.

Suppose we were able to show that observers used the mean luminance of stimuli such as those in Figure 14.2 as an indication of the range of depth in the stimulus or of surface roughness. Certainly, as the textural elements of the surface in Figure 14.2 are stretched out in depth, more shadows appear and the overall mean luminance of the display is reduced. Yet a reduction of mean luminance can result from many changes in the scene, including a reduction in overall illumination, a change of viewpoint, a change in illuminant position, or decreased surface reflectance. Thus, a pseudocue differs from a standard cue in that information provided by a pseudocue is not invariant across viewing and environmental conditions and when used can lead to misjudgments of a given object or surface property. A standard cue is one for which the observer can estimate the environmental parameters needed to interpret the raw data, and hence the observer can compute an estimate of an object or surface property independent of extraneous viewing or environmental conditions. The distinction between a standard cue and a pseudocue is one of degree; to the extent that the required environmental parameters are not available or used by the observer, the cue is less useful for estimating object or surface properties and hence is more of a "pseudocue."

In this chapter, we review experimental evidence concerning the use of such pseudocues in the perception of 3D scene properties such as roughness and depth. In the first two experiments, observers judged surface roughness of an irregular surface in which roughness was varied by scaling the range of depths of bumps and valleys. We show that observers do indeed use pseudocues such as the amount of shadow and as a result they misperceive surface roughness. We also briefly note that a similar phenomenon occurs in the perception of surface gloss. Finally, we summarize a third study in which observers judged the depth of a single bump. In this final experiment, we investigated how pseudocues might be learned and, in particular, how observers determine how much weight to give to a pseudocue in combining it with other depth cues.

## CUES AND PSEUDOCUES FOR TEXTURE ROUGHNESS

In this section we review the results of two studies (Ho et al., 2006; Ho, Maloney, & Landy, 2007) that suggest observers use pseudocues such as the amount of cast shadows as a depth cue in judgments of surface roughness. The stimuli were like those in Figure 14.2. We test whether judged roughness increases with the amount of cast shadow caused by changes in the position of the light source (Fig. 14.2C) or the position of the observer relative to the surface. Thus, we ask whether "roughness constancy" holds for this task and these viewing conditions.

### Methods

The methods are summarized in Figure 14.3. Stimuli such as those shown in Figure 14.2 were generated as follows. We began with a $20 \times 20$ array of points, $19 \times 19$ cm in size (Fig. 14.3A). First, grid intersections were randomly jittered within the grid plane (Fig. 14.3B). Next, grid intersections were randomly jittered along the $z$-axis (orthogonal to the grid plane).

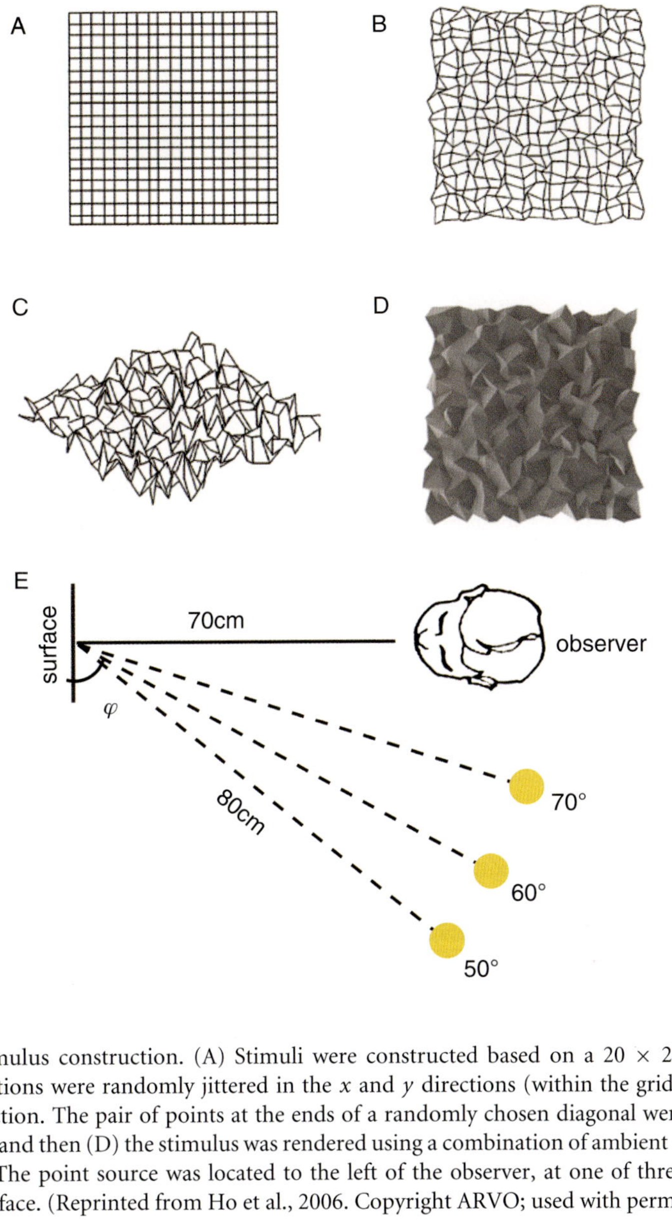


**Figure 14.3** Stimulus construction. (A) Stimuli were constructed based on a 20 × 20 grid of points. (B) Grid intersections were randomly jittered in the *x* and *y* directions (within the grid plane) and then (C) in the *z* direction. The pair of points at the ends of a randomly chosen diagonal were connected (for each grid square) and then (D) the stimulus was rendered using a combination of ambient and point-source illuminants. (E) The point source was located to the left of the observer, at one of three possible angles relative to the surface. (Reprinted from Ho et al., 2006. Copyright ARVO; used with permission.)

The *z*-values were drawn from a uniform distribution. The roughness level *r* of a given stimulus corresponded to the range of this distribution. Each grid "square" was then split into two triangles by randomly connecting one of the two "diagonals" (Fig. 14.3C). The resulting triangulation was then rendered using the RADIANCE rendering software (Larson & Shakespeare, 1996; Ward, 1994) resulting in an image like that shown in Figure 14.3D. Eight values of *r* were used, resulting in surfaces with depth ranges varying from ±0.6 to ±40 mm, as viewed from a distance of 70 cm.

For the first study we review here, the illumination environment consisted of an ambient illuminant as well as a single-point illuminant located to the left of the observer at one of three angles $\varphi$ relative to the surface (Fig. 14.3E).

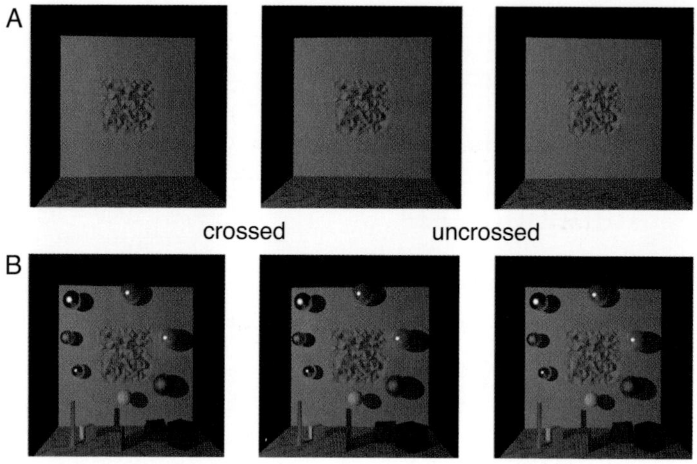


**Figure 14.4** Sample stimuli. (A) A sample stereogram for the condition with no additional context. (B) A sample stereogram for the condition in which additional objects were placed in the scene to provide cues to the position of the point source. (Reprinted from Ho et al., 2006. Copyright ARVO; used with permission.)

The bumpy surface was embedded smoothly into a wall attached to a two-dimensional (2D) textured ground surface (Fig. 14.4A). In one condition, additional context was added to the scene, that is, matte and glossy objects placed randomly about in the scene, so as to provide additional image cues to the position of the point light source (Fig. 14.4B). Stimuli were viewed on a custom stereoscope with the left and right eye's images projected onto separate cathode ray tube (CRT) displays located to the left and right of the observer.

The observer's task was a two-interval forced-choice roughness discrimination. On each trial, two stimuli were displayed in sequence. In one of the two temporal intervals, chosen randomly, a "test" stimulus was shown with a particular combination of roughness level and point-illuminant position. In the other interval a "match" stimulus was shown. The match stimulus had a different point-illuminant position and its roughness level was adjusted across trials by a staircase procedure. The observer indicated which of the two stimuli appeared to be rougher. There were interleaved staircases corresponding to several test patch roughness levels and combinations of test-match illuminant positions.

### Results: Use of Pseudocues

Figure 14.5 illustrates the analysis of the resulting data. In Figure 14.5A, the probability that an observer chose the match stimulus as appearing rougher is plotted as a function of the match stimulus roughness level for a test stimulus with roughness of $r = 2.25$ cm. The greater the rendered roughness was of the match stimulus, the more often it was perceived as rougher than the test stimulus. We fit a Weibull distribution to each such psychometric function and determined the "point of subjective equality" (PSE), the point at which we estimated the observer would judge the match stimulus to be rougher than the test stimulus 50% of the time. In other words, the PSE is an estimate of the test and match roughness levels of two surfaces under different illumination conditions that would be judged to be equally rough.

Figure 14.5B shows PSEs for one observer and one combination of test and match point-source locations ($\varphi_{\text{test}} = 70°$ and $\varphi_{\text{match}} = 50°$). For each test-patch roughness level we plot the PSE, that is, the match roughness level that, when illuminated by $\varphi_{\text{match}}$, appears as rough as the test roughness illuminated by $\varphi_{\text{test}}$. If the change in illumination position had no effect on perceived roughness, that is, if the observer

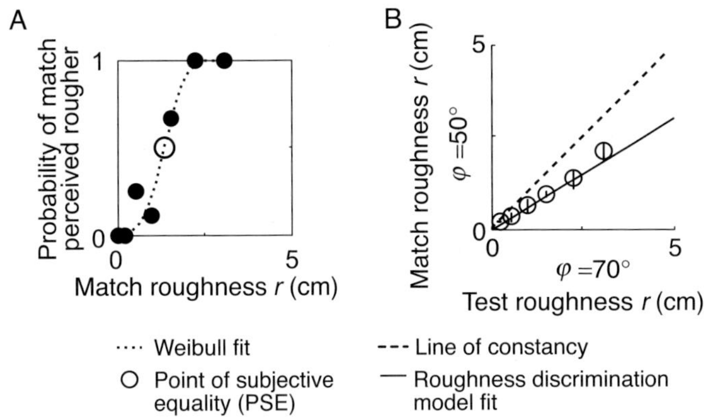


**Figure 14.5** Sample data. (A) Psychometric function for subject JG for a test patch with roughness 2.25 cm under point source $\varphi_{test} = 70°$ and match stimuli under point source $\varphi_{match} = 50°$. The open circle indicates the point of subjective equality (PSE) derived from a Weibull fit to the data (dotted line). (B) PSEs for this subject and combination of test and match illumination conditions. The dashed line indicates the line of constancy, that is, expected results for a roughness-constant observer. The solid line was fit to the data under the constraint that it pass through the origin. The slope of this line (the "PSE slope") was used to summarize each data set. (Reprinted from Ho et al., 2006. Copyright ARVO; used with permission.)

were "roughness constant" across this change in viewing conditions, then PSEs should fall roughly on the dashed identity line. Clearly, roughness constancy was not demonstrated because many PSEs fell significantly below the identity line, and a line fit to the PSEs and forced to pass through the origin had a slope significantly less than one (see Ho et al., 2006 for details on fitting).

Figure 14.6 summarizes all of our results by showing the slope of the fit PSE lines (as in Fig. 14.5B) for seven subjects and all three possible illuminant-position comparisons. The abscissa plots the PSE slope for the no-context condition (Fig. 14.4A) and the ordinate plots the corresponding PSE slope for the context condition (Fig. 14.4B). The dotted lines indicate the values of PSE slope corresponding to roughness constancy (i.e., a slope of one). Nearly all conditions resulted in slopes less than one. This means that a decrease of illuminant angle $\varphi$, corresponding to a more glancing point-source illumination and hence more cast shadows, led observers to perceive the stimulus as rougher than the identical stimulus lit with a more direct illuminant. Second, nearly all points are close to the identity line. This indicates that the additional context provided by objects in the scene was ineffective in helping subjects maintain a more constant representation of roughness. These additional objects provided cast shadows (on the ground plane) and highlights which could have provided the observer with cues to illuminant location. We hypothesized that observers would make better use of the shadow pseudocue if they had a better estimate of the pattern of illumination. Instead, the addition of these contextual cues had little effect on judgment and did not improve the degree of roughness constancy.

This suggests that the estimation of surface properties is primarily based on cues that are spatially local to the object being judged. This is consistent with the results of Hillis and colleagues (Hillis, Watt, Landy, & Banks, 2004). They examined combinations of texture and disparity cues to surface slant. The relative reliability of these two cues depends on a number of scene factors, including absolute distance to the object and the actual value of slant. As a result, for large surfaces, the weight given to each cue is determined locally and can change across the surface. They provided evidence that cue weights can indeed vary across a large

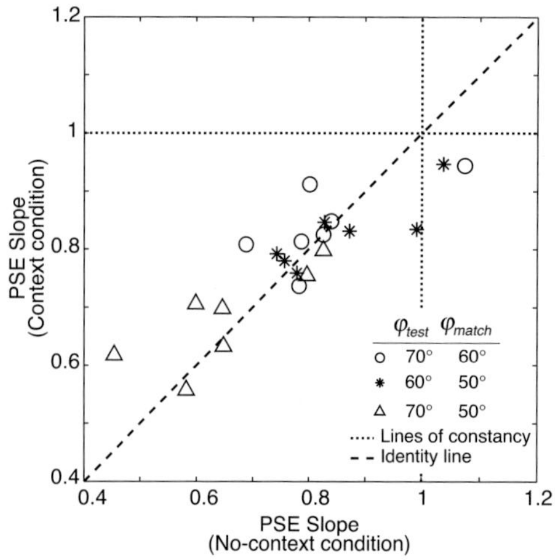


**Figure 14.6** Data from the first experiment. For each subject and illuminant comparison, we plot the point of subjective equality (PSE) slope from the no-context versus the context conditions. Different symbols indicate the illuminant comparison. Data are shown for seven subjects. The dotted lines indicate PSE slopes of one, that is, the expected result for a roughness-constant observer. The diagonal dashed identity indicates results for which the addition of context objects had no effect. (Reprinted from Ho et al., 2006. Copyright ARVO; used with permission.)

extended surface. As a result, a large planar surface with conflicting texture and disparity cues to depth appears curved as the local estimate approaches that from disparity or from texture in different regions of the stimulus.

In a subsequent study (Ho et al., 2007), we extended these results by varying the observer's viewing position relative to the rendered textured surface. The methods were similar to the study we just described. However, rather than comparing pairs of point-source locations, we compared pairs of observer viewpoints $\varphi_v$. The point-source location was fixed in the scene at $\varphi_p = 60°$. Pairs of test and match viewpoints were chosen from among those illustrated in Figure 14.7A, resulting in stimuli like those shown in Figure 14.7B.

Figure 14.7C shows a summary of the data for the four observers and the subset of viewpoint comparisons for which both viewpoints were located to the right of the point-source location (i.e., both test and match viewpoints $\varphi_v > 60°$). For this subset of viewpoints, the larger the value of $\varphi_v$ the more cast shadows are present in the image; hence, if the results of the previous experiment apply, surfaces viewed from larger viewing angles as defined here should appear rougher. Indeed, for most subjects and viewpoint pairs, PSE slopes were less than one.

## Discussion

In the two studies we have reviewed, observers displayed significant failures of roughness constancy. That is, the roughness of a surface appeared to vary with changes in the viewing conditions (change in the position of a point light source or the observer), even though there was no change in the physical rendering of the surface being judged. In all cases, apparent roughness increased with increases in the amount of visible shadow. Does this mean that the amount of visible shadow, or some related image statistic, is used by observers as a cue to 3D surface properties like roughness that contain variations in depth or, more generally, to depth itself?

To answer this question, we modeled the results as a combination of appropriate, veridical cues (disparity, contour, etc.) and putative pseudocues. The possible pseudocues we investigated included the proportion of the image in cast shadow, the mean luminance of the nonshadowed regions, the standard deviation of luminance of the nonshadowed regions, and *texture contrast* (Pont & Koenderink, 2005). These image statistics were computed for each stimulus image (resulting in the values $R_p$, $R_m$, $R_s$ and $R_c$, respectively). In addition, the veridical roughness (i.e., depth range in these experiments) was presumably signaled to the observer by disparity and other cues ($R_d$). We assumed that perceived roughness was a linear combination of the veridical cues and pseudocues:

$$R = w_d R_d + w_p R_p + w_m R_m + w_s R_s + w_c R_c, \tag{14.1}$$

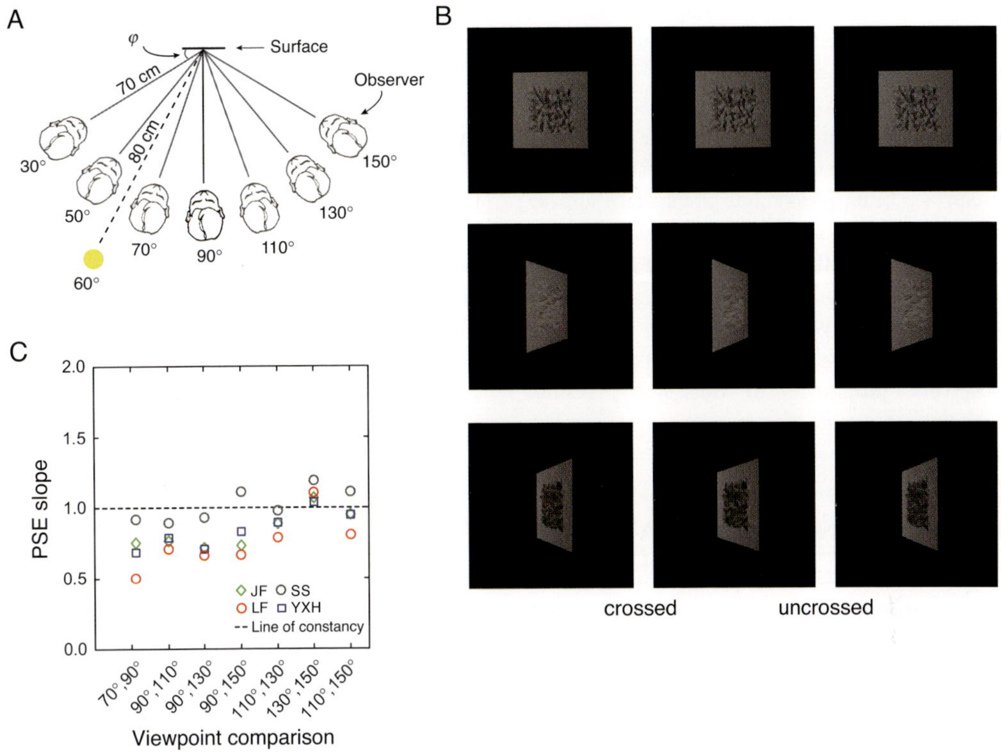


**Figure 14.7** Effect of viewpoint. (A) In this experiment, the light source position $\varphi_p$ was fixed at 60° and the viewpoint position $\varphi_v$ was varied. (B) Example stereogram stimuli. (C) Point of subjective equality (PSE) slopes for four observers and all viewpoint comparisons in which test and match viewpoints were to the right of the light source. The dashed line indicates a PSE slope of one, that is, the expected result for a roughness-constant observer. (Reprinted from Ho et al., 2007. Copyright ARVO; used with permission.)

where the values $w_i$ combine both scale factors and weights and need not sum to one. At the PSE, a second stimulus (viewed under a different lighting condition or viewpoint) has identical perceived roughness:

$$R = w_d R'_d + w_p R'_p + w_m R'_m + w_s R'_s + w_c R'_c. \tag{14.2}$$

Rearranging terms, we find

$$\Delta R_d = a_p \Delta R_p + a_m \Delta R_m + a_s \Delta R_s + a_c \Delta R_c, \tag{14.3}$$

where $a_i = -w_i/w_d$ for each pseudocue $i$ and $\Delta R_i = R_i - R'_i$. Thus, the model consisted of a regression that predicted failures of roughness constancy ($\Delta R_d$, i.e., displacements of PSEs away from the lines of constancy in Fig. 14.4B) as a linear combination of differences of the values of the pseudocues at the PSE. For almost all observers, a significant percentage of the variance in PSEs was accounted for by a subset of these pseudocues. For example, in the first study between 33% and 82% of the variance in PSEs was accounted for by a linear combination of the four candidate pseudocues (Ho et al., 2006), depending on the observer. In other words, observers did indeed appear to treat a stimulus that contained more shadows and was darker and higher in contrast as being rougher, even though that change in pseudocue resulted from changes in viewing conditions alone.

As an aside, in a third study we also identified other extraneous cues that can potentially act as pseudocues to judgments of surface properties.

In this study, observers compared pairs of surfaces that varied in bumpiness and/or degree of gloss (Ho, Landy, & Maloney, 2008). We found that the two surface properties interacted in the sense that an increase in surface gloss made the surface appear to be bumpier, and an increase in surface bumpiness made the surface appear glossier. This is another example of a failure of constancy where the percept of one property is altered when another independent property is varied. Although we did not directly investigate what particular image statistics correlated with observers' judgments in this study, results suggest that pseudocues may play a role in the perception of gloss and bumpiness.

## REWEIGHTING CANDIDATE PSEUDOCUES TO DEPTH

In the previous section, we reviewed several experiments demonstrating failures of roughness constancy across changes in viewing conditions. In particular, observers perceived stimuli as rougher when the viewpoint or pattern of illumination resulted in an image containing more cast shadows. We referred to image statistics such as the amount of cast shadow as pseudocues because such statistics vary with changes in roughness itself but also change with extraneous changes in viewing conditions or surface characteristics.

To acquire a new cue (or pseudocue), the visual system presumably needs to experience the correlation of that cue with the scene property being estimated, possibly via a "trusted" cue the visual system already uses to make that judgment. In the case of shadow or other image pseudocues, haptic input might be such a trusted cue. Arguably, for the estimation of surface roughness, manual exploration of a surface provides a more reliable estimate of surface roughness than vision and thus might be expected to dominate visual cues to roughness (Klatzky, Lederman, & Matula, 1991, 1993; Lederman & Abbott, 1981; Lederman & Klatzky, 1997). As a result, one might expect that "touch educates vision" (Berkeley, 1709).

There are at least two ways an observer might respond to changes in the relationship between two cues: recalibration and reweighting. Recalibration is needed if the estimate based on a cue becomes biased due to growth or other changes in the visual apparatus. For example, to estimate depth, binocular disparity must be scaled by an estimate of the viewing distance (i.e., based on the vergence angle) and other aspects of the viewing geometry (including the distance between the eyes: the pupillary distance, or PD). The PD increases by approximately 50% (from 4 to 6 cm) across the first 16 years of life (MacLachlan & Howland, 2002) requiring a substantial recalibration of binocular stereopsis. Reweighting should occur, on the other hand, as the relative reliability of cues changes (see Chapter 1 and Landy et al., 1995). Evidence for reweighting in response to changes in cue correlation has been found for combinations of haptic and visual depth cues (Atkins, Fiser, & Jacobs, 2001), haptic and visual cues to surface slant (Ernst, Banks, & Bülthoff, 2000), and pairs of visual cues to depth (Jacobs & Fine, 1999).

Logically, for the visual system to incorporate a new cue (or pseudocue) in its estimation of a scene property, both reweighting and recalibration must be involved. The new cue should receive a weight proportional to its reliability, which can be estimated using the degree it correlates with trusted cues. Calibration is required as well—for a new cue it is not yet *re*calibration—so that the raw cue measurement can be transformed to provide an estimate that is unbiased.

We next describe an experiment that illustrates how pseudocues, like more typical visual cues, undergo reweighting (Ho, Serwe, Trommershäuser, Maloney, & Landy, 2009). We created a correlation between a pseudocue (the amount of cast shadow) and haptic cues to depth. To provide the haptic cues we used a PHANToM 3D Touch interface (SensAble Technologies, Woburn, MA). This device does not provide realistic haptic sensory input for fine-grained surface material properties such as roughness. Therefore, we instead asked subjects to judge a larger scale scene property that potentially involves the use of similar pseudocues: the depth of an object. We determine whether this pseudocue is given greater weight in depth judgments made using vision alone after exposure to stimuli with haptic depth correlated with the shadow pseudocue.

### Methods

Participants saw and/or felt the displays in a virtual environment. The displays portrayed a gaze-normal plane with a portion of a vertically oriented circular cylinder projecting out of the plane (Fig. 14.8). In haptic conditions, observers placed their right index finger into a thimble attached to the PHANToM, which provided force feedback to the participant as the participant moved the index finger back and forth across the virtual object. The PHANToM was programmed to simulate a cylinder made of a hard, rubber-like material. The visual display consisted of a virtual image of the object (reflected in a mirror positioned above their hands), rendered so as to appear in the same location as the haptic display. The visual display was viewed binocularly with appropriate disparities using CrystalEyes 3 (Stereographics, Beverly Hills, CA) liquid-crystal shutter glasses. A small virtual sphere was displayed and updated in real time to represent the current 3D location of the index finger, although this sphere vanished whenever the observer's finger was positioned in the region of the stimulus so that the cursor itself was never a cue to object depth.

The rendered object was a 4 cm wide portion of a vertical circular cylinder and looked like a bump. The depth of the bump was determined by the curvature (the radius of the circular cylinder, only a portion of which was visible emerging from the 4×4 cm window in the background plane). The background plane and cylinder were covered in 2D texture so as to provide strong binocular disparity and texture cues to depth. In addition, the objects were rendered with a combination of an ambient and point source illuminant. The point source was located above the observer; for test stimuli the point source was located at an angle $\varphi_{test} = 45°$ above the background plane, and for match stimuli, $\varphi_{match} = 30°$. As a result, the shapes cast a curved shadow at the bottom of the cylinder (Fig. 14.8) whose size was larger for cylinders with greater depth but also for match stimuli due to the more grazing angle of illumination.

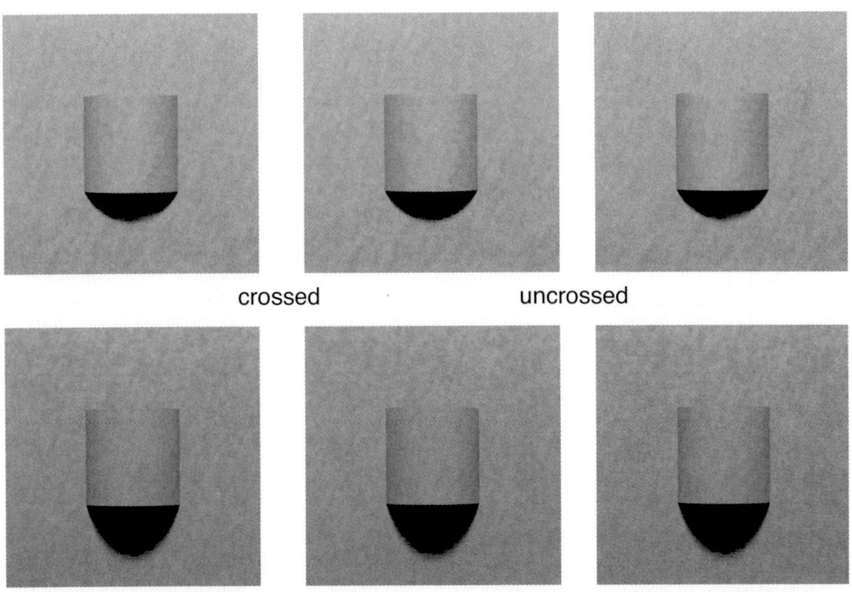


**Figure 14.8** Example stereogram stimuli from the visuohaptic experiment. (Top) Test stimulus with depth = 12 mm and point-illuminant direction $\varphi_{test} = 45°$. (Bottom) Match stimulus with the same depth and $\varphi_{match} = 30°$. (Reprinted from Ho et al., 2009; used with permission.)

A similar task and procedure was used as in the roughness experiments, although for this experiment the participant was asked to judge whether the test or match stimulus had greater depth. Each session consisted of 200 trials: 40 for each of 5 test bump depth levels. Match bump depth levels were controlled by interleaved staircases.

There were three types of sessions: visual-only, haptic-only, and visuohaptic training. In the visual-only session, objects were visible but could not be felt. These sessions allowed us to determine the extent to which a participant used the pseudocue (the size of the cast shadow). In the haptic-only session, participants could feel the objects but they were not displayed visually. These sessions were primarily used to familiarize the participants with the virtual haptic experience.

The key experimental manipulation in this study was the introduction of visuohaptic training. In visuohaptic training sessions, the rendered haptic cue was altered so that it was perfectly correlated with the shadow pseudocue. Figure 14.9 shows the proportion of the image corresponding to the cast shadow as a function of bump depth for both the test and match stimuli. For each bump depth level, we computed the average proportion of cast shadow (averaged across the test and match stimuli) and fit the resulting data with a smooth curve (dashed line). This function was then used as a lookup table to determine the amount of depth portrayed by the haptic stimuli in visuohaptic training sessions. Thus, in these sessions, a test and match stimulus were shown in succession, but the rendered haptic depth was determined by the amount of shadow in each stimulus, rather than the veridical value of depth corresponding to the disparity and texture cues in the stimulus.

The experiment was carried out over the course of 4 days, with at most a 2-day break between successive sessions. The sessions were laid out as follows (numbers in parentheses are identifying session numbers used in Fig. 14.10):

Day 1: Visual-only practice session, two visual-only sessions (1–2)
Day 2: Two visual-only sessions (3–4), one haptic-only session

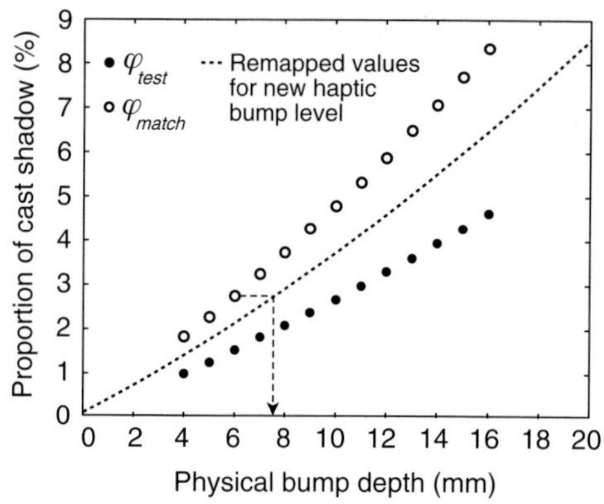


**Figure 14.9** Method of artificially correlating the haptic cue and shadow pseudocue. Plotted is the percentage of the stimulus in cast shadow as a function of bump depth (open circles: match stimuli; filled circles: test stimuli). The dashed line shows a polynomial fit to the average percentage of cast shadow for each bump depth. In visuohaptic training trials, this curve was used as a lookup table to determine the haptically rendered depth (arrows). (Reprinted from Ho et al., 2009; used with permission.)

Day 3: One visuohaptic training session (5), one visual-only session (6)
Day 4: One visuohaptic training session (7), one visual-only session (8).

### Results: Pseudocue Weights Can Change with Experience

The data from this experiment were analyzed in a manner identical to that used for the roughness experiments (Fig. 14.5), resulting in an estimated PSE slope for each session. To determine whether a subject's initial percept of depth changed with varying illumination, that is, failed to be constant across illumination conditions, we took the average of the four PSE slopes obtained for the visual-only sessions prior to visuohaptic training and compared it to a slope of one (i.e., shape constancy). Of the 12 subjects, 6 had average PSE slopes that were significantly less than one. In other words, for these subjects the pseudocue of shadow size was effective in producing a failure of size constancy across changes in the pattern of illumination.

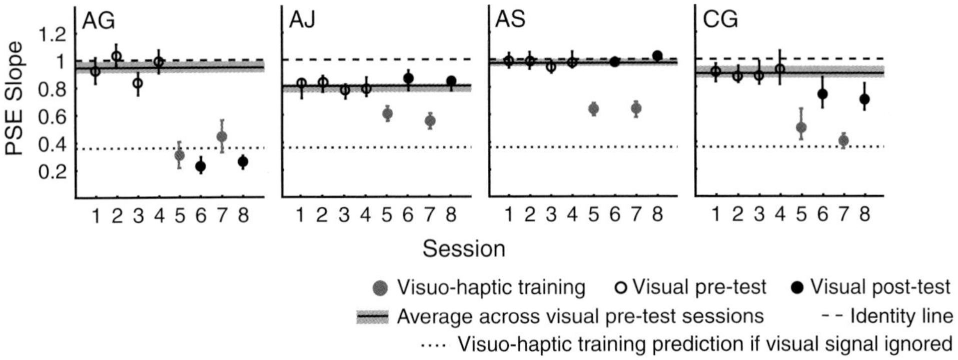


**Figure 14.10** Results of visuohaptic training. Point of subjective equality (PSE) slopes are plotted for four observers (out of the 12 observers in the study) for each session. The dashed line indicates a PSE slope of one, that is, the expected result for a roughness-constant observer. The dotted line indicates the PSE slope expected if only the haptic and/or pseudocues were used. The first four visual-only sessions (open symbols) were pretraining. The solid horizontal line and corresponding shaded 95% confidence region reflect the average PSE slopes for these first four sessions. Two of these four observers (AJ and CG) showed significant failures of depth constancy (PSE slopes < 1). All four subjects gave substantial weight to the haptic cue during visuohaptic training sessions (gray filled symbols). In subsequent visual-only sessions, some subjects (AJ and AS) reverted to their previous visual-only behavior while others (AG and CG) showed significantly less depth constancy, consistent with giving an increased weight to the shadow pseudocue as a result of visuohaptic training. (Reprinted from Ho et al., 2009; used with permission.)

For most subjects, PSE slopes were significantly smaller during visuohaptic training sessions (for example subjects, see Fig. 14.10). If a subject ignored the visual displays and responded only based on the haptic input during these sessions, this would have resulted in a PSE slope of 0.36 (dotted horizontal line in Fig. 14.10) due to the mismatch of rendered haptic depth for test and match stimuli (Fig. 14.9). Thus, most subjects gave substantial weight to the haptic cue during the visuohaptic training sessions.

The key question is whether visuohaptic training sessions resulted in an increase in the weight observers gave to the pseudocue of shadow size. An increase in this weight would imply less depth-constant performance, that is, a reduction of PSE slope. There was substantial variation in performance across subjects. Five out of 12 subjects showed a significant reduction in PSE slope after training compared to pretraining slopes (e.g., subjects AG and CG), while other subjects returned to pretraining behavior (e.g., subjects AJ and AS).

We found substantial individual differences in response to these conditions. Of the six subjects who initially showed a significant use of pseudocues (i.e., significant failure of depth constancy with pretraining PSE slopes significantly less than one), two of them increased their reliance on pseudocues after visuohaptic training. The other half of the subjects were roughly depth constant before training, and three out of these six subjects showed a significant response to pseudocues after training.

### Discussion

Individual differences are frequent when cue weights are measured in depth-cue-integration tasks. In some cases, this outcome is consistent with optimal cue integration with the individual differences stemming from differences in cue reliability across individuals (Hillis, Ernst, Banks, & Landy, 2002; Hillis et al., 2004; Knill & Saunders, 2003). In other cases, individual differences may be an indication of differences in cue correlation or suboptimal cue integration (Oruç, Maloney, & Landy, 2003). Thus, the variation across subjects of the use of pseudocues was to be expected.

Although the effect occurred in only a subset of our subjects, this experiment demonstrates that a correlation between a pseudocue and a trusted cue can result in an increase in the weight given to the pseudocue in subsequent estimates. From the optimal-integration standpoint, it is as though the correlation with the trusted cue is taken as evidence that the reliability of the pseudocue has increased. To test such a claim would require experiments in which the pseudocue is paired with cues with a range of reliabilities so as to estimate the reliability of the pseudocue based on the weight it was given (assuming optimal cue combination; see Chapter 1, Eqs. 1.1–1.2).

## CONCLUSIONS

We have provided evidence that human observers use pseudocues in the estimation of surface roughness and shape, and that the weight given to pseudocues in estimating 3D scene properties can be altered by experience, in particular if the pseudocue is highly correlated with a trusted cue (in this case, haptic cues).

The pseudocues we consider here are simple image statistics that vary with the scene property being estimated but also vary with other, irrelevant aspects of viewing conditions. We do not assume that pseudocues must be drawn from the class of image statistics. When they are, though, the use of such pseudocues can be regarded as a visual-system heuristic or trick: A correlation between a simple image statistic and a scene property is noted and then recruited as a cue to that property. These pseudocues are related to other image statistics used to estimate scene properties without solving the ill-posed inverse-optics problem. Other examples of such statistics are the use of luminance histogram skew as a cue to surface gloss (Motoyoshi, Nishida, Sharan, & Adelson, 2007) and luminance histogram moments and percentile statistics as a cue to surface lightness (Sharan, Li, Motoyoshi, Nishida, & Adelson, 2008).

Recent work indicates that the visual system combines noisy cues to form estimates that have lower variance than any of the individual cues (see Chapter 1, also Landy et al., 1995). The reduction in variance sometimes approaches the theoretical minimum for uncorrelated cues (Ernst & Banks, 2002; Landy & Kojima, 2001).

The reliability of cues changes from scene to scene (due to changes in scene content, viewing geometry, pattern of illumination, etc.) and across the life span (as the sensory apparatus matures). As a consequence, an ideal sensory system must react to changes in cue reliability by adjusting its rule of combination, giving greater or less weight to sensory cues as they become more or less reliable.

In this chapter we are concerned with how cue weights are determined. But, we are also interested in how new cues are acquired and possible errors made by the visual system while acquiring new cues. In the experiments reviewed here, it appears that the sensory systems give weight to pseudocues that result in failures of object constancy. Thus, when a pseudocue was artificially correlated with a trusted cue (haptic input), a subset of the participants apparently increased the weight of that pseudocue, resulting in more pronounced failures of depth constancy. The weighting of pseudocues need not be fixed. Rather, evidence suggests that it is dynamic and shifts with recent experiences in a similar manner to the weighting of standard depth cues when they are artificially covaried with other cues (Atkins, Jacobs, & Knill, 2003; Ernst et al., 2000; Jacobs & Fine, 1999).

Although we have only noted a handful of possible pseudocues here, there are likely many more such pseudocues that are used by the visual system to make judgments of surface and object properties. An understanding of how and when pseudocues are used could provide useful insight to how a constant representation of the visual world is—or is not—acquired.

## ACKNOWLEDGMENTS

Thanks to Sabrina Schmidt, Tim Schönwetter, and Natalie Wahl for help with data collection. This research was supported in part by National Institutes of Health grants EY16165 and

EY08266 and by the Deutsche Forschungsgemeinschaft (DFG, Emmy-Noether-Programm, grant TR 528/1-2; 1-3).

## REFERENCES

Atkins, J. E., Fiser, J., & Jacobs, R. A. (2001). Experience-dependent visual cue integration based on consistencies between visual and haptic percepts. *Vision Research, 41*, 449–461.

Atkins, J. E., Jacobs, R. A., & Knill, D. C. (2003). Experience-dependent visual cue recalibration based on discrepancies between visual and haptic percepts. *Vision Research, 43*, 2603–2613.

Backus, B. T., & Haijiang, Q. (2007). Competition between newly recruited and pre-existing visual cues during the construction of visual appearance. *Vision Research, 47*, 919–924.

Berkeley, G. (1709). An essay towards a new theory of vision. In C. M. Turbayne (Ed.), *Works on vision*. Indianapolis, IN: Bobbs-Merrill.

Burge, J., Peterson, M. A., & Palmer, S. E. (2005). Ordinal configural cues combine with metric disparity in depth perception. *Journal of Vision, 5*, 534–542.

Ernst, M. O., & Banks, M. S. (2002). Humans integrate visual and haptic information in a statistically optimal fashion. *Nature, 415*, 429–433.

Ernst, M. O., Banks, M. S., & Bülthoff, H. H. (2000). Touch can change visual slant perception. *Nature Neuroscience, 3*, 69–73.

Haijiang, Q., Saunders, J. A., Stone, R. W., & Backus, B. T. (2006). Demonstration of cue recruitment: Change in visual appearance by means of Pavlovian conditioning. *Proceedings of the National Academy of Sciences USA, 103*, 483–488.

Hillis, J. M., Ernst, M. O., Banks, M. S., & Landy, M. S. (2002). Combining sensory information: Mandatory fusion within, but not between, senses. *Science, 298*, 1627–1630.

Hillis, J. M., Watt, S. J., Landy, M. S., & Banks, M. S. (2004). Slant from texture and disparity cues: Optimal cue combination. *Journal of Vision, 4*, 967–992.

Ho, Y. X., Landy, M. S., & Maloney, L. T. (2006). How direction of illumination affects visually perceived surface roughness. *Journal of Vision, 6*, 634–648.

Ho, Y. X., Landy, M. S., & Maloney, L. T. (2008). Conjoint measurement of gloss and surface texture. *Psychological Science, 19*, 196–204.

Ho, Y. X., Maloney, L. T., & Landy, M. S. (2007). The effect of viewpoint on perceived visual roughness. *Journal of Vision, 7*(1):1, 1–16.

Ho, Y. X., Serwe, S., Trommershäuser, J., Maloney, L. T., & Landy, M. S. (2009). The role of visuohaptic experience in visually perceived depth. *Journal of Neurophysiology, 101*, 2789–2801.

Jacobs, R. A., & Fine, I. (1999). Experience-dependent integration of texture and motion cues to depth. *Vision Research, 39*, 4062–4075.

Kaufman, L. (1974). *Sight and mind*. New York, NY: Oxford University Press.

Kellman, P. J., & Arterberry, M. E. (1998). *The cradle of knowledge: Development of perception in infancy*. Cambridge, MA: MIT Press.

Kellman, P. J., & Arterberry, M. E. (2006). Infant visual perception. In D. Kuhn & R. S. Siegler (Eds.), *Handbook of child psychology, Volume 2. Cognition, perception, and language*. Hoboken, NJ: Wiley.

Klatzky, R. L., Lederman, S. J., & Matula, D. E. (1991). Imagined haptic exploration in judgments of object properties. *Journal of Experimental Psychology: Learning, Memory, and Cognition, 17*, 314–322.

Klatzky, R. L., Lederman, S. J., & Matula, D. E. (1993). Haptic exploration in the presence of vision. *Journal of Experimental Psychology: Human Perception and Performance, 19*, 726–743.

Knill, D. C., & Saunders, J. A. (2003). Do humans optimally integrate stereo and texture information for judgments of surface slant? *Vision Research, 43*, 2539–2558.

Landy, M. S., & Kojima, H. (2001). Ideal cue combination for localizing texture-defined edges. *Journal of the Optical Society of America A: Optics, Image Science, and Vision, 18*, 2307–2320.

Landy, M. S., Maloney, L. T., Johnston, E. B., & Young, M. (1995). Measurement and modeling of depth cue combination: In defense of weak fusion. *Vision Research, 35*, 389–412.

Larson, G. W., & Shakespeare, R. (1996). *Rendering with radiance: The art and science of lighting and visualization*. San Francisco, CA: Morgan Kaufmann Publishers, Inc.

Lederman, S. J., & Abbott, S. G. (1981). Texture perception: Studies of intersensory organization using a discrepancy paradigm, and visual versus tactual psychophysics. *Journal of Experimental Psychology: Human Perception and Performance, 7*, 902–915.

Lederman, S. J., & Klatzky, R. L. (1997). Relative availability of surface and object properties during early haptic processing. *Journal of Experimental Psychology: Human Perception and Performance, 23*, 1680–1707.

MacLachlan, C., & Howland, H. C. (2002). Normal values and standard deviations for pupil diameter and interpupillary distance in subjects aged 1 month to 19 years. *Ophthalmic and Physiological Optics, 22*, 175–182.

Motoyoshi, I., Nishida, S., Sharan, L., & Adelson, E. H. (2007). Image statistics and the perception of surface qualities. *Nature, 447*, 206–209.

Necker, L. A. (1832). Observations on some remarkable optical phaenomena seen in Switzerland; and on an optical phaenomenon which occurs on viewing a figure of a crystal or geometrical solid. *The London and Edinburgh Philosophical Magazine and Journal of Science, 1*(5), 329–337.

Oruç, I., Maloney, L. T., & Landy, M. S. (2003). Weighted linear cue combination with possibly correlated error. *Vision Research, 43*, 2451–2468.

Pont, S. C., & Koenderink, J. J. (2005). Bidirectional texture contrast function. *International Journal of Computer Vision, 62*, 17–34.

Sharan, L., Li, Y. Z., Motoyoshi, I., Nishida, S., & Adelson, E. H. (2008). Image statistics for surface reflectance perception. *Journal of the Optical Society of America A: Optics, Image Science, and Vision, 25*, 846–865.

Ward, G. J. (1994). The RADIANCE lighting simulation and rendering system. *Computer Graphics, 28*, 459–472.

# CHAPTER 15

# Optimality Principles Apply to a Broad Range of Information Integration Problems in Perception and Action

*Melchi M. Michel, Anne-Marie Brouwer, Robert A. Jacobs, and David C. Knill*

## INTRODUCTION

A common approach to understanding human perception is to compare people's perceptual behaviors to those of computational models known as "ideal observers" (Barlow, 1959; Geisler, 2004; Green & Swets, 1966; Knill & Richards, 1996; Marr, 1982). When designing an ideal observer, a scientist makes assumptions about prior beliefs relevant to the task, about information sources providing data used during task performance, and about the costs of different types of errors. Ideal observers combine prior beliefs, data, and the costs of errors to choose actions optimally. Consequently, they perform as well as possible on a task given the assumptions built into the model.

Using the performance of an ideal observer as a "gold standard" or benchmark for human performance often leads to interesting insights. If a person performs a task at the same level as an ideal observer, then we have an explanation for the person's behavior: The person is behaving optimally because he or she is using and combining all relevant information in an optimal manner. If a person's performance is worse than that of an ideal observer, then this suggests that the person has perceptual or cognitive bottlenecks (e.g., limited working memory capacity or attentional resources) preventing better performance. Additional experimentation is often needed to identify these bottlenecks. Lastly, if a person's performance exceeds that of an ideal observer, then this suggests that the assumptions built into the model are too restrictive. It may be, for example, that the person is using information sources that are not available to the model. A scientist may consider designing a new, more complex ideal observer in this case.

As discussed in nearly all the chapters in this book, scientists are interested in using ideal observers to characterize how people combine sensory information based on multiple perceptual cues. These cues might arise from a common sensory modality or from different modalities. For example, an observer attempting to determine the curvature of a surface may have access to visual cues based on visual texture, binocular disparity, and shading, as well as to haptic cues obtained by manually exploring the surface.

Among the most important findings on this topic is that people tend to combine information based on different cues in a statistically optimal manner (see Chapter 1). Specifically, their perceptual judgments tend to match those of an ideal observer that estimates the value of a scene property as a weighted average of estimates based on individual cues. Moreover, the weight associated with a cue is related to the reliability of the cue, where the reliability of a cue is inversely proportional to the variance of the distribution of a scene property given a cue's value (e.g., Battaglia, Jacobs, & Aslin, 2003; Ernst & Banks, 2002, Jacobs, 1999; Johnston, Cumming, & Landy, 1994; Knill & Saunders, 2003; Landy, Maloney, Johnston, & Young, 1995; Maloney & Landy, 1989; Young, Landy, & Maloney, 1993). Because of the ubiquity of this ideal observer in the perceptual-sciences literature, it is henceforth referred to as the "standard ideal observer."

Consider, for example, a standard ideal observer attempting to estimate the curvature of a surface that is both seen and touched. Information about the surface's curvature is provided by a visual stereo cue and by a haptic cue. Suppose that the visual stereo cue provides precise or highly diagnostic information in the sense that it indicates that the curvature lies within a narrow range, but the haptic cue provides imprecise information meaning that it indicates that the curvature lies within a broad range. In this case, the standard ideal observer will form its estimate of curvature as a weighted average of the estimate based on the visual cue and the estimate based on the haptic cue. The stereo cue will be regarded as more reliable and, thus, the curvature estimate based on this cue will be assigned a larger weight. In contrast, the haptic cue will be regarded as less reliable; the estimate based on the haptic cue will be assigned a smaller weight.

To date, most studies have considered simple tasks in which a person estimates a continuous quantity (e.g., surface slant or curvature) based on two sensory cues (e.g., visual stereo and haptic cues). Under these conditions, the standard ideal observer is adequate in the sense that its predictions typically match people's judgments. This chapter describes two research projects that evaluated whether people's judgments are predicted by those of the standard ideal observer in more complex situations. By considering more complex situations, these projects expanded the scope of the standard ideal observer in new directions that had not been previously explored.

The first project, conducted by Michel and Jacobs (2008), examined how people learn to combine information from arbitrary visual features when performing a set of perceptual discrimination tasks. This project challenged the standard ideal observer in several ways. First, the standard ideal observer has nearly always been applied to tasks requiring judgments based on conventional perceptual cues such as those listed in undergraduate textbooks (e.g., visual cues such as shading, texture gradients, binocular disparity, motion parallax, familiar size, etc.), which are highly familiar to people. Does the standard ideal observer still predict people's judgments when information sources are arbitrary visual features that must be learned? Second, the standard ideal observer has typically been applied to tasks with very few sensory cues, perhaps two or three. Does this observer provide a good model of people's judgments on larger tasks such as ones with twenty information sources? Finally, the standard ideal observer as typically used in the scientific literature emphasizes the content of different information sources in the context of a single task. A limitation of this viewpoint is that it does not stress the possibility that people's sensory integrations are strongly shaped by the task they are currently performing. Do people modify the way they combine information from multiple sources when different sources are reliable on different tasks?

The second project, conducted by Brouwer and Knill (2007, 2009), examined how people combine location information from vision and memory in a sensorimotor task. This project also challenged the standard ideal observer in interesting ways. A recurring question in the field of Cognitive Science is the extent to which mental or neural processes overlap. For example, do perception and memory share common principles of operation, or does each operate in its own way? To date, the perceptual sciences have considered cue combination only in situations where information sources are sensory signals. What would happen, however, if people were placed in a task in which they could combine sensory information with information from short-term memory? Would the standard ideal observer still provide a good model of people's judgments if its notion of an information source was suitably expanded to include memory? If so, does that mean that people evaluate the reliability of an information source in the same manner regardless of whether the source is perception or memory?

## INTEGRATION OF ARBITRARY FEATURES WHEN PERFORMING A SET OF PERCEPTUAL DISCRIMINATION TASKS

As mentioned earlier, we examined how people learn to combine information from arbitrary visual features in a set of perceptual discrimination tasks (Michel & Jacobs, 2008). Visual stimuli were linear combinations of an underlying set of visual "basis" features or primitives. These basis features are illustrated in Figure 15.1. At first glance, these features should seem to be arbitrary texture blobs. In fact, they are not completely arbitrary. They were created using an optimization procedure that yielded features which are orthogonal to each other (if features are written as vectors of pixel values, then the vectors are orthogonal to each other), relatively smooth (the optimization procedure minimized the sum of the Laplacian across each image), and equally salient (feature luminance-contrast values were normalized based on a feature's spatial frequency content).

Subjects performed a set of binary classification tasks. The prototype for each class was a linear combination of the basis features. The linear coefficients for class $A$ were randomly set to either 1.0 or $-1.0$. The coefficients for class $B$ were the negative of the coefficients for class $A$. In addition, a matrix $K$ was added to each prototype where $K$ consisted of the background luminance plus an arbitrary image constructed in the null space of the basis feature set (the addition of this arbitrary matrix prevented the

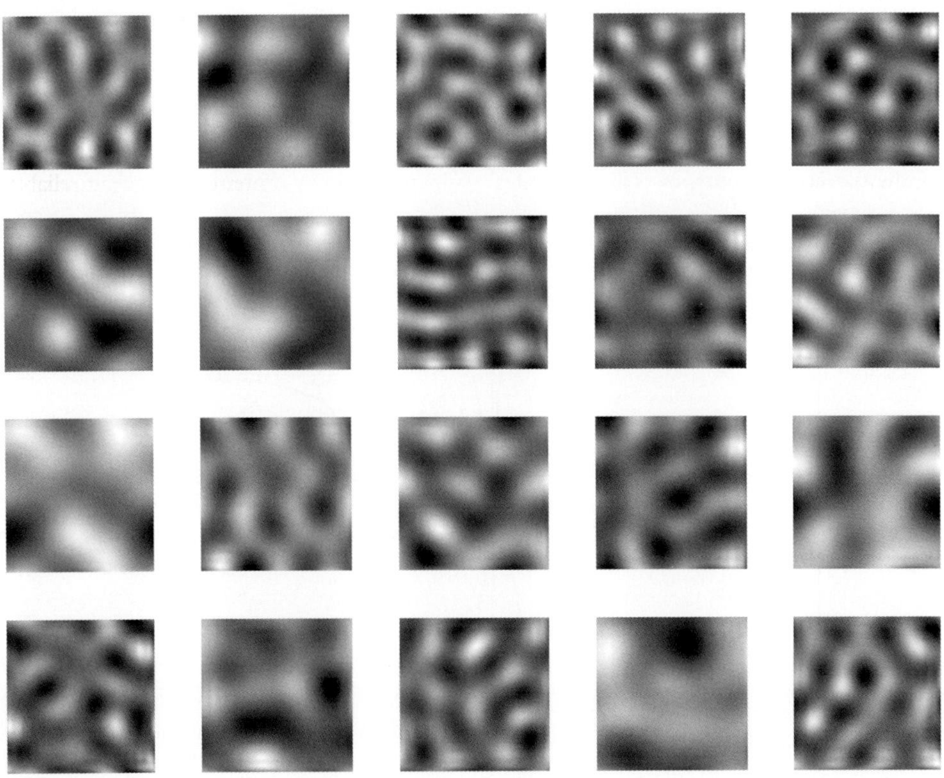

**Figure 15.1** The 20 visual basis features used to construct the visual stimuli.

prototypes from appearing as contrast-reversed versions of the same image). In summary, a prototype was computed using the equation:

$$\text{prototype} = K + \sum_i c_i F_i$$

where $F_i$ is basis feature $i$ and $c_i$ is its corresponding linear coefficient.

Exemplars from a class were created by randomly perturbing the linear coefficients $c_i$ defining the prototype for that class. This was done using the equation:

$$\text{exemplar} = K + \sum_i (c_i + \varepsilon_i) F_i$$

where $\varepsilon_i$ is a random sample from a normal distribution with mean zero and variance $\sigma_i^2$. This variance is referred to as a feature's noise variance. Importantly, each feature had its own noise variance, and the magnitude of this variance determined the reliability of a feature. Features with small noise variances tended to have coefficient values near one of the class prototypes. Therefore, these features were highly diagnostic of whether an exemplar belonged to class *A* or *B*. In contrast, features with large noise variances tended to have coefficient values far from the class prototypes. These features were less diagnostic of an exemplar's class membership.

This general idea is schematically illustrated in Figure 15.2. Consider a binary classification task where each prototype and exemplar contains two features, denoted *x1* and *x2*. The horizontal and vertical axes in the graphs in Figure 15.2 correspond to these two features. The black and gray dots in each graph represent the prototypes for classes *A* and *B*, respectively, and the black solid and gray dashed circles represent the spread of exemplars around these prototypes. In the leftmost graph, features *x1* and *x2* have equal noise variances, meaning that the features are equally reliable predictors of class membership. The diagonal line is the optimal linear discriminant dividing the two classes. In the middle graph, feature *x*1 has a small noise variance, whereas feature *x2* has a large noise variance. In this case, *x1* is a reliable feature and *x2* is an unreliable feature. The optimal discriminant estimates class membership by primarily using feature *x1*. This situation is reversed in the rightmost graph. Here, feature *x1* has a large noise variance, meaning that it is an unreliable feature, and feature *x2* has a small noise variance, meaning that it is a reliable feature. The optimal discriminant estimates class membership by primarily using feature *x2*.

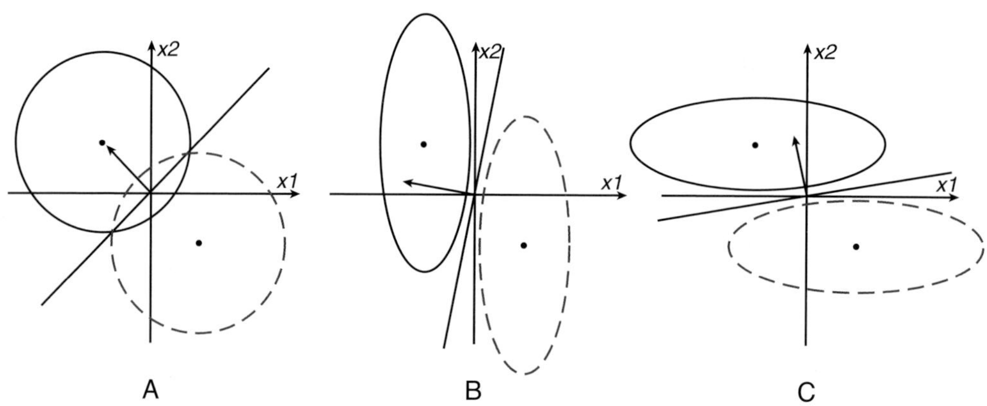


**Figure 15.2** A schematic illustration of two classes of stimuli in a two-dimensional feature space. In the leftmost graph, the two features have equal noise variances. In the middle graph, feature *x1* has a smaller noise variance than feature *x2*. In the rightmost graph, feature *x1* has a larger noise variance than feature *x2*. The optimal linear discriminant dividing the two classes is shown in each graph.

Each trial of the experiment began with the presentation of a fixation square, followed by an exemplar, referred to as a test stimulus, followed by the prototypes of classes *A* and *B*. Subjects were instructed to decide which of the two prototypes had appeared in the test stimulus, and they responded by pressing the key corresponding to the selected prototype. Subjects received immediate auditory feedback after every trial indicating the correctness of their response. In addition, after every 15 trials, a printed message appeared on the screen indicating their (percent correct) performance on the previous 15 trials.

Each subject performed two classification tasks, Task 1 on days 1–3 (trials 1–3600) and Task 2 on days 4–6 (trials 3601–7200). Importantly, the exemplars (but not the prototypes) were manipulated across the two tasks. This was accomplished by modifying the feature noise variances. In Task 1, half the features were randomly chosen to serve as reliable features for determining class membership. These features had a small noise variance ($\sigma^2 = 1$). The remaining features served as unreliable features and were assigned a large noise variance ($\sigma^2 = 25$). In Task 2, the roles of the two sets of features were swapped such that the reliable features were made unreliable, and the unreliable features were made reliable. Subjects were not explicitly informed about the switch from Task 1 to Task 2.

Our prediction was that subjects would learn to integrate information from the basis features based on the relative reliabilities of these features. Consequently, we expected subjects to successfully track the reliable versus unreliable features during the course of the experiment. When performing Task 1, we expected subjects would make their visual judgments on the basis of half the features—the reliable features—and ignore the remaining features. When performing Task 2, we expected subjects to flip their use of each feature. That is, we expected subjects' judgments to be based on the newly reliable features (the features that were previously ignored) and to ignore the newly unreliable features (the features that were previously the basis of subjects' judgments).

To evaluate this prediction, we needed a way of assessing the degree to which a subject used each feature throughout the course of training. In the vision sciences, classification images have become a popular method to estimate the stimulus components that an observer uses when classifying an exemplar as belonging to one of two classes (e.g., Abbey & Eckstein, 2002; Ahumada, 1996; Gold, Sekuler, & Bennett, 2004; Lu & Liu, 2006; Neri & Heeger, 2002; Neri, Parker, & Blakemore, 1999). Classification images are typically computed as follows (Ahumada, 1967, 2002). On each trial, a test stimulus is created by corrupting a prototype with random pixel noise sampled from a mean-zero normal distribution. The observer classifies the test stimulus as belonging to either class *A* or *B*. At the end of the experiment, the researcher correlates the noise added on each trial with the observer's classification. This is achieved by computing the difference between the average noise added to a test stimulus classified as belonging to class *A* and the average noise added to a test stimulus classified as belonging to class *B*. This difference is the observer's classification image.

Although commonly used in the vision sciences, this method of calculating classification images has shortcomings that make it undesirable in many circumstances. These shortcomings arise from the enormous dimensionality of the stimulus space. Calculating a classification image when stimuli are represented within a $128 \times 128$ pixel space, for example, requires calculating $128^2 = 16,384$ parameters. Consequently, thousands of experimental trials are required to obtain a reasonable classification image for a single observer. Previous work suggested that the correlation of the resulting images with mathematically optimal classification images is generally quite low (Gold et al., 2004). One possibility is that this low correlation is due to poor estimates of observers' classification images as a result of a paucity of data items and, thus, poor sampling of the stimulus space. Several researchers have attempted to ameliorate this problem by restricting the final analysis to select portions of the classification image (e.g., Gold et al., 2004), by averaging across regions of the image (e.g., Abbey & Eckstein, 2002;

Abbey, Eckstein, & Bochud, 1999), or by using a combination of these methods (e.g., Chauvin, Worsley, Schyns, Arguin, & Gosselin, 2005). Such measures work by effectively reducing the dimensionality of the stimulus space so that instead of calculating regression coefficients for each pixel, researchers calculate a much smaller number of coefficients for various linear combinations of pixels. Essentially, these researchers consider the noise in pixel space but perform their analyses in terms of a lower dimensional basis space.

In our study, we simplified this process by specifying this lower dimensional basis space explicitly and a priori (see Li, Levi, & Klein, 2004, and Olman & Kersten, 2004, for related approaches). In addition to its simplicity, this approach has several advantages over alternative methods for estimating classification images. First, by specifying the bases in advance, we can limit the added noise to the subspace spanned by these bases, ensuring that the noise is white and densely sampled in this subspace, and ensuring that only features within the spanned subspace contribute to the observer's decisions (because all stimulus variance is contained within this subspace). Second, because we specify the bases in advance, we can select these bases in an intelligent way, representing only those features that observers are likely to find useful in making discriminations, such as those features that contain information relevant to the task (i.e., features that vary across the stimulus classes). Finally, this approach makes it possible to manipulate the variance of the noise added to different features and, thus, to vary the reliabilities of these features. This allows us to investigate how observers combine information from different features using methods similar to those that have been used in studying perceptual cue combination.

We computed a subject's classification image at each session of the experiment as follows. On each trial, a subject viewed an exemplar defined by a set of 20 linear coefficients in the space of our visual basis features, and the subject judged whether the exemplar belonged to class *A* or *B*. The subject's responses were modeled using logistic regression (see Michel & Jacobs, 2008, for details). The input to a regressor was a set of linear coefficients defining an exemplar. The regressor's output was an estimate of the probability that the subject judged the exemplar as belonging to class *A*. Maximum-likelihood estimates of a logistic regressor's parameter values were found using the iterative reweighted least-squares procedure and a Bernoulli response-likelihood function. These parameter estimates indicate the extent to which each feature in the set of basis features was used by a subject when making a classification judgment. Because they indicate the stimulus features a subject used for classification, these parameter estimates are a subject's classification image.

The mathematically optimal (in a maximum-likelihood sense) classification image was also found via logistic regression. In this case, the input to the regressor was the linear coefficients defining an exemplar, and the output was the true probability that the exemplar belonged to class *A*. Because the two classes were defined as normal distributions, it was possible to define the true probabilities, and it was also possible to find the optimal parameter values of the logistic regressor. These parameter values are the classification image of an optimal or "ideal" observer.

We evaluated each subject's performance at multiple points during the experiment by comparing a subject's classification image with the ideal classification image. Let $w_{subj}$ and $w_{ideal}$ be vectors denoting a subject's classification image and the ideal classification image, respectively. A subject's "template correlation" is the normalized dot-product of these two vectors:

$$\text{template correlation} = \frac{w_{subj}^T \, w_{ideal}}{\left\| w_{subj} \right\| \, \left\| w_{ideal} \right\|}.$$

This quantity is large if the subject's and ideal classification images are highly similar, meaning that the subject performed in a near-optimal manner. If this quantity is small, then the subject's performance was far from optimal.

The results are shown in Figure 15.3. The four graphs in the figure correspond to the

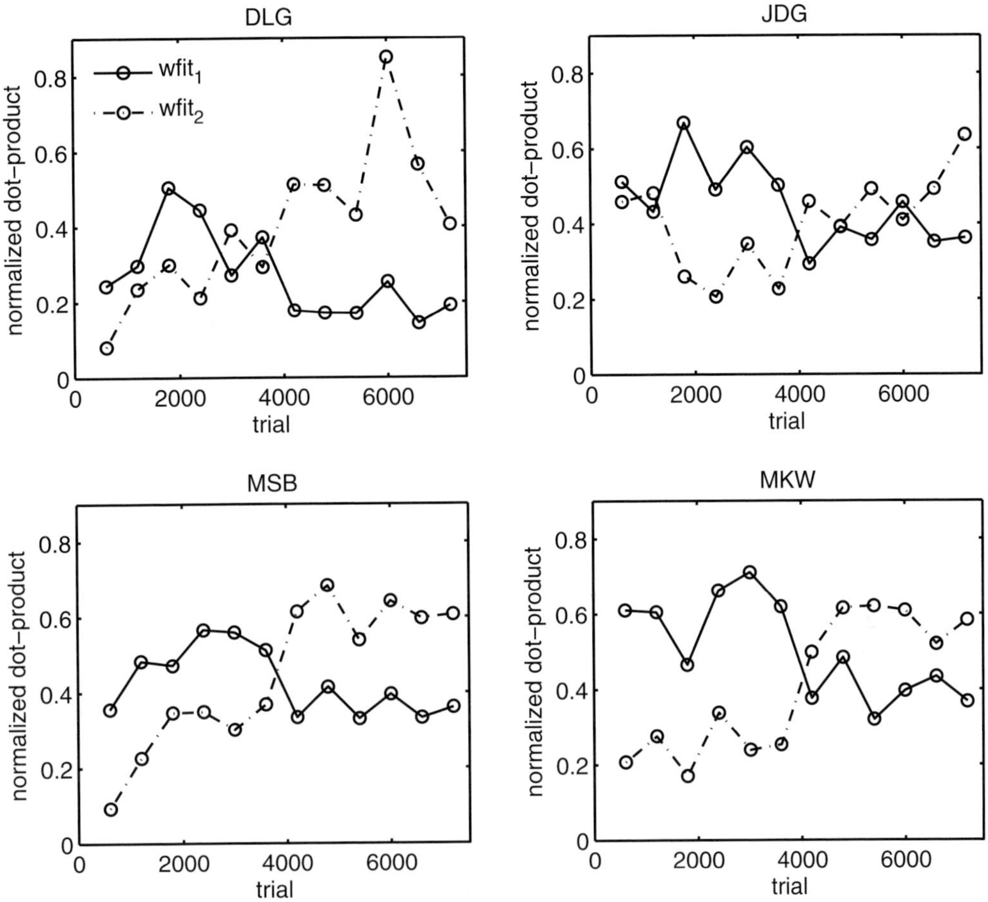


**Figure 15.3** The template correlations or normalized dot-products for each of the four subjects as a function of the trial number.

four subjects. The horizontal axis of each graph plots the trial number. The vertical axis plots a subject's template correlation. The data points correspond to a subject's average correlation across pairs of experimental sessions. Recall that subjects were trained on two tasks: During the first half of the experiment, they performed Task 1 (one set of reliable and unreliable features), and they performed Task 2 during the second half of the experiment (the reliable and unreliable features were swapped). The solid line in each graph shows a subject's template correlation when the ideal classification image was based on Task 1 (denoted $wfit_1$), and the dotted line shows the correlation when the ideal classification image was based on Task 2 ($wfit_2$).

All four subjects had significantly larger template correlations based on the ideal classification image for Task 1 during the first half of training, and larger correlations based on the ideal classification image for Task 2 during the second half of training. Clearly, subjects successfully tracked the reliabilities of the visual basis features by tracking the noise variances of these features, and they preferentially used the reliable features when performing each task.

This result suggests that an expanded perspective on the standard ideal observer for cue combination is warranted. As discussed earlier, the standard ideal observer is nearly always applied to the combination of information based on conventional perceptual cues that are frequently studied in the perceptual sciences and are highly familiar to people. The experiment reported here suggests that the standard ideal observer is also applicable to the combination of information based on arbitrary visual features that must be learned. This is important because there is much uncertainty in the perceptual sciences about the cues or information sources underlying people's judgments, and because people seem to be able to learn to use new cues in an experience-dependent manner (Chapter 6; Haijiang, Saunders, Stone, & Backus, 2006; Michel & Jacobs, 2007). In addition, the standard ideal observer is typically used to combine information based on two or three cues. The experiment reported here suggests that the observer is also applicable when there are 20 cues. If so, then the observer can scale to larger and more realistic perceptual settings. Lastly, the standard ideal observer is typically used to analyze the content of information sources in the context of a single task. The experiment reported here suggests that people can combine information from multiple sources differently on different tasks depending on the statistical structures of those tasks. That is, people's cue combinations are task dependent.

In summary, the experiment indicates that the standard ideal observer has significantly greater applicability than the current perceptual sciences literature would lead one to believe. For instance, it suggests that the notion of an "information source" needs to be expanded beyond conventional perceptual cues. But how far can this notion be pushed? Is it limited to perceptual features? Or can it include nonperceptual information sources such as memory? This topic is the focus of the second project described in this chapter.

## INTEGRATION OF VISION AND MEMORY IN A SENSORIMOTOR TASK

The second research project examined how people combine position information from vision and memory while reaching for a target (Brouwer & Knill, 2007, 2009). A key question addressed by this project is: Do people integrate position information in visual short-term memory (VSTM) with online visual information to plan hand movements? On the one hand, there are reasons they should not. First, some experiments have suggested that the accuracy of VSTM is poor. For example, it has been found that the visual system cannot retain detailed visual information across saccades (Henderson & Hollingworth, 2003; Irwin, 1991). Second, combining information from online perception with information from VSTM may require the use of coordinate transformations across viewpoints. Such transformations are known to be prone to noise (Schlicht & Schrater, 2007). Third, the world is often nonstationary, meaning that the properties of an object (such as its position) can change without warning. In this case, information about the past stored in VSTM may be irrelevant to current performance on a task. Lastly, why store and use information in VSTM when it is easy to simply look at the world?

On the other hand, there are good reasons that one should integrate information in VSTM with online visual information. First, the accuracy of online visual information is poor in the visual periphery. It may be possible to compensate for the poor quality of peripheral information using information from VSTM. In addition, we know from the field of statistics that optimal integration of information from different sources may aid performance on a task, and it will never diminish performance.

The apparatus used in the experiment is illustrated on the left side of Figure 15.4. Subjects viewed a display of a scene and were able to interact with the objects in the display. The scene was rendered from left-eye and right-eye viewpoints, and subjects viewed the display stereoscopically through liquid crystal display (LCD) shutter glasses. In addition, the three-dimensional position and pose of a subject's finger were recorded. A "virtual" finger was rendered in the display at the position and orientation of a subject's real finger.

As illustrated on the right side of Figure 15.4, a scene initially consisted of a cross located at the bottom of the workspace; a square object and

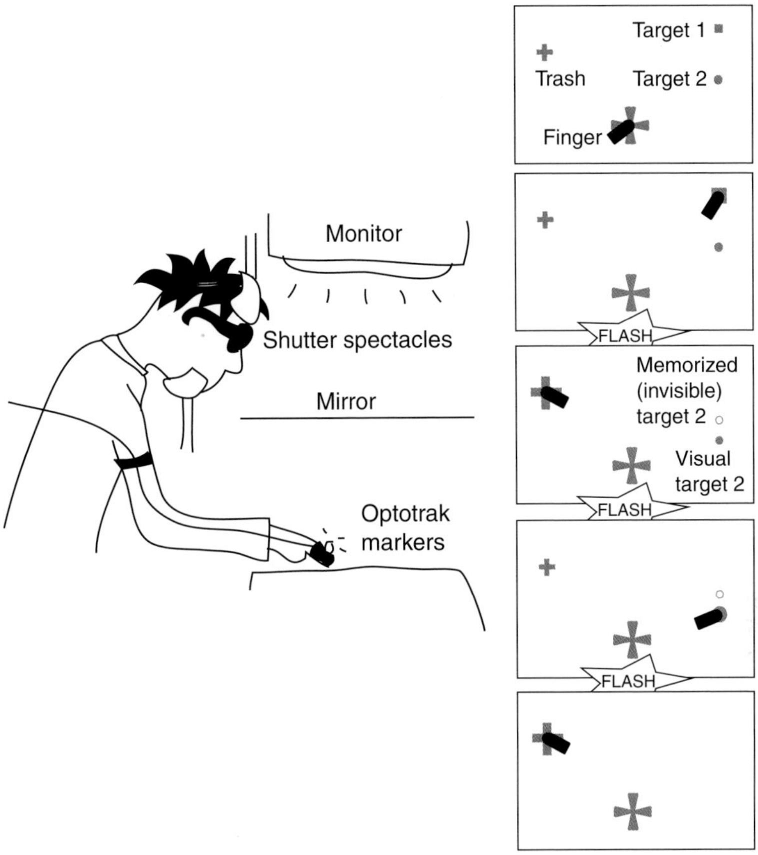


**Figure 15.4** On the left is a schematic illustration of the experimental apparatus. On the right is a schematic illustration of an experimental trial.

a circular object, referred to as Targets 1 and 2, respectively, located at random locations on the workspace's right side; and a Trash Bin located on the workspace's left side. A subject started a trial by touching the cross with the finger. The subject then touched Target 1. On touching the target, it "magnetically" stuck to the finger. The subject next started to move Target 1 toward the Trash Bin. During this movement, a masking flicker was presented, rendering the whole screen successively black for two frames and white for two frames. On two-thirds of trials, nothing changed during the flicker, but on one-third of trials, Target 2 shifted either 1 cm up or down. When the subject touched Target 1 to the Trash Bin, it disappeared. The subject then moved the finger from the Trash Bin to Target 2. During this movement, a flicker was again presented. Subjects picked up Target 2 and moved it to the Trash Bin.

Of all trials, perhaps the most important were those on which Target 2 was perturbed up or down. On these trials, there were two sources of information about Target 2's position that a subject could use when moving the finger from the Trash Bin to Target 2. One source of information was the online visual percept of Target 2's new location. The other source was the memory of Target 2's old location prior to the perturbation. The experiment was designed to evaluate how people integrate information from these two sources.

Ten subjects participated in the experiment, and each subject performed 12 blocks of trials. Each block consisted of 92 trials. For half the trials in a block, Targets 1 and 2 were displayed with a high contrast. They were displayed with a low contrast for the remaining trials. At each level of contrast, there were 30 trials in which Target 2 was unperturbed, 8 trials in which it was perturbed upward, and 8 trials in which it was perturbed downward.

The eye movements of 4 of 10 subjects were recorded. When moving the finger from the Trash Bin to Target 2, these subjects tended to first fixate at or near the Trash Bin, to then start moving their fingers from the Trash Bin to Target 2, and, lastly, to move their eyes from the Trash Bin to Target 2. Notably, during the first 206 ms of the movement of the finger, subjects were fixating the Trash Bin and, thus, the only online visual information about the position of Target 2 was information from the visual periphery. Because of the poor quality of information from the visual periphery, we predicted that subjects would make large use of position information from VSTM during this time period.

To evaluate this prediction, the relative weights that subjects' assigned to online visual information and to information from VSTM were estimated. Let $Y(t)$ denote the vertical position of a subject's finger at time $t$ during the movement from the Trash Bin to Target 2. Let $Y_{vis}$ denote the vertical position of Target 2, and let $Y_{mem}$ denote Target 2's position prior to any perturbation of Target 2 that might have occurred during a trial. That is, $Y_{mem} = Y_{vis}$ on trials in which Target 2 was unperturbed. But on trials in which Target 2 was perturbed, $Y_{mem}$ is the position before the perturbation and $Y_{vis}$ is the position after the perturbation. It was assumed that $Y(t)$ could be estimated by the following linear equation:

$$Y(t) = (W_{vis}(t) \times Y_{vis}) + (W_{mem}(t) \times Y_{mem}) + K + \text{noise}$$

where $W_{vis}(t)$ and $W_{mem}(t)$ are time-dependent linear coefficients and $K$ is a constant. The relative contribution of the memorized position of Target 2 at time $t$ is

$$W_{mem}(t)/(W_{mem}(t) + W_{vis}(t)).$$

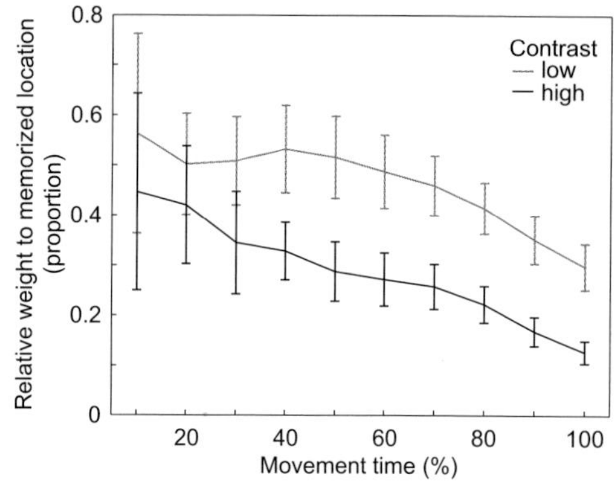


**Figure 15.5** Subjects' average relative contribution of the memorized position as a function of the movement time (error bars show standard errors of the means).

The relative contribution of position information from online visual information is one minus this quantity.

Figure 15.5 shows subjects' average relative contribution of the memorized position as a function of the movement time. Finger position is more correlated with remembered target location in the first half of subjects' movements. This is sensible because early portions of a movement presumably reflect motor planning based on remembered location and because online visual information of Target 2's position came from the periphery toward the start of a movement and, thus, was low quality during this time period. At the end of a movement, subjects fixated Target 2, meaning that online visual information was higher quality and, thus, subjects relied more on this online visual information. In addition, Figure 15.5 reveals that subjects used the memorized position more when Target 2 was low contrast than when it was high contrast. Again, this is sensible because subjects used memorized position more when visual information was low quality, and they used memorized position less when visual information was high quality.

Figure 15.6 shows subjects' vertical errors at the end of a movement from the Trash Bin to Target 2 as a function of the value of the perturbation that took place on a trial.

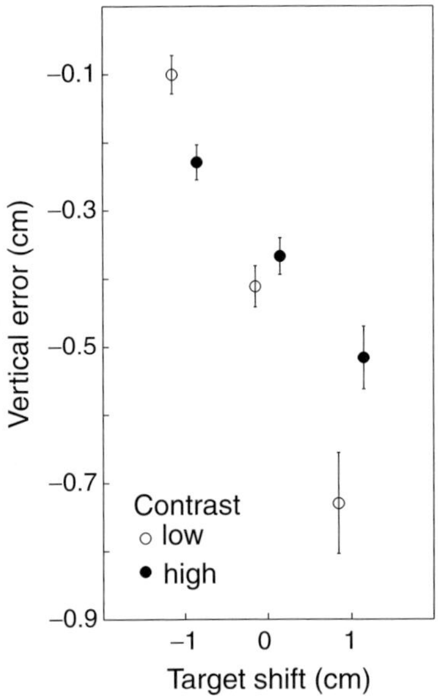


**Figure 15.6** Subjects' average vertical errors at the end of a movement from the Trash Bin to Target 2 as a function of the value of the perturbation that took place on a trial (error bars show standard errors of the means).

When there was no perturbation, subjects tended to moderately undershoot Target 2. When Target 2 was perturbed downward, the undershoot of Target 2 was smaller, and when Target 2 was perturbed upward, the undershoot of Target 2 was larger. Thus, relative to unperturbed targets, subjects hit perturbed targets in the direction of where they used to be, suggesting that memorized position played an important role in subjects' movements. As expected, this effect was stronger for low-contrast targets than for high-contrast targets.

Taken as a whole, the results strongly suggest that people used information from memory more when visual information was poor, and they used information from memory less when visual information was good. That is, subjects evaluated the relative reliabilities of information from memory and online visual information at each moment in time and used each information source based on that source's relative reliability. If so, then this suggests that the scope of the standard ideal observer needs to be expanded. The observer has always been applied to tasks in which people combine information based on multiple perceptual cues. But the experiment reported here indicates that the observer has broader applicability; it also provides a useful model of people's behaviors when combining information from perception with information from memory.

## SUMMARY AND CONCLUSIONS

The perceptual-sciences literature contains many articles reporting experiments in which subjects made perceptual judgments based on information provided by two cues. It has often been found that subjects' judgments based on both cues matched those of the standard ideal observer. Consequently, the observer has provided an important conceptual framework explaining subjects' cue combinations.

To date, however, the scope of the standard ideal observer has been limited. This chapter has described two research projects suggesting that an expanded perspective on the standard ideal observer is warranted. The observer is applicable to tasks involving arbitrary perceptual signals that need to be learned, not just conventional perceptual cues that are highly familiar; to tasks involving many information sources, not just two sources; to multitask settings in which different cue combinations are optimal for different tasks, not just single-task settings; and to tasks involving information stored in memory, not just tasks in which information is based on perception.

In general, ideal-observer analysis is useful because it forces scientists to think deeply about the information available to a person during task performance. Information sources might be familiar perceptual cues, novel features, or a combination of the two. If novel features are important, then scientists are confronted with the question of how people might learn new perceptual features. Similarly, information sources might be perception, memory, or some combination. If memory is important, then scientists studying perception and action will need to think about how the properties of memory, such as limited short-term memory capacity, influence task performance. Lastly, information sources are likely to be task dependent; which sources are relevant and reliable will vary from task to task. Scientists will therefore need to study how people rapidly and accurately determine the useful information sources for the tasks that they are currently performing. By identifying and examining task-dependent information sources, ideal-observer analysis quickly leads scientists to a broad range of exciting and challenging questions about human cognition.

## REFERENCES

Abbey, C. K., & Eckstein, M. P. (2002). Classification image analysis: Estimation and statistical inference for two-alternative forced-choice experiments. *Journal of Vision, 2*, 66–78.

Abbey, C. K., Eckstein, M. P., & Bochud, F. O. (1999). Estimation of human-observer templates for 2 alternative forced choice tasks. *Proceedings of SPIE, 3663*, 284–295.

Ahumada, A. J. (1967). *Detection of tones masked by noise: A comparison of human observers with digital-computer-simulated energy detectors of varying bandwidths.* Unpublished doctoral dissertation, University of California, Los Angeles.

Ahumada, A. J. (1996). Perceptual classification images from vernier acuity masked by noise. *Perception, 25*, 18.

Ahumada, A. J. (2002). Classification image weights and internal noise level estimation. *Journal of Vision, 2*, 121–131.

Barlow, H. B. (1959). Possible principles underlying the transformation of sensory messages. In W. Rosenblith (Ed.), *Sensory communication* (pp. 217–234). Cambridge, MA: MIT Press.

Battaglia, P. W., Jacobs, R. A., & Aslin, R. N. (2003). Bayesian integration of visual and auditory signals for spatial localization. *Journal of the Optical Society of America A, 20*, 1391–1397.

Brouwer, A-M., & Knill, D. C. (2007). The role of memory in visually guided reaching. *Journal of Vision, 7*(5):6, 1–12.

Brouwer, A-M., & Knill, D. C. (2009). Humans use visual and remembered information about object location to plan pointing movements. *Journal of Vision, 9*(1):24, 1–19.

Chauvin, A., Worsley, K. J., Schyns, P. G., Arguin, M., & Gosselin, F. (2005). Accurate statistical tests for smooth classification images. *Journal of Vision, 5*, 659–667.

Ernst, M. O., & Banks, M. S. (2002). Humans integrate visual and haptic information in a statistically optimal fashion. *Nature, 415*, 429–433.

Geisler, W. S. (2004). Ideal observer analysis. In L. M. Chalupa & J. S. Werner (Eds.), *The visual neurosciences* (Vol. 1, pp. 825–837). Cambridge, MA: MIT Press.

Gold, J. M., Sekuler, A. B., & Bennett, P. J. (2004). Characterizing perceptual learning with external noise. *Cognitive Science, 28*, 167–207.

Green, D. M., & Swets, J. A. (1966). *Signal detection theory and psychophysics.* New York, NY: Wiley.

Haijiang, Q., Saunders, J. A., Stone, R. W., & Backus, B. T. (2006). Demonstration of cue recruitment: Change in visual appearance by means of Pavlovian conditioning. *Proceedings of the National Academy of Science USA, 103*, 483–488.

Henderson, J. M., & Hollingworth, A. (2003). Global transsaccadic change blindness during scene perception. *Psychological Science, 14*, 493–497.

Irwin, D. E. (1991). Information integration across saccadic eye movements. *Cognitive Psychology, 23*, 420–456.

Jacobs, R. A. (1999). Optimal integration of texture and motion cues to depth. *Vision Research, 39*, 3621–3629.

Johnston, E. B., Cumming, B. G., & Landy, M. S. (1994). Integration of motion and stereopsis cues. *Vision Research, 34*, 2259–2275.

Knill, D. C., & Richards, W. (Eds.). (1996). *Perception as Bayesian inference.* Cambridge, England: Cambridge University Press.

Knill, D. C., & Saunders, J. (2003). Do humans optimally integrate stereo and texture information for judgments of surface slant? *Vision Research, 43*, 2539–2558.

Landy, M. S., Maloney, L. T., Johnston, E. B., & Young, M. (1995). Measurement and modeling of depth cue combination: In defense of weak fusion. *Vision Research, 35*, 389–412.

Li, R. W., Levi, D. M., & Klein, S. A. (2004). Perceptual learning improves efficiency by re-tuning the decision "template" for position discrimination. *Nature Neuroscience, 7*, 178–183.

Lu, H., & Liu, Z. (2006). Computing dynamic classification images from correlation maps. *Journal of Vision*, *6*, 475–483.

Maloney, L. T., & Landy, M. S. (1989). A statistical framework for robust fusion of depth information. In W. A. Pearlman (Ed.), *Visual Communications and Image Processing IV: Proceedings of the SPIE*, *1199*, 1154–1163. SPIE: Bellingham, WA.

Marr, D. (1982). *Vision*. New York, NY: Freeman.

Michel, M. M., & Jacobs, R. A. (2007). Parameter learning but not structure learning: A Bayesian network model of constraints on early perceptual learning. *Journal of Vision*, *7*(1):4, 1–18.

Michel, M. M., & Jacobs, R. A. (2008). Learning optimal integration of arbitrary features in a perceptual discrimination task. *Journal of Vision*, *8*(2):3, 1–16.

Neri, P., & Heeger, D. J. (2002). Spatiotemporal mechanisms for detecting and identifying image features in human vision. *Nature Neuroscience*, *5*, 812–816.

Neri, P., Parker, A. J., & Blakemore, C. (1999). Probing the human stereoscopic system with reverse correlation. *Nature*, *401*, 695–698.

Olman, C., & Kersten, D. (2004). Classification objects, ideal observers, and generative models. *Cognitive Science*, *28*, 227–240.

Schlicht, E. J., & Schrater, P. R. (2007). Impact of coordinate transformation uncertainty on human sensorimotor control. *Journal of Neurophysiology*, *97*, 4203–4217.

Young, M. J., Landy, M. S., & Maloney, L. T. (1993). A perturbation analysis of depth perception from combinations of texture and motion cues. *Vision Research*, *33*, 2685–2696.

# SECTION III

# Introduction to Section III: Neural Implementation

This third section of the book summarizes both behavioral evidence and computational work concerned with the neural encoding of uncertainty and the use of estimates of uncertainty for cue combination. It consists of two main parts. The first four chapters of Section III introduce neurophysiological insights into cue combination. The final three chapters describe computational models of how the nervous system might implement the cue-combination approaches discussed in Sections I and II. While Sections I and II focus on framing the problems that a human needs to solve for effective cue integration and discussing the optimal solutions to these problems, the chapters in this section ask how the nervous system implements such algorithms.

The first four chapters of Section III review experiments designed to determine the algorithm used by the nervous system to perform cue integration. Fetsch, Gu, DeAngelis, and Angelaki ask how the estimation of self-motion is implemented in the nervous system. They present single-cell and behavioral data from nonhuman primates in a visual/vestibular cue-integration task and compare both to predictions of the optimal linear cue-combination model. Buneo, Apker, and Shi ask which brain areas might be involved in combining visual and somatic cues to limb position in the control of arm movements. Rowland, Stein, and Stanford discuss models of the integration of visual and auditory cues in the cat superior colliculus. Welchman reviews the cortical coding of individual depth cues and discusses functional magnetic resonance imaging (fMRI) experiments that look for the cortical representation of cue-integrated depth. These chapters reflect substantial progress in our understanding of cue combination in the brain.

The last three chapters of Section III present some of the leading theories of the neural implementation of cue combination. Natarajan and Zemel describe a neural model of dynamic cue combination in a distributed population of neurons. The chapter focuses on the integration of information from cues over time. Ma, Beck, and Pouget describe a model of optimal Bayesian cue combination that can be computed easily by spiking neurons with Poisson firing statistics. In the final chapter, Denève and Lochmann interpret contextual modulation of visual receptive fields from a Bayesian perspective. They propose a model of how nonlinear cue combination effects may arise from neural mechanisms. These theoretical studies suggest a number of ways in which neurons might encode uncertainty and use that information to control cue integration.

# CHAPTER 16

## Self-Motion Perception: Multisensory Integration in Extrastriate Visual Cortex

*Christopher R. Fetsch, Yong Gu, Gregory C. DeAngelis, and Dora E. Angelaki*

### INTRODUCTION

The accurate perception of self-motion is essential for spatial orientation, navigation, and motor planning. Estimating our instantaneous direction of translation, or heading, is a particularly relevant multisensory problem because it requires cross-modal integration even under ordinary conditions. In addition, as we will summarize in this chapter, heading perception is a useful model for studying the neural basis of multisensory integration for two main reasons. First, there are well-defined brain structures that receive both visual and vestibular signals related to self-motion (e.g., macaque areas MSTd and VIP). Second, the problem is amenable to study using a standard "fine" psychophysical discrimination task, for which there are already well-established behavioral and neurophysiological analysis methods.

### VISUAL AND VESTIBULAR SELF-MOTION CUES: WHY INTEGRATE?

It has long been recognized that visual cues provide a rich source of information about heading direction (Gibson, 1950; Warren, 2003). As we move through the environment, the resulting pattern of full-field retinal motion (known as optic flow) can be used to estimate heading, for instance, by calculating the position of the focus of radial expansion. Typically, however, the motion of the retinal image is confounded by movements of the eyes and head (Banks, Ehrlich, Backus, & Crowell, 1996; Crowell, Banks, Shenoy, & Andersen, 1998; Royden, Banks, & Crowell, 1992; Royden, Crowell, & Banks, 1994) and by motion of other objects in the visual field (Gibson, 1954; Royden & Hildreth, 1996; Warren & Saunders, 1995). An extensive literature has been devoted to the mechanisms by which we might compensate for eye/head rotation during translational self-motion, either from retinal or extraretinal signals (reviewed by Warren, 2003). However, this represents only one class of ambiguities in the optic flow field, and it does not address the issue of self- versus object motion.

A more general solution to the limitations of optic flow would be to make use of inertial signals that specify the actual motion of the head in space, such as from the vestibular otolith organs (Benson, Spencer, & Stott, 1986; Fernandez & Goldberg, 1976a, 1976b; Guedry, 1974).[1] The otoliths behave much like linear accelerometers,

[1] Other modalities, such as somatosensation and proprioception, may contribute to heading perception under some conditions. However, our working assumption has been that the vestibular system is the primary nonvisual modality involved in heading perception, based in part on experiments in which monkeys were greatly impaired in a vestibular heading discrimination task after labyrinthectomy (Gu, DeAngelis, & Angelaki, 2007).

and otolith afferents (and their downstream targets) exhibit directional selectivity that could in principle be used to guide heading judgments. Indeed, with a sensory organ that signals real inertial motion, one might ask why the nervous system should rely on visual information at all. Part of the answer is that even a reliable linear accelerometer has shortcomings, such as the inability to encode constant-velocity motion and the inability to distinguish between translation and tilt relative to gravity (due to Einstein's equivalence principle). The latter problem could be resolved using angular velocity signals from the semicircular canals (Angelaki, McHenry, Dickman, Newlands, & Hess, 1999; Angelaki, Shaikh, Green, & Dickman, 2004; Merfeld, Zupan, & Peterka, 1999), but the properties of the canals render this strategy ineffective during low-frequency motion or static tilts. In fact, in the absence of visual cues, linear acceleration is often misperceived as tilt (the somatogravic illusion; Previc, Varner, & Gillingham, 1992; Wolfe & Cramer, 1970). This illusion can be quite dangerous for aviators, who feel compelled to pitch the nose downward to compensate for a nonexistent upward tilt, when in fact what they experienced was linear inertial acceleration.

In summary, both the visual and vestibular systems are limited in their ability to signal self-motion unambiguously. A sensible approach for heading estimation would thus be to combine visual and vestibular information when necessary to overcome the limitations of each modality on its own. Furthermore, as discussed in a later section ("Near-Optimal Cue Integration in a Heading Discrimination Task"), this cross-modal integration in general improves perceptual performance.

## BEHAVIORAL EVIDENCE FOR VISUAL–VESTIBULAR INTERACTIONS IN SELF-MOTION PERCEPTION

The earliest studies of visual–vestibular interactions focused mainly on the phenomenon of vection. First reported by Ernst Mach in 1875, vection is the illusory perception of self-motion induced by visual motion (Berthoz, Pavard, & Young, 1975; Brandt, Dichgans, & Koenig, 1972; Dichgans & Brandt, 1978; Howard, 1982; Mach, 1875). The illusion is typically evoked after several seconds of viewing constant-velocity rotation of an optokinetic pattern (circular vection; Fig. 16.1A) or an expanding, contracting, or laminar optic flow field (linear vection; Fig. 16.1B).

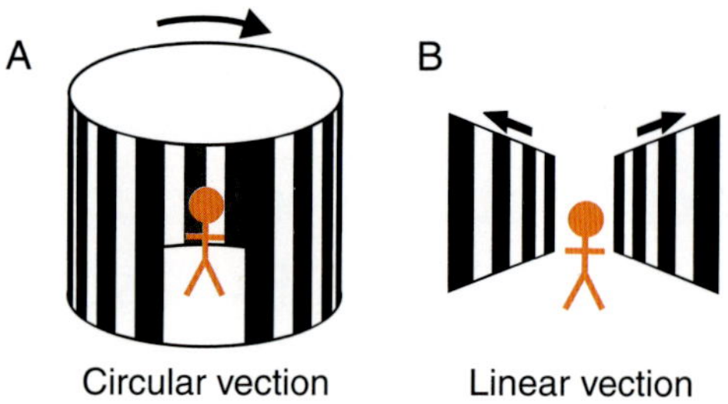


**Figure 16.1** Schematic of typical stimuli used to elicit vection. (A) Optokinetic "drum" chamber in which a pattern on the chamber walls rotates around a stationary observer, causing circular vection (illusory self-rotation). (B) Translating patterns projected in the peripheral visual field (after Berthoz et al., 1975), causing linear vection in the forward direction (observer is facing into the page).

Although not traditionally studied within an ideal-observer cue-combination framework, vection can be thought of as a case of "visual capture" in a cue-conflict condition. Under steady-state (constant-velocity) conditions, the vestibular system is telling the brain that there is no self-motion (or at least is agnostic about it), because afferent responses decay to baseline after several seconds (Büttner & Waespe, 1981; Fernandez & Goldberg, 1976a; Si, Angelaki, & Dickman, 1997). Meanwhile, the visual system signals that there is indeed self-motion, under the reasonable assumption that full-field retinal motion is usually indicative of self-motion (i.e., the probability of the entire visual scene moving across the retina while you are stationary is very small). According to any reliability-based combination rule, the brain should reconcile these conflicting signals by giving a high weight to the visual cue, which is reliable in the sense that its speed and contrast are suprathreshold.

In contrast, the vestibular cue is unreliable in the sense of being ambiguous or uninformative, and thus it should be given a low weight. The result would be visual capture and the illusion of self-motion.[2]

There has been considerable debate (e.g., Howard & Heckmann, 1989; Probst, Straube, & Bles, 1985; Tarita-Nistor, Gonzalez, Spigelman, & Steinbach, 2006; Telford & Frost, 1993; Zacharias & Young, 1981) as to which stimulus parameters are necessary and/or sufficient to produce vection (i.e., the factors that determine whether visual or vestibular cues dominate the percept of self-motion). It seems likely that some of the discrepancies in the literature could be resolved within the context of an ideal-observer or optimal-integration framework, but to our knowledge no one has attempted to apply such a model to the problem. For example, most early studies did not use a behavioral task that allowed measurement of cue reliability from task performance. Instead, subjects were often asked to make a verbal or joystick report of their perceived motion (either a simple yes-no detection task or an analog speed-estimation task), without well-isolated single-cue conditions or systematic changes in cue reliability.

A more recent study by Ohmi (1996) used a different approach, asking subjects to report their perceived direction rather than speed (or presence/absence) of self-motion. This and another study by the same group (Telford, Howard, & Ohmi, 1995) were some of the first attempts to isolate the contributions of visual and vestibular cues for heading perception (somatosensory/proprioceptive cues were also studied, but they will not be discussed here). Subjects were seated on a cart that was wheeled down a corridor using a rail and pulley system. Vertical bars were hung from the ceiling to provide an optic flow field, which subjects viewed through a pair of helmet-mounted cameras and monitors. Because actual cart motion was necessary to produce the optic flow, the visual and vestibular cues were isolated by using either subthreshold (0.005 G; "visual condition") or suprathreshold accelerations (0.05 G; "visual–vestibular condition"). Vestibular stimulation alone was achieved by turning off the room lights in the high-acceleration condition. Heading angle (in head- and body-centered coordinates) was varied across trials, and following each trial the subjects' task was to align an unseen pointer (15 cm rod mounted on a vertical shaft in front of the subject) by hand in the direction of their perceived self-motion direction. In the first part of the experiment, optic flow and inertial motion were always congruent (heading angle varied between 0°, ±5°, ±10°, ±15°, and ±20° relative to straight forward), while in the second part a conflict was introduced by changing the initial angular position of the head and body (0°, +30°, +150°, or +180°) while keeping the cameras facing forward.

The results of this experiment showed that the precision of heading estimates was greater in the visual condition (average standard deviation $\approx$ 5.8°) compared to the vestibular condition (SD $\approx$ 8.9°). Performance improved slightly in the combined visual–vestibular condition (SD $\approx$ 5.0°), but this difference was not statistically significant. Interestingly, when cues were in conflict, subjects' reports were completely determined by either the visual or the vestibular cue, depending on the magnitude of the conflict. With a conflict of 30°, heading estimates were aligned with the visual cue, whereas with a conflict of 180° their estimates followed the vestibular cue (Ohmi, 1996).

A similar conflict dependence on visual–vestibular integration has been reported for vertical linear self-motion (Wright, DiZio, & Lackner, 2005) and horizontal (yaw) rotation (Zacharias & Young, 1981). Other factors such as the amplitude (Wright et al., 2005) and frequency (Zacharias & Young, 1981; but see Probst et al. 1985) of vestibular stimulation were proposed to influence the combination weights.

[2]An alternative view is that vection stimuli are not cue-conflict conditions at all, because the response of the acceleration-sensitive vestibular afferents (i.e., a constant firing rate) is consistent with the visual cue. We would argue that constant-velocity motion in one direction for many seconds is a highly unnatural stimulus, and that the resulting vestibular input is more likely to be interpreted by the brain as zero self-motion. This distinction may be largely semantic, however.

These studies, as well as the study by Ohmi (1996), have concluded that visual–vestibular interactions entail nonlinearities, such that the cues are combined with relative weights determined by, among other things, the magnitude of the conflict between them. Alternatively, it could be that a linear combination rule still applies, and that the relative reliability (and thus the cue weights) are changing with conflict magnitude or other stimulus parameters. The question of linear versus nonlinear integration needs to be evaluated on a case-by-case basis, taking into consideration the conditions and assumptions outlined in Chapter 1 (see also Chapter 2 for a discussion of linear and nonlinear models).

Regardless of the specifics, the behavioral evidence described up to this point suggests that human self-motion perception makes use of both visual and vestibular cues. Many unanswered questions remain, and it is clear that the field could benefit from a more rigorous theoretical treatment such as one provided by ideal-observer models. Later in the chapter, we will review recent work that attempts to apply such a model to psychophysical and neurophysiological measurements in monkeys performing a heading discrimination task. First, we will summarize what was previously known about the interplay between visual and vestibular signals in the brain.

## NEUROPHYSIOLOGICAL STUDIES OF VISUAL–VESTIBULAR CONVERGENCE

In parallel with the early studies of vection and visual–vestibular interactions in perception, several labs investigated the neuronal convergence of visual and vestibular signals that could mediate these interactions. Putative visual–vestibular convergence has been reported as early as one or two synapses from the vestibular periphery, in the brainstem vestibular nuclei (Daunton & Thomsen, 1979; Henn, Young, & Finley, 1974; Robinson, 1977; Waespe & Henn, 1977) and vestibulo-cerebellum (Markert, Büttner, Straube, & Boyle, 1988; Waespe, Büttner, & Henn, 1981; Waespe & Henn, 1981). However, responses to visual (optokinetic) stimuli within these subcortical circuits are more likely related to gaze stabilization and eye movements (optokinetic nystagmus [OKN], vestibulo-ocular reflex [VOR], and/or smooth pursuit) rather than self-motion perception per se. This conclusion is supported by recent experiments (Bryan & Angelaki, 2009) showing a lack of optic-flow responsiveness in the vestibular and deep cerebellar nuclei when animals were required to fixate a head-fixed target (suppressing OKN).

At higher stages of processing, several interconnected cortical areas have traditionally been recognized as "vestibular cortex" (Fukushima, 1997), and they are believed to receive multiple sensory inputs (visual, vestibular, and somatosensory/proprioceptive in particular). These areas include the parieto-insular vestibular cortex (PIVC; Grüsser, Pause, & Schreiter, 1990a), area 2v (Schwarz & Fredrickson, 1971), and area 3a (Odkvist, Schwarz, Fredrickson, & Hassler, 1974). In addition to vestibular responsiveness, neurons in PIVC (Grüsser, Pause, & Schreiter, 1990b) and 2v (Büttner & Buettner, 1978) were reported to show an influence of visual/optokinetic stimulation, similar to subcortical structures. However, none of these areas have been conclusively demonstrated to respond to naturalistic optic flow simulating observer translation, as one would expect from an area involved in self-motion perception. In fact, preliminary evidence indicates that PIVC and 2v neurons are insensitive to brief (2-second) optic-flow stimuli with a Gaussian velocity profile (Chen, Angelaki, & DeAngelis, 2010 and unpublished observations), despite the usefulness of these stimuli for estimating heading (Gu, Angelaki, & DeAngelis, 2008; see later discussion).

These findings raise doubts about the involvement of traditional vestibular cortical areas in visual–vestibular integration for heading perception. Recent work points instead toward areas better known for their responses to optic flow, specifically the dorsal medial superior temporal area (MSTd; Duffy & Wurtz, 1991, 1995; Tanaka et al., 1986; Tanaka & Saito, 1989) and ventral intraparietal area (VIP; Bremmer,

Duhamel, Ben Hamed, & Graf, 2002; Schaafsma & Duysens, 1996). MSTd and VIP stand out as good candidates for the processing of optic flow to subserve heading perception because *(a)* they have large receptive fields and selectivity for complex optic flow patterns that simulate self-motion, *(b)* they show some compensation for shifts of the focus of expansion due to pursuit eye movements (Bradley, Maxwell, Andersen, Banks, & Shenoy, 1996; Page & Duffy, 1999; Zhang, Heuer, & Britten, 2004), and *(c)* they have been causally linked to heading perception in microstimulation studies (Britten & van Wezel, 1998; Zhang & Britten, 2003). Most important, MSTd and VIP contain neurons sensitive to physical translation in darkness (Bremmer, Klam, Duhamel, Ben Hamed, & Graf, 2002; Bremmer, Kubischik, Pekel, Lappe, & Hoffmann, 1999; Duffy, 1998). This suggests the presence of vestibular signals that may be useful for heading perception, and thus the potential for integration with visual (optic flow) signals.[3]

The discovery of vestibular translation responses in MSTd, first reported by Duffy (1998), was surprising because this area is traditionally considered part of extrastriate visual cortex. Duffy used a projector and screen mounted on a motorized sled (Fig. 16.2A) to present three main stimulus conditions: optic flow alone ("visual"), inertial motion alone ("vestibular"), and combined optic flow and inertial motion ("combined"). Movement trajectories were limited to the horizontal plane (Fig. 16.2B), and firing rate was analyzed during the constant-velocity portion of a trapezoidal velocity profile (Fig. 16.2C). The results of this study revealed a wide variety of visual–vestibular interactions, including enhancement and suppression of responses relative to single-cue conditions, as well as changes in cells' preferred direction with anticongruent stimulation.

Building upon these findings, we (Gu, Watkins, Angelaki, & DeAngelis, 2006) used a custom-built virtual reality system (Fig. 16.2D) to examine the spatial tuning of MSTd neurons in three dimensions (Fig. 16.2E), and with a Gaussian stimulus velocity profile (Fig. 16.2F) that is well suited for activating the otolith organs. Naturalistic optic flow stimuli (Fig. 16.2G) were generated by moving a virtual "camera" through a 3D cloud of triangles plotted in a virtual workspace. Similar to Duffy (1998), tuning was measured under three stimulus conditions: visual only, vestibular only, and a combined condition in which the optic flow and platform motion were synchronized to within 1 ms using a predictive algorithm. We found that about 60% of MSTd neurons showed significant tuning for both visual and vestibular heading cues, and that the preferred headings of these cells were distributed throughout 3D space (Gu et al., 2006).

Interestingly, MSTd neurons seemed to fall into one of two categories (Fig. 16.3): *congruent* cells, for which the visual and vestibular heading preferences were nearly matched (Fig. 16.3A), and *opposite* cells, which have preferred headings roughly 180° apart (Fig. 16.3B). Partly because of this subpopulation of incongruent cells, heading tuning overall was not stronger under combined visual–vestibular stimulation. This result was initially interpreted as evidence against the hypothesis that MSTd combines visual and vestibular cues to encode heading more robustly (Gu et al., 2006). However, the animals in this study were passively fixating a target, rather than performing a behavioral task that required them to report their perception of self-motion. In addition, the lack of a measurable increase in tuning strength under the combined condition may have been due to the use of high-coherence optic flow stimuli, which are more effective at driving MSTd neurons than our physical motion stimulus. Indeed, combined responses tended to be dominated by the visual cue and were difficult to distinguish from visual responses (Fig. 16.3).

In a follow-up study (Fetsch, Wang, Gu, DeAngelis, & Angelaki, 2007), we tested whether visual and vestibular heading signals in MSTd share a common reference frame. Figure 16.4 shows the 3D tuning for two example neurons in the vestibular (A) and visual (B) conditions. The tuning for each cell was measured at three

[3]The vestibular origin of these responses was later confirmed by experiments in which MSTd cells were no longer tuned during inertial motion following bilateral labyrinthectomy (Gu et al., 2007; Takahashi et al., 2007).

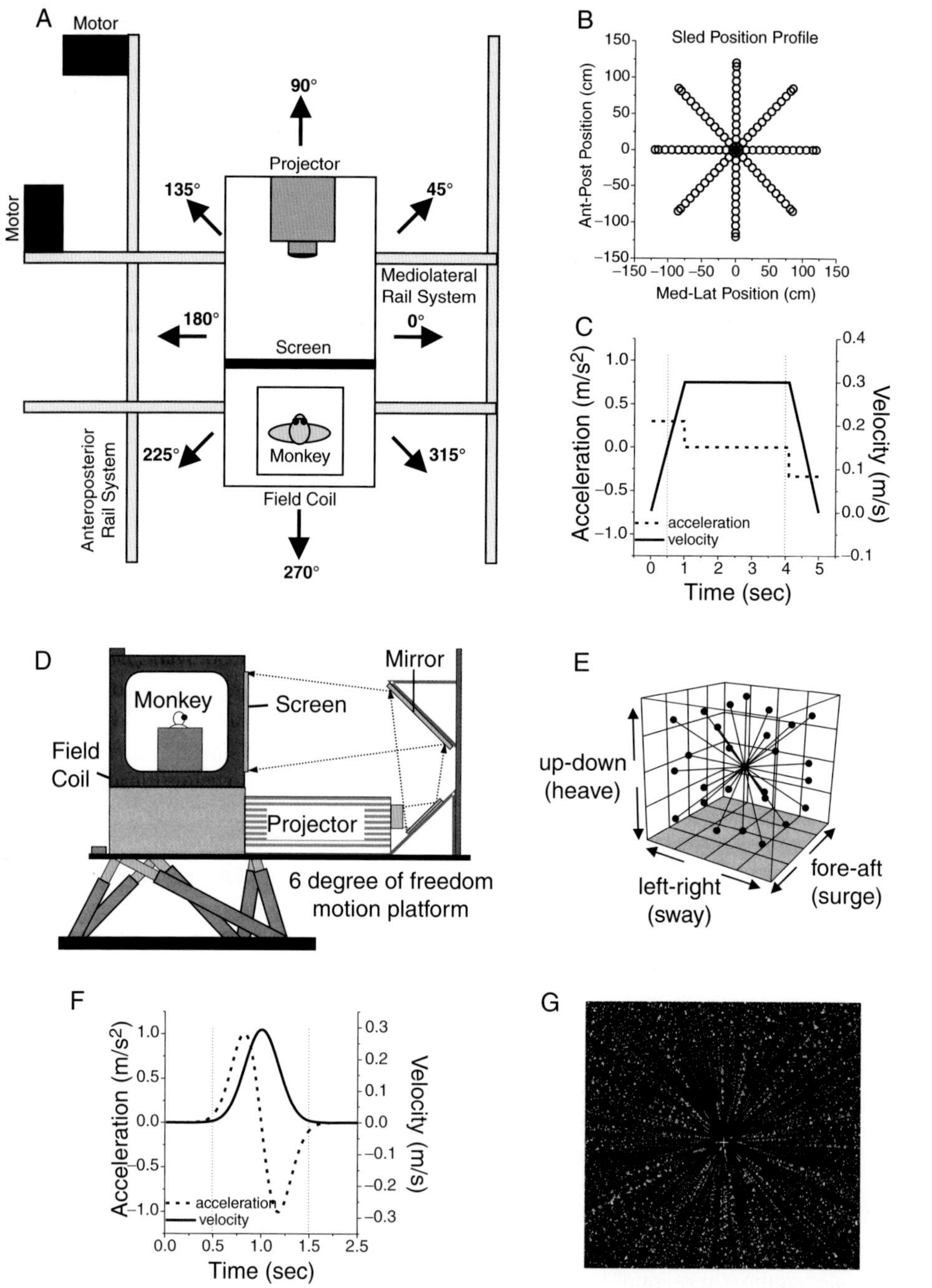


**Figure 16.2** Apparatus and stimuli used to examine visual–vestibular interactions in rhesus monkeys. (A) Motorized sled system, (B) position profile, and (C) velocity and acceleration profiles used by Duffy (reproduced with permission from Duffy, 1998). (D) Three-dimensional virtual reality system, (E) heading trajectories (reproduced with permission from Gu et al., 2006), (F) velocity and acceleration profiles used by Gu et al. (2006), and (G) example optic flow stimulus. The image in (G) was created by overlaying five sequential screen captures from the actual flow field (generated with OpenGL) during simulated forward motion.

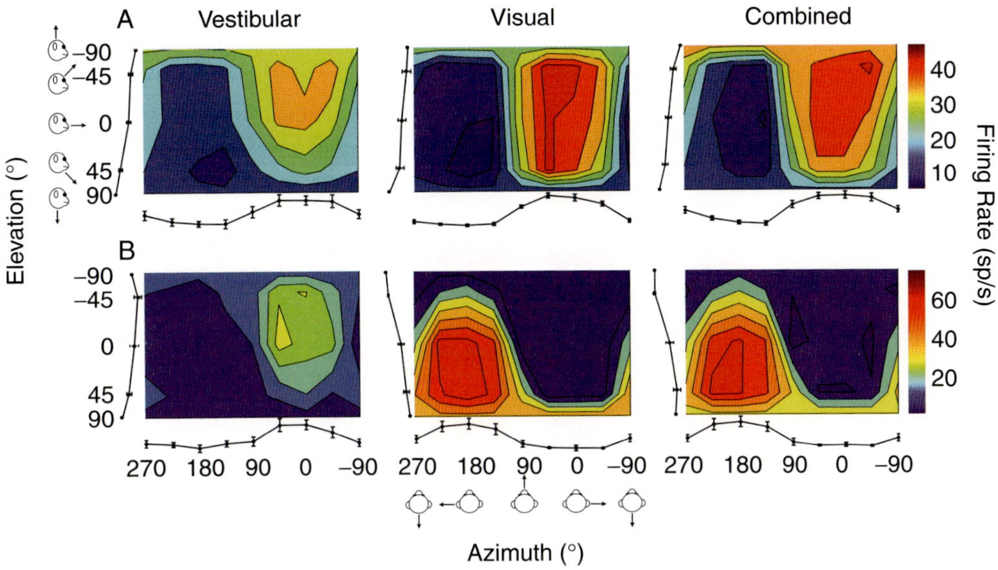


**Figure 16.3** Three-dimensional heading tuning functions of two example MSTd neurons, a "congruent" cell (A) and an "opposite" cell (B). Firing rate (grayscale) is plotted as a function of the azimuth (abscissa) and elevation (ordinate) of the heading trajectory. For each cell, tuning was measured in three stimulus conditions: vestibular (inertial motion only), visual (optic flow only), and combined visual–vestibular stimulation.

different eye positions, and these curves were compared with a cross-correlation technique to determine whether they shifted with eye position (indicating an eye-centered reference frame) or remained stable across eye positions (a head-centered frame). We found that visual tuning was primarily eye centered (Figs. 16.4B and 16.4C, red bars), whereas vestibular tuning was closer to head centered (Figs. 16.4A and 16.4C, black bars). The lack of a common reference frame for visual and vestibular signals might seem to cast doubt on the ability of this area to perform sensory integration for heading perception. However, computational modeling suggests that sensory signals need not explicitly occupy a common reference frame for integration to occur (Avillac, Denève, Olivier, Pouget, & Duhamel, 2005; Denève, Latham, & Pouget, 2001). Consistent with the predictions of this neural network model, the reference frame of MSTd neurons during combined stimulation varied as a function of the relative strength of visual and vestibular tuning (visual–vestibular ratio, or VVR, defined as the ratio of the maximum visual response to the maximum vestibular response, after subtracting spontaneous firing rate from each). Specifically, combined reference frames varied from intermediate to eye centered as VVR increased (Fig. 16.4D, blue diamonds).

## NEAR-OPTIMAL CUE INTEGRATION IN A HEADING DISCRIMINATION TASK

### Behavioral Results

In the monkey studies described earlier (Fetsch et al., 2007; Gu et al., 2006), subjects were not required to perform any task with the stimuli but merely to fixate a stationary fixation point. To probe the neural basis of cue integration for heading perception, neural activity should be measured and/or manipulated in the context of a behavioral task that requires the subject to report his or her perception of self-motion. Thus, in a subsequent study (Gu et al., 2008), monkeys were trained to indicate their perceived heading

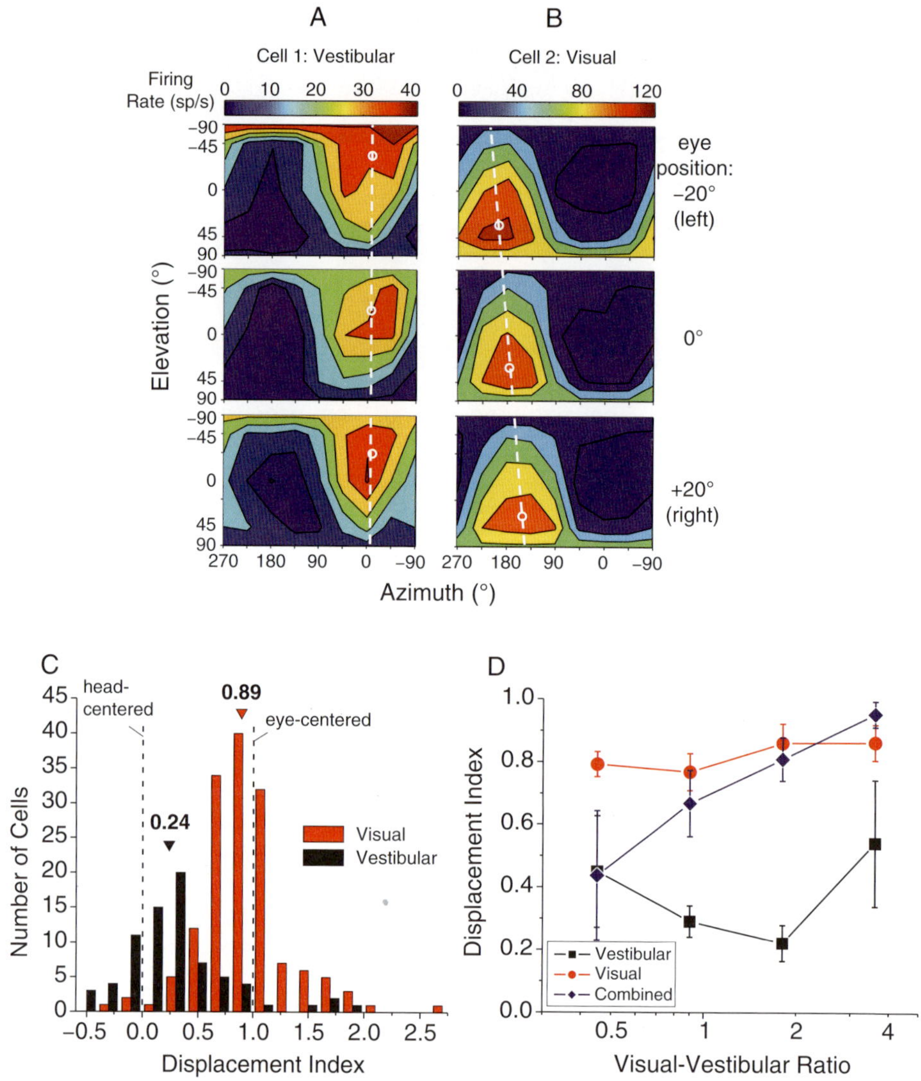


**Figure 16.4** Reference frames of visual and vestibular heading signals in MSTd. Tuning functions are plotted (in head-centered coordinates) for two example cells in the vestibular (A) and visual (B) conditions, measured separately at three static eye positions along the horizontal meridian: –20° (top), 0° (middle), and +20° (bottom). The dashed white line connects the preferred heading in each case, to illustrate the horizontal shift (or lack thereof) of the tuning function across eye positions. (C) Histogram of displacement index (DI) values for MSTd neurons tested in the vestibular (black bars) and visual (red bars) conditions. DI is defined as the angular shift of the tuning function normalized by the change in eye position; thus, a value of 0 indicates a head- (or body-) centered reference frame and 1 indicates an eye-centered frame. (D) Summary of the relationship between DI and the relative strength of visual and vestibular single-cue tuning (visual–vestibular ratio, or VVR). DI values from all neurons with significant tuning in each condition (vestibular N = 66, visual N = 103, combined N = 86) were grouped by VVR in four log-spaced bins, and then averaged to produce each data point (± SEM). (Reproduced with permission from Fetsch et al., 2007.)

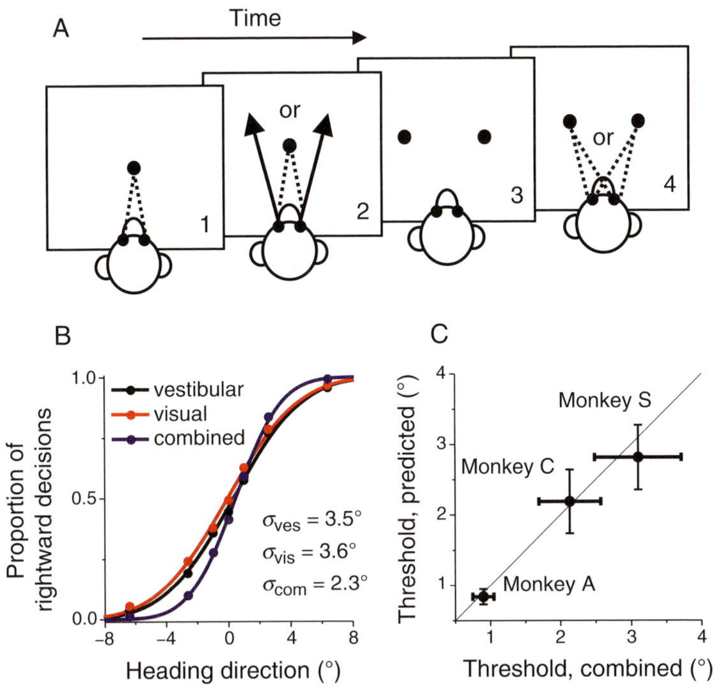


**Figure 16.5** Heading discrimination task. (A) After fixating a visual target (panel 1), the monkey experiences forward motion (real and/or simulated with optic flow) with a small leftward or rightward component (panel 2, solid arrows). After the fixation point is extinguished (panel 3), he reports his perceived heading ("left" or "right") by making a saccadic eye movement to one of two choice targets (panel 4). (B) Average psychometric functions for one animal under unimodal (vestibular: black curve; visual: red curve) and bimodal (blue curve) conditions. Psychophysical threshold was defined as the standard deviation ($\sigma$) of the fitted cumulative Gaussian. (Reproduced with permission from Gu et al., 2008.) (C) Comparison between observed thresholds in the combined condition and predicted thresholds assuming statistically optimal cue integration (Eq. 16.1). Data are shown for three animals.

relative to straight ahead in a two-alternative forced-choice task (Fig. 16.5A). This task enabled us to ask some fundamental questions that had remained unaddressed: *(1)* Can monkeys integrate visual and vestibular cues to improve heading discrimination performance? *(2)* Is this improvement statistically optimal in a Bayesian or maximum-likelihood sense? and *(3)* Can the activity of MSTd neurons account for the behavioral improvement?

This study used the same motion system as in Figure 16.2D and the same three stimulus conditions (visual, vestibular, combined), except that the heading angles during the task were limited to a small range around straight forward. Psychometric functions were plotted as the proportion of rightward choices as a function of heading angle (negative = leftward, positive = rightward) and fit with a cumulative Gaussian (Wichmann & Hill, 2001). The standard deviation ($\sigma$) of the fitted function was taken as the psychophysical threshold, corresponding to the heading at which the subject was approximately 84% correct.

The prediction from standard optimal-integration models (e.g., Alais & Burr, 2004; Ernst & Banks, 2002; Knill & Saunders, 2003; also see Chapter 1) was that the threshold in the combined condition would be lower than the best single-cue threshold, as given by

$$\sigma^2_{comb} = \frac{\sigma^2_{vis}\sigma^2_{ves}}{\sigma^2_{vis} + \sigma^2_{ves}}. \tag{16.1}$$

To maximize the predicted improvement, the reliability of the cues (as measured by thresholds in the single-cue conditions) was matched by adjusting the motion coherence of the display.[4] Average psychometric functions for one animal are plotted in Figure 16.5B. The vestibular (black symbols and curve) and visual (red) functions are nearly overlapping, with thresholds of 3.5° and 3.6°, respectively. In the combined condition (blue), the monkey's heading threshold was substantially smaller (2.3°), as evidenced by the steeper slope of the psychometric function. For all three animals tested, the combined thresholds were significantly lower than the best single-cue threshold (Gu et al., 2008), and very similar to the optimal prediction from Eq. 16.1 (unity line, Fig. 16.5C).

### Neurophysiological Results

Having established near-optimal cue integration behavior in macaques (Figs. 16.5B and 16.5C), we recorded from single neurons in area MSTd while monkeys performed the heading discrimination task (Gu et al., 2008). Figures 16.6A and 16.6B show the tuning curves from two example neurons tested with heading directions evenly spaced in the horizontal plane. The neuron in Figure 16.6A preferred leftward (negative) headings for both stimuli and was classified as a congruent cell. In contrast, the neuron in Figure 16.6B preferred leftward headings under the visual condition (red line) and rightward headings under the vestibular condition (black line), and it was classified as an opposite cell.

Figures 16.6C and 16.6D show the tuning of the same example neurons shown in A and B, respectively, over the much narrower range of headings sampled during discrimination. For the congruent cell (Fig. 16.6C), heading tuning became steeper in the combined condition, whereas for the opposite cell (Fig. 16.6D) it became flatter. To allow direct comparisons between neuronal and behavioral sensitivity, we used signal detection theory (ROC analysis; Bradley, Skottun, Ohzawa, Sclar, & Freeman, 1987; Britten, Shadlen, Newsome, & Movshon, 1992; Green & Swets, 1966) to quantify the ability of an ideal observer to discriminate heading based on the activity of a single neuron (Figs. 16.6E and 16.6F, symbols). As with the psychometric data, we fitted these "neurometric" data with cumulative Gaussian functions (Figs. 16.6E and 16.6F, smooth curves) and defined the neuronal threshold as the standard deviation of the Gaussian. For the congruent neuron (Fig. 16.6E), the neuronal threshold was smallest in the combined condition (blue symbols and lines), indicating that the neuron could discriminate smaller variations in heading when both cues were provided. In contrast, for the opposite neuron (Fig. 16.6F), the reverse was true: The neuron became less sensitive in the presence of both cues (blue symbols and lines).

The effect of visual–vestibular congruency on neuronal sensitivity in the combined condition held across the population of neurons. To summarize this effect, we defined a congruency index (CI) as the product $R_{\text{visual}} \times R_{\text{vestibular}}$, where each $R$ is the correlation coefficient between firing rate and heading angle for the respective single-cue tuning functions. This index ranges from +1 (when visual and vestibular tuning functions have a consistent slope, e.g. Fig. 16.6C) to −1 (when they have opposite slopes; Fig. 16.6D). Neurons with flat tuning around 0° for either cue will have a CI near zero. We then computed, for each neuron, the ratio of the neuronal threshold in the combined condition to the threshold expected if neurons combine cues optimally according to Eq. 16.1. A significant correlation was seen between the ratio of combined to predicted thresholds and CI (Fig. 16.7A), such that neurons with large positive CIs (congruent cells, cyan symbols) had thresholds close to the optimal prediction (ratios near unity). Thus, neuronal thresholds for congruent MSTd cells followed a pattern similar to the monkeys' behavior. In contrast, combined thresholds for opposite cells (Fig. 16.7A, magenta symbols) were generally much higher than predicted from optimal cue integration, indicating that these neurons

[4]That this matching is important is illustrated by the studies of Telford et al. (1995) and Ohmi (1996), in which visual and vestibular precision were too discrepant to allow the detection of such a small predicted improvement from cue integration (with any reasonable sample size).

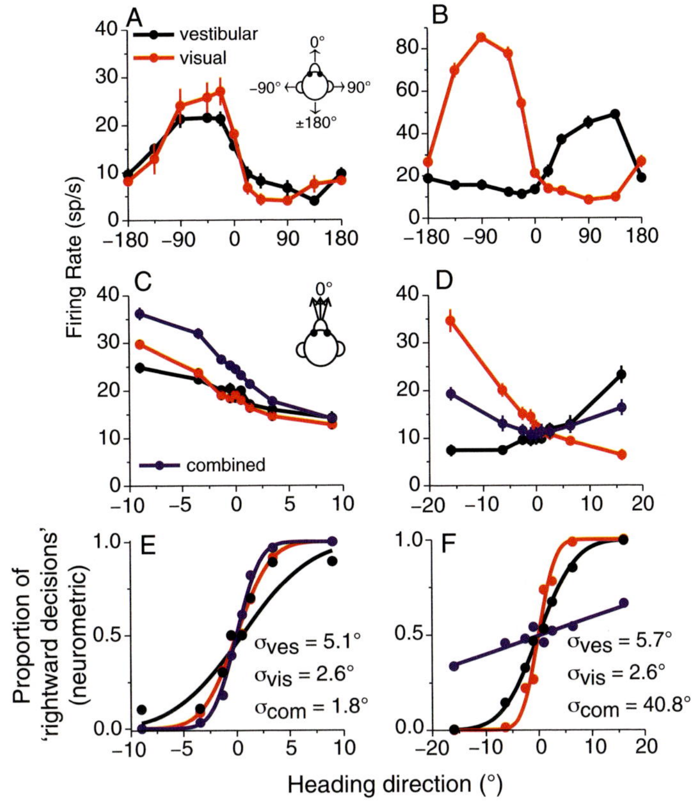


**Figure 16.6** Heading sensitivity in area MSTd. (A and B) Heading tuning curves of two example neurons with congruent (A) and opposite (B) visual–vestibular heading preferences. Note the different scale of the ordinate in (B). (C and D) Responses of the same neurons to the narrow range of heading stimuli presented while the monkey performed the discrimination task. (E and F) Neurometric functions computed by ROC analysis from the firing rate data plotted in (C) and (D). Smooth curves show best-fitting cumulative Gaussian functions. (Reproduced with permission from Gu et al., 2008.)

became less sensitive during cue combination. Lastly, Figures 16.7B and 16.7C summarize the neuronal thresholds across stimulus conditions, confirming that congruent cells (7B) became more sensitive (lower thresholds) in the combined condition versus the single-cue conditions, whereas opposite cells (7C) did not.

### Correlations with Behavioral Choice

If monkeys rely on area MSTd for heading discrimination, the results of Figure 16.7 suggest that they selectively monitor the activity of congruent cells and not opposite cells. To test this hypothesis, we used the data from the recording experiments (Gu, DeAngelis, & Angelaki, 2007; Gu et al., 2008) to compute choice probabilities, or CPs (Britten, Newsome, Shadlen, Celebrini, & Movshon, 1996). CPs are computed by ROC analysis similar to neuronal thresholds, except the ideal observer is asked to determine the monkey's *choice* (rather than the heading) from the firing rate of the neuron. Neurons are first assigned a preferred heading direction (right or left) based on the slope of the tuning function around 0° for a given stimulus condition (separate CPs are computed for visual, vestibular, and combined trials). Responses are then sorted based on whether the monkey chose the preferred or nonpreferred (null) heading on a given trial. An ROC curve is generated from the comparison of the preferred and null response distributions, and the area under the

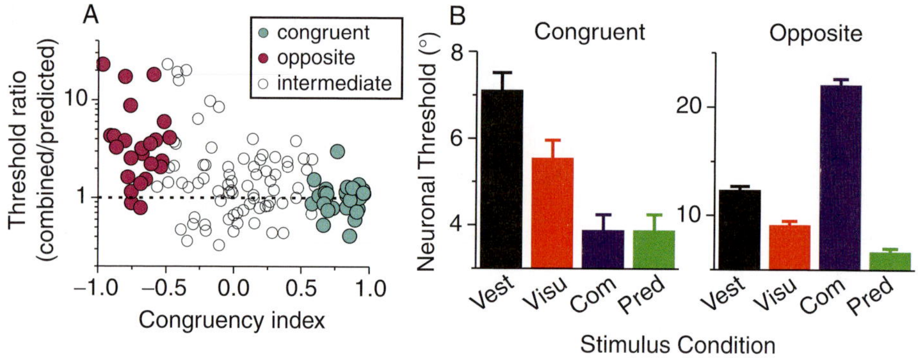


**Figure 16.7** (A) Neuronal sensitivity under cue combination as a function of visual–vestibular congruency. The ordinate in this scatter plot represents the ratio of the threshold measured in the combined condition to the prediction from optimal cue integration. The abscissa represents the congruency index (CI) of heading tuning for visual and vestibular responses. Neurons are color coded by congruency classification: cyan for "congruent" cells (CI significantly greater than zero), magenta for "opposite" cells (CI significantly less than zero), and unfilled circles for "intermediate" cells (CI was not significantly different from zero). The dashed horizontal line indicates where the threshold in the combined condition is equal to the prediction. (B and C) Average neuronal thresholds (geometric mean ± geometric SEM) in the vestibular (black), visual (red), and combined (blue) conditions. The optimal prediction from Eq. 16.1 is shown by the green bars. Cells were separated by congruency classification (B, congruent cells; C, opposite cells; note the different vertical scale between the two panels). The average combined threshold was less than the single-cue thresholds ($p < 0.001$) and very similar to the prediction ($p = 0.9$) for congruent cells, but not for opposite cells. (Reproduced with permission from Gu et al., 2008.)

ROC curve is the CP (the probability that an ideal observer would correctly identify the choice that was made based on the neuronal firing rates). Thus, CPs quantify the relationship between trial-to-trial fluctuations in neural firing rates and the monkeys' perceptual decisions. A CP significantly greater than 0.5 indicates that the monkey tended to choose the neuron's preferred heading (leftward or rightward) when the neuron fires more strongly. Such a result is thought to reflect a functional link between the neuron and perception (Britten et al., 1996; Krug, 2004; Parker & Newsome, 1998).

Notably, although MSTd is classically considered visual cortex, CPs in the vestibular condition were significantly larger than 0.5 (mean = 0.55) irrespective of congruency (Fig. 16.8A; Gu et al., 2007). In contrast, perhaps surprisingly, CPs in the visual and combined conditions were smaller on average (0.52 in both cases) and were strongly dependent on congruency (Fig. 16.8B and 16.8C). Specifically, congruent cells tended to have CPs greater than 0.5 and opposite cells tended to have CPs less than or near 0.5. Neurons with a significant CP < 0.5 paradoxically increase their firing rates when the monkey chooses their nonpreferred direction. For opposite cells, this paradoxical result leads to an interesting interpretation. Recall that CPs are simply ROC values based on the comparison of two firing rate distributions, and whether a given CP is greater or less than 0.5 depends on the assignment of preferred and null directions to the two distributions. Thus, if the *visual* CP for an opposite cell is less than 0.5, this same value would become greater than 0.5 if expressed relative to the cell's *vestibular* preference. One interpretation of this finding is that visual responses may be decoded relative to the vestibular preference of the neurons. In other words, when the cell happens to fire more strongly, the monkey tends to choose the preferred vestibular heading of the cell, which for opposite cells is the nonpreferred visual heading (see also the Discussion of Gu et al., 2008). Regardless of the interpretation of CPs <0.5,

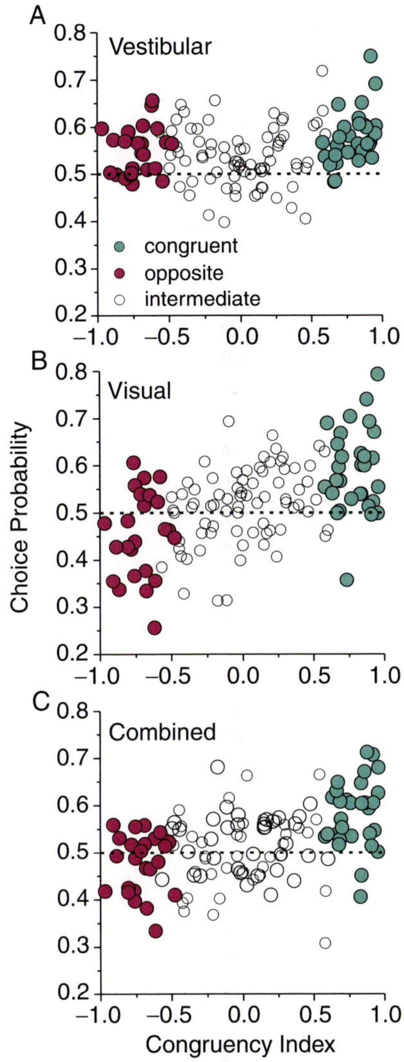


**Figure 16.8** Correlations between MSTd responses and perceptual decisions. Choice probability (CP) data are plotted as a function of congruency index for each MSTd neuron tested in the vestibular (A), visual (B), and combined (C) conditions. Color indicates congruency classification as in Figure 16.7. (Reproduced with permission from Gu et al., 2008.)

it is clear that CPs in the combined condition were greater for congruent versus opposite cells (Fig. 16.8C, compare cyan vs. magenta symbols). This is consistent with the idea that the animals may have selectively monitored this subpopulation of congruent cells to achieve near-optimal cue integration.[5]

In summary, by simultaneously monitoring neural activity and behavior, it has been possible to study neural mechanisms of multisensory processing under conditions in which cue integration is known to take place perceptually. In addition to demonstrating near-optimal cue integration by monkeys, a population of neurons has been identified in area MSTd that could account for the improvement in psychophysical performance under cue combination. These findings implicate area MSTd in sensory integration for heading perception and establish a model system for studying the detailed mechanisms by which neurons combine different sensory signals. However, because the reliability of the visual and vestibular cues was not varied in these experiments, they could not address whether monkeys and MSTd neurons dynamically reweight these cues, as predicted by optimal cue-integration schemes. The next set of experiments was designed to test this very important prediction of optimal cue integration.

## EFFECTS OF CUE RELIABILITY

As a first step to investigate how cue reliability modulates visual–vestibular cue integration, an experiment was performed in which the reliability (motion coherence) of the visual cue was varied during neural recordings in passively fixating animals (Morgan, DeAngelis, & Angelaki, 2008). Without assuming any particular decoding scheme to translate MSTd responses into psychophysical estimates, this study asked a more basic physiological question: What is the mathematical rule by which MSTd neurons combine their visual and vestibular inputs? Specifically, we asked whether bimodal responses in MSTd are well fit by weighted linear sums of unimodal responses, or whether a nonlinear

[5] The function of opposite cells remains a mystery and the topic of ongoing research. One hypothesis is that the difference in activity between populations of congruent and opposite cells could be used to help distinguish object motion from self-motion.

combination rule is required. We also asked whether the weights that neurons apply to these cues change with the relative reliability of the two cues.[6]

We measured unimodal tuning curves using 8 evenly spaced directions (45° apart) in the horizontal plane, as well as bimodal responses to the 64 possible combinations of these 8 vestibular and visual headings, including 8 congruent and 56 incongruent (cue-conflict) presentations. Unimodal tuning curves are shown for an example congruent cell in Figure 16.9 along the left ordinate (visual) and abscissa (vestibular). For the bimodal stimuli, where each response is associated with both a vestibular heading and a visual heading, responses have been illustrated as two-dimensional contour maps with vestibular heading along the abscissa and visual heading along the ordinate (Fig. 16.9).

At 100% coherence, bimodal responses often more strongly reflected the visual unimodal tuning preference, as indicated by the horizontal band of high firing rates (Fig. 16.9A). Lowering the coherence to 50% and 25% (Fig. 16.9B and 16.9C) reduced the peak-to-trough modulation of the visual heading tuning curve, while at the same time revealed a transition from visual dominance to vestibular dominance in the bimodal responses. Specifically, the presence of a clear symmetric peak at 50% coherence suggests well-matched visual and vestibular contributions to the bimodal response (Fig. 16.9B). As visual coherence was further reduced to 25%, vestibular dominance is observed, with the bimodal response taking the form of a vertical band aligned with the vestibular heading preference (Fig. 16.9C).

Bimodal responses were adequately fit by a weighted linear sum of responses from the

[6]Note the distinction between the weights discussed here (in the context of a single neuron computing a weighted sum of its inputs) and the behavioral "weights" often used to describe psychophysical measurements during cue-conflict experiments (e.g., Alais & Burr, 2004; Ernst & Banks, 2002; Landy, Maloney, Johnston, & Young, 1995; Young, Landy, & Maloney, 1993). Although related, they describe very different quantities, and the relationship between them depends on the specific population readout mechanisms involved.

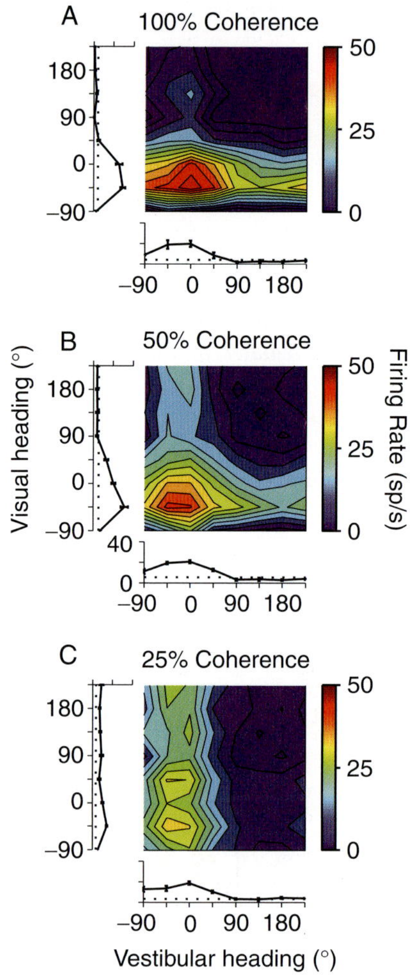


**Figure 16.9** Comparison of unimodal and bimodal tuning for a congruent MSTd cell, tested at three motion coherences. Color maps show mean firing rates as a function of vestibular and visual headings in the bimodal condition (including all 64 possible combinations of 8 visual headings and 8 vestibular headings at 45° intervals). Tuning curves along the left and bottom margins show mean (± SEM) firing rates versus heading for the unimodal visual and vestibular conditions, respectively. (A) Bimodal responses at 100% coherence are visually dominated. (B) Bimodal responses at 50% coherence show a balanced contribution of visual and vestibular cues. (C) At 25% coherence, bimodal responses appear to be dominated by the vestibular input. (Reproduced with permission from Morgan et al., 2008.)

vestibular and visual conditions, with visual and vestibular weights describing the strength of the contributions of each unimodal input to the bimodal response (Morgan et al., 2008). Given that the relative influence of the two cues on the bimodal response changes with motion coherence (Fig. 16.9), an important question then arises: Do the weights remain fixed as coherence changes, such that the decreased visual influence on the bimodal tuning is simply due to weaker visual signals at lower coherences? Or do the weights themselves change with the relative reliability of the two cues? The results from the fits to the linear model support the latter possibility: As compared to 100% coherence, vestibular weights at 50% coherence shifted toward larger values (Fig. 16.10A), and visual weights shifted toward smaller values (Fig. 16.10B). For cells recorded at all three coherence levels, a monotonic relationship is observed in which visual weights increase and vestibular weights decrease with increasing motion coherence (Fig. 16.10C and 16.10D). This result suggests that the multisensory combination rule used by MSTd neurons is not fixed—these cells appear to modify their combination rule when the quality of the sensory information changes.

One limitation of the study by Morgan et al. (2008) is that we presented different motion coherences in separate blocks of trials; thus, we cannot examine the temporal dynamics of cue reweighting. It is also important to measure reweighting in an animal performing

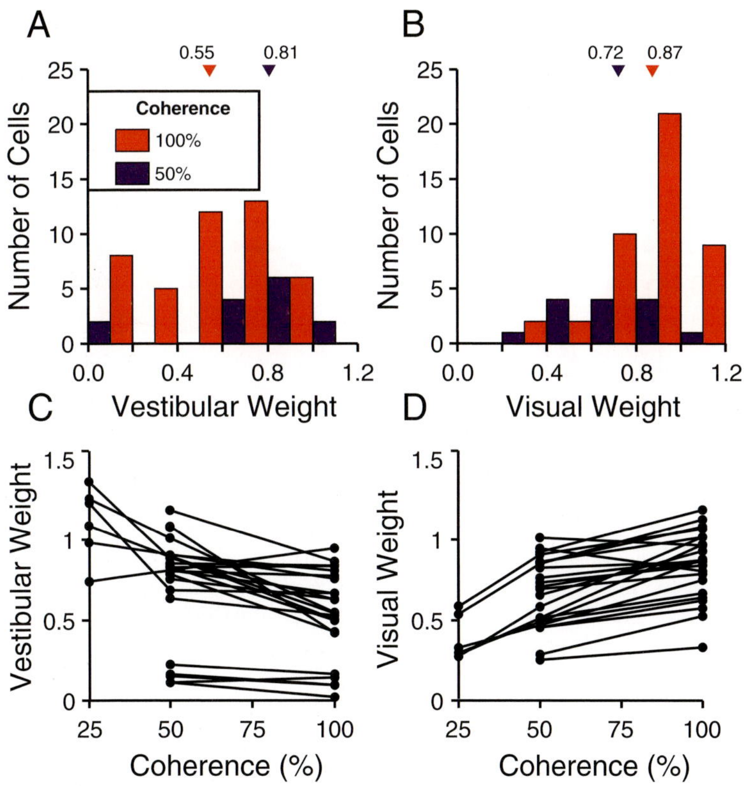


**Figure 16.10** Dependence of vestibular and visual weights on visual motion coherence. Vestibular and visual weights for each MSTd neuron were derived from linear fits to bimodal responses like those in Figure 16.9. (A and B) Histograms of vestibular and visual weights computed from data at 100% (red) and 50% (blue) coherence. Triangles are plotted at the medians. (C and D) Vestibular and visual weights are plotted as a function of motion coherence. (Reproduced with permission from Morgan et al., 2008.)

the discrimination task rather than passively fixating. For these reasons, we tested for behavioral evidence of dynamic (trial-by-trial) cue reweighting in both humans and monkeys (Fetsch, Turner, DeAngelis, & Angelaki, 2009). This study applied a standard "perturbation" analysis (e.g., Alais & Burr, 2004; Ernst & Banks, 2002; Landy, Maloney, Johnston, & Young, 1995; Young, Landy, & Maloney, 1993) to our heading-discrimination task, in which a small conflict angle (Δ) was introduced between the heading specified by visual and vestibular cues (Fig. 16.11A). The relative reliability of the cues was varied across trials by randomly interleaving multiple levels of motion coherence (changing visual reliability while keeping vestibular reliability constant).

Psychometric functions for a single monkey subject are plotted for the single-cue conditions in Fig. 16.11B. Note that the two coherence levels shown here were chosen such that the visual thresholds would be smaller (high coherence) or larger (low coherence) than the vestibular threshold. In this case, the vestibular threshold was 2.8°, and the visual thresholds were 7.3° and 1.0° for 12% and 96% coherence, respectively. From these threshold values, predicted (maximum-likelihood, ML)

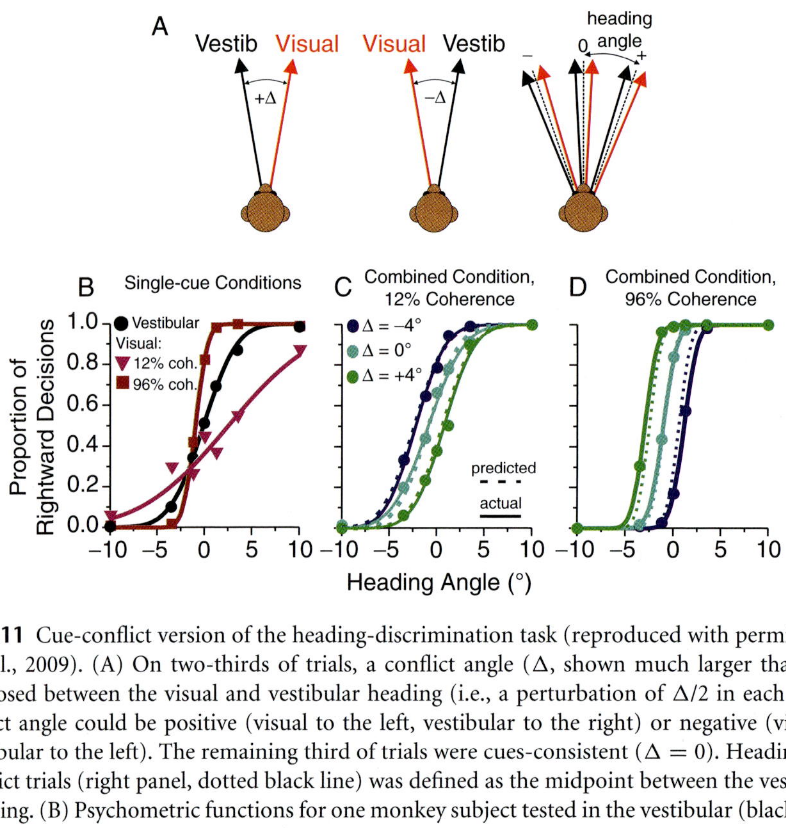


**Figure 16.11** Cue-conflict version of the heading-discrimination task (reproduced with permission from Fetsch et al., 2009). (A) On two-thirds of trials, a conflict angle (Δ, shown much larger than to scale) was interposed between the visual and vestibular heading (i.e., a perturbation of Δ/2 in each direction). The conflict angle could be positive (visual to the left, vestibular to the right) or negative (visual to the right, vestibular to the left). The remaining third of trials were cues-consistent ($\Delta = 0$). Heading angle on these conflict trials (right panel, dotted black line) was defined as the midpoint between the vestibular and visual heading. (B) Psychometric functions for one monkey subject tested in the vestibular (black curve and circles) and visual condition at two coherence levels (12%: light magenta curve and triangles; 96%: dark red curve and squares). (C) Combined condition data at 12% coherence, plotted separately for the three conflict angles: $\Delta = -4°$, 0°, +4° (blue, cyan, and green curves, respectively). The leftward shift of the blue curve and rightward shift of the green curve indicate vestibular dominance (high vestibular weight, low visual weight), as predicted by the relative single-cue thresholds (Eq. 16.2; optimal predictions shown by the dashed curves). (D) Same as (C), but for 96% coherence. Here the PSEs shift in the opposite direction, indicating visual dominance (as predicted).

weights[7] are computed as

$$w_{vis}(ML) = \frac{1/\sigma_{vis}^2}{1/\sigma_{vis}^2 + 1/\sigma_{ves}^2}$$

$$w_{ves}(ML) = \frac{1/\sigma_{ves}^2}{1/\sigma_{vis}^2 + 1/\sigma_{ves}^2}. \qquad (16.2)$$

Because the high- and low-coherence visual thresholds straddled the vestibular threshold (Fig. 16.11B), the behavior in the combined condition was expected to show visual dominance in one case and vestibular dominance in the other. Specifically, the predicted vestibular weights were 0.85 (12% coherence) and 0.12 (96% coherence), equivalent to visual weights of 0.15 and 0.88, respectively.

We compared the predicted weights to "actual" weights derived from the combined-condition data (Figs. 16.11C and 16.11D) as follows. Separate psychometric functions are plotted for the three conflict conditions: $+\Delta$ (defined as visual to the right, vestibular to the left), $-\Delta$ (vice versa), and $\Delta = 0$ (no conflict). For a given coherence level, the shifts of the point of subjective equality (PSE, defined as the mean of the fitted cumulative Gaussian) were normalized by the magnitude of the perturbation ($|\Delta|/2$) to compute the actual weights that subjects assigned to each cue (Alais & Burr, 2004; Ernst & Banks, 2002; Landy et al., 1995). For example, when $\Delta$ is positive (left panel in Fig. 16.11A, green curves in Figs. 16.11C and 16.11D), a rightward shift of the PSE corresponds to high vestibular weight, while a leftward shift corresponds to a low vestibular weight (and vice versa for $-\Delta$, blue curves). The actual vestibular weights for this subject were 0.87 (12% coherence) and 0.0 (96% coherence), a reasonably close match with the prediction of 0.85 and 0.12.

[7]Again, be wary of the distinction between these behavioral weights and the neuronal weights depicted in Figure 16.10. More work is needed to fully understand the link between the two quantities, although it is notable that optimal behavioral reweighting does not necessarily require changes in neuronal weights (Ma, Beck, Latham, & Pouget, 2006), even though this is what we observed in MSTd (Fig. 16.10; Morgan et al., 2008).

Figure 16.12 summarizes the predicted and actual weights for five human (A) and five monkey (B) subjects. While some subjects' weights were very close to the optimal predictions, on average both humans and monkeys appear to overweight the vestibular cue (or underweight the visual cue). This modest but systematic deviation from strict optimality remains to be explained by future studies. Although the details are beyond the scope of this chapter, one possible explanation involves causal inference (Körding et al., 2007; see also Chapter 2). Causal-inference models predict that apparent biases can arise when subjects infer separate causes for the two cues, an inference that should occur more often as conflict magnitude increases (Körding et al., 2007). However, we did not observe systematic differences in the size of the deviation from optimality (i.e., the degree of vestibular "bias") when conflict magnitude ($|\Delta|$) was varied between 2.5° and 5° in humans (Fig. 16.12A, compare orange and purple traces) and from 2° to 6° in monkeys (data not shown), even though this range extended well above the smallest single-cue thresholds. It might be the case that larger conflict angles are necessary to probe causal aspects of multisensory integration in our task.

It also remains to be seen whether and how neurons dynamically reweight sensory signals according to their reliability. One way to test this would be to record from an area such as MSTd while the monkey performed the task and to carry out a similar reweighting analysis as in Figure 16.11 using neurometric functions (computed via ROC analysis) instead of psychometric functions. If such an analysis revealed that MSTd neurons show near-optimal cue reweighting with changes in reliability, it would further support a role for these cells in visual–vestibular integration for heading perception and could contribute to our understanding of the neural mechanisms of statistical inference in multisensory processing.

## CONCLUSION

In this chapter we have attempted to summarize decades of work on visual–vestibular cue

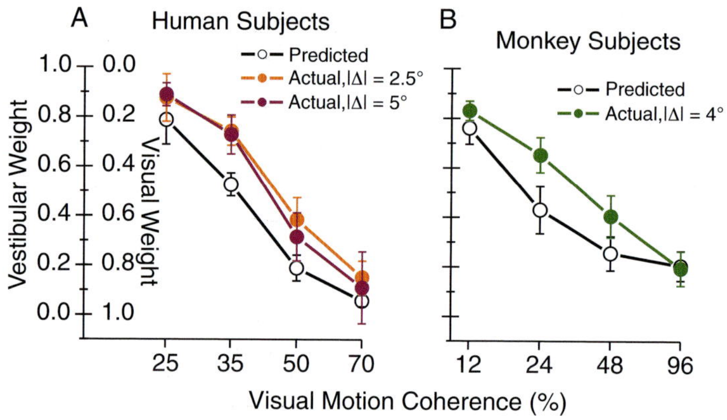


**Figure 16.12** Summary of predicted and actual cue weights (reproduced with permission from Fetsch et al., 2009). Average vestibular weight (1 – visual weight) is plotted as a function of visual motion coherence for five human subjects (A) and five monkey subjects (B). Error bars represent ±SEM across subjects. Predicted weights (open symbols) were computed from Eq. 16.2 using single-cue thresholds, and actual weights (filled symbols) were computed from the shift of the PSE relative to the magnitude of cue conflict (see Figs. 16.11B–16.11D and text). For human subjects, actual weights are shown for two different conflict magnitudes (|Δ|): 2.5° (orange) and 5° (purple).

integration for self-motion perception and its possible neuronal substrates. This field has evolved from a focus on illusions and eye movements to a number of theoretically grounded psychophysical/neurophysiological studies from several laboratories. The application of ideal-observer models and Bayesian decision theory to the problem of visual–vestibular integration should continue to shed new light on how the brain effortlessly solves the inherently multisensory problems of spatial orientation and navigation through complex environments.

More generally, future studies using experimental approaches like the ones presented here will contribute to our understanding of how sensory uncertainty is represented by neural populations, and how probabilistic quantities are combined and read out by downstream decision-making circuits. A major unanswered question is whether the activity of multisensory cortical areas such as MSTd reflects the full conditional probability distributions over the stimuli, which are required for Bayesian computations (Knill & Pouget, 2004). Recent theoretical efforts (Beck et al., 2008; Jazayeri & Movshon, 2006; Ma, Beck, Latham, & Pouget, 2006; see also Chapter 21) have described elegant and biologically plausible solutions to the problem of probabilistic coding and decision making. It is now up to the experimentalists to design studies that are rigorous and incisive enough to put their predictions to the test.

## REFERENCES


Alais, D., & Burr, D. (2004). The ventriloquist effect results from near-optimal bimodal integration. *Current Biology, 14,* 257–262.

Angelaki, D. E., McHenry, M. Q., Dickman, J. D., Newlands, S. D., & Hess, B. J. (1999). Computation of inertial motion: Neural strategies to resolve ambiguous otolith information. *Journal of Neuroscience, 19,* 316–327.

Angelaki, D. E., Shaikh, A. G., Green, A. M., & Dickman, J. D. (2004). Neurons compute internal models of the physical laws of motion. *Nature, 430,* 560–564.

Avillac, M., Denève, S., Olivier, E., Pouget, A., & Duhamel, J. R. (2005). Reference frames for representing visual and tactile locations in parietal cortex. *Nature Neuroscience, 8,* 941–949.

Banks, M. S., Ehrlich, S. M., Backus, B. T., & Crowell, J. A. (1996). Estimating heading during real and simulated eye movements. *Vision Research, 36,* 431–443.

Beck, J. M., Ma, W. J., Kiani, R., Hanks, T., Churchland, A. K., Roitman, J., . . . Pouget, A. (2008). Probabilistic population codes for Bayesian decision making. *Neuron, 60,* 1142–1152.

Benson, A. J., Spencer, M. B., & Stott, J. R. (1986). Thresholds for the detection of the direction of whole-body, linear movement in the horizontal plane. *Aviation, Space, and Environmental Medicine, 57,* 1088–1096.

Berthoz, A., Pavard, B., & Young, L. R. (1975). Perception of linear horizontal self-motion induced by peripheral vision (linearvection) basic characteristics and visual-vestibular interactions. *Experimental Brain Research, 23,* 471–489.

Bradley, A., Skottun, B. C., Ohzawa, I., Sclar, G., & Freeman, R. D. (1987). Visual orientation and spatial frequency discrimination: a comparison of single neurons and behavior. *Journal of Neurophysiology, 57,* 755–772.

Bradley, D. C., Maxwell, M., Andersen, R. A., Banks, M. S., & Shenoy, K. V. (1996). Mechanisms of heading perception in primate visual cortex. *Science, 273,* 1544–1547.

Brandt, T., Dichgans, J., & Koenig, E. (1972). Perception of self-rotation (circular vection) induced by optokinetic stimuli. *Pflügers Archiv, 332*(Suppl. 332), R398.

Bremmer, F., Duhamel, J. R., Ben Hamed, S., & Graf, W. (2002). Heading encoding in the macaque ventral intraparietal area (VIP). *European Journal of Neuroscience, 16,* 1554–1568.

Bremmer, F., Klam, F., Duhamel, J. R., Ben Hamed, S., & Graf, W. (2002). Visual-vestibular interactive responses in the macaque ventral intraparietal area (VIP). *European Journal of Neuroscience, 16,* 1569–1586.

Bremmer, F., Kubischik, M., Pekel, M., Lappe, M., & Hoffmann, K. P. (1999). Linear vestibular self-motion signals in monkey medial superior temporal area. *Annals of the New York Academy of Sciences, 871,* 272–281.

Britten, K. H., Newsome, W. T., Shadlen, M. N., Celebrini, S., & Movshon, J. A. (1996). A relationship between behavioral choice and the visual responses of neurons in macaque MT. *Visual Neuroscience, 13,* 87–100.

Britten, K. H., Shadlen, M. N., Newsome, W. T., & Movshon, J. A. (1992). The analysis of visual motion: A comparison of neuronal and psychophysical performance. *Journal of Neuroscience, 12,* 4745–4765.

Britten, K. H., & van Wezel, R. J. (1998). Electrical microstimulation of cortical area MST biases heading perception in monkeys. *Nature Neuroscience, 1,* 59–63.

Bryan, A. S., & Angelaki, D. E. (2009). Optokinetic and vestibular responsiveness in the macaque rostral vestibular and fastigial nuclei. *Journal of Neurophysiology, 101,* 714–720.

Büttner, U., & Buettner, U. W. (1978). Parietal cortex (2v) neuronal activity in the alert monkey during natural vestibular and optokinetic stimulation. *Brain Research, 153,* 392–397.

Büttner, U., & Waespe, W. (1981). Vestibular nerve activity in the alert monkey during vestibular and optokinetic nystagmus. *Experimental Brain Research, 41,* 310–315.

Chen, A., Angelaki, D. E., & DeAngelis, G. C. (2010). Macaque parieto-insular vestibular cortex: responses to self-motion and optic flow *Journal of Neuroscience, 30,* 3022-3042.

Crowell, J. A., Banks, M. S., Shenoy, K. V., & Andersen, R. A. (1998). Visual self-motion perception during head turns. *Nature Neuroscience, 1,* 732–737.

Daunton, N., & Thomsen, D. (1979). Visual modulation of otolith-dependent units in cat vestibular nuclei. *Experimental Brain Research, 37,* 173–176.

Denève, S., Latham, P. E., & Pouget, A. (2001). Efficient computation and cue integration with noisy population codes. *Nature Neuroscience, 4,* 826–831.

Dichgans, J., & Brandt, T. (1978). Visual-vestibular interaction: Effects on self-motion perception and postural control. In R. Held, H. W. Leibowitz, & H. L. Teuber (Eds.), *Handbook of sensory physiology, Vol. 8. Perception* (pp. 756–804). Berlin, Germany: Springer-Verlag.

Duffy, C. J. (1998). MST neurons respond to optic flow and translational movement. *Journal of Neurophysiology, 80,* 1816–1827.

Duffy, C. J., & Wurtz, R. H. (1991). Sensitivity of MST neurons to optic flow stimuli. II. Mechanisms of response selectivity revealed by small-field stimuli. *Journal of Neurophysiology, 65,* 1346–1359.

Duffy, C. J., & Wurtz, R. H. (1995). Response of monkey MST neurons to optic flow stimuli with shifted centers of motion. *Journal of Neuroscience, 15,* 5192–5208.

Ernst, M. O., & Banks, M. S. (2002). Humans integrate visual and haptic information in a statistically optimal fashion. *Nature, 415,* 429–433.

Fernandez, C., & Goldberg, J. M. (1976a). Physiology of peripheral neurons innervating otolith organs of the squirrel monkey. I. Response to static tilts and to long-duration centrifugal force. *Journal of Neurophysiology, 39*, 970–984.

Fernandez, C., & Goldberg, J. M. (1976b). Physiology of peripheral neurons innervating otolith organs of the squirrel monkey. II. Directional selectivity and force-response relations. *Journal of Neurophysiology, 39*, 985–995.

Fetsch, C. R., Turner, A. H., DeAngelis, G. C., & Angelaki, D. E. (2009). Dynamic re-weighting of visual and vestibular cues during self-motion perception. *Journal of Neuroscience, 27*, 700–712.

Fetsch, C. R., Wang, S., Gu, Y., DeAngelis, G. C., & Angelaki, D. E. (2007). Spatial reference frames of visual, vestibular, and multimodal heading signals in the dorsal subdivision of the medial superior temporal area. *Journal of Neuroscience, 27*, 700–712.

Fukushima, K. (1997). Corticovestibular interactions: Anatomy, electrophysiology, and functional considerations. *Experimental Brain Research, 117*, 1–16.

Gibson, J. J. (1950). *The perception of the visual world.* Boston, MA: Houghton-Mifflin.

Gibson, J. J. (1954). The visual perception of objective motion and subjective movement. *Psychological Review, 61*, 304–314.

Green, D. M., & Swets, J. A. (1966). *Signal detection theory and psychophysics.* New York, NY: Wiley.

Grüsser, O. J., Pause, M., & Schreiter, U. (1990a). Localization and responses of neurones in the parieto-insular vestibular cortex of awake monkeys (Macaca fascicularis). *Journal of Physiology, 430*, 537–557.

Grüsser, O. J., Pause, M., & Schreiter, U. (1990b). Vestibular neurones in the parieto-insular cortex of monkeys (Macaca fascicularis): Visual and neck receptor responses. *Journal of Physiology, 430*, 559–583.

Gu, Y., Angelaki, D. E., & DeAngelis, G. C. (2008). Neural correlates of multisensory cue integration in macaque MSTd. *Nature Neuroscience, 11*, 1201–1210.

Gu, Y., DeAngelis, G. C., & Angelaki, D. E. (2007). A functional link between area MSTd and heading perception based on vestibular signals. *Nature Neuroscience, 10*, 1038–1047.

Gu, Y., Watkins, P. V., Angelaki, D. E., & DeAngelis, G. C. (2006). Visual and nonvisual contributions to three-dimensional heading selectivity in the medial superior temporal area. *Journal of Neuroscience, 26*, 73–85.

Guedry, F. E. (1974). Psychophysics of vestibular sensation. In H. H. Kornhuber (Ed.), *Handbook of sensory physiology, Vol. 6, Pt. 2. Vestibular System. Part 2: Psychophysics, applied aspects and general interpretations.* (pp. 3–154). New York, NY: Springer-Verlag.

Henn, V., Young, L. R., & Finley, C. (1974). Vestibular nucleus units in alert monkeys are also influenced by moving visual fields. *Brain Research, 71*, 144–149.

Howard, I. P. (1982). *Human visual orientation.* New York, NY: John Wiley.

Howard, I. P., & Heckmann, T. (1989). Circular vection as a function of the relative sizes, distances, and positions of two competing visual displays. *Perception, 18*, 657–665.

Jazayeri, M., & Movshon, J. A. (2006). Optimal representation of sensory information by neural populations. *Nature Neuroscience, 9*, 690–696.

Knill, D. C., & Pouget, A. (2004). The Bayesian brain: The role of uncertainty in neural coding and computation. *Trends in Neurosciences, 27*, 712–719.

Knill, D. C., & Saunders, J. A. (2003). Do humans optimally integrate stereo and texture information for judgments of surface slant? *Vision Research, 43*, 2539–2558.

Körding, K. P., Beierholm, U., Ma, W. J., Quartz, S., Tenenbaum, J. B., & Shams, L. (2007). Causal inference in multisensory perception. *PLoS ONE, 2*, e943.

Krug, K. (2004). A common neuronal code for perceptual processes in visual cortex? Comparing choice and attentional correlates in V5/MT. *Philosophical Transactions of the Royal Society of London B: Biological Sciences, 359*, 929–941.

Landy, M. S., Maloney, L. T., Johnston, E. B., & Young, M. (1995). Measurement and modeling of depth cue combination: In defense of weak fusion. *Vision Research, 35*, 389–412.

Ma, W. J., Beck, J. M., Latham, P. E., & Pouget, A. (2006). Bayesian inference with probabilistic population codes. *Nature Neuroscience, 9*, 1432–1438.

Mach, E. (1875). *Grundlinien der Lehre von den Bewegungsempfindungen.* Leipzig, Germany: W. Engelmann.

Markert, G., Büttner, U., Straube, A., & Boyle, R. (1988). Neuronal activity in the flocculus of the alert monkey during sinusoidal optokinetic stimulation. *Experimental Brain Research, 70*, 134–144.

Merfeld, D. M., Zupan, L., & Peterka, R. J. (1999). Humans use internal models to estimate gravity and linear acceleration. *Nature, 398*, 615–618.

Morgan, M. L., DeAngelis, G. C., & Angelaki, D. E. (2008). Multisensory integration in macaque visual cortex depends on cue reliability. *Neuron, 59*, 662–673.

Odkvist, L. M., Schwarz, D. W., Fredrickson, J. M., & Hassler, R. (1974). Projection of the vestibular nerve to the area 3a arm field in the squirrel monkey (saimiri sciureus). *Experimental Brain Research, 21*, 97–105.

Ohmi, M. (1996). Egocentric perception through interaction among many sensory systems. *Brain Research Cognitive Brain Research, 5*, 87–96.

Page, W. K., & Duffy, C. J. (1999). MST neuronal responses to heading direction during pursuit eye movements. *Journal of Neurophysiology, 81*, 596–610.

Parker, A. J., & Newsome, W. T. (1998). Sense and the single neuron: Probing the physiology of perception. *Annual Review of Neuroscience, 21*, 227–277.

Previc, F. H., Varner, D. C., & Gillingham, K. K. (1992). Visual scene effects on the somatogravic illusion. *Aviation, Space, and Environmental Medicine, 63*, 1060–1064.

Probst, T., Straube, A., & Bles, W. (1985). Differential effects of ambivalent visual-vestibular-somatosensory stimulation on the perception of self-motion. *Behavioural Brain Research, 16*, 71–79.

Robinson, D. A. (1977). Linear addition of optokinetic and vestibular signals in the vestibular nucleus. *Experimental Brain Research, 30*, 447–450.

Royden, C. S., Banks, M. S., & Crowell, J. A. (1992). The perception of heading during eye movements. *Nature, 360*, 583–585.

Royden, C. S., Crowell, J. A., & Banks, M. S. (1994). Estimating heading during eye movements. *Vision Research, 34*, 3197–3214.

Royden, C. S., & Hildreth, E. C. (1996). Human heading judgments in the presence of moving objects. *Perception and Psychophysics, 58*, 836–856.

Schaafsma, S. J., & Duysens, J. (1996). Neurons in the ventral intraparietal area of awake macaque monkey closely resemble neurons in the dorsal part of the medial superior temporal area in their responses to optic flow patterns. *Journal of Neurophysiology, 76*, 4056–4068.

Schwarz, D. W., & Fredrickson, J. M. (1971). Rhesus monkey vestibular cortex: A bimodal primary projection field. *Science, 172*, 280–281.

Si, X., Angelaki, D. E., & Dickman, J. D. (1997). Response properties of pigeon otolith afferents to linear acceleration. *Experimental Brain Research, 117*, 242–250.

Takahashi, K., Gu, Y., May, P. J., Newlands, S. D., DeAngelis, G. C., & Angelaki, D. E. (2007). Multimodal coding of three-dimensional rotation and translation in area MSTd: Comparison of visual and vestibular selectivity. *Journal of Neuroscience, 27*, 9742–9756.

Tanaka, K., Hikosaka, K., Saito, H., Yukie, M., Fukada, Y., & Iwai, E. (1986). Analysis of local and wide-field movements in the superior temporal visual areas of the macaque monkey. *Journal of Neuroscience, 6*, 134–144.

Tanaka, K., & Saito, H. (1989). Analysis of motion of the visual field by direction, expansion/contraction, and rotation cells clustered in the dorsal part of the medial superior temporal area of the macaque monkey. *Journal of Neurophysiology, 62*, 626–641.

Tarita-Nistor, L., Gonzalez, E. G., Spigelman, A. J., & Steinbach, M. J. (2006). Linear vection as a function of stimulus eccentricity, visual angle, and fixation. *Journal of Vestibular Research: Equilibrium and Orientation, 16*, 265–272.

Telford, L., & Frost, B. J. (1993). Factors affecting the onset and magnitude of linear vection. *Perception and Psychophysics, 53*, 682–692.

Telford, L., Howard, I. P., & Ohmi, M. (1995). Heading judgments during active and passive self-motion. *Experimental Brain Research, 104*, 502–510.

Waespe, W., Büttner, U., & Henn, V. (1981). Visual-vestibular interaction in the flocculus of the alert monkey. I. Input activity. *Experimental Brain Research, 43*, 337–348.

Waespe, W., & Henn, V. (1977). Neuronal activity in the vestibular nuclei of the alert monkey during vestibular and optokinetic stimulation. *Experimental Brain Research, 27*, 523–538.

Waespe, W., & Henn, V. (1981). Visual-vestibular interaction in the flocculus of the alert monkey. II. Purkinje cell activity. *Experimental Brain Research, 43*, 349–360.

Warren, W. H. (2003). Optic Flow. In L. M. Chalupa & J. S. Werner (Eds.), *The visual neurosciences* (Vol. 2, pp. 1247–1259). Cambridge, MA: MIT Press.

Warren, W. H., & Saunders, J. A. (1995). Perceiving heading in the presence of moving objects. *Perception, 24,* 315–331.

Wichmann, F. A., & Hill, N. J. (2001). The psychometric function: I. Fitting, sampling, and goodness of fit. *Perception and Psychophysics, 63,* 1293–1313.

Wolfe, J. W., & Cramer, R. L. (1970). Illusions of pitch induced by centripetal acceleration. *Aerospace Medicine, 41,* 1136–1139.

Wright, W. G., DiZio, P., & Lackner, J. R. (2005). Vertical linear self-motion perception during visual and inertial motion: more than weighted summation of sensory inputs. *Journal of Vestibular Research: Equilibrium and Orientation, 15,* 185–195.

Young, M. J., Landy, M. S., & Maloney, L. T. (1993). A perturbation analysis of depth perception from combinations of texture and motion cues. *Vision Research, 33,* 2685–2696.

Zacharias, G. L., & Young, L. R. (1981). Influence of combined visual and vestibular cues on human perception and control of horizontal rotation. *Experimental Brain Research, 41,* 159–171.

Zhang, T., & Britten, K. H. (2003). *Microstimulation of area VIP biases heading perception in monkeys.* Program No. 339.9. 2003 Neuroscience Abstract Viewer/Itinerary Planner. New Orleans, LA: Society for Neuroscience.

Zhang, T., Heuer, H. W., & Britten, K. H. (2004). Parietal area VIP neuronal responses to heading stimuli are encoded in head-centered coordinates. *Neuron, 42,* 993–1001.

# CHAPTER 17

## Probing Neural Correlates of Cue Integration

*Christopher A. Buneo, Gregory Apker, and Ying Shi*

### INTRODUCTION

Ideal-observer models have provided a useful framework for investigating cue integration during a variety of behaviors. Despite a large and accumulating body of theoretical and psychophysical work in support of such models, investigations into the neural underpinnings of cue integration have not generally examined the predictions of *optimal* cue integration. The one exception is the elegant work of Angelaki, DeAngelis, and colleagues (Chapter 16), who have probed some of these predictions in neural structures involved in self-motion perception. Optimal or not, there are several reasons why neural correlates of cue integration might be expected to differ across neural structures. The first concerns the nature of the cues themselves, which, depending on the structure, can be multisensory or both sensory and motor based, possibly necessitating different integration strategies. Second, the density of anatomical projections from unimodal brain areas to a given multimodal one can differ substantially, which may place constraints on the weighting and reweighting of sensory and/or motor cues. Lastly, differences in how optimality is defined in perceptual versus action-based integration may affect how this integration manifests in sensory versus motor structures.

As a result, we will review neural correlates of cue integration in two distinct neural systems (one perceptual, the other sensorimotor), both in nonhuman primates. The first involves structures involved with the integration of somatic and visual cues during visually guided reaching. As with most behavioral neurophysiology, these studies focus on analyses of spiking activity (i.e., the mean firing rate of extracellular action potentials). However, it has become increasingly clear that analyses of other "nonspiking" signals such as local field potentials (LFPs) can provide important additional insights into the neural mechanisms of perceptual and motor processes, including cue integration. Thus, we will also review recent work conducted in a system where LFP modulations have been observed during integration, that is, the audiovisual perceptual system. At that point we will also discuss the combined analysis of spikes and LFPs as a potentially fruitful avenue for investigations into the neural correlates of cue integration.

### CUE INTEGRATION: NEURAL SUBSTRATES AND MECHANISMS

Where in the brain does cue integration occur? Traditionally, only a few areas have been implicated in multisensory integration. By far the most well-studied of these is the superior colliculus (SC) in the midbrain. Most of this impressive body of work has been performed in cats and has been reviewed extensively elsewhere

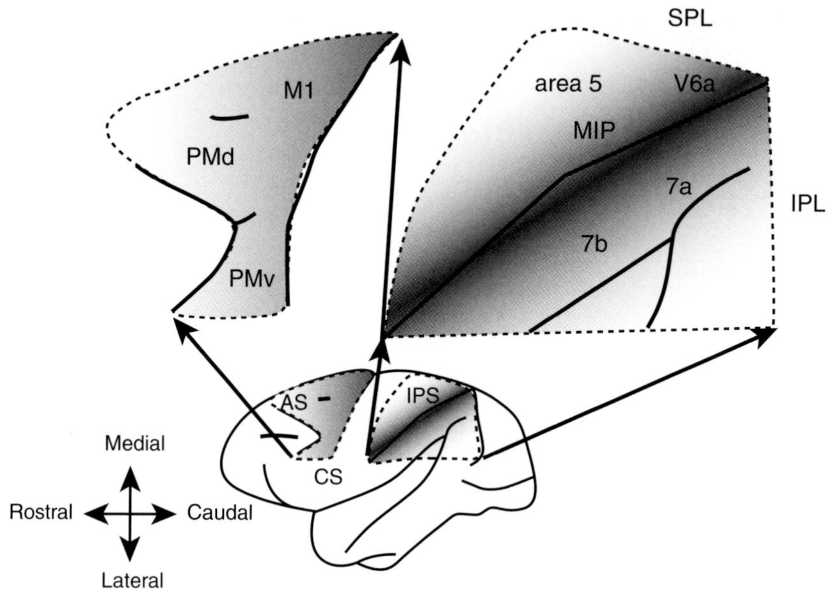


**Figure 17.1** Lateral view of the rhesus macaque monkey brain with parts of the frontal and parietal lobes highlighted and expanded. Shaded regions indicate the banks of sulci. AS, arcuate sulcus; CS, central sulcus; IPL, inferior parietal lobule; IPS, intraparietal sulcus; SPL, superior parietal lobule.

(Stein & Stanford, 2008); therefore, we will touch only briefly on this work. More recently the range of multisensory areas has expanded to include areas previously thought to be unisensory; in fact, it has been argued that most, if not all, of the cerebral cortex might be multisensory in nature (Ghazanfar & Schroeder, 2006). For example, in nonhuman primates several areas have been implicated in the integration of somatic information with visual information near the body (Fig. 17.1) including the SC, putamen, ventral premotor cortex (PMv), and the following parietal areas: 5, 7, the medial intraparietal area (MIP), and the ventral intraparietal area (VIP) (Duhamel, Colby, & Goldberg, 1998; Graziano, Cooke, & Taylor, 2000; Graziano & Gross, 1993; Graziano, Gross, Taylor, & Moore, 2004; Graziano, Yap, & Gross, 1994; Groh & Sparks, 1996). Some of these areas (e.g., VIP and PMv) also respond to auditory signals, making them trimodal, similar to areas in and around the superior temporal sulcus (STS). Still other areas have been implicated in the integration of auditory and visual cues such as the lateral intraparietal area (LIP) and the ventrolateral prefrontal cortex (Mazzoni, Bracewell, Barash, & Andersen, 1996; Sugihara, Diltz, Averbeck, & Romanski, 2006).

Within these multimodal areas, neural correlates of cue integration have been shown to manifest in several ways. In important early work investigating multisensory integration at the neuronal level, Stein and colleagues evaluated the responses of cat SC neurons to visual, somatosensory, and auditory stimuli (reviewed by Stein & Stanford, 2008). Chiefly, their findings indicated that multimodal responses were generally greater than corresponding unimodal responses. In fact, simultaneous presentation of two relatively weak unimodal stimuli typically resulted in multimodal responses that were greater than the sum of the unimodal responses. This effect was referred to as "superadditivity" and suggested a nonlinear sensory-integration scheme. Interestingly, the strength of the superadditivity was inversely related to the strength of the stimuli; that is, the weaker the unimodal stimuli, the more nonlinear the multimodal integration. This property was termed "the principle of inverse effectiveness." Subsequent studies established superadditivity as a ubiquitous neural correlate of cue integration. However, these properties were only observed for stimuli that were below perceptual threshold. As stimulus strength moved to threshold levels and beyond, multimodal responses were no longer superadditive but were more consistent with a linear summation of unimodal responses (Stanford, Quessy, & Stein, 2005). This observation, along with other recent evidence from single-unit studies suggests that while superadditivity may play an important role in perception, it is not the sole mechanism underlying cue integration (Stanford & Stein, 2007).

Other correlates of cue integration have also been observed at the level of single neurons, most recently in nonhuman primates. For instance, in a heading detection task, Gu, Angelaki, and DeAngelis (2008) showed that neurons in the dorsal medial superior temporal area (MSTd) with congruent, or nearly congruent, preferred directions for vestibular and visual heading, were most strongly correlated with perceptual estimations of heading. Interestingly, congruence did not necessarily produce a summation of unimodal activity levels. In fact, in general, the congruent cells demonstrated a *subadditive* combination of unimodal responses. However, greater congruence did predict how strongly these cells correlated with behavior (Gu et al., 2008). This represented a major advance in our understanding of the neural mechanisms of cue integration because it established a strong link between neural activity and behavior.

What types of responses would one expect of neurons involved in *optimal* cue integration? Several behavioral studies have demonstrated that both humans and monkeys integrate sensory cues in a nearly Bayes-optimal manner. Applications of probabilistic approaches to neural coding suggest that multimodal population activity would also be considered Bayes optimal if the population response approximated a weighted sum of the population response to unimodal inputs (Ma & Pouget, 2008). These ideas have also been extended to the single-unit level. For example, one model predicts that, under the assumption of Poisson spiking statistics, the optimal response of a single neuron involved in cue integration may be the weighted sum of its responses to unimodal stimuli (Ma & Pouget, 2008) (Fig. 17.2A). An important corollary to this is that firing rates of multimodal cells may demonstrate varying degrees of additivity. The observations of subadditivity made by Gu et al. (2008) are consistent with this weighted-sum prediction and therefore represent one of the first demonstrations of a link between Bayes-optimal behavior and single-unit activity.

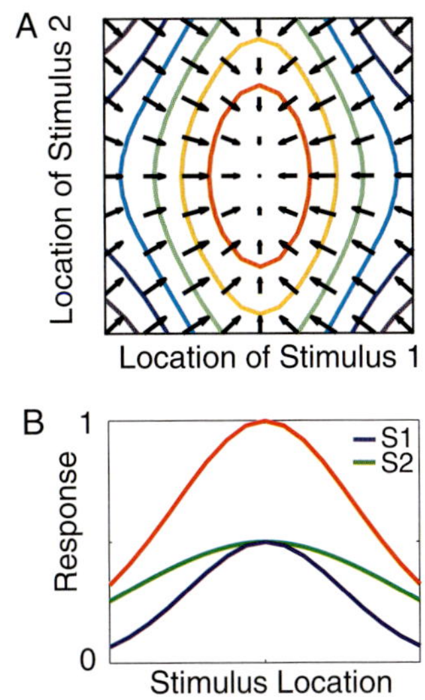


**Figure 17.2** (A) Idealized neural responses to two unimodal stimuli under the assumption that the bimodal response is the sum of the unimodal responses. Response magnitude is indicated by colored contours. The superimposed vector field (black arrows) converges toward the peak of the response field. (B) Red curve: diagonal slice passing through the peak of the response field in (A). Blue curve: idealized response to Stimulus 1. Green curve: idealized response to Stimulus 2.

The aforementioned observations were strengthened by a similar study of bimodal MSTd neurons in which coherence of visual feedback was varied (Morgan, DeAngelis, & Angelaki, 2008). As visual coherence decreased, responses were increasingly biased by vestibular responses, demonstrating that cue reliability affected integration, as has been observed behaviorally. Observations of Bayes-optimal integration appear to extend beyond the combination of two or more unimodal signals to the integration of single modalities over time. For example, it has recently been shown that during information accumulation, neurons in LIP encode probability distributions that can accurately predict an animal's behavior (Beck et al., 2008).

Predicted manifestations of optimal cue integration at the single-cell level also have implications for understanding the encoding of spatial information in different reference frames. The unimodal tuning curves shown in Figure 17.2B are depicted as being aligned in space; that is, their peak responses are associated with the same stimulus location. As a result, responses to two simultaneously delivered unimodal inputs are predicted to result in an integrated tuning curve with a peak response that is associated with the same location. This would be expected if the two unimodal inputs were encoding information in the same spatial reference frame. For example, recent experiments in area 5 have shown that even in the absence of visual input some neurons encode the position of the arm with respect to the direction of gaze. This implies that somatic and visual information about arm position are encoded in the same eye-centered reference frame in this area (Buneo & Andersen, 2003), which results in responses similar to those shown in Figure 17.2B. However, unimodal inputs are often encoded in different reference frames. This leads to unimodal tuning curves that appear shifted with respect to one another (i.e., the peaks are not aligned) and an integrated curve that lies intermediate to the two unimodal curves. This phenomenon has been observed in several cortical areas, including area 5, LIP, and VIP (Buneo, Jarvis, Batista, & Andersen, 2002; Duhamel, Bremmer, Ben Hamed, & Grof, 1997; Stricanne, Andersen, & Mazzoni, 1996). Note that these apparent shifts do not invalidate the optimal integration hypothesis; in fact, it has been argued that such "intermediate" response fields are a natural by-product of this process (Denève, Latham, & Pouget, 2001; Denève & Pouget, 2004; Pouget, Denève, & Duhamel, 2002).

## CUE INTEGRATION DURING VISUALLY GUIDED REACHING: WHAT IS THE PROBLEM?

Before discussing neural correlates of cue integration in the arm movement system, it would be helpful to review how cue integration fits into the overall scheme of visually guided reaching (Fig. 17.3). The computations involved in this behavior necessarily involve a comparison of target position with hand position and thus can potentially involve solving two problems in cue integration. One is in determining target position, a process that though typically visually based can also involve multisensory integration, as in estimating the position of a buzzing fly from visual and auditory cues. As discussed elsewhere in this volume, this is a perceptual problem with the goal being to integrate noisy sensory information in order to reduce variability in the estimate of target position (e.g., see Chapter 1).

The other cue-integration problem involves determining hand position. Hand-position estimation is required for initial movement planning and for correcting movement errors online. It is also required for associating visual and proprioceptive feedback at the end of movement with previous motor commands (efference copy), the so-called credit-assignment problem. This is required for transforming sensory errors into a format that can be used to correct motor commands, a critical aspect of motor learning (Jordan & Rumelhart, 1992). Thus, while these two cue-integration problems are similar, hand-position estimation differs from target-position estimation in that it involves the integration of motor "cues" with sensory cues.

Cue integration during target- and hand-position estimation must address either implicity or explicitly the "reference-frame problem." That is, targets and hand positions are initially encoded in the brain in the natural reference

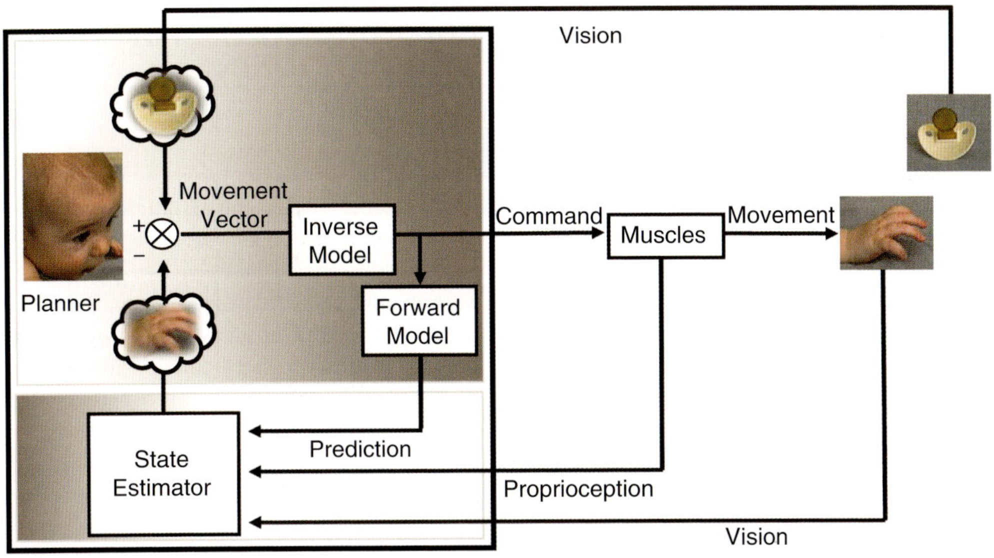


**Figure 17.3** Flow diagram of the various computations involved in visually guided reaching.

frames of the sensors. In many circumstances these frames will differ, that is, while target position is typically encoded in visual or "eye-centered" coordinates, reaches are often initiated with the hand out of view, suggesting a proprioceptive or "body-centered" reference frame for hand-position coding. It has been suggested that this problem is simplified by transforming hand position into the same reference frame used to encode target position or vice versa (Flanders, Helms-Tillery, & Soechting, 1992). In the presence of vision this would likely be "eye-centered" coordinates, though in other contexts a body-centered frame could be used (Buneo et al., 2002; McIntyre, Stratta, & Lacquaniti, 1997, 1998). However, recent modeling and neurophysiological studies have demonstrated that explicit coordinate transformations are not necessary for optimal cue integration to occur (Gu et al., 2008; Pouget et al., 2002), though such computations might still be beneficial in certain contexts. Thus, it is unclear whether the "state estimator" shown in Figure 17.3 is involved in both coordinate transformations *and* cue integration and, if so, whether these computations involve the same or different neural structures/networks.

The question of what is optimized during reaching is also relevant to this discussion. Various schemes have been proposed, including the minimization of jerk (Hogan & Flash, 1987), minimization of torque change (Uno, Kawato, & Suzuki, 1989), and minimization of energy (Soechting, Buneo, Herrmann, & Flanders, 1995), among others. More recently it has been proposed that many known characteristics of reaching movements (as well as saccadic eye movements) are best explained by an optimization process that seeks to minimize endpoint variance (Harris & Wolpert, 1998). In this context, estimation of hand position during reaching (in part a control problem) becomes a cue-integration problem analogous to that of estimating target position and integration of noisy sensory and motor cues functions to minimize variability in reach endpoint position.

Given these observations, which arm-movement-related areas are best suited for probing optimal cue integration? One consideration should be the relative strength with which unimodal inputs are represented within a given area. That is, the densities of anatomical connections from unimodal areas to a given multimodal area are often variable and relatively unequal, which may place limitations on the extent to which these unimodal inputs can be weighted in a given task (Apker, Shi, & Buneo, 2009). For example, dorsal area 5, while reportedly multimodal, appears to be dominated by somatic input while the adjacent MIP appears to represent visual and somatic signals more equally (Caminiti, Ferraina, & Johnson, 1996; Colby & Duhamel, 1991). Note also that the previously described predictions presume that cue integration will manifest neurally as changes in the mean firing rates of neurons in a given area. However, neural correlates of optimal integration could manifest as a synchronous activation of two or more areas that are largely devoted to either visual or somatic processing. Examples of network-level correlates of cue integration are discussed later in this chapter.

While the predictions of the optimal-integration hypothesis at the single-cell level are relatively straightforward, testing these predictions neurophysiologically can be challenging, especially in the arm-movement system. This is due to the difficulty in providing "natural" visual cues about limb position in isolation of concomitant somatic cues. In other words, whereas visual and auditory cues for objects extrinsic to the body do on occasion occur in isolation, visual cues about arm position never occur naturally without concomitant somatic input. This imposes limitations on experimental paradigms designed to probe optimal cue integration in this system and on the interpretation of the resulting data. As a result, studies of the neural mechanisms of multisensory integration for arm movements to date have not explicitly examined whether integration at the single-cell level conforms to principles of optimality. Instead, these studies have focused on whether neurons encode both visual and somatic signals and/or on whether these signals are encoded in a common reference frame. Still, these studies do hint at which areas could contribute to optimal integration and how that integration might manifest neurally. Work related to integration during static positioning of the arm (posture activity) and during movement is discussed in the sections that follow.

## CUE INTEGRATION FOR STATIC ARM POSITIONING

### Area 5/MIP

Graziano and colleagues have studied the visual and proprioceptive coding of static limb position in area 5 in a paradigm where the unseen limb was passively varied between two positions in a horizontal plane (Graziano et al., 2000). In these experiments, animals also viewed a fake monkey arm that could be placed in positions that were either congruent or incongruent with the real arm. Variations in discharge due to manipulations of the unseen or "felt" arm were attributed to somatic signals, whereas variations due to the fake "seen" arm were interpreted as being related to visual information about limb position. Approximately one-half of the recorded neurons were modulated by manipulation of the unseen arm, in agreement with previous studies in this area (Buneo et al., 2002; Georgopoulos, Caminiti, & Kalaska, 1984; Lacquaniti, Guigon, Bianchi, Ferraina, & Caminiti, 1995). Although almost no cells responded to manipulations of the seen arm only, 27% of recorded neurons responded to both the seen and unseen arm. Despite the fact that only approximately one-quarter of area 5 neurons responded to both stimuli, these effects were statistically significant at the population level.

These findings have been interpreted as evidence that area 5 is involved in integrating visual and somatic signals. It should be noted, however, that in this study animals were not required to make a perceptual judgment nor were they required to actively control the position of their limbs to perform a particular motor task; thus, it is unclear if the fake arm was perceived by the animals as a visual signal regarding the position of their limb. In addition, although modulations were significant across the population, changing the felt position of the limb resulted in an approximately 25% change in the responsiveness of neurons in this area, whereas modulation by the seen arm position was only on the order of 5%–10%. This is not what one would expect of areas strongly involved in multisensory cue integration for arm movements. Lastly, since animals were not required to actively maintain their limb position and in fact had their limbs passively placed in position, the contribution of motor processes (efference copy) to position coding was not addressed in this experiment.

### PMv

Graziano, Gross, and colleagues have also studied the integration of visual and proprioceptive signals in PMv (Graziano, 1999; Graziano, Hu, & Gross, 1997; Graziano et al., 1994). In their experimental paradigm, small spheres (positioned along the horizontal) were moved toward the arm, which was held fixed in one of two horizontal positions. In an initial experiment, the animals could see their arms as well as the visual stimuli. Neurons in this area responded preferentially to the sight of one of the stimuli moving toward the arm. These neurons also had tactile receptive fields and responded to changes in arm position as well; thus, these cells were multimodal (visual, tactile, proprioceptive). When arm position was varied between the two horizontal positions, the peak response of the neuron changed such that it was associated with the position of a different visual stimulus in space, but the same stimulus position with respect to the arm. In other words, the visual receptive fields of these cells appeared to move with the arm or were "arm centered." This could only be accomplished via the convergence of visual signals with proprioceptive signals regarding arm position. Note, however, that the visual stimulus driving the cell in this case was a visual stimulus regarding object (sphere) position, not arm position. Thus, this result demonstrates that PMv integrates visual information regarding *extrinsic* objects with somatic information (which is inherently intrinsic to the body).

The experiment just described did not address the integration of intrinsic somatic information with intrinsic visual information (i.e., visual information about body parts). In a subsequent experiment, Graziano and colleagues partially addressed this issue by blocking vision of the arm (reviewed in Graziano, 1999). When view of the arm was blocked, it was reported that movements of the receptive field were reduced, suggesting these neurons also integrate visual information about arm position. This phenomenon was examined further by varying the position of a fake monkey arm, as described earlier for area 5. On average, the visual receptive fields moved almost to the same extent as when the real arm was moved, supporting the idea that these neurons encode intrinsic visual stimuli. However, due to the small number of neurons tested in this latter paradigm as well as the presence of concurrent extrinsic and intrinsic visual stimuli, it is difficult to reliably gauge the extent to which PMv neurons are modulated by intrinsic visual and somatic signals. In addition, arm position was varied passively in this study as well, thus the contribution of efference copy to limb position coding in these neurons is unclear.

### Other Multimodal Areas

Similar multimodal arm cells have been reported in parietal areas 7b and the putamen (Graziano & Gross, 1993, 1996). However, in these areas the tendency for visual receptive fields to move with the arm is less common. Whereas up to 67% of multimodal neurons in PMv reportedly have visual receptive fields that are "modulated" by arm position, only 20%–25% of cells in the putamen exhibit this property and apparently no cells in 7b do. Although many VIP cells are multimodal and stimulation in this area can produce arm movements (Thier & Andersen, 1998), the nature of multimodal integration for the limb has not been well characterized in this area. However, VIP neurons with tactile receptive fields on the face and visual receptive fields near the head do not, in general, appear to encode spatial information in a single body-part-centered reference frame. That is, tactile receptive fields in these neurons are somatotopic or "head centered," and visual receptive fields are widely distributed between retinotopic (i.e., eye-centered) and head-centered coordinates (Avillac, Denève, Olivier, Pouget, & Duhamel, 2005). This suggests that if VIP does integrate visual and somatic information about the arm, it does so in a manner that is different than that in PMv.

## CUE INTEGRATION DURING ARM MOVEMENT

### Area 5

The integration of visual and somatic limb position signals in area 5 has been studied more recently during the production and sustained maintenance of motor output (Buneo & Andersen, 2003). In these experiments, monkeys made reaching movements from each of four horizontally arranged initial hand positions to each of four horizontally arranged targets (located above or below the array of initial hand positions). The initial hand positions and target positions were sampled in two different workspaces that corresponded to different horizontal gaze positions. Movements were performed with or without visual information regarding initial hand position. The following was observed: first, the combination of initial hand position and target position for which the cells responded best was generally the same for each workspace. Thus, these neurons had a preferred hand position and target position in eye-centered coordinates, rather than body-or world-centered coordinates. Furthermore, this was true even though the animal could not see its hand during the behavioral epoch under examination and had in fact not received a visual update of its hand position for several hundred milliseconds. These findings confirm previous results that a code for hand position in eye coordinates exists in the PPC (Buneo et al., 2002), and they additionally demonstrate that this code exists even in the absence of vision, suggesting that it results from the transformation of somatic signals from body- to eye-centered coordinates.

Another principal finding from this experiment was that allowing vision of the hand prior to movement did *not* affect the coding of hand position in most cells. That is, only 10% of the neurons were modulated by visual information about the hand at the starting position, a number less than would be predicted by the results of Graziano and colleagues (2000). However, as with the latter study, there were limitations to this more "active" paradigm as well. In this experiment, animals were required to continually push a button that corresponded to the required initial hand position. The combination of tactile, proprioceptive, and force feedback experienced during this button press, as well as the continuously generated motor output, likely provided a very reliable somatic estimate of limb position. As a result, visual signals may have been *relatively* unreliable and consequently not weighted very strongly in this task, resulting in only small differences between the "vision" and "no vision" conditions. Thus, despite the fact that few cells were modulated by vision in this task, the results were not necessarily inconsistent with a role for area 5 in optimally integrating motor and sensory information to estimate limb position. This logic would only hold true, however, if the visual and proprioceptive signals were perceptually equivalent during this task, which seems unlikely for the reasons mentioned earlier. Experiments described next are designed to examine integration in a context where visual and somatic feedback should be more equally relevant, that is, during the maintenance of positions held in free space.

### 7a

The few studies that have examined arm-movement-related responses in this area in the presence and absence of vision have not focused explicitly on limb vision but visual responsiveness in general. That is, responses were studied under conditions of complete darkness (no visual stimuli at all) versus full vision (MacKay & Riehle, 1992), or under conditions where arm vision was unavailable but responses to visual stimuli presented alone or as reach targets were assessed (Battaglia-Mayer, Mascaro, & Caminiti, 2007). These studies also do not support a strong role for vision in the encoding of dynamic limb position and velocity in area 7a. For example, although some reach-related neurons in this area are visually responsive, these responses appear to be relatively independent of movement-related activity in these neurons (Battaglia-Mayer et al., 2007). That is, the responses of these neurons generally did not differentiate between movements to visual targets and movements to memorized locations. Thus, these results, as well as the results described earlier for area 5 under static and dynamic conditions, suggest that arm-movement-related neurons in these areas do not strongly encode the visually perceived position of the limb.

### PMv

As indicated earlier, PMv neurons encode spatial information about the locations of extrinsic objects, as well as somatically derived information about the static position of the limb. Although limitations in the experimental design have made elucidating the role of intrinsic visual information about static limb position more difficult, recent studies of active movements generally support the idea that this information is encoded by PMv neurons. When animals are trained to make arm movements under conditions that dissociate movement of the effector from the corresponding visual feedback of that movement, activity in PMv appears to be better correlated with the visually perceived movement rather than the actual movement (Schwartz, Moran, & Reina, 2004). This appears to indicate that PMv neurons are strongly involved in signaling visual feedback of the moving limb. However, other studies have shown that PMv neurons do not strongly encode information on the particular arm (left or right) that will be used to make a given movement (Hoshi & Tanji, 2002) but instead reflect the visual motion of the hand in a limb-independent manner (Ochiai, Mushiake, & Tanji, 2005). Thus, although PMv neurons may represent both visual and somatic information about the limb, this information does not appear to be integrated in a straightforward manner in this area.

## PROBING OPTIMAL CUE INTEGRATION FOR THE ARM

As indicated earlier, although it is difficult to test some predictions of the optimal-integration hypothesis in the arm movement system, it is possible to assess whether multimodal activity is correlated with the reliabilities of unimodal inputs. One approach to studying this latter prediction is to alter artificially the relative reliability of the unimodal cues, as Angelaki and colleagues have done in their studies of self-motion (Morgan et al., 2008; see also Chapter 16). Alternatively, one can take advantage of "natural" variations in the reliability of unimodal cues. For example, the precision of somatic and visual information varies as a function of arm configuration, leading to a relative weighting of these signals during the estimation of static limb position that is both position and direction dependent. For example, when human subjects are required to localize the endpoint of one arm with their other arm using only somatic cues or a combination of somatic and visual cues, the following is observed: *(1)* localization on the basis of somatic signals alone is more precise for positions closer to the body (implying vision should be weighted less for these locations), and *(2)* proprioceptive localization is more precise in depth than in azimuth (radial direction with respect to the shoulder), and vice versa for vision (van Beers, Sittig, & van der Gon, 1998; van Beers, Wolpert, & Haggard, 2002). These findings are summarized graphically in Figure 17.4. Differences in precision as a function of position can be gleaned from the relative

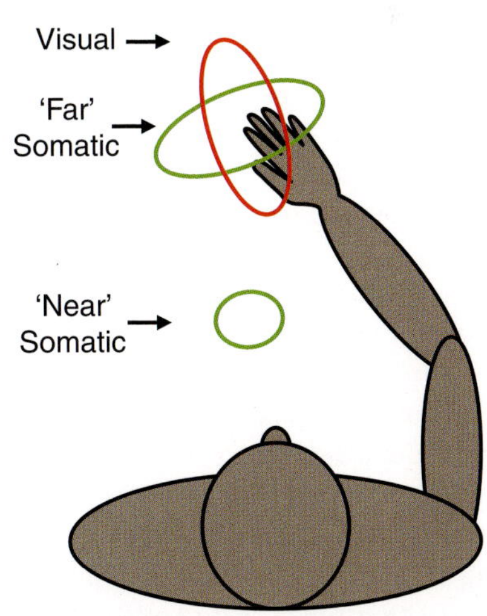


**Figure 17.4** Direction and position-dependent precision of somatic and visual localization. Adapted from van Beers et al. (2002).

sizes of the "near" and "far" somatic ellipses; direction dependence can be appreciated from the elongated shapes of the "far" somatic and visual ellipses.

The work of van Beers and colleagues leads to some testable predictions regarding optimal cue integration in arm-movement-related areas of the brain. As mentioned earlier, cells in most arm-movement-related areas of the brain exhibit static positional discharge that is spatially tuned; that is, cells have preferred limb positions and nonpreferred positions, with the activity across the sampled positions approximating a gradient in two-dimensional (Georgopoulos et al., 1984) or three-dimensional space (Kettner, Schwartz, & Georgopoulos, 1988). The work of van Beers and colleagues suggests that cells with preferred limb positions located farther from the body should be modulated more by concurrent visual input of the limb than cells with preferred positions located closer to the body, reflecting the decreased precision of somatic information at more extended arm positions. As a precursor to such an experiment, we are currently assessing the activity of neurons in the surface cortex of the PPC as the arm is held at various positions with respect to the body. In this experiment, activity is mapped at each position under conditions where visual and somatic input are concurrently available ("somatic + visual") as well as in the absence of visual input ("somatic"), controlled via a virtual-reality system (Shi & Buneo, 2009). To date, analysis has focused on changes in peak response magnitude induced by viewing the arm. While more than half the cells in this region appear to be modulated by static limb position, only 10% of the neurons appear to differentiate between somatic and somatic + visual conditions. Even more surprisingly, very few of these latter cells are also tuned to position and very few cells overall show a significant interaction between position and sensory conditions. Moreover, the presence of vision appears to interfere with the coding of limb position even in populations of purely position-tuned cells (Apker et al., 2009). Nevertheless, few cells in the surface cortex of the PPC appear to be modulated by the sight of the limb during static holding. This implies that this area does not receive strong input from areas devoted to the visual processing of body parts and is therefore not likely to be the primary site of integration for the arm.

## SUMMARY

In the parietal areas that have been examined thus far, visual information about arm position does not appear to be strongly represented. This is true even under conditions where visual input is expected to have a strong effect, that is, during the maintenance of static positions in free space. Note that the finding that cells in area 5/MIP encode hand position in eye-centered coordinates is not incongruent with this idea. That is, such a coding scheme is still possible via coordinate transformations of somatic signals. Note also that the aforementioned findings do not mean that cells in this area are not visually responsive. An anatomical basis exists for visual information to flow into both the superior and inferior parietal lobules (Caminiti et al., 1996) and moderate to strong responses to visual stimuli have been well documented in these areas (Andersen & Buneo, 2002, 2003; Buneo & Andersen, 2006). The relatively weak evidence for multisensory integration of visual and somatic arm-position information is therefore surprising, given the history of recordings in the PPC (Andersen, Snyder, Bradley, & Xing, 1997). Visual input to these areas may primarily convey information about extrinsic objects such as reach targets, rather than information about arm position. However, it is also possible that visual information about arm position will be more evident when it is needed for online control of limb movements rather than simply during the maintenance of static arm position. Lastly, most of the recordings performed in the superior parietal lobule have focused on surface cortex (area 5) with smaller numbers of neurons being recorded in MIP. The relatively strong visual responsiveness of neurons in this area and its reported involvement in eye-centered coding of spatial information suggests this area (or the adjacent V6A) could still exhibit responses more consistent with the predictions of areas involved in multisensory cue integration.

Regarding other areas, the putamen also does not appear to be a strong candidate area for optimal cue integration. PMv certainly appears to be the most visually driven of the areas we have discussed, but the results of Hoshi and Tanji (2002) suggest that somatic and visual responses are not integrated in a manner that one would expect of areas involved in optimal integration, though clearly more experiments are needed in the area. However, cells in the *dorsal* premotor cortex (PMd) exhibit responses that could point to a role in visuosomatic integration for the arm. PMd neurons encode information about both the static position and configuration of the limb (Pesaran, Nelson, & Andersen, 2006; Scott, Sergio, & Kalaska, 1997) and the area is known to receive visual input via the parietal lobe (Caminiti et al., 1996). In addition, and in contrast to PMv, PMd strongly encodes information on the arm that will be used to make a given movement (Hoshi & Tanji, 2000).

## CUE INTEGRATION: EVIDENCE FROM NONSPIKING ACTIVITY DURING AUDIOVISUAL INTEGRATION

The previous sections focused on neural correlates of cue integration in the arm-movement system, with an emphasis on changes in mean firing rates under unimodal versus multimodal conditions. In recent years, there has been an upsurge in interest in other aspects of neural coding, such as temporal coding in trains of action potentials (spikes) and in local field potentials (LFPs). In the case of LFPs, this interest has been driven by the relative ease with which these signals can be recorded, their observed relation to various motor and sensory phenomenon (Fries, Reynolds, Rorie, & Desimone, 2001; Lakatos et al., 2005; Liu & Newsome, 2006; Pesaran, Pezaris, Sahani, Mitra, & Andersen, 2002; Sanes & Donoghue, 1993; Scherberger, Jarvis, & Andersen, 2005), and the fact that LFPs appear to be better correlated with the fMRI BOLD signal than spiking activity (Logothetis, Guggenberger, Peled, & Pauls, 1999; Logothetis, Pauls, Oeltermann, Trinath, & Augath, 2000). As a result it has been proposed that LFPs provide a critical link between spikes and behavior (Buzsaki & Draguhn, 2004). Here we review some recent literature on changes in LFPs during visual-auditory cue integration in the auditory cortex and STS. It will be shown that an analysis of LFPs both within and across brain areas may provide insights into the neural mechanisms of cue integration that are not attainable through analysis of mean firing rates alone.

### LFPs

What exactly are LFPs? LFPs reflect the bulk movement of extracellular currents arising from a local neuronal ensemble. More specifically, LFPs are a summation signal of excitatory and inhibitory potentials generated near the dendrites (i.e., nonspiking activity). This is in contrast to extracellularly recorded action potentials, which are thought to arise largely from the soma or axon hillock of pyramidal or stellate cells (Humphrey & Schmidt, 1990) and reflect the output of a cortical column (Mitzdorf, 1985). Although it is certainly possible to elicit spikes in the absence of concomitant changes in LFPs, the opposite is also true. When LFP modulations and changes in spiking occur at the same time, it suggests a role for LFPs in driving spiking activity, whereas LFP modulations in the absence of changes in action-potential frequency suggest a more modulatory role for LFPs (Lakatos, Chen, O'Connell, Mills, & Schroeder, 2007). Evidence for a modulatory role is supported by the finding of LFP modulations with no concurrent spiking activity in the auditory cortex during the simultaneous presentation of somatosensory and auditory stimuli (Lakatos et al., 2007). Evidence for a driving role for LFPs is supported by the observation that LFP modulations are often accompanied by corresponding increases and decreases in spiking activity in the same cortical site (Fu et al., 2004; Gail, Brinksmeyer, & Eckhorn, 2004; Schroeder et al., 2001).

LFPs can be decomposed into their constituent frequency bands via various mathematical transforms, and it has been argued that these different bands represent distinct neural processes; that is, low-frequency bands may reflect the input in a local cortical microcolumn, whereas high-frequency bands may reflect local processing within that column (Chandrasekaran & Ghazanfar, 2009; Gray, Konig, Engel, & Singer, 1989; Lakatos et al., 2005; Liu & Newsome, 2006). The role of this oscillatory activity in multisensory integration is only beginning to be unraveled. The discussion that follows highlights some key findings in this area from recordings in and around the STS, the region in which these effects have been best characterized (Lakatos et al., 2007).

### Modulation of LFPs during Cue Integration

Ghazanfar, Maier, Hoffman, and Logothetis (2005) reported enhancement and suppression of raw LFPs in the core and lateral belt regions of auditory cortex when monkeys viewed the faces of other monkeys vocalizing. This was in comparison to responses recorded during the presentation of facial and vocal signals alone. In the core and lateral belt regions 73% and 89% of the sites, respectively, showed such neural correlates of multisensory integration (enhancement, suppression, or both) (Ghazanfar et al., 2005). Interestingly enhancement and suppression of multiunit spiking activity was much less common (35% and 40%, respectively), pointing to the idea that neural correlates of cue integration may be more evident in nonspiking than spiking activity.

More recently it has been reported that the manifestation of multisensory integration of facial and vocal signals in the auditory cortex differs for the different frequency bands present in the LFP signal (Chandrasekaran & Ghazanfar, 2009). LFPs were subjected to spectral analysis, and the power of the underlying frequency components was analyzed. The frequency bands typically analyzed, that is, theta (4–8 Hz), alpha (8–14 Hz), and gamma bands (>40 Hz), exhibited differing degrees of multisensory integration in response to the combined presentation of faces and voices. Gamma-band activity in particular showed the most consistent effects, being enhanced under most conditions, relative to the presentation of unimodal stimuli. Since gamma-band activity is thought to represent local processing in a cortical microcolumn (Liu & Newsome, 2006), these results suggest that enhancement of the gamma band of LFPs might be a strong neural correlate of multisensory integration.

In the study of Chandrasekaran and Ghazanfar (2009), the relative timing of the unimodal inputs strongly influenced the extent of multisensory integration in the LFP alpha band. That is, the tendency for enhancement in this frequency band depended upon the "time to voice," that is, the natural temporal offset between observed mouth movements and the voice. The importance of the relative timing of unimodal inputs in multisensory integration was illustrated more dramatically in a recent paper by Lakatos and colleagues (2007). These authors showed that the phase of ongoing neural oscillations in the primary auditory cortex could be reset by the presentation of a somatosensory stimulus. As a result, subsequent auditory responses could be enhanced or suppressed depending on where they occurred with respect to the reset oscillations. This result indicates that temporal factors are likely more complex and more important in multisensory integration than previous work has suggested (Meredith, Nemitz, & Stein, 1987).

### Interareal Synchrony

As described earlier, cue integration can manifest neurally as changes in multisensory response fields derived from mean firing rates, changes in the amplitude of raw LFP signals, or as changes in power within certain frequency bands of the LFP. These results are all consistent with the idea that multisensory cue integration is achieved via the convergence of inputs from largely unimodal areas onto higher order multisensory areas, which may subsequently be fed back to lower level unisensory areas (Bauer, 2008). However, some aspects of cue integration could also be achieved via lateral interactions between unimodal areas (Bauer, 2008). A recent study has provided evidence for such a mechanism from an analysis of the LFP "coherence," a measure of the linear correlation between the frequency components of two signals that has been used to quantify synchrony between areas. Presentation of combined auditory and visual looming signals (i.e., signals indicating the rapid approach of potentially harmful objects) was shown to result in increased gamma-band coherence between sites in the auditory cortex and the STS, relative to the case where only unimodal signals were presented (Maier, Chandrasekaran, & Ghazanfar, 2008). The result is particularly compelling because these authors had previously shown that the perception of looming signals is enhanced when visual and auditory signals are presented together (Maier, Neuhoff, Logothetis, & Ghazanfar, 2004). Taken together, these results suggest that interareal synchronization might prove to be a useful probe for some aspects of cue integration, particularly if such synchrony can be shown to covary with behavioral measures of integration (Bauer, 2008).

### Future Directions

Analysis of LFPs has proven to be very useful for studying multisensory interactions in the auditory cortex and STS of nonhuman primates. Combined study of LFPs and simultaneously recorded spiking activity may prove to be even more fruitful, as such analyses in other systems have identified subtle aspects of neural coding that could not be inferred by studying these signals separately (Monosov, Trageser, & Thompson, 2008; Nielsen, Logothetis, & Rainer, 2006). This approach will likely by useful not only for studying higher order sensory areas but also for the study of areas involved in transforming such sensory information into plans for movement.

## ACKNOWLEDGMENTS

This work was supported by the National Science Foundation, Science Foundation Arizona, and the Arizona Biomedical Research Commission.

## REFERENCES

Andersen, R. A., & Buneo, C. A. (2002). Intentional maps in posterior parietal cortex. *Annual Review of Neuroscience, 25,* 189–220.

Andersen, R. A., & Buneo, C. A. (2003). Sensory-motor integration in the posterior parietal cortex. In A. Segal, R. A. Andersen, H. J. Freund, & D. D. Spencer (Eds.), *Advances in neurology: The parietal lobes* (Vol. 93, pp. 159–179). Philadelphia, PA: Lippincott, Williams and Wilkins.

Andersen, R. A., Snyder, L. H., Bradley, D. C., & Xing, J. (1997). Multimodal representation of space in the posterior parietal cortex and its use in planning movements. *Annual Review of Neuroscience, 20,* 303–330.

Apker, G. A., Shi, Y., & Buneo, C. A. (2009, October). *The role of visual and somatic signals in the decoding of limb position in area 5.* Program No. 355.25, 2009 Neuroscience Meeting Planner. Chicago, IL: Society for Neuroscience. Online.

Avillac, M., Denève, S., Olivier, E., Pouget, A., & Duhamel, J. R. (2005). Reference frames for representing visual and tactile locations in parietal cortex. *Nature Neuroscience, 8,* 941–949.

Battaglia-Mayer, A., Mascaro, M., & Caminiti, R. (2007). Temporal evolution and strength of neural activity in parietal cortex during eye and hand movements. *Cerebral Cortex, 17,* 1350–1363.

Bauer, M. (2008). Multisensory integration: A functional role for inter-area synchronization? *Current Biology, 18,* R709–R710.

Beck, J. M., Ma, W. J., Kiani, R., Hanks, T., Churchland, A. K., Roitman, J., . . . Pouget, A. (2008). Probabilistic population codes for Bayesian decision making. *Neuron, 60,* 1142–1152.

Buneo, C. A., & Andersen, R. A. (2003, November). *The role of area 5 somatosensory input in visuomotor transformations for reaching.* Program No. 14.1, 2003 Neuroscience Meeting Planner. New Orleans, LA: Society for Neuroscience. Online.

Buneo, C. A., & Andersen, R. A. (2006). The posterior parietal cortex: Sensorimotor interface for the planning and online control of visually guided movements. *Neuropsychologia, 44,* 2594–2606.

Buneo, C. A., Jarvis, M. R., Batista, A. P., & Andersen, R. A. (2002). Direct visuomotor transformations for reaching. *Nature, 416,* 632–636.

Buzsaki, G., & Draguhn, A. (2004). Neuronal oscillations in cortical networks. *Science, 304,* 1926–1929.

Caminiti, R., Ferraina, S., & Johnson, P. B. (1996). The sources of visual information to the primate frontal lobe: A novel role for the superior parietal lobule. *Cerebral Cortex, 6*, 319–328.

Chandrasekaran, C., & Ghazanfar, A. A. (2009). Different neural frequency bands integrate faces and voices differently in the superior temporal sulcus. *Journal of Neurophysiology, 101*, 773–788.

Colby, C. L., & Duhamel, J. R. (1991). Heterogeneity of extrastriate visual areas and multiple parietal areas in the macaque monkey. *Neuropsychologia, 29*, 517–537.

Denève, S., Latham, P. E., & Pouget, A. (2001). Efficient computation and cue integration with noisy population codes. *Nature Neuroscience, 4*, 826–831.

Denève, S., & Pouget, A. (2004). Bayesian multisensory integration and cross-modal spatial links. *Journal of Physiology-Paris, 98*, 249–258.

Duhamel, J. R., Bremmer, F., Ben Hamed, S., & Grof, W. (1997). Spatial invariance of visual receptive fields in parietal cortex neurons. *Nature, 389*, 845–848.

Duhamel, J. R., Colby, C. L., & Goldberg, M. E. (1998). Ventral intraparietal area of the macaque: Congruent visual and somatic response properties. *Journal of Neurophysiology, 79*, 126–136.

Flanders, M., Helms-Tillery, S. I., & Soechting, J. F. (1992). Early stages in a sensorimotor transformation. *The Behavioral and Brain Sciences, 15*, 309–362.

Fries, P., Reynolds, J. H., Rorie, A. E., & Desimone, R. (2001). Modulation of oscillatory neuronal synchronization by selective visual attention. *Science, 291*, 1560–1563.

Fu, K. M. G., Shah, A. S., O'Connell, M. N., McGinnis, T., Eckholdt, H., Lakatos, P., ... Schroeder, C. E. (2004). Timing and laminar profile of eye-position effects on auditory responses in primate auditory cortex. *Journal of Neurophysiology, 92*, 3522–3531.

Gail, A., Brinksmeyer, H. J., & Eckhorn, R. (2004). Perception-related modulations of local field potential power and coherence in primary visual cortex of awake monkey during binocular rivalry. *Cerebral Cortex, 14*, 300–313.

Georgopoulos, A. P., Caminiti, R., & Kalaska, J. F. (1984). Static spatial effects in motor cortex and area 5: Quantitative relations in a two-dimensional space. *Experimental Brain Research, 54*, 446–454.

Ghazanfar, A. A., Maier, J. X., Hoffman, K. L., & Logothetis, N. K. (2005). Multisensory integration of dynamic faces and voices in rhesus monkey auditory cortex. *Journal of Neuroscience, 25*, 5004–5012.

Ghazanfar, A. A., & Schroeder, C. E. (2006). Is neocortex essentially multisensory? *Trends in Cognitive Sciences, 10*, 278–285.

Gray, C. M., Konig, P., Engel, A. K., & Singer, W. (1989). Oscillatory responses in cat visual cortex exhibit inter-columnar synchronization which reflects global stimulus properties. *Nature, 338*, 334–337.

Graziano, M. S. (1999). Where is my arm? The relative role of vision and proprioception in the neuronal representation of limb position. *Proceedings of the National Academy of Sciences USA, 96*, 10418–10421.

Graziano, M. S., Cooke, D. F., & Taylor, C. S. (2000). Coding the location of the arm by sight. *Science, 290*, 1782–1786.

Graziano, M. S., & Gross, C. G. (1993). A bimodal map of space: Somatosensory receptive fields in the macaque putamen with corresponding visual receptive fields. *Experimental Brain Research, 97*, 96–109.

Graziano, M. S., & Gross, C. G. (1996). Multiple pathways for processing visual space. In T. Inui & J. L. McClelland (Eds.), *Attention and performance XVI* (pp. 181–207). Cambridge, MA: MIT Press.

Graziano, M. S., Gross, C. G., Taylor, C. S. R., & Moore, T. (2004). Multisensory neurons for the control of defensive movements. In G. Calvert, C. Spence, & B. E. Stein (Eds.), *The handbook of multisensory processes* (pp. 443–452). Cambridge, MA: MIT Press.

Graziano, M. S., Hu, X. T., & Gross, C. G. (1997). Visuospatial properties of ventral premotor cortex. *Journal of Neurophysiology, 77*, 2268–2292.

Graziano, M. S., Yap, G. S., & Gross, C. G. (1994). Coding of visual space by premotor neurons. *Science, 266*, 1054–1057.

Groh, J. M., & Sparks, D. L. (1996). Saccades to somatosensory targets. III. Eye-position-dependent somatosensory activity in primate superior colliculus. *Journal of Neurophysiology, 75*, 439–453.

Gu, Y., Angelaki, D. E., & DeAngelis, G. C. (2008). Neural correlates of multisensory cue integration in macaque MSTd. *Nature Neuroscience, 11*, 1201–1210.

Harris, C. M., & Wolpert, D. M. (1998). Signal-dependent noise determines motor planning. *Nature, 394*, 780–784.

Hogan, N., & Flash, T. (1987). Moving gracefully - quantitative theories of motor coordination. *Trends in Neurosciences, 10,* 170–174.

Hoshi, E., & Tanji, J. (2000). Integration of target and body-part information in the premotor cortex when planning action. *Nature, 408,* 466–470.

Hoshi, E., & Tanji, J. (2002). Contrasting neuronal activity in the dorsal and ventral premotor areas during preparation to reach. *Journal of Neurophysiology, 87,* 1123–1128.

Humphrey, D. R., & Schmidt, E. M. (1990). Extracellular single-unit recording methods. In A. A. Boulton, G. B. Baker, & C. H. Vanderwolf (Eds.), *Neurophysiological techniques: Applications to neural systems* (pp. 1–59). Clifton, NJ: Humana Press.

Jordan, M. I., & Rumelhart, D. E. (1992). Forward models: Supervised learning with a distal teacher. *Cognitive Science, 16,* 307–354.

Kettner, R. E., Schwartz, A. B., & Georgopoulos, A. P. (1988). Primate motor cortex and free arm movements to visual targets in three-dimensional space. III. Positional gradients and population coding of movement direction from various movement origins. *Journal of Neuroscience, 8,* 2938–2947.

Lacquaniti, F., Guigon, E., Bianchi, L., Ferraina, S., & Caminiti, R. (1995). Representing spatial information for limb movement: Role of area 5 in the monkey. *Cerebral Cortex, 5,* 391–409.

Lakatos, P., Chen, C. M., O'Connell, M. N., Mills, A., & Schroeder, C. E. (2007). Neuronal oscillations and multisensory interaction in primary auditory cortex. *Neuron, 53,* 279–292.

Lakatos, P., Shah, A. S., Knuth, K. H., Ulbert, I., Karmos, G., & Schroeder, C. E. (2005). An oscillatory hierarchy controlling neuronal excitability and stimulus processing in the auditory cortex. *Journal of Neurophysiology, 94,* 1904–1911.

Liu, J., & Newsome, W. T. (2006). Local field potential in cortical area MT: Stimulus tuning and behavioral correlations. *Journal of Neuroscience, 26,* 7779–7790.

Logothetis, N. K., Guggenberger, H., Peled, S., & Pauls, J. (1999). Functional imaging of the monkey brain. *Nature Neuroscience, 2,* 555–562.

Logothetis, N. K., Pauls, J., Oeltermann, A., Trinath, T., & Augath, M. (2000). The relationship of LFPS, MUA and SUA to the BOLD fMRI signal. *Proceedings of the Society for Neuroscience, 26,* 820.

Ma, W. J., & Pouget, A. (2008). Linking neurons to behavior in multisensory perception: A computational review. *Brain Research, 1242,* 4–12.

MacKay, W. A., & Riehle, A. (1992). Planning a reach: Spatial analysis by area 7a neurons. In G. Stelmach & J. Requin (Eds.), *Tutorials in motor behavior 2.* New York, NY: Elsevier.

Maier, J. X., Chandrasekaran, C., & Ghazanfar, A. A. (2008). Integration of bimodal looming signals through neuronal coherence in the temporal lobe. *Current Biology, 18,* 963–968.

Maier, J. X., Neuhoff, J. G., Logothetis, N. K., & Ghazanfar, A. A. (2004). Multisensory integration of looming signals by Rhesus monkeys. *Neuron, 43,* 177–181.

Mazzoni, P., Bracewell, R. M., Barash, S., & Andersen, R. A. (1996). Spatially tuned auditory responses in area LIP of macaques performing delayed memory saccades to acoustic targets. *Journal of Neurophysiology, 75,* 1233–1241.

McIntyre, J., Stratta, F., & Lacquaniti, F. (1997). Viewer-centered frame of reference for pointing to memorized targets in three-dimensional space. *Journal of Neurophysiology, 78,* 1601–1618.

McIntyre, J., Stratta, F., & Lacquaniti, F. (1998). Short-term memory for reaching to visual targets: Psychophysical evidence for body-centered reference frames. *Journal of Neuroscience, 18,* 8423–8435.

Meredith, M. A., Nemitz, J. W., & Stein, B. E. (1987). Determinants of multisensory integration in superior colliculus neurons. I. Temporal factors. *Journal of Neuroscience, 7,* 3215–3229.

Mitzdorf, U. (1985). Current source-density method and application in cat cerebral cortex: Investigation of evoked potentials and EEG phenomena. *Physiological Reviews, 65,* 37–100.

Monosov, I. E., Trageser, J. C., & Thompson, K. G. (2008). Measurements of simultaneously recorded spiking activity and local field potentials suggest that spatial selection emerges in the frontal eye field. *Neuron, 57,* 614–625.

Morgan, M. L., DeAngelis, G. C., & Angelaki, D. E. (2008). Multisensory integration in macaque visual cortex depends on cue reliability. *Neuron, 59,* 662–673.

Nielsen, K. J., Logothetis, N. K., & Rainer, G. (2006). Dissociation between local field potentials and spiking activity in macaque inferior temporal cortex reveals diagnosticity-based encoding of complex objects. *Journal of Neuroscience, 26,* 9639–9645.

Ochiai, T., Mushiake, H., & Tanji, J. (2005). Involvement of the ventral premotor cortex in controlling image motion of the hand during performance of a target-capturing task. *Cerebral Cortex, 15*, 929–937.

Pesaran, B., Nelson, M. J., & Andersen, R. A. (2006). Dorsal premotor neurons encode the relative position of the hand, eye, and goal during reach planning. *Neuron, 51*, 125–134.

Pesaran, B., Pezaris, J. S., Sahani, M., Mitra, P., & Andersen, R. A. (2002). Temporal structure in neuronal activity during working memory in macaque parietal cortex. *Nature Neuroscience, 5*, 805–811.

Pouget, A., Denève, S., & Duhamel, J. R. (2002). A computational perspective on the neural basis of multisensory spatial representations. *Nature Reviews Neuroscience, 3*, 741–747.

Sanes, J. N., & Donoghue, J. P. (1993). Oscillations in local-field potentials of the primate motor cortex during voluntary movement. *Proceedings of the National Academy of Sciences USA, 90*, 4470–4474.

Scherberger, H., Jarvis, M. R., & Andersen, R. A. (2005). Cortical local field potential encodes movement intentions in the posterior parietal cortex. *Neuron, 46*, 347–354.

Schroeder, C. E., Lindsley, R. W., Specht, C., Marcovici, A., Smiley, J. F., & Javitt, D. C. (2001). Somatosensory input to auditory association cortex in the macaque monkey. *Journal of Neurophysiology, 85*, 1322–1327.

Schwartz, A. B., Moran, D. W., & Reina, G. A. (2004). Differential representation of perception and action in the frontal cortex. *Science, 303*, 380–383.

Scott, S. H., Sergio, L. E., & Kalaska, J. F. (1997). Reaching movements with similar hand paths but different arm orientations. II. Activity of individual cells in dorsal premotor cortex and parietal area 5. *Journal of Neurophysiology, 78*, 2413–2426.

Shi, Y., & Buneo, C. A. (2009, October). *Integration of somatic and visual cues for arm position in the posterior parietal cortex.* Program No. 355.28, 2009 Neuroscience Meeting Planner, Chicago, IL: Society for Neuroscience. Online.

Soechting, J. F., Buneo, C. A., Herrmann, U., & Flanders, M. (1995). Moving effortlessly in 3-dimensions: Does Donder's law apply to arm movement. *Journal of Neuroscience, 15*, 6271–6280.

Stanford, T. R., Quessy, S., & Stein, B. E. (2005). Evaluating the operations underlying multisensory integration in the cat superior colliculus. *Journal of Neuroscience, 25*, 6499–6508.

Stanford, T. R., & Stein, B. E. (2007). Superadditivity in multisensory integration: Putting the computation in context. *Neuroreport, 18*, 787–792.

Stein, B. E., & Stanford, T. R. (2008). Multisensory integration: Current issues from the perspective of the single neuron. *Nature Reviews Neuroscience, 9*, 255–266.

Stricanne, B., Andersen, R. A., & Mazzoni, P. (1996). Auditory signals are transformed to eye-centered coordinates in posterior parietal cortex. *Journal of Neurophysiology, 76*, 2071–2075.

Sugihara, T., Diltz, M. D., Averbeck, B. B., & Romanski, L. M. (2006). Integration of auditory and visual communication information in the primate ventrolateral prefrontal cortex. *Journal of Neuroscience, 26*, 11138–11147.

Thier, P., & Andersen, R. A. (1998). Electrical microstimulation distinguishes distinct saccade-related areas in the posterior parietal cortex. *Journal of Neurophysiology, 80*, 1713–1735.

Uno, Y., Kawato, M., & Suzuki, R. (1989). Formation and control of optimal trajectory in human multijoint arm movement. Minimum torque-change model. *Biological Cybernetics, 61*, 89–101.

van Beers, R. J., Sittig, A. C., & van der Gon, J. J. D. (1998). The precision of proprioceptive position sense. *Experimental Brain Research, 122*, 367–377.

van Beers, R. J., Wolpert, D. M., & Haggard, P. (2002). When feeling is more important than seeing in sensorimotor adaptation. *Current Biology, 12*, 834–837.

# CHAPTER 18

# Computational Models of Multisensory Integration in the Cat Superior Colliculus

*Benjamin A. Rowland, Barry E. Stein, and Terrence R. Stanford*

The ability to orient rapidly and accurately toward potentially important environmental events is essential for survival. The superior colliculus (SC), a midbrain structure serving this function, is highly conserved across species and is a principal site where sensory inputs are translated into the motor commands required to orient the eyes, ears, head, and/or body toward salient stimuli (for reviews, see Hall & Moschovakis, 2004; Sparks & Jay, 1986; Stein, 1984; Stein & Meredith 1993; Vanegas, 1984). Neurons within the deep layers of the SC are multisensory and respond to visual, auditory, and somatosensory stimuli located within similar circumscribed regions of space, forming overlapping topographic sensory maps. These sensory maps are in register with corresponding motor maps that move the eyes, ears, head, and body. As a result, sensory events will activate a region of the SC and initiate a motor response that orients the animal to it. This organization is elegant in its simplicity.

Understanding the biophysical bases of how the SC integrates inputs from multiple sensory modalities can give us insight into how the brain has evolved to solve the problems inherent in multisensory integration. Here we summarize four theoretical models that provide different perspectives on multisensory integration in the SC and compare their predictions to empirical data to complement the more theoretical approaches to understanding this phenomenon described in other chapters (see Chapters 2, 10, and 13).

Activity at different loci within the SC sensory maps can be conceptualized as competitors for access to a motor apparatus that is able to produce only one movement vector at a time (Arai, McPeek, & Keller, 2004; Horwitz & Newsome, 2001; Kim & Basso, 2008; McPeek & Keller, 2001, 2004). Although the exact mechanisms for resolving this competition are unknown, evidence suggests that greater levels of activity at certain loci, or greater increases in the amount of activity, increase the likelihood of a motor response being initiated to that location (Carello & Krauzlis, 2004; McPeek & Keller, 2004). Theoretically, the simultaneous activation of independent modality-specific inputs to a multisensory neuron should evoke more activity than when either channel alone is active; that is, multisensory neurons should respond more vigorously to a cross-modal stimulus than to either of its modality-specific components (see Stanford, Quessy, & Stein, 2005). This has been observed empirically, is called "multisensory enhancement" (Meredith & Stein, 1983), and is a typical feature of multisensory neurons in the SC: Spatially and temporally concordant sensory cues (e.g., auditory and visual) usually evoke significantly more impulses than does a single-modality stimulus alone (Meredith & Stein, 1986a, b). Conversely, when the same two stimuli are presented at disparate locations, such that one lies beyond the (excitatory) receptive field, the stimulus within the receptive field often evokes significantly fewer impulses than if it had been presented alone—a phenomenon termed "multisensory depression" (Kadunce, Vaughan, Wallace, Benedek, & Stein, 1997; Meredith & Stein 1983). These physiological observations are paralleled in SC-mediated orientation behaviors: Spatiotemporally concordant cross-modal stimuli generate more accurate responses than the constituent modality-specific stimuli, and spatially disparate but synchronous cross-modal stimuli generate less accurate responses (Stein, Huneycutt, & Meredith, 1988).

The basic computational principles underlying multisensory enhancement and depression are simple and intuitive: When integrating two sensory estimates of the location of an event, responses are more robust when their actual locations are concordant and less robust when they are discordant. However, the underlying computations and biophysical bases of this phenomenon are unknown and can potentially be quite complicated. Any number of mathematical operations (e.g., summation, multiplication) could produce enhancement, and while simple competitive interactions (e.g., lateral inhibition) might be the basis for multisensory depression, the substrate for this is currently unknown.

## BIOLOGICALLY INSPIRED MODELS OF MULTISENSORY INTEGRATION

While the essential multisensory phenomena have been well characterized in both behavior and physiology, the biophysical computations that underlie multisensory integration are poorly understood. Recently, however, there have been a number of attempts to model multisensory integration on the basis of findings from single neurons in the cat SC (Anastasio, Patton, & Belkacem-Boussaid, 2000; Patton & Anastasio, 2003; Rowland, Stanford, & Stein, 2007). The wealth of data from the cat SC provides a number of specific biological constraints that favor some model elements and preclude others. Primary among these are two key empirical observations. The first, termed "inverse effectiveness," refers to the fact that the magnitude of multisensory enhancement is inversely proportional to the efficacies of the modality-specific stimuli that compose the cross-modal event (Meredith & Stein, 1986b; Stein, Stanford, Ramachandran, Perrault, & Rowland, 2009). Functionally, the concept of inverse effectiveness suggests that the benefits of multisensory integration should be greatest when weakly effective cues are combined and increasingly less pronounced as the modality-specific cues themselves become more salient. This has been observed empirically (Fig. 18.1). Behavioral manifestations of inverse effectiveness have been observed for both stimulus detection and reaction time in many species (Corneil & Munoz, 1996; Frens, Van Opstal, & Van der Willigen, 1995; Gielen, Schmidt, & Van den Heuvel, 1983; Goldring, Dorris, Corneil, Ballantyne, & Munoz, 1996; Hughes, Reuter-Lorenz, Nozawa, & Fendrich, 1994; Jiang, Jiang, & Stein, 2002; Meredith & Stein, 1983; Perrott, Saberi, Brown, & Strybel, 1990; Wilkinson, Meredith, & Stein, 1996). Mechanistically, inverse effectiveness, and the particular way in which it manifests in the responses of single SC neurons, dictates that specific computational elements be incorporated into any plausible model (see later discussion).

The second and perhaps the most constraining empirical observation for developing a realistic model is that multisensory integration in the cat SC is dependent on input from particular regions of the ipsilateral association cortex, the anterior ectosylvian sulcus (AES), and the rostrolateral suprasylvian sulcus (rLS). Behaviorally, when AES and rLS are temporarily deactivated, ablated, or even ablated early in development, animals fail to show substantially enhanced orienting performance to coincident visual-auditory stimuli, despite retaining the ability to see and hear stimuli at each location (Jiang et al., 2002; Wilkinson et al., 1996). These behavioral observations are paralleled by neurophysiological observations: Deactivating these regions eliminates SC multisensory enhancement in single SC neurons (Alvarado, Stanford, Rowland, Vaughan, & Stein, 2009; Alvarado, Vaughan, Stanford, & Stein, 2007; Jiang, Wallace, Jiang, Vaughan, & Stein, 2001; Stein, Wallace,

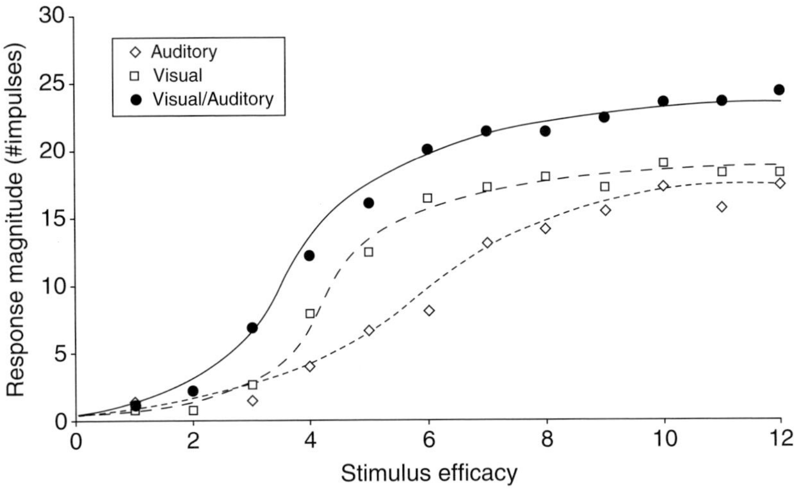


**Figure 18.1** A visual-auditory neuron showing multisensory enhancement. This neuron was stimulated with visual, auditory, and visual-auditory stimuli with different intensities (x-axis). The response of this neuron to each stimulus is presented on the y-axis. Spatiotemporally concordant cross-modal stimuli evoked larger responses than component modality-specific stimuli. (From Perrault, Vaughan, Stein, and Wallace (2005); used with permission.)

Stanford, & Jiang, 2002). Crucially, however, multisensory enhancement is abolished without eliminating the SC neuron's capacity to respond to each of its modality-specific inputs; that is, the SC neuron remains multisensory, but it loses the ability to integrate inputs from the different senses. As discussed later in this chapter, implementing this dependence of multisensory integration on this broader cortico-collicular circuit into a biologically plausible model is nontrivial.

## FOUR SPECIFIC MODELS OF SC MULTISENSORY INTEGRATION

Here we describe four models. Each model endeavors to account for essential characteristics of multisensory integration within the SC. Models 1–3 are analytical models, each incorporating elements of the former but also evolving in an attempt to better incorporate the aforementioned empirical observations to explain multisensory enhancement. Model 4, a network model, incorporates the same key empirical observations as does Model 3, but with an entirely different implementation and also accounts for multisensory depression. The key features of each model, along with the insights and physiological predictions they provide, are discussed in turn in the sections that follow.

### Model 1: A Quasilinear Model

The most intuitive model to assume of any circuit for multisensory integration is that it behaves in an almost linear fashion; that is, the receiving neuron simply sums its inputs and passes this sum through some transfer function (e.g., linear, sigmoidal) to produce its output (Fig. 18.2). The empirical results showing that multisensory integration is nonlinearly dependent on inputs from AES suggests that such a model cannot explain the empirical observations of multisensory integration in the SC.

***Details*** Assume that a bisensory neuron receives input from four sources: visual and auditory inputs from upstream, non-AES areas ($V_u$ and $A_u$) and their modality-matched inputs from the downstream AES ($V_d$ and $A_d$). Each input is taken to represent the net input from topographically aligned populations in each respective region and is assigned an analog value

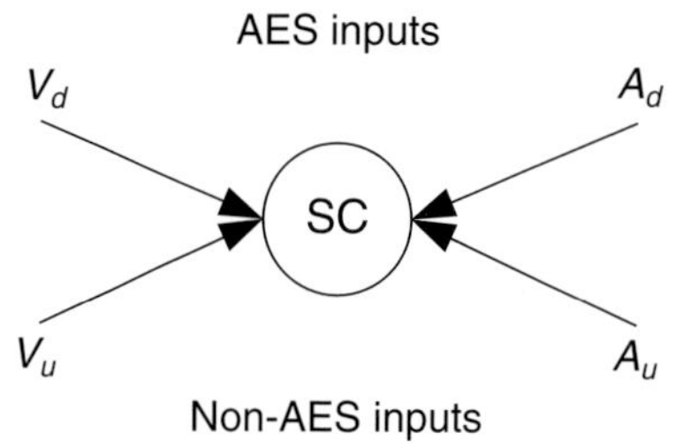


**Figure 18.2** A quasi-linear model in which a single SC neuron receives visual ($V$) and auditory ($A$) input from AES-derived ($V_d$, $A_d$) and non-AES ($V_u$, $A_u$) sources. The neuron simply sums up its net input and passes the result through a sigmoidal nonlinearity.

that represents its strength or efficacy. High input values correspond to strong or potent stimuli, whereas very low values are assigned to simulate weak or absent stimuli (i.e., to model spontaneous activity). If a neuron $k$ simply sums its inputs and transduces them to an output using a sigmoidal transfer function, the equation describing its output is simply:

$$O_k = S(V_u + A_u + V_d + A_d, \alpha, \gamma, \phi), \tag{18.1}$$

$$S(x, a, b, c) = \frac{a}{1 + \exp(b(-x - c))}, \tag{18.2}$$

where $\alpha$, $\gamma$, and $\phi$ act as scaling parameters in this equation.

***Insights*** Though simple, this model can account for some of the key physiological properties of SC multisensory neurons. In particular, the model produces both multisensory enhancement and inverse effectiveness. Inverse effectiveness is implemented by the sigmoidal transfer function, which is initially supralinear and transitions to sublinear with increasing values of input. As a result, the response to combinations of weak, near-threshold unisensory inputs is generally superadditive, whereas those to stronger stimulus combinations tend toward subadditivity. Though successful at accounting for some important features of SC multisensory integration, the model fails to capture the effects of AES deactivation; when either or both (auditory, visual) AES inputs are removed, the model's behavior does not change substantially. Both the unisensory and multisensory responses are reduced by the same magnitude, but multisensory enhancement is still evident and has in fact increased in proportionate magnitude. Thus, a simple linear model, which treats all inputs equally regardless of their source (e.g., AES, non-AES) does not have provision for altering multisensory enhancement independent of unisensory responsiveness.

### Model 2: A Modulation Model

The model of Patton and Anastasio (2003) represents a significant evolution and has a great amount of explanatory power in describing SC multisensory integration (see Anastasio et al., 2000; Patton & Anastasio, 2003). Another benefit of this model is that it specifies how its underlying architecture may be formed by unsupervised learning rules during development (see also Anastasio, 2009). The essential insight of this model is that the cortex-dependent nature of multisensory integration in the SC may be thought of in the context of gain modulation. The fundamental assumption of this Modulation Model is that descending inputs from AES form close relationships with inputs derived from other areas that carry signals belonging to a different sensory modality. Thus, for example, a visual input from AES might make a close contact with an auditory input from the inferior colliculus, or an auditory input from AES might make a close contact with an input from a primary visual area (Fig. 18.3). Critically, the AES inputs in this model function as modulators, meaning that they act to change the strength (i.e., the synaptic weight) of the non-AES inputs. When simulating a response to a cross-modal stimulus, each input is activated, and the cortical modulation inputs provide an additional "boost" to the ascending inputs that they contact. Removal of the modulators also removes their enhancing influence.

***Details*** In this model, individual SC neurons receive input from multiple "primary" (i.e., non-AES) and "modulatory" (i.e., AES)

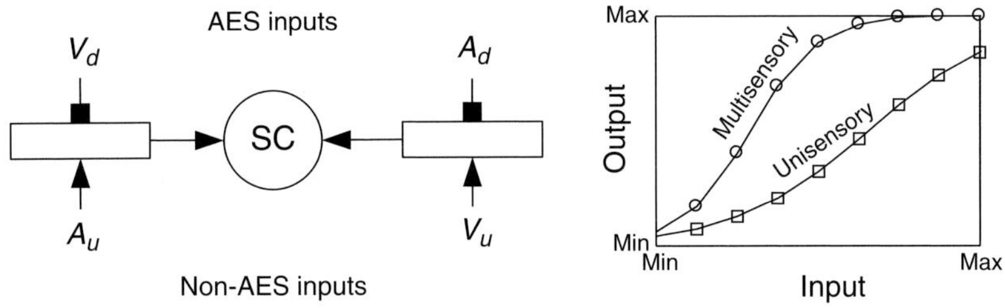


**Figure 18.3** A schematic of a modulation model in which a single SC neuron receives input from multiple sensory sources (conventions the same as Fig. 18.2). The AES inputs are drawn with square connectors to indicate that they modulate the activity of the non-AES input with which they are matched. These matches are established between AES inputs and non-AES inputs derived from different sensory modalities. The unisensory and multisensory responses (assuming that unisensory inputs had equivalent efficacy) are displayed on the right.

inputs. Using the aforementioned conventions, the value of each primary input ($V_u$, $A_u$) and modulatory input ($V_d$, $A_d$) is the sum ($r$) of 20 binary random inputs, where the probability that each variable takes value 1 is $p_{Ix}$. This probability varies depending on whether the input is primary or modulatory, and whether it is driven (by a sensory source of its specific modality) or spontaneous (not driven). For simplicity the individual inputs are assumed to be independent, and the probability that an input takes a specific value $r$ is binomially distributed. The binomial distribution is used only for convenience. Expressed mathematically, each input $I_x$ (where $I$ is either $V$ or $A$, and $x$ is either $u$ or $d$, indicating non-AES ["up"] sources or AES-derived ["down"] sources) is defined according to the associated probability of activation ($p_{Ix}$) as follows:

$$P[I_x = r] = \frac{20!}{r!(20-r)!} p_{Ix}^r (1 - p_{Ix})^{20-r}. \tag{18.3}$$

Spontaneous activity (present in channels in which no stimulus is presented) is modeled with low activation rates. The output of a single neuron $k$ in the SC ($O_k$) is calculated by summing the net input and passing the result through a sigmoid function,

$$O_k = S\left(\sum_j w_{kj} x_j, \alpha, \gamma, \phi\right), \tag{18.4}$$

where the sigmoid function $S(\ldots)$ is defined above (Eq. 18.2), $w_{kj}$ is the weight of the connection from non-AES input unit $j$ to SC unit $k$, and $x_j$ represents the input units activity. The activity of AES inputs is seen in the computation of this weight value,

$$w_{kj} = u_{kj} + \sum_i v_{ijk} y_i, \tag{18.5}$$

where $u_{kj}$ is the unmodulated weight of this connection, $y_i$ represents the activity of AES input $i$, and $v_{ijk}$ represents the strength of the modulation. As a consequence, AES afferents modulate non-AES inputs that are derived from different sensory sources.

***Insights*** Like the linear model, this model produces multisensory enhancement with superadditive, additive, and subadditive regions, with weakly effective stimuli typically generating superadditive integration and strongly effective stimuli generating subadditive integration (i.e., inverse effectiveness). Here, multisensory enhancement is attributable to the nonlinear nature of the transfer function and the nonlinear, multiplicative interaction between non-AES inputs and AES inputs from different sensory modalities. When the cortical deactivation is simulated by removing the modulatory influence of AES, the enhancement effect of the AES on non-AES inputs is lost because of the loss of the "boost" provided by their multiplicative interaction. The multisensory response magnitude is substantially reduced as a consequence, and at the lowest stimulus efficacy values multisensory enhancement is eliminated.

### Model 3: A Synergy Model

The model of Rowland, Stanford, and Stein (2007) follows the work of Patton and Anastasio (2003) but begins with a different premise, which is that the AES inputs do not directly target SC inputs derived from other sources in a cross-modal fashion (e.g., an AES visual projection onto a non-AES auditory input), but rather target each other by forming close contacts (i.e., clustering) on the membranes of their recipient SC neurons (Fig. 18.4). In this model, the AES inputs to an SC neuron are computationally segregated from inputs from other sources by having different dendritic target regions. The model assumes both AMPA and NMDA receptors are present in every dendritic region, and it assumes that as a consequence inputs clustering in the same region interact nonlinearly. AES inputs from different sensory modalities are presumed to target proximal dendrites, and so the currents and membrane potential changes they introduce affect one another to produce a nonlinear amplification. The non-AES inputs are computationally segregated from one another and other inputs because they contact distal dendrites, whose smaller diameter is assumed to limit interactions. The net consequence is that inputs derived from different AES subregions interact synergistically through AMPA and NMDA receptors on their SC targets, but inputs from non-AES sources do not. The final critical component of this model is that all inputs also contact a population of inhibitory interneurons, which also project to SC multisensory neurons. This configuration causes the output of the SC neuron to be dependent on the balance of excitation delivered directly by excitatory afferents (amplified within the neuron) and the offsetting shunting inhibition carried by the population of inhibitory interneurons.

***Details*** Originally the authors provided an algebraic form of the model that makes the relationships between the presumed underlying computations and the model behavior simple and obvious. They also reduced a bisensory neuron to a four-compartment architecture in which one compartment represents proximal areas of its dendrites receiving converging input from multiple modality-specific AES subregions;

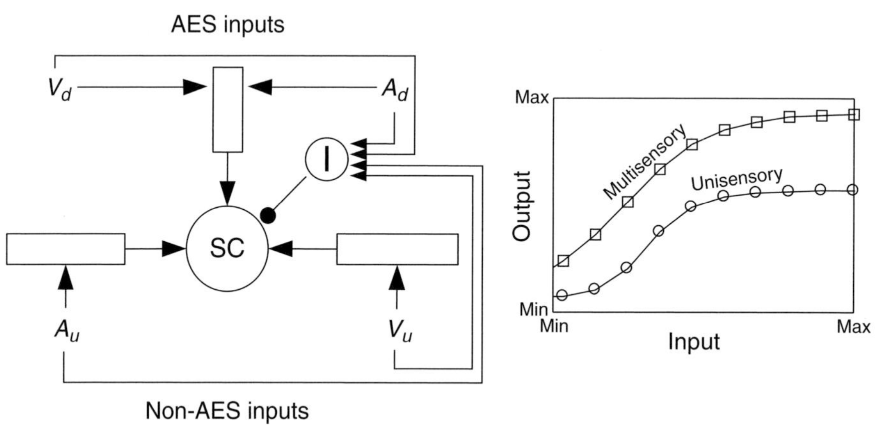


**Figure 18.4** Schematic of a model of SC multisensory integration based on synergy between AES inputs (conventions the same as Fig. 18.2). All inputs project to the SC multisensory output neuron and to a common population of inhibitory interneurons ($I$), which project inhibitory connections to the output neuron (drawn with a closed circle to indicate inhibition). Each dendritic compartment (rectangles) implements a nonlinear sigmoidal function on its inputs. The inhibition is applied at the somatic compartment (circle). The unisensory and multisensory responses are displayed on the right.

two compartments represent dendritic regions that each receive input from a different non-AES sensory region; and a fourth compartment that represents the soma, which sums all of these inputs and implements the neuron's transfer function. The authors assumed the transfer function to be a nonsaturating logarithmic function in the range of sensory responses. Each dendritic compartment sums its inputs and passes the sum through a nonlinear transfer function, which is assumed to be quadratic when stimulus efficacy is weak. The quadratic transfer function for each dendritic compartment is an appropriate model for the transform implemented by clusters of AMPA and NMDA receptors at low input levels. These assumptions permit algebraic simplifications that demonstrate the model's effectiveness in replicating empirical results, although it requires strict limitations on the scaling of input values (e.g., their values must be between 1 and 2). The equation describing the output of SC neuron $k$ in the model is

$$O_k = \theta \log \left[ \phi (V_u^2 + A_u^2 + (V_d + A_d)^2) / (V_u + A_u + V_d + A_d) \right], \tag{18.6}$$

where $\theta$ and $\phi$ are scaling parameters. A more sophisticated version of this model would combine the constraints regarding the scaling of input values and the quadratic dendritic transfer functions into a saturating transfer function for each dendrite. This form of the model produces equivalent results as the aforementioned, but it is slightly more advanced:

$$O_k = \theta \log \left[ \phi \frac{\left( \begin{array}{l} (1+S(V_u,\alpha,\beta,\gamma)) \\ +(1+S(A_u,\alpha,\beta,\gamma)) \\ +2(1+S(V_d+A_d,\alpha,\beta,\gamma)) \end{array} \right)}{\left( \begin{array}{l} (1+S(V_u)+1 \\ +S(A_u)+1+S(V_d) \\ +1+S(A_d)) \end{array} \right)} \right]. \tag{18.7}$$

***Insights*** When the circuit is intact, this model produces the same response trends and relationships as the Modulation Model mentioned earlier, although its architecture relies on fundamentally different assumptions regarding the underlying anatomy and physiology. It diverges from the Modulation Model in that the multisensory response does not saturate at the same level as the unisensory response, which is a closer match to the available physiological data. Similarly, when cortex is deactivated, the unisensory and multisensory responses become nearly equivalent over the entire dynamic range. This too matches the physiological data. The model makes one additional prediction, that deactivation of only a single unisensory subregion of the AES would be sufficient to eliminate multisensory integration. This prediction is consistent with some very recent empirical findings (Alvarado et al., 2009).

### Model 4: A Network Model

The model of Cuppini, Ursino, Magosso, Rowland, and Stein (2009) involves an architecture in which the SC and each of its inputs are represented by topographically organized (one-dimensional) arrays of units. Within each input array, competitive interactions result in a shaped population response that is approximately Gaussian (Fig. 18.5). Each input array projects to both the SC array in a topographic fashion (resulting in overlapping topographic maps) and also several distinct populations of interneurons, which selectively project to each other and to the SC multisensory neurons. This projection scheme produces a balance of excitation, inhibition, and disinhibition (through interneuron interactions) that determines the responses of SC neurons. Like the synergy model described earlier, this model also includes an assumption that AMPA and NMDA receptors are present on SC neurons, AES and non-AES inputs are computationally segregated on the dendrites of SC neurons, and non-AES inputs derived from different sensory modalities are also segregated from each other. Critical to this model is the assumption that, when intact, the AES almost completely controls the activity of SC neurons, muting the non-AES inputs by virtue of its strong inhibitory influence. In this respect, the model represents an architecture in which the AES has evolved to subsume the functions previously

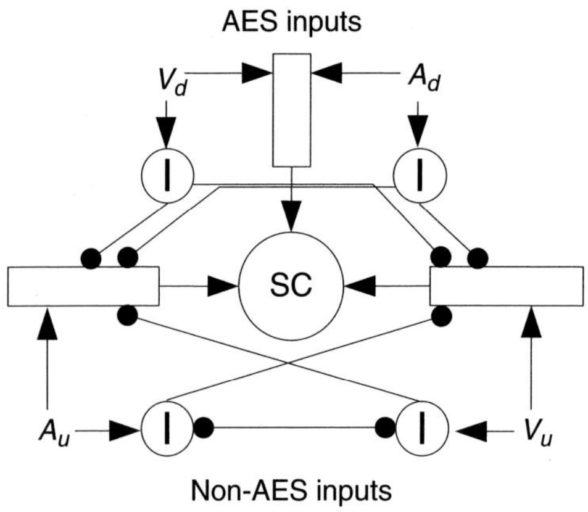


**Figure 18.5** Schematic of a network model of SC multisensory integration (all conventions are the same as Fig. 18.2). Input populations are represented as single units, while in reality they are topographically organized arrays of units. AES inputs contact dendrites of the SC multisensory output neuron directly and also inhibitory interneuron populations which specifically send inhibitory input to the dendritic compartments (rectangles) stimulated by non-AES inputs. Non-AES inputs target different dendritic compartments as well as their own subsets of the interneuron populations. Interneuron populations contacted by the non-AES inputs inhibit one another and the dendritic compartments contacted by excitatory non-AES inputs of other sensory modalities.

implemented by non-AES inputs. Only in the absence of AES input (e.g., when AES is deactivated) are the influences of non-AES inputs seen on multisensory SC neurons. Non-AES inputs are functionally engaged in a type of "winner-take-all" competition due to their computational segregation on the dendrites of SC neurons and the interaction between the inhibitory interneuron populations contacted by each.

***Details*** In the model, each SC output unit receives input from multiple units in topographically organized areas representing AES and non-AES sources and populations of inhibitory interneurons that also receive input from those regions. The output of each unit in the network (including those belonging to the input, interneuron, and SC output populations) is computed by numerical simulation of a differential equation with an associated time constant and forcing function represented by its net input. In other words, the net input to unit $k(Z_k)$ is transformed to its output $(O_k)$ using the following equation:

$$\tau \frac{\partial O_k}{\partial t} = -O_k + S(Z_k, \alpha, \gamma, \beta), \qquad (18.8)$$

where $\tau$ is a time constant.

Each input unit is simulated as having a spatially restricted Gaussian receptive field that shares some overlap with those of their neighbors. Additionally, input units extend lateral inhibitory influences to other neurons in their originating area. The net effect of this arrangement is that a given stimulus generates a pattern of population activity in each sensitive input region that is shaped like a "Mexican hat" function.

There are four distinct populations of interneurons, each receiving their (weighted) excitatory input from a different sensory source (i.e., $V_u$, $A_u$, $V_d$, and $A_d$). The interneurons receiving excitatory input from AES sources receive input from only their respective sources and project to inhibit areas of the multisensory neuron receiving excitatory input from non-AES sources. Interneurons receiving input from non-AES sources project to inhibit each other as well. In this way, inhibitory influences driven by AES sources tend to silence the effects of inputs from non-AES sources when active. When not active, inhibitory influences from non-AES sources tend to select one or the other channel to provide the primary excitatory activity to the SC.

Multisensory output neurons in the SC receive excitatory sensory inputs from AES and non-AES sources, from each other, and from the various and multiple interneuron populations. The weights connecting each area are arranged in topographic format, so that units responding to the same areas of space are likely to be coactivated, while units responding to different areas of space are likely to compete with one another for activation. Each neuron is modeled as composed of four compartments, one receiving only AES input, two receiving excitatory input from either the visual or auditory non-AES areas, and a fourth representing the soma. The compartment receiving input from different subregions of AES is not inhibited. However, each compartment receiving input from a non-AES source is inhibited by both interneuron populations receiving input from AES and the interneuron population receiving input from the non-AES source representing the other sensory modality. For example, the compartment receiving excitatory input from the non-AES visual channel receives inhibitory input from the interneuron populations responding to the AES visual channel, the AES auditory channel, and the non-AES auditory channel. The multisensory output neurons also interact with one another via lateral connections. The strength of these influences obeys a Mexican Hat function.

***Insights*** When the full circuit is intact, the behavior of this model is equivalent to that of the single-neuron models described earlier. Furthermore, when simulating the effects of AES deactivation, the model behaves similarly to the Modulation Model. It also produces the same results when a single unisensory subregion of AES is deactivated. However, while the results are similar, the mechanism by which this model implements the dependency of multisensory integration on an apparent synergy between cortico-collicular inputs is fundamentally different. Because AES afferents obscure (via inhibitory interneurons) the influences of modality-specific inputs originating elsewhere, loss of one AES subregion (visual or auditory) is equivalent to the loss of a multisensory signal. The neuron will still respond to the other (i.e., the deactivated) sensory modality when the appropriate stimulus is presented in isolation, however, because the respective non-AES input is intact and the nondeactivated AES input would not be stimulated in that circumstance. When all AES inputs are deactivated, only the influence of non-AES inputs is seen, and their interaction is mutually inhibitory (i.e., competitive) through the interneuron complex.

## NEW DIRECTIONS

Here we have summarized four modeling approaches to the implementation of multisensory integration in the SC. Although each model produces some of the same response patterns, and many of these patterns mimic those seen empirically, they have fundamentally different biophysical assumptions. The presence of multiple possible models not only encourages conceptual creativity, but more important, provides a theoretical basis for future experiments. We now outline the limitations of these models and our current appreciation of the work that needs to be done to come to a consensus regarding the essential biophysical computations that underlie multisensory integration in this circuit.

A principal limitation of each of these models is that, while they attempt to capture the essential biophysical computations underlying multisensory integration, they rely on changes in the responses of SC neurons to different stimulus configurations and infer through them how the inputs must have changed. Obviously there are several neural processing stages that intervene between stimulus transduction and delivery of the signal to the multisensory neuron SC, but the outputs of these multistage transformations that provide the inputs to the model are poorly understood. As a consequence, current modeling efforts must include many assumptions about the inputs. Fortunately, modern technology has provided experimentalists the means to conduct simultaneous recordings from the SC and multiple input regions. Efforts to resolve many of these issues are currently underway.

Another limitation is that most of these modeling efforts have been directed at reproducing the behaviors of a theoretical "canonical neuron": a single set of relationships between presumed inputs and observed outputs derived from the behavior of a large population of observed neurons presented with stimuli tailored to their specific receptive fields. Actual physiological responses are often variable, in ways that the theoretician and empiricist might wish that they were not. The sources of variability are numerous and difficult to control; for example, while a model typically assumes a linear relationship between stimulus intensity and efficacy (i.e., the response of the neuron to the stimulus), this is not always the case because SC neurons appear to have (among other things) contrast-sensitivity response profiles that are nonlinear. A complete, yet succinct model must not only account for the responses of a "canonical" neuron but also for the empirically observed variance in the data.

Another recent empirical finding that impacts the present research is that multisensory enhancement is not uniform over the time course of the response. Rowland and colleagues (Rowland, Quessy, Stanford, & Stein, 2007; Rowland & Stein, 2007, 2008) examined the temporal profile of the multisensory response as compared to the expected unisensory response magnitudes at each moment in time. This study found that superadditive computations were typically evident early in the response, while it was "ramping up" (i.e., when the initial response magnitude was weakest). These superadditive computations were sometimes "washed out" by additive computations found later in the response, so that the entire response reflected an overall additive computation. While this observation is consistent with inverse effectiveness, it also suggests that in cases where the overall computation was found to be superadditive, the "extra impulses" may have been generated during periods of the response when the neuron was responding at or near threshold levels. These observations may breathe new life into continuous-time quasilinear models such as the integrate-and-fire neuron, which, by virtue of their thresholding behavior, permit subthreshold inputs to interact synergistically to evoke impulses when the responses are near threshold. Of course, these observations do not mean that the mechanisms specified in the described models are not also in place (for example, the slow time constant governing the operation of NMDA channels may account for the long windows in which multisensory interactions may occur), nor do they explain the nonlinear dependency of these computations on inputs from AES, but they certainly add a new wrinkle to attempts at deriving the simplest possible computational model to describe SC multisensory integration.

## ACKNOWLEDGMENTS

The authors thank Tom Anastasio for help in revising the manuscript. This work was supported by NIH grants NS036916 and EY016716.

## REFERENCES

Alvarado, J. C., Stanford, T. R., Rowland, B. A., Vaughan, J. W., & Stein, B. E. (2009). Multisensory integration in the superior colliculus requires synergy among corticocollicular inputs. *Journal of Neuroscience, 29*, 6580–6592.

Alvarado, J. C., Vaughan, J. W., Stanford, T. R., & Stein, B. E. (2007). Multisensory versus unisensory integration: Contrasting modes in the superior colliculus. *Journal of Neuroscience, 97*, 3193–3205.

Anastasio, T. J. (2009). *Tutorial on neural systems modeling.* Sunderland, MA: Sinauer.

Anastasio, T. J., Patton, P. E., & Belkacem-Boussaid, K. (2000). Using Bayes rule to model multisensory enhancement in the superior colliculus. *Neural Computation, 12*, 1165–1187.

Arai, K., McPeek, R. M., & Keller, E. L. (2004). Properties of saccadic responses in monkey when multiple competing visual stimuli are present. *Journal of Neurophysiology, 91*, 890–900.

Carello, C. D., & Krauzlis, R. J. (2004). Manipulating intent: Evidence for a causal role of the superior colliculus in target selection. *Neuron, 43*, 575–583.

Corneil, B. D., & Munoz, D. P. (1996). The influence of auditory and visual distractors on human orienting gaze shifts. *Journal of Neuroscience, 16*, 8193–8207.

Cuppini, C., Ursino, M., Magosso, E., Rowland, B. A., & Stein, B. E. (2009). Multisensory integration in superior colliculus (SC) neurons: A computational study. *International Multisensory Research Forum Abstract, 10*, 184.

Frens, M. A., Van Opstal, A. J., & Van der Willigen, R. F. (1995). Spatial and temporal factors determine auditory-visual interactions in human saccadic eye movements. *Perception and Psychophysics, 57*, 802–816.

Gielen, S. C., Schmidt, R. A., & Van den Heuvel, P. J. (1983). On the nature of intersensory facilitation of reaction time. *Perception and Psychophysics, 34,* 161–168.

Goldring, J. E., Dorris, M. C., Corneil, B. D., Ballantyne, P. A., & Munoz, D. P. (1996). Combined eye-head gaze shifts to visual and auditory targets in humans. *Experimental Brain Research, 111,* 68–78.

Hall, W. C., & Moschovakis, A. (2004). *The superior colliculus: New approaches for studying sensorimotor integration.* Boca Raton, FL: CRC Press.

Horwitz, G. D., & Newsome, W. T. (2001). Target selection for saccadic eye movements: Prelude activity in the superior colliculus during a direction-discrimination task. *Journal of Neurophysiology, 86,* 2543–2558.

Hughes, H. C., Reuter-Lorenz, P. A., Nozawa, G., & Fendrich, R. (1994). Visual-auditory interactions in sensorimotor processing: Saccades versus manual responses. *Journal of Experimental Psychology: Human Perception and Performance, 20,* 131–153.

Jiang, W., Jiang, H., & Stein, B. E. (2002). Two corticotectal areas facilitate multisensory orientation behavior. *Journal of Cognitive Neuroscience, 14,* 1240–1255.

Jiang, W., Wallace, M. T., Jiang, H., Vaughan, J. W., & Stein, B. E. (2001). Two cortical areas mediate multisensory integration in superior colliculus neurons. *Journal of Neurophysiology, 85,* 506–522.

Kadunce, D. C., Vaughan, J. W., Wallace, M. T., Benedek, G., & Stein, B. E. (1997). Mechanisms of within- and cross-modality suppression in the superior colliculus. *Journal of Neurophysiology, 78,* 2834–2847.

Kim, B., & Basso, M. A. (2008). Saccade target selection in the superior colliculus: A signal detection theory approach. *Journal of Neuroscience, 28,* 2991–3007.

McPeek, R. M., & Keller, E. L. (2001). Short-term priming, concurrent processing, and saccade curvature during a target selection task in the monkey. *Vision Research, 41,* 785–800.

McPeek, R. M., & Keller, E. L. (2004). Deficits in saccade target selection after inactivation of superior colliculus. *Nature Neuroscience, 7,* 757–763.

Meredith, M. A., & Stein, B. E. (1983). Interactions among converging sensory inputs in the superior colliculus. *Science, 221,* 389–391.

Meredith, M. A., & Stein, B. E. (1986a). Spatial factors determine the activity of multisensory neurons in cat superior colliculus. *Brain Research, 365,* 350–354.

Meredith, M. A., & Stein, B. E. (1986b). Visual, auditory, and somatosensory convergence on cells in superior colliculus results in multisensory integration. *Journal of Neurophysiology, 56,* 640–662.

Patton, P. E., & Anastasio, T. J. (2003). Modeling cross-modal enhancement and modality-specific suppression in multisensory neurons. *Neural Computation, 15,* 783–810.

Perrott, D. R., Saberi, K., Brown, K., & Strybel, T. Z. (1990). Auditory psychomotor coordination and visual search performance. *Perception and Psychophysics, 48,* 214–226.

Rowland, B. A., Quessy, S., Stanford, T. R., & Stein, B. E. (2007). Multisensory integration shortens physiological response latencies. *Journal of Neuroscience, 27,* 5879–5884.

Rowland, B. A., Stanford, T. R., & Stein, B. E. (2007). A model of the neural mechanisms underlying multisensory integration in the superior colliculus. *Perception, 36,* 1431–1443.

Rowland, B. A., & Stein, B. E. (2007). Multisensory integration produces an initial response enhancement. *Frontiers in Integrative Neuroscience, 1,* 4.

Rowland, B. A., & Stein, B. E. (2008). Temporal profiles of response enhancement in multisensory integration. *Frontiers in Neuroscience, 2,* 218–224.

Sparks, D. L., & Jay, M. F. (1986). The functional organization of the primate superior colliculus: A motor perspective. *Progress in Brain Research, 64,* 235–241.

Stanford, T. R., Quessy, S., & Stein, B. E. (2005). Evaluating the operations underlying multisensory integration in the cat superior colliculus. *Journal of Neuroscience, 25,* 6499–6508.

Stein, B. E. (1984). Development of the superior colliculus. *Annual Review of Neuroscience, 7,* 95–125.

Stein, B. E., Huneycutt, W. S., & Meredith, M. A. (1988). Neurons and behavior: The same rules of multisensory integration apply. *Brain Research, 448,* 355–358.

Stein, B. E., & Meredith, M. A. (1993). *The merging of the senses.* Cambridge, MA: The MIT Press.

Stein, B. E., Stanford, T. R., Ramachandran, R., Perrault, T. J., Jr., & Rowland, B. A. (2009). Challenges in quantifying multisensory integration: Alternative criteria, models, and inverse effectiveness. *Experimental Brain Research, 198*, 113–126.

Stein, B. E., Wallace, M. W., Stanford, T. R., & Jiang, W. (2002). Cortex governs multisensory integration in the midbrain. *Neuroscientist, 8*, 306–314.

Vanegas, H. (1984). *Comparative neurology of the optic tectum.* New York, NY: Plenum Press.

Wilkinson, L. K., Meredith, M. A., & Stein, B. E. (1996). The role of anterior ectosylvian cortex in cross-modality orientation and approach behavior. *Experimental Brain Research, 112*, 1–10.

# CHAPTER 19

## Decoding the Cortical Representation of Depth

*Andrew E. Welchman*

Everyday decisions and actions depend on knowledge of the three-dimensional (3D) structure of the environment. To compute robust and reliable estimators of depth, the brain takes advantage of multiple visual cues that are diagnostic of depth structure (Chapter 1) as well as internalized information about the environment's statistics (Chapters 9 and 11). The brain's flexibility in exploiting these signals is remarkable. For example, an observer can gain a vivid impression of depth from both a sparse collection of seemingly random dots (Julesz, 1971; Wallach & O'Connell, 1953) and a flat, pictorially rich painting. This sophistication at the input level (multiple routes to depth) is matched by the range of different behaviors dependent upon depth information (multiple functional outputs). Together, this complexity poses a significant challenge when seeking to investigate empirically the sequence of neural computations that enable depth estimation.

This chapter aims to review advances in elucidating functional specialization for depth processing by the human brain while recognizing the complexity of the problem. I start by discussing the conceptual and methodological challenges faced when investigating the neural circuits that process depth signals. I then review evidence for the specialization of different cortical areas in processing individual depth cues, and finally I discuss work examining the representation of 3D structure from a combination of signals. The tenet of the chapter is that linking functional magnetic resonance imaging (fMRI) recordings with psychophysical measurements provides a strong basis from which to test the cortical representation of 3D structure.

### CONCEPTUALIZING THE FUNCTIONAL ARCHITECTURE OF DEPTH PROCESSING

Evaluating the role played by a particular cortical area in depth estimation necessitates considering what is being processed (i.e., the input), how it is encoded (i.e., the representation) and why it is being processed (i.e., the output). Consider, for example, measuring the neural response when an observer views a disparity-defined shape depicted in a random-dot stereogram. What would this response reveal about the underlying cortical process? In particular, does the response correspond to low-level disparity statistics, an estimate of depth yielded by the disparity cue (but not other cues), or a full estimate of shape based on integrating the available sensory signals with prior knowledge? Moreover, what is the purpose of the representation? Among other things, disparity can be used to break camouflage (Julesz, 1971), estimate albedo (Blake & Bülthoff, 1990), or grasp an object (Watt & Bradshaw, 2002). Thus, does the observed response pertain to a single functional use, a subset of possible tasks, or act as generic representation exploitable for multiple purposes? Managing the complexity of different inputs, representations, and outputs requires a conceptual framework within which to address the problem of depth estimation (Landy, Maloney, Johnston, & Young, 1995).

To conceptualize the cortical organization of depth processing, I will suppose a continuum of scenarios bounded by two unlikely extremes (Fig. 19.1). At one extreme there might be no specialization, with the gamut of different cues (e.g., binocular disparity, motion, perspective, etc.) processed by common, distributed neural circuits followed by outputs to areas specialized for different functional purposes (e.g., control a grasp, judge shape, etc.). At the other extreme, there might be a wholly modular system in which individual depth cues are processed independently and the outputs used opportunistically to perform a given task (e.g., make a judgment of shape). (Note, under both of these schemes, modularity is assumed at the output level in that different functional outputs involve relatively independent neural processes.)

Neither the "distributed" nor the "modular" extreme scenarios would seem satisfactory. An absence of specialization would not benefit from the distinct computational advantages that arise from modularity when dealing with signals subject to different constraints (Marr, 1976). Moreover, the practicalities of simultaneously encoding signals at different spatial scales might make this scheme unwieldy. For example, consider the contrast between texture and disparity. Exploiting texture signals is likely to involve neurons that pool signals from large portions of an image; in contrast, highly localized spatial encoding is often more appropriate for disparity. Accordingly, psychophysical results point to a large degree of independence in the processing of texture and disparity signals (Hillis, Watt, Landy, & Banks, 2004). On the other hand, extreme modular specialization would necessitate redundancy at higher levels of the visual system, whereby similar operations would be performed in parallel at considerable energetic cost. Empirically, there is little evidence to suggest the existence of cortical areas wholly specialized for the processing of a particular depth cue. For example, neurons sensitive to disparity are found throughout visual and parietal cortices (Orban, Janssen, & Vogels, 2006; Parker, 2007) and beyond (Georgieva, Peeters, Kolster, Todd, & Orban, 2009).

The prospect for investigations of depth-cue processing is thus one in which a degree of specialization is expected at the level of individual cues within particular areas (or subareas) of cortex. Moreover, the different functional purposes to which information is put might further differentiate processing. Within this continuum, two different perspectives have

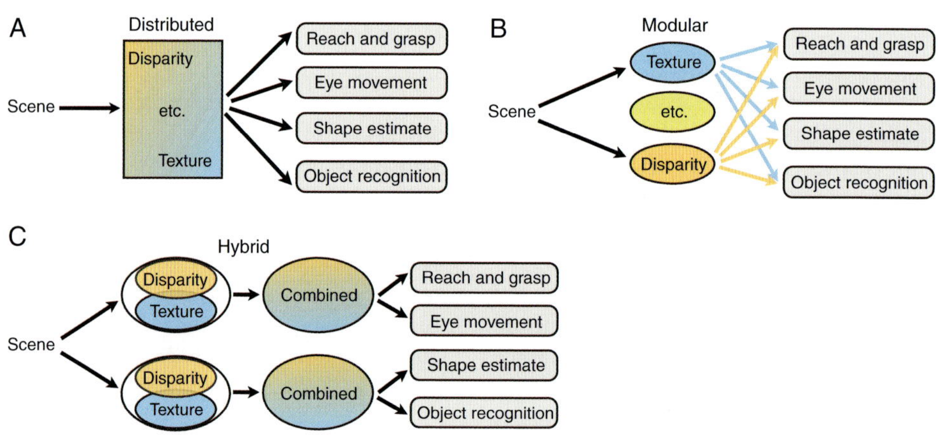


**Figure 19.1** Schematic illustrations of different schemes for the processing of depth signals. (A) and (B) represent the "strong" and "weak" fusion models discussed by Landy et al. (1995). (C) represents a hybrid scenario. Note that modularity is assumed at the output level under all three schemes.

been proposed on the brain's use of disparity signals. One view suggests a relatively early functional distinction between disparity processing in the ventral and dorsal visual streams and proposes that dorsal activity supports action-type behavior (visual orientation and navigation) while ventral processing computes 3D shape (Parker, 2007). The alternative view emphasizes the similarities between cortical responses at the dorsal and ventral ends of the processing streams, and it suggests an important role for interactions between pathways (Orban et al., 2006). The relative scarcity of studies investigating responses to disparity in particular, and other depth cues more generally, means that these approaches are necessarily working hypotheses, rather than strong theories. The challenge for empirical investigation is thus to identify the extent to which functional specialization for particular *(1)* cues and *(2)* tasks is observed.

## OPPORTUNITIES AND CHALLENGES WHEN USING FMRI TO INVESTIGATE DEPTH PROCESSING

In this chapter I focus on the use of fMRI in human adults to provide a valuable technique to link brain activity with the estimation of 3D structure. While fMRI responses are an indirect measure of neural activity and have general limitations (Heeger & Ress, 2002), they offer a promising means of extending understanding of depth processing. Moreover, by integrating psychophysical tasks with concurrent fMRI measures, it is possible to address the challenge of considering both the visual inputs and the behavioral outputs when identifying the cortical networks responsible for depth-cue processing. For instance, ideal-observer methods can be applied that relate trial-by-trial variations in the fMRI signal to variations in perceptual judgments (Chandrasekaran, Canon, Dahmen, Kourtzi, & Welchman, 2007). The approach of integrating neural measures with behavioral assays was pioneered in the awake behaving macaque (Parker & Newsome, 1998), and it is elegantly espoused by Fetsch and colleagues in this volume (Chapter 16). Using human fMRI has the advantage that the participants are (generally) easier to train, facilitating data acquisition. Nevertheless, there are a number of challenges and limitations of the fMRI technique that should be borne in mind when studying depth-cue processing.

First, to make an inference about the functional processing within a given area of cortex, the classical approach to fMRI requires that a contrast be made between the activities evoked by different stimulus conditions. A basic starting point is often to establish that an area responds to a visual signal (e.g., stimulus on vs. stimulus off). However, asking more detailed questions about the processing within an area requires more sophisticated contrasts. Consider investigating whether an area encodes 3D structure from a cue such as shading. The choice of test stimulus might be obvious (a shading pattern that evokes a depth percept); however, it is often difficult to select an appropriate null stimulus. Ideally, the experimenter would choose a contrasting stimulus that has the same image features but does not give rise to a depth percept. In practice this is very difficult to achieve, so forms of spatial scrambling of the image features are often employed (e.g., Kanwisher, Chun, McDermott, & Ledden, 1996). This approach has been successful when localizing cortical activity related to high-level visual features; however, low-level image differences can constitute a concern.

Second, if the low-level image features differ between "depth" and "nondepth" stimuli, it can be difficult to determine whether an fMRI response relates to low-level feature differences or the depth percept. Yet the low-level feature differences are presumably responsible for determining whether a 3D structure is perceived. Thus, it can be problematic to draw a distinction between the representation of low-level features and the representation of depth structure. One approach is to randomize the images (e.g., type of texture or reflectance map) as much as possible and look for consistency in fMRI responses across common depth structure despite dramatic changes in the visual features of the input. This approach can be successful, provided that images that appear radically different do not share the same underlying structure (Fleming, Torralba, & Adelson, 2004).

A third, related issue concerns the near impossibility of "isolating" a single depth cue because, by so doing, other cues are unwittingly placed into conflict with the cue under study. For instance, consider a random-dot stereogram. The phenomenology of seeing depth from random black and white dots suggests a compelling means of studying depth perception using a "pure disparity" stimulus. However, such viewing conditions often create large cue conflicts: Random-dot patterns specify that the viewed surface is flat (i.e., there is no texture gradient or element-size cue), in contrast to the disparity information. Similarly, "isolating" the shading cue, for example, often involves participants viewing stimuli binocularly with the effect that the brain receives very good evidence that the viewed surface is flat. Thus, studying the cortical basis of depth estimation by adding or subtracting individual cues can be misleading. Steps can be taken to minimize the impact of cue conflicts either by tailoring the stimuli (Hillis et al., 2004) or by using parametric manipulations of a particular cue to investigate how cortical responses vary in line with changes in that cue while any cue conflicts remain broadly constant.

Fourth, constraints are imposed by the sensitivity and resolution with which fMRI data are acquired. The basic unit of fMRI measurement is crude (voxels are typically $3 \times 3 \times 3$ mm in size) in relation to individual neurons such that a single voxel measurement pools the activity of (at least) hundreds of thousands of neurons. Thus, it is easy to fail to detect important processing performed within an area, particularly if computations are performed by a small number of neurons (Scannell & Young, 1999). Moreover, limited fMRI resolution may fail to differentiate the processing of different depth signals that occurs within the same voxels. For instance, two cues, such as disparity and motion, might be processed independently within the same cortical area by different subsets of neurons. By averaging the responses of these subpopulations, the voxel response might appear identical when the different depth cues are presented. This could be taken to suggest a convergence of depth signals, when in actuality information is processed in parallel and follows different routes through the cortex (Ponce, Lomber, & Born, 2008). Later, I describe one approach (fMRI adaptation) that can help to mitigate this limitation of fMRI resolution.

Finally, insight into depth processing is often limited by fMRI analysis methods. Data treatment often involves fairly extensive spatial smoothing, exacerbating the problem of differentiating the convergence of depth signals from separate encoding by independent neuronal subpopulations described earlier. Moreover, fMRI activity within a particular region of cortex is often treated as equivalent, and thus it is quantified on the basis of the grand average (i.e., univariate) response. Adopting multivariate analysis methods for fMRI data provides a promising development that exploits the complexity of the data. Nevertheless, these methods are fallible. In particular, multivariate analysis tools can prove overly powerful for fMRI data sets with limited exemplars, suggesting the presence of signals that are not encoded by the brain area under study (i.e., a false positive). Similarly, multivariate analysis methods might exploit features of a data set unintended by the experimenter, producing a null result for the experimental question under test (i.e., a miss). These limitations should be considered and where possible addressed, when using multivariate methods. In the next section. I describe results using high-resolution imaging and multivariate analysis. Further developments in data acquisition and the use of other advanced methods or nonlinear algorithms offer further potential to extend insights into depth processing.

## THE BRAIN'S PROCESSING OF INDIVIDUAL DEPTH CUES

In this section I review evidence for functional specialization in the processing of depth information by considering work that looks at signals individually (disparity, motion, shading, and texture). This separation into easy-to-label cues is unlikely to map directly to the brain's approach to exploiting this information, so the aim of this section is not to pinpoint the "disparity area" or the "texture area." Rather, by considering neural responses to the different cues, the aim is to identify the different types of computation that might be supported in different parts of the visual processing hierarchy.

### Binocular Disparity

Of all the visual depth cues, the brain's processing of binocular disparity has been studied most extensively. Electrophysiological recordings in the primary visual cortex of the cat began in the 1960s (Barlow, Blakemore, & Pettigrew, 1967), and subsequent work in the primate brain has revealed responses across the visual hierarchy (Cumming & DeAngelis, 2001; Orban et al., 2006; Parker, 2007). Cortical areas of particular interest are V2 (Thomas, Cumming, & Parker, 2002), V3 (Adams & Zeki, 2001; Poggio, Gonzalez, & Krause, 1988), V4 (Hinkle & Connor, 2005; Tanabe, Umeda, & Fujita, 2004), MT/V5 (DeAngelis & Newsome, 1999; Krug, Cumming, & Parker, 2004; Palanca & DeAngelis, 2003; Uka & DeAngelis, 2006), and regions of the temporal cortex (Janssen, Vogels, & Orban, 2000; Uka, Tanaka, Yoshiyama, Kato, & Fujita, 2000) and parietal cortex (Taira, Tsutsui, Jiang, Yara, & Sakata, 2000). Results from human and monkey brain-imaging studies have suggested particularly strong responses to disparity signals in dorsal visual areas (Backus, Fleet, Parker, & Heeger, 2001; Tsao et al., 2003). Figure 19.2 illustrates the arrangement of visually responsive areas on a flat-map representation of the posterior portion of a human participant's left and right cortices.

The study by Backus and colleagues (2001) is notable for providing the first link between perceptual judgments and the magnitude of the fMRI response to disparity in the human brain.

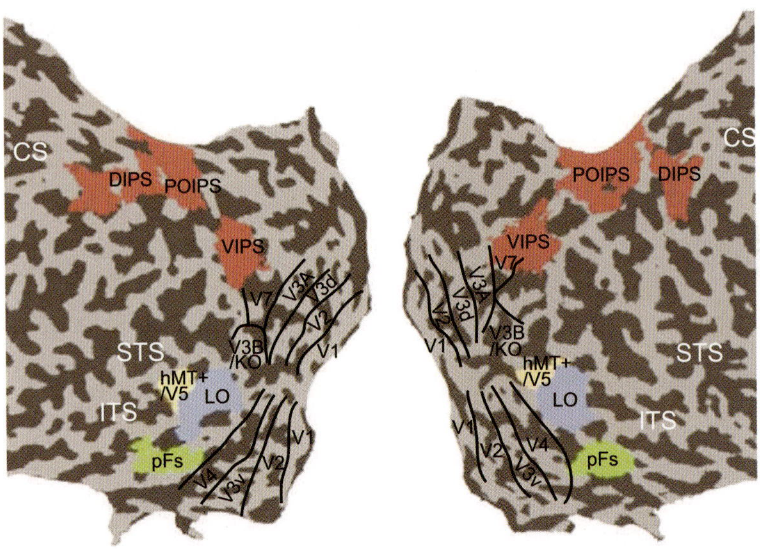


**Figure 19.2** Regions of interest within the visual and parietal cortices on a flattened representation of the cortex. The left and right portions of the figure show posterior sections of the left and right cerebral hemispheres cut along the calcarine sulcus. Dark gray areas depict sulci; light gray areas depict gyri. Major sulci are labeled as follows: STS, superior temporal sulcus; ITS, inferior temporal sulcus; CS, central sulcus. Functional activation maps for a single subject are overlaid to show the early retinotopic regions, V3B/KO, hMT+/V5 (yellow), LOC (comprising the regions labeled pFs [green] and LO [blue]) and three-dimensional shape-related areas in the parietal cortex (burgundy: VIPS, POIPS, DIPS). These areas were identified using standard independent localizer methods (see Preston, Kourtzi, & Welchman, 2008). (Adapted with permission from Preston et al., 2008.)

Using parametric manipulations of disparity, they were able to show that once disparities became too large to be perceptually useful, there was a corresponding drop in the fMRI response. In particular, increasing disparity to the point where disparity discrimination performance dropped to chance was associated with decreased fMRI responses in early (V1, V2) and dorsal visual areas (V3, V3A, human motion complex: hMT+/V5).

A similar parametric approach was taken by Chandrasekaran and colleagues (2007) to investigate the relationship between fMRI responses and the perception of disparity-defined 3D shape. The study used random-dot patterns (Fig. 19.3A) to ensure that the 3D structure of the display was only apparent after global binocular correspondence had been established. To test for cortical areas whose activity related to processing of disparity signals for 3D shape perception, shapes were systematically degraded to measure the effects on both fMRI response and perceptual discrimination. Specifically, the spatial integrity of the disparity-defined shapes was parametrically manipulated by randomly relocating the spatial positions of dots with a given disparity in the display (Fig. 19.3A). This affected observers' performance in judging the global 3D shape (Fig. 19.3B) while keeping the histogram of dot disparities unchanged.

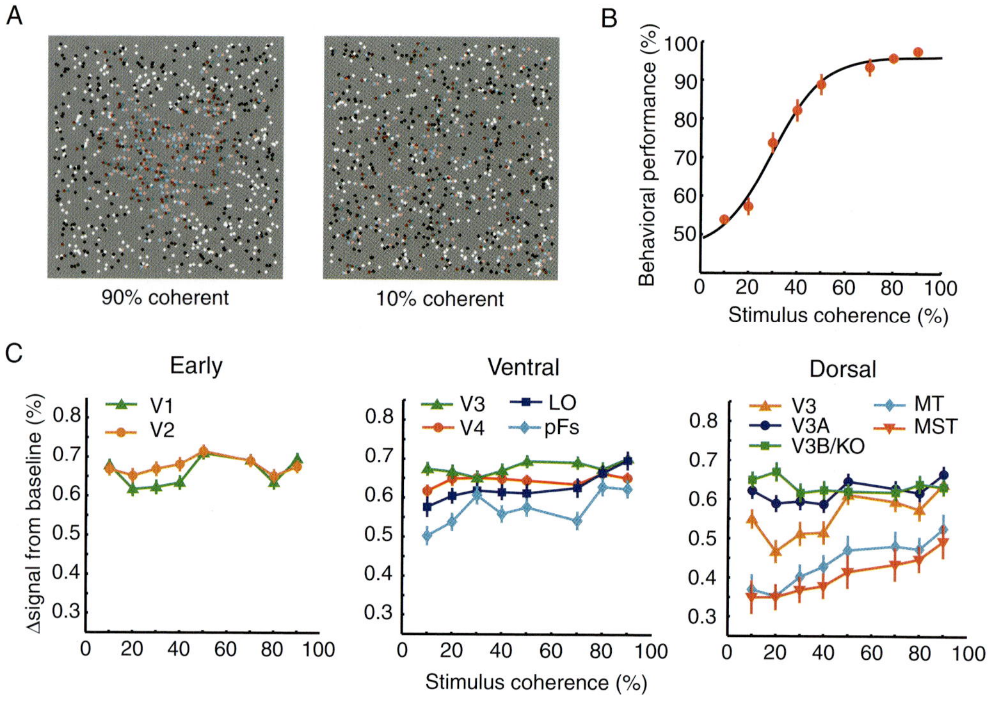


**Figure 19.3** (A) Examples of random-dot stimuli (for anaglyphic viewing) depicting the same three-dimensional (3D) shape at different levels of coherence. Coherence was manipulated by randomly relocating dot pairs throughout the display. The left side stimulus illustrates 10% shuffling (90% of dots in their original location). The right side stimulus depicts 90% shuffling. Participants were instructed to decide whether the 3D shape had a horizontal or vertical axis of symmetry. (B) Mean psychophysical performance ($n = 10$) in discriminating the axis of symmetry at different levels of stimulus coherence. Error bars depict the between-subjects SEM. (C) Mean functional magnetic resonance imaging (fMRI) response as a function of stimulus coherence in the early, ventral, and dorsal visual areas. The fMRI response corresponds to the percentage change from a fixation baseline. Error bars depict the between-subjects SEM. (Adapted with permission from Chandrasekaran et al., 2007.)

The experimental logic of Chandrasekaran et al.'s (2007) study was that reliable perceptual judgments of disparity-defined shape would be associated with strong fMRI responses in areas that encode disparity signals for 3D shape. The study demonstrated different patterns of results in different cortical areas. In particular, responses in early visual areas were largely unaffected by the manipulation of shape coherence (Fig. 19.3C). This suggests a local processing of disparity signals in early areas that is blind to the global coherence of the shape. In contrast, responses in higher ventral (lateral occipital, or LO) and dorsal (hMT+/V5) areas increased significantly as the shapes became more coherent, suggesting the encoding of more extensive surfaces important for shape judgments. Further support for a link between activity in these areas and perceptual judgments of 3D shape was provided by significant correlations between individual observers' psychophysical judgments and individual mean fMRI responses.

In addition to regions in the visual cortex, Chandrasekaran and colleagues (2007) considered disparity-related fMRI responses in three regions along the intraparietal sulcus (IPS). In contrast to the increases in fMRI responses observed in hMT+/V5 and LO, activity along the IPS was found to decrease as shape coherence increased and perceptual judgments became more reliable. Analyzing participants' response times suggested that the most parsimonious explanation for this discrepancy was that fMRI responses along the IPS related to the difficulty of the perceptual task, rather than the computation of disparity structure (although see Georgieva et al., 2009, for an alternative view).

While correlating average perceptual judgments with mean fMRI responses suggests a link between neural activity and behavior, this coupling is more compelling if provided on a trial-by-trial basis. The approach of exploiting between-trial variation is well established in macaque electrophysiology (Britten, Shadlen, Newsome, & Movshon, 1992), and it was adopted by Chandrasekaran et al. (2007) for the analysis of a subset of fMRI responses. In particular, they asked whether it was possible to determine the 3D shape viewed by a participant based only on fMRI responses within a particular area of cortex. Using the distributions of fMRI responses obtained across trials for different types of 3D shape (horizontal vs. vertical axis of symmetry), they computed receiver operating characteristic (ROC) curves, revealing fMRI responses diagnostic of the viewed shape in cortical areas V3, V3B/KO, hMT+/V5, and LO. This analysis did not allow them to dissociate the stimulus from its perceptual interpretation (Bradley, Chang, & Andersen, 1998), because wholly ambiguous stimuli were not employed. However, the idea of predicting the viewed stimulus given only the fMRI response has been explored more thoroughly in subsequent work using machine-learning fMRI data analysis.

To test the relationship between fMRI responses and the perception of disparity-defined depth, Preston and colleagues (Preston, Li, Kourtzi, & Welchman, 2008) used a low-level stimulus manipulation to affect whether observers were able to perceive disparity-defined depth structure. They used random-dot stereograms (RDSs) to render planes with different disparities and altered the visibility of the disparity-defined form by manipulating the contrast of the dots presented to the two eyes (Fig. 19.4A). In cases where the contrast of the dots presented to each eye was the same (correlated RDS: a white dot in the left eye matches a white dot in the right eye), observers had no difficulty in determining the depth position of a target plane. However, reversing the contrast of dots in the two eyes (anticorrelated RDS: a black dot in the left eye matches a white dot in the right eye) abolished the perception of disparity-defined depth (Cogan, Kontsevich, Lomakin, Halpern, & Blake, 1995; Cumming, Shapiro, & Parker, 1998). Nevertheless, the disparity information contained in anticorrelated RDS stimuli is encoded by neurons in primary visual cortex of the macaque (Cumming & Parker, 1997), and the stimuli can drive eye movements (Masson, Busettini, & Miles, 1997). Thus, examining responses evoked by correlated and anticorrelated random-dot stimuli provides a useful means of identifying disparity responses

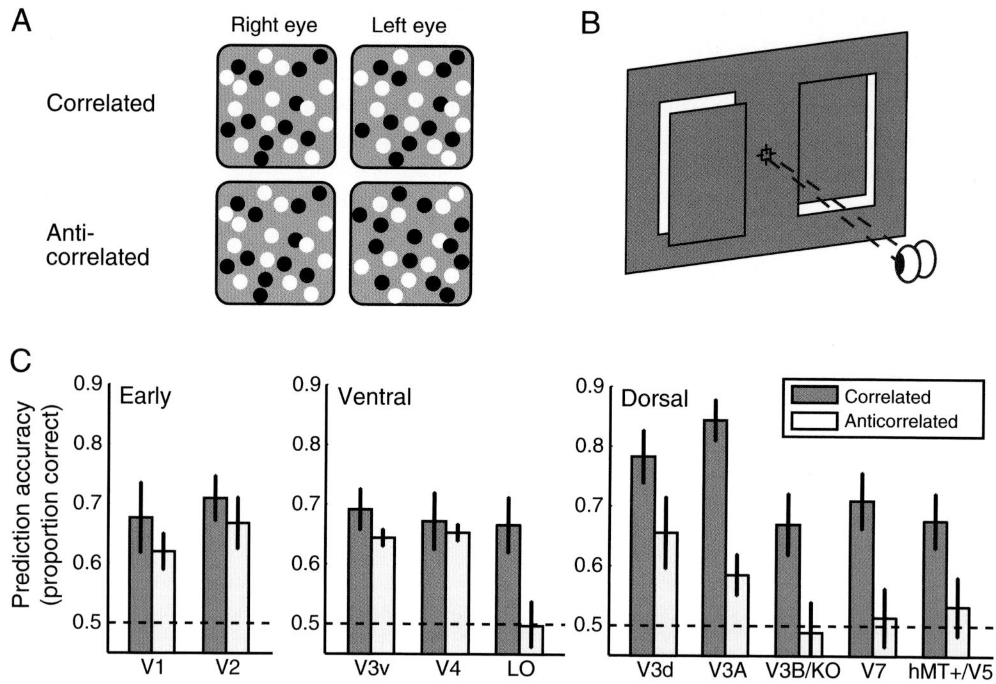


**Figure 19.4** (A) A cartoon random-dot-pattern stereogram illustrating correlated or anticorrelated dots. Free-fusing the stereo pairs by crossing the eyes yields a percept of a square in front of the background for the correlated pattern. The same disparities are contained in the anticorrelated pattern; however, the contrast polarity of dots in the two eyes is reversed, with the effect that there is no reliable impression of a disparity-defined surface. (B) Participants were presented with a pair of planes—one on either side of the fixation point. One plane had crossed disparity (here illustrated as the plane on the left), the other uncrossed disparity (the plane on the right). A machine-learning algorithm (linear classifier) was trained to associate the stimulus configuration (left-near, right-far vs. left-far, right near) with the pattern of functional magnetic resonance imaging (fMRI) activity evoked in cortical regions of interest. (C) The mean prediction accuracy of a classifier trained to discriminate near and far depth positions. Dark bars represent performance of the classifier using fMRI responses evoked by correlated stimuli, and white bars represent performance for anticorrelated stimuli. The dotted horizontal lines depict chance performance (0.5 accuracy). Error bars depict the SEM across subjects ($n = 8$). (Adapted with permission from Preston et al., 2008.)

that are related to perceptual judgments (see also Bridge & Parker, 2007).

Preston et al. (2008) manipulated stimulus correlation to test for areas that contained information about depth structure only when observers could perceive the disparity-defined structure of the stimuli. They investigated a basic property of disparity encoding: whether a target is positioned near (crossed disparity) or far (uncrossed disparity) with respect to the fixation point (Fig. 19.4B). Measuring the fMRI responses evoked by crossed versus uncrossed disparities using both correlated and anticorrelated stimuli allowed them to determine which cortical areas represent disparity signals that are constrained by matching features with the same luminance contrast between the eyes. Based on results from neurophysiology, neurons sensitive to crossed and uncrossed disparities are closely colocated within cortex (DeAngelis & Newsome, 1999). Therefore, a standard fMRI analysis that compared responses to targets in front of versus behind the fixation point would be unlikely to yield reliably different responses because neurons selective to near and far stimuli would be colocated within the same voxels. Thus, Preston et al. designed their study for multivariate data analysis. These methods work by extracting and pooling weak biases for stimulus features (e.g., near or far depth positions) that are distributed across the population of voxels rather than relying on the independent responses of individual voxels (Cox & Savoy, 2003; Haynes & Rees, 2006; Kamitani & Tong, 2005; Norman, Polyn, Detre, & Haxby, 2006).

Preston et al. trained a support vector machine (SVM) to associate the pattern of fMRI responses evoked by random-dot stereograms that depicted depth positions behind or in front of the fixation plane. This method is a standard approach taken in machine learning to classify different patterns of data through supervised learning from exemplars (Vapnik, 1995). Then, using an independent data set, they tested how well the SVM classifier could determine what the participant had been looking at on every trial, based only on their fMRI data. The classifier's performance in discriminating whether the subject had viewed a near or far stimulus thus provided an index of the information contained in a particular region of cortex.

Decoding accuracies suggested a differential pattern of responses for correlated and anticorrelated stimuli across the visual hierarchy. The classifier's ability to predict the viewed stimulus was significantly above chance across the visual cortex when subjects viewed correlated stimuli (Fig. 19.4C). This is consistent with previous imaging and neurophysiological data that show disparity-selective responses widespread throughout cortex. However, the same was not true for anticorrelated stimuli. In early visual areas the classifier could also decode the disparity signals contained in anticorrelated stimuli. This is consistent with electrophysiological recordings in suggesting dissociation between early cortical responses and the perception of disparity-defined depth (Cumming & Parker, 1997). Results in higher areas were somewhat surprising in that activity in intermediate areas in the ventral stream (V3v, V4), like early visual cortex, supported similar decoding performance for correlated and anticorrelated stimuli. In contrast, responses in higher ventral lateral occipital (LO) area supported significant decoding of correlated, but not anticorrelated, stimuli. This suggests that, like perceptual judgments, responses in LO are selective for binocular matches that involve similar features in the two eyes.

Intriguingly, the pattern observed in ventral area LO was similar to that seen throughout the dorsal visual stream (Fig. 19.4C). The question therefore arises of where the selectivity for correlated features in area LO originates. In particular, fMRI responses to anticorrelated stimuli do not appear to be progressively attenuated as information travels through intermediate ventral areas (V3v, V4) to terminate in LO. Rather, attenuation in the response to anticorrelated stimuli seems to be a property of the dorsal stream, suggesting that responses in LO may derive from activity in dorsal areas. This notion is necessarily speculative, because fMRI does not reveal the nature of the intracortical interactions that give rise to responses in different cortical areas. It is therefore possible that Preston et al.'s fMRI measures and analysis do not capture the important contributions to disparity processing made by intermediate ventral areas. Nevertheless, it is reassuring to note agreement between their findings and neurophysiological recordings in inferior temporal cortex (analogous to LO), where responses to anticorrelated stimuli are not observed (Janssen, Vogels, Liu, & Orban, 2003). Recordings from area V4 of the macaque suggest that responses to anticorrelated stimuli are attenuated (Kumano, Tanabe, & Fujita, 2008; Tanabe et al., 2004) which appears at odds with the human fMRI results; however, this discrepancy may relate to the noncorresponding nomenclature between humans and macaques for the dorsal V4 recording sites used by Fujita and colleagues (see Preston et al. for a detailed discussion of this issue).

While these results suggest representations of perceptually useful disparity signals in both higher ventral (LO) and dorsal (V3A, V3B/KO, V7, hMT+/V5) visual areas, further experiments by Preston et al. suggested differences between the encoding in ventral and dorsal areas. Using parametric disparity manipulations (Fig. 19.5A), they investigated how well a detector (built from a system of one-against-one binary SVM classifiers) could determine the specific depth of the viewed stimulus based on fMRI activity. The interest in this analysis was to determine the extent to which detectors show a "tuned" response, mispredicting stimuli with similar disparities more frequently than stimuli differing by a large amount of disparity. Figure 19.5B shows example detector outputs for different cortical regions of interest (V1, V3A, LO). For all the cortical regions of interest examined, detectors preferred the stimulus they had been trained to detect (i.e., curves peak at zero difference between the stimulus that evoked the fMRI test pattern and the disparity predicted by the classifier). However, the specificity of the responses differed between areas, with dorsal areas showing sharper pattern-based tuning than the detectors that relied on signals from ventral LO. This decoding analysis suggests a dorsal representation of disparity that is more closely related to the specific disparity signals than that in higher ventral cortex.

Further evidence for a distinction between the representation of disparity signals in dorsal and ventral cortex came from considering the performance of detectors trained to distinguish "near" from "far" depth positions as a function of the difference in disparity between the test stimuli (Fig. 19.5C). Specifically, for each possible disparity difference between the test planes (6, 12, 18, 24, 30 arcmin) classifiers were built to determine whether the viewed stimulus was in front of or behind the fixation plane. In the majority of visual areas considered, classification accuracy increased as a function of the disparity step size. However, classification accuracy in LO was unaffected by the disparity difference—that is, performance was similar whether the disparity planes were located close to the fixation point (±3 arcmin) or far away (±15 arcmin). This result, in conjunction with the analysis of pattern-based tuning widths, suggests that area LO may represent depth in a categorical manner to reflect depth configurations (i.e., surfaces in front or behind their neighbors) to support the invariant recognition of objects across different positions in depth. In contrast, the metric-type activity in dorsal areas (V3A and V7) may be more appropriate for judgments requiring fine positional discriminations and the fine control of body movements.

In summary, neural responses to binocular disparity are widespread throughout visually responsive cortex. fMRI results have highlighted the strong disparity modulation of dorsal visual areas (V3A, V7), suggesting a degree of specialization for disparity signals. Dorsal responses appear selective for the specific disparity content of presented stimuli, in contrast to higher ventral cortex (LO) where responses appear more categorical in nature. While activity in both dorsal and ventral areas is commensurate with the use of disparity signals for perceptual judgments, different types of representation (metric vs. configural) may be employed to subserve different types of computation (positional information for movement control vs. more invariant signals for recognition).

### Depth Structure from Motion

In common with binocular disparity, the statistical coherence of seemingly uninformative moving random dots can provide a compelling impression of 3D structure, even in the absence of other cues (Wallach & O'Connell, 1953). To examine specialization for the use of motion signals for depth, fMRI studies have typically contrasted patterns of motion consistent with a 3D structure with motion that depicts a 2D structure. The logic of this approach is that the difference between "depth" and "non-depth" configurations reveals the functional signatures of depth estimation. This localization approach suggests a large network of cortical areas engaged by structure-from-motion stimuli. For instance, contrasting fMRI activity evoked by the movement of 3D versus 2D structures reveals activity in ventral LO, dorsal areas (V3A, V3B/KO, hMT+/V5), and regions along the IPS (Orban, Sunaert, Todd, Van Hecke, & Marchal, 1999; Vanduffel, Tootell, Schoups, & Orban, 2002). Moreover, instructing participants to attend to 3D motion (rather than other stimulus attributes) results in higher fMRI responses in

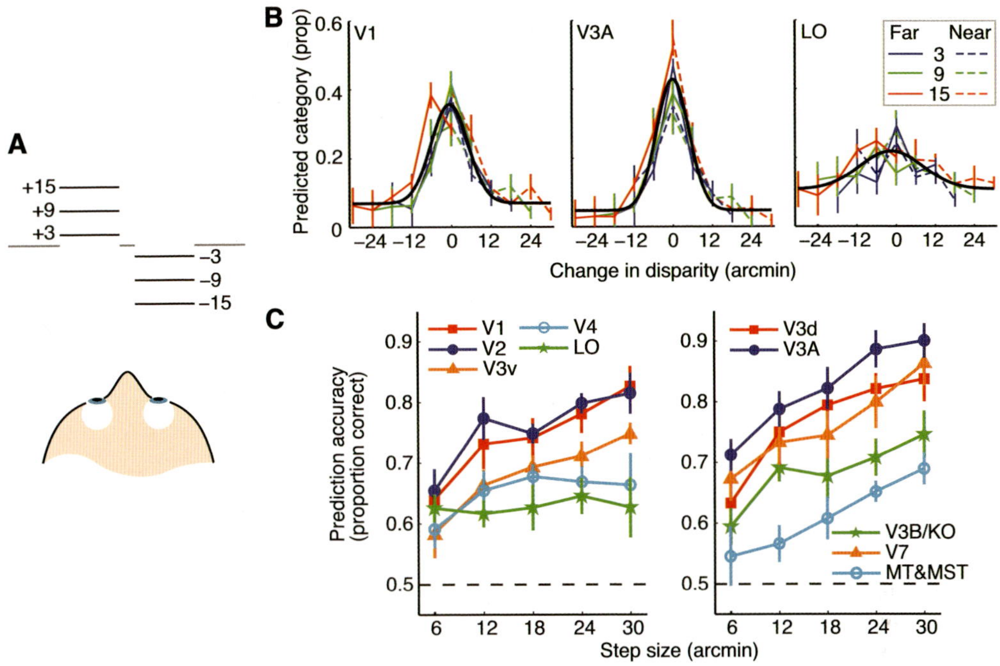


**Figure 19.5** (A) A cartoon illustrating disparity-defined planes with different magnitudes of disparity with respect to the fixation plane. The stimulus configuration was as illustrated in Figure 19.4B. The disparities presented to the left and right of fixation were equal and opposite. (B) Functional magnetic resonance imaging (fMRI) pattern-based tuning curves for three sample areas: early (V1), dorsal (V3A), and ventral (LO). The proportion of predictions made to each of the stimulus disparity values is expressed in terms of the disparity difference between the viewed stimulus and the prediction made by the SVM-based detector. Each series corresponds to predictions made for activity evoked by a different disparity stimulus. The solid black line shows the best-fitting Gaussian to the data. Random predictions would correspond to a proportion of 0.167. Error bars depict the between-subjects SEM ($n = 8$). (C) Mean prediction accuracy for a crossed versus uncrossed disparity discrimination as a function of the disparity difference (step size) between the two sets of presented stimuli. The dotted horizontal lines show chance performance. Error bars depict the SEM across subjects ($n = 8$). (Adapted with permission from Preston et al., 2008.)

these areas (Peuskens et al., 2004). fMRI results obtained from both anesthetized and awake macaques have suggested higher activity for the movement of 3D structures in the ventral, dorsal, and parietal areas (Durand et al., 2007; Sereno, Trinath, Augath, & Logothetis, 2002).

This apparently widely distributed encoding of 3D structure from motion is somewhat difficult to interpret. Are all these areas involved in the computation of shape from motion, and if so, what contribution is made by each? Motion signals per se tend to evoke vigorous neural responses, so it is important to ensure that the stimulus sets that are contrasted to isolate the key signatures of depth processing are equated for their motion energy. One means of ensuring that (at least) the distribution of local motion signals is constant between conditions is to use a random-dot-defined structure contrasted against a scrambled version of the same stimulus. Using this approach, Murray, Olshausen, and Woods (2003) reported that an area anterior to V3B/KO in dorsal visual cortex (labeled superior lateral occipital) was the only region where activity increased when motion depicted 3D structure. This perhaps suggests a more confined role for dorsal-occipital cortex in extracting shape information from motion signals. However, this conclusion is tempered by the limited number of cortical regions considered by this study, raising the possibility that important contributions made elsewhere may have been missed (e.g., Vanduffel et al., 2002). At present, therefore, there are a large number of candidate areas in both the ventral and dorsal stream involved in extracting 3D structure from motion signals. Future parametric investigations that are linked to behavioral judgments may provide the means to delineate the functional computations carried out within each of these areas.

### Shape from Texture and Shading

The preceding sections on disparity and motion processing have implicated common sites of cortical activation in ventral and dorsal cortical areas. This might be expected from computational considerations (disparity is frozen motion, or, motion defrosted disparity, depending on your perspective) and psychophysical results that suggest common processing of these signals (e.g., Nawrot & Blake, 1989). It is of considerable interest, therefore, to determine cortical responses to other, less-related sources of depth information such as texture and shading cues.

Initial studies of fMRI responses to structures defined by shading and texture cues suggested widespread responses in dorsal, ventral, and parietal areas. Specifically, two studies addressed the use of shading and texture cues, respectively, by contrasting fMRI responses when participants were instructed to attend to different features of a stimulus. This approach suggested activity related to texture judgments along the IPS (Shikata et al., 2001), whereas judgments based on shading resulted in stronger activations in dorsal, ventral, and parietal areas (Taira, Nose, Inoue, & Tsutsui, 2001). One region likely to exploit information about 3D structure is the ventral lateral occipital complex (LOC: comprising area LO and the more anterior posterior fusiform sulcus, or pFs) known to be involved in object processing (Kourtzi & Kanwisher, 2001). Two studies have suggested that the LOC responds more vigorously to 3D shapes defined by shading cues than similar-image objects with 2D structures (Kourtzi, Erb, Grodd, & Bülthoff, 2003; Moore & Engel, 2001), implying a preference for volumetric object representations informed by shading information in the LOC.

Further evidence for a functional distinction between the processing of shading and texture information was provided by Georgieva, Todd, Peeters, and Orban (2008). While 3D objects depicted by variations of shading or texture can provide a compelling impression of 3D structure, their complex nature means that low-level feature differences need to be taken into account when contrasting stimuli that do, and do not, support estimates of depth. Thus, Georgieva and colleagues employed a comprehensive set of control stimuli designed to target low-level feature differences. When they contrasted fMRI responses to texture-defined 3D stimuli with control images, they localized widespread activity in ventral (LO), dorsal (V3B/KO, V7), and parietal (vIPS, poIPS, dIPS) areas. However, comparable contrasts for 3D structures defined by shading only revealed activations in a ventral region (in the vicinity of LO). This is intriguing in suggesting a restricted role for shading information processing 3D structure. In particular, Georgieva et al. highlighted the functional importance of texture signals for tasks involving both shape judgments and controlling actions, and they suggested this could explain extensive activations for texture signals in ventral and dorsal areas. In contrast, shading information, though useful for judging shape, would be of limited use for controlling actions, commensurate with activity more restricted to ventral cortical areas. An interesting test of this hypothesis would be to contrast responses to texture signals during tasks that make differential use of shape judgments versus movement responses.

## THE BRAIN'S COMBINATION OF VISUAL DEPTH CUES

The preceding review has highlighted activity in ventral area LO, higher dorsal visual areas (V3B/KO, V7), and along the IPS, in relation to the processing of disparity-, motion-, or texture-defined 3D structures. This suggests cortical areas in which information from different depth cues may converge, but it does not imply that signals are combined. In this section I consider evidence for areas that, like everyday perceptual judgments, respond on the basis of combining different sources of depth information, rather than relying on individual cues.

Single-cell recordings from the macaque support the fMRI evidence (reviewed earlier) that different depth signals converge in common cortical areas. In particular, recordings from parietal cortex (the caudal intraparietal sulcus, roughly corresponding to V7/vIPS in the human) have identified neurons that encode the tilt (i.e., orientation in the frontal plane) of a receding surface whether that surface is defined by a dot pattern, a grid, or disparity rendered in a random-dot stereogram (Tsutsui, Sakata, Naganuma, & Taira, 2002). Similarly, recordings from ventral cortex (TEs in inferior temporal cortex, roughly analogous to LO in the human) suggest similarities in the tilt-selective response of neurons to surfaces defined by disparity and texture slant cues (Liu, Vogels, & Orban, 2004). However, because neither study considered responses when two types of depth signal were available concurrently, this work does not allow inferences to be made about the combination of depth signals.

One approach to investigating the commonalities in the processing of different depth cues is to compare the pattern of fMRI activation evoked when participants view stimuli defined by different depth cues. In particular, studies have sought to identify the intersection of activity evoked by different cues, based on the logic that the areas commonly activated by different cues should be those where information converges. For instance, fMRI in macaques using stimuli defined by texture, shading, and motion yielded overlapping activations for different cues in MT/V5, along the superior temporal sulcus, the fundus of the temporal sulcus, and along the IPS (Sereno et al., 2002). A subsequent monkey fMRI study provided detailed tests of disparity and motion cues to 3D structure, and it suggested a more limited area of overlap in posterior and anterior intraparietal areas (Durand et al., 2007). Finally, a human fMRI study by Tyler, Likova, Kontsevich, and Wade (2006) tested for similarities in the response to edges defined by different types of disparity, motion, and luminance. This study highlighted activity in the dorsal, kinetic occipital (KO) area as a location that responds to depth structure defined by different types of information; thus, it is a candidate site for the computation of 3D structure from different cues.

These results suggest a convergence of signals in cortical areas that might combine cues; however, based on current understanding of cue combination (Chapter 1), it is problematic to equate or contrast the depth evoked by different cues directly. As discussed in the section on the challenges of using fMRI, presenting depth structure defined by a random-dot pattern entails a conflict between texture cues to structure and disparity information. Moreover, it is commonly observed that individuals differ in the weights they assign to different cues, meaning that, without concurrent measures of perception, it is difficult to make inferences about areas that encode structure on the basis of combined cues.

To counter these concerns, Welchman, Deubelius, Conrad, Bülthoff, and Kourtzi (2005) conducted a concurrent fMRI-psychophysical study that sought to identify areas that process structure from a combination of cues. Rather than contrasting one cue against another based on the logic of isolating individual cues, the study took a perturbation approach (Landy et al., 1995), measuring how a small change in an individual cue affected both behavioral and fMRI responses. This enabled the correlation between cue and percept changes to be broken, allowing tests for areas involved in cue combination.

Participants were asked to judge the 3D shape of a hinged plane, described to them as looking like an "open book" (Fig. 19.6A). This stimulus consisted of two planes slanted in depth in which horizontal disparity and perspective cues provided information about the magnitude of slant. On every trial, participants compared two, sequentially presented stimuli and decided which looked more "open" (or, more technically, which hinged plane had the larger dihedral angle). To assess the brain's combination of the

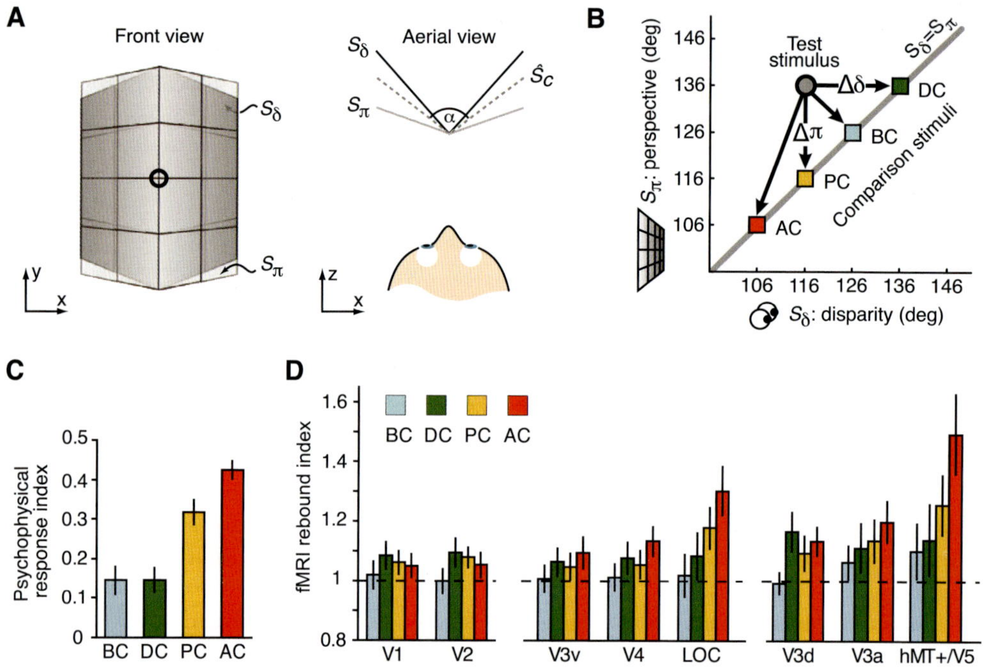


**Figure 19.6** (A) A cartoon of the stimulus used to study cue combination. Participants judged the "openness" of a hinged plane with dihedral angle ($\alpha$). The shape was defined by disparity and perspective cues, where the dihedral angle specified by disparity ($S_\delta$) was smaller than that specified by perspective ($S_\pi$). Participants combined the cues, perceiving a shape intermediate between that defined by disparity and perspective ($\hat{S}_c$). (B) An illustration stimulus space for dihedral angles specified by disparity and perspective. The diagonal line indicates consistent-cue shapes. The inconsistent-cue test stimulus (circular marker) was paired with consistent-cue comparison stimuli (square markers). Pairs of stimuli could differ along one cue dimension (DC, disparity change condition; PC, perspective change conditions), the cues could change in equal and opposite directions (BC, balanced change condition), or both cues could change in the same direction (AC, all change condition). (C) Psychophysical performance in judging dihedral angle expressed the change in estimated dihedral angle between the test and comparison stimuli. The response index corresponds to the absolute difference in the proportion of "more open" responses from the PSE. Zero indicates the test and comparison stimuli have the same perceived dihedral angle (on average); 0.5 would indicate a perfectly reliable difference in the estimated dihedral angles of the test and comparison stimuli. Error bars show the between-subject SEM ($n = 11$). (D) Functional magnetic resonance imaging (fMRI) responses in each condition and region of interest expressed as a rebound index. This index corresponds to the peak fMRI response in a given condition divided by the peak fMRI response evoked in the baseline condition (test stimulus shown twice). A value of 1 indicates an adapted response (i.e., no difference from that obtained when viewing the same stimulus twice). Values above 1 indicate fMRI sensitivity to changes in the stimulus. Error bars (normalized SEM) incorporate the error estimates of both numerator and denominator. (Adapted with permission from Welchman et al., 2005.)

dihedral angles specified by disparity ($S_\delta$) and perspective ($S_\pi$), a slight conflict was introduced between the two cues, such that they specified different angles. Using a two-interval forced-choice paradigm, the perceived shape ($\hat{S}_c$) of this cue-conflict test stimulus (i.e., $S_\delta \neq S_\pi$) was assessed though comparison with a range of stimuli in which the angles specified by disparity and perspective were the same ($S_\delta = S_\pi$). The PSE from the resultant psychometric function provided a measure of the perceived dihedral angle ($\hat{S}_c$) of the cue-conflict test stimulus. The weights assigned to disparity ($w_\delta$) and perspective ($w_\pi$) cues could then be determined by assuming psychophysical judgments correspond to a weighted combination of the component (experimentally controlled) cues,

$$\hat{S}_c = w_\delta S_\delta + w_\pi S_\pi, \qquad (19.1)$$

where the weights sum to one (Landy et al., 1995),

$$w_\delta + w_\pi = 1. \qquad (19.2)$$

Note that the design of this study does not remove cue conflicts. The comparison stimuli used in the study were "consistent" inasmuch as disparity and perspective specified the same slant, while other cues (accommodation, blur, shading, etc.) did not vary in a manner appropriate for a physical object. The approach was therefore one of minimizing the impact of conflict with other cues by *(a)* ensuring that the weight given to other cues would not be high (i.e., a long fixation distance [78 cm] and a small [~3.6 cm] depth range were used); and *(b)* making parametric variations of individual cues, rather than pitting one cue-inconsistent stimulus against another (i.e., the study did not compare a zero disparity "perspective" stimulus against a zero perspective random-dot "disparity" stimulus).

The two-interval psychophysical design used by Welchman et al. formed the basis of an fMRI-adaptation paradigm that tested for neural responses to combined cues. In particular, an event-related adaptation procedure was used that capitalizes on neural adaptation and repetition-suppression effects whereby neural activity is lower for stimuli that have been viewed recently than for stimuli that have not (Grill-Spector & Malach, 2001; Kourtzi & Kanwisher, 2001). The logic of this approach is that showing the same stimulus twice ("test-test") results in an adapted fMRI response, whereas pairing the test stimulus with a stimulus that engages a different set of neurons ("test-comparison") will not produce an adapted response. The difference in the fMRI response between these two conditions ("the rebound effect") thus acts as an index of the sensitivity of the underlying neural population to differences between the test and comparison stimuli.

To illustrate the logic underlying the experiment, consider the following example. If the test and comparison stimuli differed in their component cues (disparity and perspective) but engaged the same neural population (e.g., a selectivity for generally book-shaped stimuli), no rebound effect would be observed despite differences in stimuli. Conversely, if the stimuli selectively engage different neural populations, a rebound effect would be observed relative to the adapted baseline response. The selectivity of the underlying neural population could take different forms: it could relate to the disparity cue, or the perspective cue, or an estimate of shape based on combined cues. If only consistent-cue stimuli had been used, it would be impossible to decouple changes in the component cues from changes in the percept. However, the inconsistent-cue test stimulus broke the correlation between cue changes and percept changes. In particular, if the disparity and perspective cues changed in opposite directions between the test and comparison stimuli, this would result in a small change in the perceived shape as observers' judgments rely on the combination of the disparity and perspective signals. Thus, the selectivity of the neural response could be inferred by characterizing differences between test and comparison stimuli in terms of *(1)* simple changes in individual cues, or *(2)* the change in perceived shape that results from the combination of component cues.

The first experiment in the study involved collecting data for a fixed set of test-comparison pairs. As illustrated in Figure 19.6B, these conditions consisted of isolated changes in individual cues ("Disparity Change," "Perspective Change") and conditions in which both cues changed simultaneously ("Balanced Change," "All Change"). To test which cortical areas process cue-based information, the adapted (test-test) fMRI response was compared against responses evoked when the test-reference stimuli differed in only one cue. Changes in the disparity cue evoked significant activity changes in early and intermediate visual areas (V1, V2, V3, V3a, V4), consistent with other studies on disparity processing (see review in preceding section). Similarly, changes in the perspective cue evoked widespread significant activity changes in early (V1, V2) and dorsal (V3, V3a) areas with marginal effects in ventral V3 and V4. These significant responses do not imply that, for instance, V1 computes slant from perspective per se. Rather, the computation of perspective slant involves a hierarchy of visual responses. If this result had been observed throughout all visual areas, it would be trivial (i.e., changing a stimulus evokes a response). However, a different pattern of results was observed in higher visual areas. Specifically, changing the perspective cue, but not the disparity cue, evoked significant responses in the LOC and hMT+/V5. This might imply that these areas are not sensitive to disparity; however, the preceding discussion of disparity processing suggests this is not the case. Interestingly, the lack of strong sensitivity to disparity changes was consistent with observers' psychophysical judgments, where estimated shape was more reliant on the perspective cue than the disparity information.

To examine the relationship between 3D shape estimation and fMRI responses, the change in perceived shape between the test and comparison stimuli was computed for each condition and compared with fMRI rebound responses in different cortical areas. As shown in Figure 19.6C, this comparison suggested a link between perceptual judgments based on combined cues and fMRI responses in higher visual areas (LOC, hMT+/V5) but not in earlier visual areas (confirmed by statistical tests). As an additional line of evidence, between-subject differences in the weight given to the disparity and perspective cues were exploited. Specifically, subjects were placed in one of three groups depending on the extent to which their shape judgments were informed by disparity. These three groups of subjects showed different patterns of psychophysical judgment and had corresponding differences in fMRI responses in higher areas. This relationship was confirmed using regression analyses that related individual subjects' fMRI responses to their psychophysical judgments of shape. In particular, significant relationships between combined-cue shape perception and fMRI responses were observed in LOC and hMT+/V5, but not in early areas.

To test further the hypothesis that higher areas compute estimated shape on the basis of combined cues, Welchman et al. conducted an additional experiment in which stimuli were tailored for individual participants according to their cue weights. Specifically, by measuring the weights given to disparity and perspective cues, they tested for fMRI adaptation to perceived shape using stimuli that differed in their component cues but were reported to have a similar 3D shape (Hillis, Ernst, Banks, & Landy, 2002).

The logic behind this experiment was that participants would be able to perceive a change in shape when component cues were changed individually (i.e., the test and comparison stimuli differed only in perspective or disparity); however, when those same cue changes occurred concurrently, there would be little change in the perception, and thus no fMRI rebound effect. To achieve this, participants performed a psychophysical experiment inside the scanner (before collecting fMRI data) that provided a measure of cue weights. This enabled a stimulus to be constructed in which the two cues changed in opposite directions, with the result that the perceived shape of the test stimulus was similar to a cue-consistent comparison ($S_{cc}$). In particular, given a consistent-cue stimulus in which the dihedral angle specified by disparity and perspective was the same,

$$\hat{S}_{cc} = S_{\delta} = S_{\pi}, \tag{19.3}$$

an inconsistent-cue stimulus ($S_{ci}$) could be constructed in which the dihedral angles specified by disparity ($\delta$) and perspective ($\pi$) differed from the consistent-cue signal in opposite directions

$$\hat{S}_{ci} = w_{\delta}\delta + w_{\pi}\pi \tag{19.4}$$

such that, when combined using weighted averaging, perceived shape was similar to the consistent-cue stimulus

$$\hat{S}_{cc} \approx \hat{S}_{ci}. \tag{19.5}$$

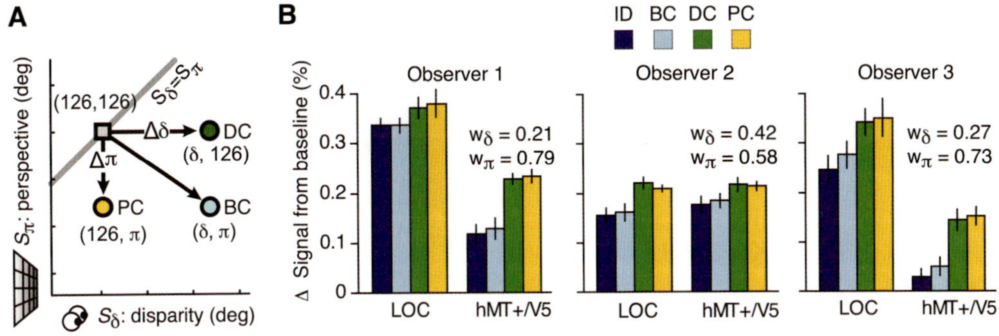


**Figure 19.7** (A) An illustration of the design for the second test of cue combination. In this experiment, the inconsistent-cue test stimuli reflected an individual's cue weights ($w_\pi$, $w_\delta$). The inconsistent-cue stimulus for the balanced change (BC) condition was constructed (following psychophysical measurements) so that perceived dihedral angle was very similar to the consistent-cue reference (square marker on the diagonal, $S_\delta = S_\pi = 126°$). The inconsistent-cue stimuli for the disparity change (DC) and perspective change (PC) conditions consisted of the individual cue changes required for the balanced change inconsistent-cue stimulus. The logic of the experiment was that cue changes would be perceptible when made in isolation, but not when both cues changed in opposite directions simultaneously. (B) Mean functional magnetic resonance imaging (fMRI) response in the LOC and hMT+/V5 for three individual subjects. fMRI response in the balanced change condition (light blue bars) was very similar to the adapted response obtained from showing the reference stimulus twice (dark blue bars). However, increases in the fMRI response were obtained when cues changed individually (green and yellow bars). Each individual's cue weights are shown on the figure. (Adapted with permission from Welchman et al., 2005.)

An illustration of the design is provided in Figure 19.7A. The change in perceived shape should be minimal when the consistent-cue dihedral angle (indicated by the gray square box, $S_\delta = S_\pi = 126°$) is paired with a stimulus in which disparity and perspective cues change in opposite directions (blue circle marker, where the angles specified by disparity ($\delta$) and perspective ($\pi$) depend on cue weights).

The experiment tested for fMRI responses to changes in individual cues (that resulted in an obvious change of shape) and changes in both cues concurrently (producing little change in perceived shape). Based on the logic of fMRI adaptation, areas engaged in 3D shape perception from combined cues should show an adapted response when both cues changed concurrently, owing to the perceptual similarity of the test and reference 3D shapes (balanced change, or BC, condition should match the identical, or ID, condition). However, these areas should show increased responses when the individual cue changes were made due to differences in perceived 3D shape (DC: disparity change, and PC: perspective change conditions). fMRI responses in the higher visual areas were consistent with these predictions (Fig. 19.7B). The results from two experiments therefore suggest fMRI responses in LOC and hMT+/V5 change in line with the perception of shape based on combined cues.

While these results suggest the combination of disparity and perspective depth cues, on the basis of the population-level response measured by fMRI, it is not possible to determine whether individual neurons within an area respond on the basis of cue combination, or whether subpopulations within an area carry information about the two cues independently. However, even if disparity and perspective signals are encoded separately, it is intriguing that the response magnitude of these subpopulations in LOC and hMT+/V5 seems to vary in accordance with the 3D shape percept. Based on findings published subsequent to this study (Georgieva et al., 2008; Preston et al., 2008; Tyler et al., 2006), it would be informative to have also considered activity in V3B/KO and V7 to assess their role in cue combination (unfortunately, they were not independently localized). As will be discussed next, recent evidence suggests these areas may play an important role in depth estimation from different cues.

## ESTIMATING DEPTH BY TAKING PRIOR KNOWLEDGE INTO ACCOUNT

So far, I have considered the process of depth estimation in a bottom-up manner, discussing the importance of different cues and their combination in estimating 3D structure. Yet individual cues alone are ambiguous, and they can conflict with one another, so prior knowledge is important when estimating depth structure (e.g., see Chapters 1, 9, 11, and 12). The final study I discuss considered one form of this internalized knowledge about the environment, examining the role of short-term adaptive effects in guiding the interpretation of ambiguous sensory signals (Preston, Kourtzi, & Welchman, 2009). The goal of the study was to investigate the brain regions involved in interpreting depth structure when sensory input remains ambiguous but 3D shape perception is guided by adaptation.

Preston and colleagues used two classic bistable stimuli: *(1)* a Mach card (Mach, 1886) that gives rise to two competing depth percepts: either "convex" (like viewing the covers of a book) or "concave" (like viewing the internal pages of a book) (Fig. 19.8A); *(2)* the kinetic depth effect (KDE) (Wallach & O'Connell, 1953) in which observers perceive either the interior (convex) or exterior (concave) surface of a rotating half-cylinder (Fig. 19.8B). By adding *(1)* disparity to the Mach card and *(2)* texture and shading to the KDE cylinder, the stimuli were disambiguated sufficiently so that observers' perceptual judgments were stable.

The study examined how the processing of a bistable probe stimulus was affected by a preceding period of adaptation to a disambiguated stimulus. In particular, consistent with a range of psychophysical studies on depth adaptation (Berends, Liu, & Schor, 2005; Bergman & Gibson, 1959; Blakemore & Julesz, 1971; Knapen & van Ee, 2006; Kohler & Emery, 1947; Taya, Sato, & Nakamizo, 2005), the study exploited repulsive after-effects, whereby adapting to a convex shape made it more likely that observers would interpret the ambiguous stimulus as concave, and vice versa.

Psychophysical measures of adaptation provided evidence for an asymmetry in the observers' judgments whereby there was a larger change in the estimated shape following adaptation to a convex stimulus than following adaptation to a concave stimulus (Fig. 19.8C). The fMRI adaptation data collected concurrently with the psychophysical data provided evidence for similar asymmetric adaptation effects in higher dorsal areas (V3B/KO, V7, vIPS, dIPS), suggesting a relationship between fMRI responses and perceptual judgments based on two quite different types of stimulus (Fig. 19.8D).

In addition to data obtained for the Mach card and KDE stimuli with a short adaptation paradigm, two further experiments were conducted in which fMRI measurements were obtained during prolonged viewing of bistable stimuli, and when observers viewed less ambiguous stimuli. Results from these two further experiments suggested a shift in the network of fMRI responses; highly ambiguous stimuli involved enhanced activity in parietal and frontal regions, whereas less ambiguous stimuli produced enhanced responses in ventral cortex. Intriguingly, the commonalities between these two networks were centered on the junction between dorsal visual cortex and posterior parietal cortex (V3B/KO, V7, vIPS). Together, these results suggest a confined ensemble of areas intricately involved in the estimation of 3D shape structure from both monocular and binocular depth cues.

The short-term adaptive effects exploited by Preston et al.'s (2009) study most likely involve a change in sensory encoding (Stocker & Simoncelli, 2005) that provides a means of internalizing information about the environment at short timescales. It is an interesting question for future research to determine whether the same cortical circuits are involved when the brain estimates depth by combining sensory input with long-term internalized statistical regularities

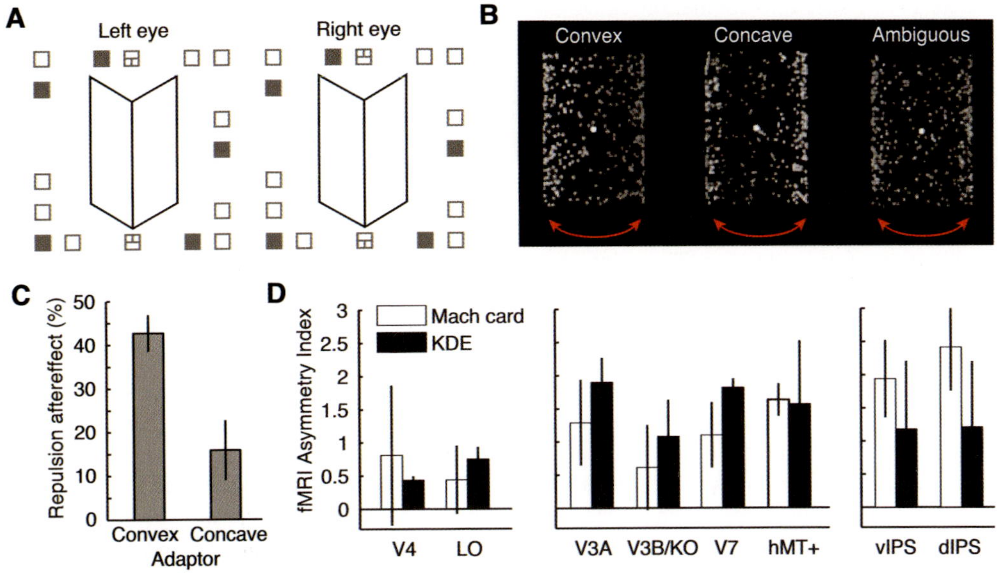


**Figure 19.8** (A) An illustration of the Mach card stimulus. Prolonged viewing of one-half of the stereo pair illustrates the alternation of convex and concave depth interpretations. The study involved studying the effects of adapting to a stimulus that had been disambiguated through the addition of binocular disparity (cross-fuse the stereo pair). (B) Illustrations of the KDE stimulus. The stimulus rotated around its vertical axis to depict the exterior or interior surface of a cylinder. Texture and shading cues disambiguated the stimulus (left, center), while the ambiguous stimulus was a shuffled version of the convex and concave stimuli (right). The arrows depict rotation in depth. (C) Psychophysical measure of the repulsion aftereffect produced by adapting to either a convex or a concave Mach card stimulus. The data express change in the psychophysical response after adaptation relative to baseline measures without adaptation. There was a larger change in the interpretation of the ambiguous Mach card following adaptation to a convex stimulus. Error bars show between-subjects SEM. (D) Functional magnetic resonance imaging (fMRI) response expressed as an asymmetry index that contrasts the fMRI rebound effect following exposure to convex or concave adaptors. A value of zero corresponds to an equal effect of the two types of adaptor, whereas values above zero indicate stronger effects of convex adaptors. In line with perceptual judgments, an asymmetry in the fMRI responses was observed. This was most marked in the higher dorsal areas, and it was similar for the results of experiments using the Mach card involving disparity, or the KDE experiment involving shading and texture cues. Error bars depict normalized SEM. (Adapted with permission from Preston et al., 2009.)

(Mamassian & Goutcher, 2001; Mamassian, Landy, & Maloney, 2002), learning (Bülthoff, Bülthoff, & Sinha, 1998; Sinha & Poggio, 1996), and sensory recalibration (Adams, Graf, & Ernst, 2004).

## SUMMARY

In this chapter I have sought to review progress in understanding the brain's processing and combination of signals related to 3D structure. I have focused on the use of fMRI as a means of obtaining data from multiple cortical areas simultaneously, as well as its suitability for designing paradigms that include concurrent measures of perception. This approach is not without its challenges and limitations, and it needs to be complemented by investigating depth processing and cue combination at the level of individual neurons (Chapters 16–18) and detailed computational models (Chapters 20 and 21). However, an approach based on parametric stimulus manipulation, concurrent measures of perception, and a theoretical understanding of cue combination clearly has great potential to advance understanding of depth processing in the human brain.

What conclusions can be drawn about the architecture of depth processing in the human brain? In particular, where does the cortical implementation sit between the "modular" and "distributed" extreme scenarios outlined at the start of this chapter? The widespread responses to a range of depth cues (disparity, motion, texture) that have been observed throughout ventral, dorsal, and parietal cortical areas might suggest a less specialized, "distributed" processing architecture. However, from experiments that have targeted the use of these signals for the perception of 3D structure, a slightly more confined ensemble of areas is suggested. In particular, within the dorsal stream, higher visual areas (V3B/KO, V7) appear to prefer perceptually relevant disparity signals and process depth information from both binocular and monocular cues. Activity in higher ventral area LO also appears to be consistent with perception, although intriguingly, intermediate ventral areas do not have response properties that are strongly suggestive of hierarchical processing that terminates in LO. Rather, it is possible that LO obtains its depth information from activity in the dorsal stream. Such a cross-link might reasonably be supposed on the basis that signals originally important for controlling action were subsequently corralled into areas specialized for object recognition (on either an evolutionary or developmental basis).

One possibility is that the function of higher dorsal areas is to produce a generic depth map that is invariant to the particular cue that specifies depth and is exploitable for multiple purposes. Yet the different demands imposed by tasks such as controlling movements or recognizing objects might impose different type of representations. Rather, higher dorsal responses may reflect a halfway specialization for signals whose full resolution depends on activity in higher ventral areas or parietal cortex. Specifically, integrating structural information with information about surface properties may be important when recognizing objects invariant to the particular viewing situation. In contrast, lower variance estimators that result from combining independent signals will provide the best foundation for the control of action. The observation of "metric" versus "categorical" depth coding in dorsal areas versus ventral LO (Preston et al., 2008) is suggestive of this distinction.

Finally, this review has been concerned almost entirely with studying the representation of depth signals for perceptual judgments of shape. Understanding links between fMRI responses for depth signals and judgments of material properties and the control of (MRI compatible) actions are, as yet, largely untested. The development of novel fMRI paradigms and advances in data acquisition (e.g., high resolution) and analysis (e.g., multivariate techniques) provides an exciting basis for future developments.

## ACKNOWLEDGMENTS

This work was supported by the Biotechnology and Biological Sciences Research Council (grant C520620A) and the Birmingham University Imaging Centre. I am indebted to Julia Trommershäuser, Mike Landy, and two other readers for their thoughtful critiques of an earlier draft of this manuscript.

## REFERENCES

Adams, D. L., & Zeki, S. (2001). Functional organization of macaque V3 for stereoscopic depth. *Journal of Neurophysiology, 86*, 2195–2203.

Adams, W. J., Graf, E. W., & Ernst, M. O. (2004). Experience can change the "light-from-above" prior. *Nature Neuroscience, 7*, 1057–1058.

Backus, B. T., Fleet, D. J., Parker, A. J., & Heeger, D. J. (2001). Human cortical activity correlates with stereoscopic depth perception. *Journal of Neurophysiology, 86*, 2054–2068.

Barlow, H. B., Blakemore, C., & Pettigrew, J. D. (1967). The neural mechanism of binocular depth discrimination. *Journal of Physiology, 193*, 327–342.

Berends, E. M., Liu, B. X., & Schor, C. M. (2005). Stereo-slant adaptation is high level and does not involve disparity coding. *Journal of Vision, 5*, 71–80.

Bergman, R., & Gibson, J. J. (1959). The negative aftereffect of the perception of a surface slanted in the 3rd dimension. *American Journal of Psychology, 72,* 364–374.

Blake, A., & Bülthoff, H. H. (1990). Does the brain know the physics of specular reflection? *Nature, 343,* 165–168.

Blakemore, C., & Julesz, B. (1971). Stereoscopic depth aftereffect produced without monocular oues. *Science, 171,* 286–288.

Bradley, D. C., Chang, G. C., & Andersen, R. A. (1998). Encoding of three- dimensional structure-from-motion by primate area MT neurons. *Nature, 392,* 714–717.

Bridge, H., & Parker, A. J. (2007). Topographical representation of binocular depth in the human visual cortex using fMRI. *Journal of Vision, 7*(14):15, 1–14.

Britten, K. H., Shadlen, M. N., Newsome, W. T., & Movshon, J. A. (1992). The analysis of visual motion: A comparison of neuronal and psychophysical performance. *Journal of Neuroscience, 12,* 4745–4765.

Bülthoff, I., Bülthoff, H. H., & Sinha, P. (1998). Top-down influences on stereoscopic depth-perception. *Nature Neuroscience, 1,* 254–257.

Chandrasekaran, C., Canon, V., Dahmen, J. C., Kourtzi, Z., & Welchman, A. E. (2007). Neural correlates of disparity-defined shape discrimination in the human brain. *Journal of Neurophysiology, 97,* 1553–1565.

Cogan, A. I., Kontsevich, L. L., Lomakin, A. J., Halpern, D. L., & Blake, R. (1995). Binocular disparity processing with opposite-contrast stimuli. *Perception, 24,* 33–47.

Cox, D. D., & Savoy, R. L. (2003). Functional magnetic resonance imaging (fMRI) "brain reading": detecting and classifying distributed patterns of fMRI activity in human visual cortex. *Neuroimage, 19,* 261–270.

Cumming, B. G., & DeAngelis, G. C. (2001). The physiology of stereopsis. *Annual Review of Neuroscience, 24,* 203–238.

Cumming, B. G., & Parker, A. J. (1997). Responses of primary visual cortical neurons to binocular disparity without depth perception. *Nature, 389,* 280–283.

Cumming, B. G., Shapiro, S. E., & Parker, A. J. (1998). Disparity detection in anticorrelated stereograms. *Perception, 27,* 1367–1377.

DeAngelis, G. C., & Newsome, W. T. (1999). Organization of disparity-selective neurons in macaque area MT. *Journal of Neuroscience, 19,* 1398–1415.

Durand, J. B., Nelissen, K., Joly, O., Wardak, C., Todd, J. T., Norman, J. F., Janssen, P., Vanduffel, W., & Orban, G. A. (2007). Anterior regions of monkey parietal cortex process visual 3D shape. *Neuron, 55,* 493–505.

Fleming, R. W., Torralba, A., & Adelson, E. H. (2004). Specular reflections and the perception of shape. *Journal of Vision, 4,* 798–820.

Georgieva, S. S., Peeters, R., Kolster, H., Todd, J. T., & Orban, G. A. (2009). The processing of 3D shape from disparity in the human brain. *Journal of Neuroscience, 29,* 727–742.

Georgieva, S. S., Todd, J. T., Peeters, R., & Orban, G. A. (2008). The extraction of 3D shape from texture and shading in the human brain. *Cerebral Cortex, 18,* 2416–2438.

Grill-Spector, K., & Malach, R. (2001). fMR-adaptation: A tool for studying the functional properties of human cortical neurons. *Acta Psychologica, 107,* 293–321.

Haynes, J. D., & Rees, G. (2006). Decoding mental states from brain activity in humans. *Nature Reviews Neuroscience, 7,* 523–534.

Heeger, D. J., & Ress, D. (2002). What does fMRI tell us about neuronal activity? *Nature Reviews Neuroscience, 3,* 142–151.

Hillis, J. M., Ernst, M. O., Banks, M. S., & Landy, M. S. (2002). Combining sensory information: Mandatory fusion within, but not between, senses. *Science, 298,* 1627–1630.

Hillis, J. M., Watt, S. J., Landy, M. S., & Banks, M. S. (2004). Slant from texture and disparity cues: Optimal cue combination. *Journal of Vision, 4,* 967–992.

Hinkle, D. A., & Connor, C. E. (2005). Quantitative characterization of disparity tuning in ventral pathway area V4. *Journal of Neurophysiology, 94,* 2726–2737.

Janssen, P., Vogels, R., Liu, Y., & Orban, G. A. (2003). At least at the level of inferior temporal cortex, the stereo correspondence problem is solved. *Neuron, 37,* 693–701.

Janssen, P., Vogels, R., & Orban, G. A. (2000). Three-dimensional shape coding in inferior temporal cortex. *Neuron, 27,* 385–397.

Julesz, B. (1971). *Foundations of cyclopean perception.* Chicago, IL: University of Chicago.

Kamitani, Y., & Tong, F. (2005). Decoding the visual and subjective contents of the human brain. *Nature Neuroscience, 8,* 679–685.

Kanwisher, N., Chun, M. M., McDermott J., & Ledden, P. J. (1996). Functional imagining of human visual recognition. *Brain Research Cognitive Brain Research, 5*, 55–67.

Knapen, T., & van Ee, R. (2006). Slant perception, and its voluntary control, do not govern the slant aftereffect: Multiple slant signals adapt independently. *Vision Research, 46*, 3381–3392.

Kohler, W., & Emery, D. A. (1947). Figural after-effects in the 3rd dimension of visual space. *American Journal of Psychology, 60*, 159–201.

Kourtzi, Z., Erb, M., Grodd, W., & Bülthoff, H. H. (2003). Representation of the perceived 3-D object shape in the human lateral occipital complex. *Cerebral Cortex, 13*, 911–920.

Kourtzi, Z., & Kanwisher, N. (2001). Representation of perceived object shape by the human lateral occipital complex. *Science, 293*, 1506–1509.

Krug, K., Cumming, B. G., & Parker, A. J. (2004). Comparing perceptual signals of single V5/MT neurons in two binocular depth tasks. *Journal of Neurophysiology, 92*, 1586–1596.

Kumano, H., Tanabe, S., & Fujita, I. (2008). Spatial frequency integration for binocular correspondence in macaque area V4. *Journal of Neurophysiology, 99*, 402–408.

Landy, M. S., Maloney, L. T., Johnston, E. B., & Young, M. (1995). Measurement and modeling of depth cue combination: In defense of weak fusion. *Vision Research, 35*, 389–412.

Liu, Y., Vogels, R., & Orban, G. A. (2004). Convergence of depth from texture and depth from disparity in macaque inferior temporal cortex. *Journal of Neuroscience, 24*, 3795–3800.

Mach, E. (1886). *The analysis of sensations.* New York, NY: Dover.

Mamassian, P., & Goutcher, R. (2001). Prior knowledge on the illumination position. *Cognition, 81*, B1–B9.

Mamassian, P., Landy, M. S., & Maloney, L. T. (2002). Bayesian modeling of visual perception. In R. P. N. Rao, B. A. Olshausen, & M. S. Lewicki (Eds.), *Probabilistic models of the brain* (pp. 13–60). Cambridge, MA: MIT Press.

Marr, D. (1976). Early processing of visual information. *Philosophical Transactions of the Royal Society of London B: Biological Sciences, 275*, 483–519.

Masson, G. S., Busettini, C., & Miles, F. A. (1997). Vergence eye movements in response to binocular disparity without depth perception. *Nature, 389*, 283–286.

Moore, C., & Engel, S. A. (2001). Neural response to perception of volume in the lateral occipital complex. *Neuron, 29*, 277–286.

Murray, S. O., Olshausen, B. A., & Woods, D. L. (2003). Processing shape, motion and three-dimensional shape-from-motion in the human cortex. *Cerebral Cortex, 13*, 508–516.

Nawrot, M., & Blake, R. (1989). Neural integration of information specifying structure from stereopsis and motion. *Science, 244*, 716–718.

Norman, K. A., Polyn, S. M., Detre, G. J., & Haxby, J. V. (2006). Beyond mind-reading: Multi-voxel pattern analysis of fMRI data. *Trends in Cognitive Sciences, 10*, 424–430.

Orban, G. A., Janssen, P., & Vogels, R. (2006). Extracting 3D structure from disparity. *Trends in Neurosciences, 29*, 466–473.

Orban, G. A., Sunaert, S., Todd, J. T., Van Hecke, P., & Marchal, G. (1999). Human cortical regions involved in extracting depth from motion. *Neuron, 24*, 929–940.

Palanca, B. J., & DeAngelis, G. C. (2003). Macaque middle temporal neurons signal depth in the absence of motion. *Journal of Neuroscience, 23*, 7647–7658.

Parker, A. J. (2007). Binocular depth perception and the cerebral cortex. *Nature Reviews Neuroscience, 8*, 379–391.

Parker, A. J., & Newsome, W. T. (1998). Sense and the single neuron: Probing the physiology of perception. *Annual Review of Neuroscience, 21*, 227–277.

Peuskens, H., Claeys, K. G., Todd, J. T., Norman, J. F., Van Hecke, P., & Orban, G. A. (2004). Attention to 3-D shape, 3-D motion, and texture in 3-D structure from motion displays. *Journal of Cognitive Neuroscience, 16*, 665–682.

Poggio, G. F., Gonzalez, F., & Krause, F. (1988). Stereoscopic mechanisms in monkey visual cortex: Binocular correlation and disparity selectivity. *Journal of Neuroscience, 8*, 4531–4550.

Ponce, C. R., Lomber, S. G., & Born, R. T. (2008). Integrating motion and depth via parallel pathways. *Nature Neuroscience, 11*, 216–223.

Preston, T. J., Kourtzi, Z., & Welchman, A. E. (2009). Adaptive estimation of three-dimensional structure in the human brain. *Journal of Neuroscience, 29*, 1688–1698.

Preston, T. J., Li, S., Kourtzi, Z., & Welchman, A. E. (2008). Multivoxel pattern selectivity for perceptually relevant binocular disparities in the human brain. *Journal of Neuroscience, 28,* 11315–11327.

Scannell, J. W., & Young, M. P. (1999). Neuronal population activity and functional imaging. *Proceedings of the Royal Society B: Biological Sciences, 266,* 875–881.

Sereno, M. E., Trinath, T., Augath, M., & Logothetis, N. K. (2002). Three-dimensional shape representation in monkey cortex. *Neuron, 33,* 635–652.

Shikata, E., Hamzei, F., Glauche, V., Knab, R., Dettmers, C., Weiller, C., & Büchel, C. (2001). Surface orientation discrimination activates caudal and anterior intraparietal sulcus in humans: An event-related fMRI study. *Journal of Neurophysiology, 85,* 1309–1314.

Sinha, P., & Poggio, T. (1996). Role of learning in three-dimensional form perception. *Nature, 384,* 460–463.

Stocker, A. A., & Simoncelli, E. P. (2005). Constraining a Bayesian model of human visual speed perception. In Y. Weiss, B. Schölkopf, & J. Platt (Eds.), *NIPS* (pp. 1291–1298). Cambridge, MA: MIT Press.

Taira, M., Nose, I., Inoue, K., & Tsutsui, K. (2001). Cortical areas related to attention to 3D surface structures based on shading: An fMRI study. *Neuroimage, 14,* 959–966.

Taira, M., Tsutsui, K. I., Jiang, M., Yara, K., & Sakata, H. (2000). Parietal neurons represent surface orientation from the gradient of binocular disparity. *Journal of Neurophysiology, 83,* 3140–3146.

Tanabe, S., Umeda, K., & Fujita, I. (2004). Rejection of false matches for binocular correspondence in macaque visual cortical area V4. *Journal of Neuroscience, 24,* 8170–8180.

Taya, S., Sato, M., & Nakamizo, S. (2005). Stereoscopic depth aftereffects without retinal position correspondence between adaptation and test stimuli. *Vision Research, 45,* 1857–1866.

Thomas, O. M., Cumming, B. G., & Parker, A. J. (2002). A specialization for relative disparity in V2. *Nature Neuroscience, 5,* 472–478.

Tsao, D. Y., Vanduffel, W., Sasaki, Y., Fize, D., Knutsen, T. A., Mandeville, J. B., ... Tootell, R. B. (2003). Stereopsis activates V3A and caudal intraparietal areas in macaques and humans. *Neuron, 39,* 555–568.

Tsutsui, K., Sakata, H., Naganuma, T., & Taira, M. (2002). Neural correlates for perception of 3D surface orientation from texture gradient. *Science, 298,* 409–412.

Tyler, C. W., Likova, L. T., Kontsevich, L. L., & Wade, A. R. (2006). The specificity of cortical region KO to depth structure. *Neuroimage, 30,* 228–238.

Uka, T., & DeAngelis, G. C. (2006). Linking neural representation to function in stereoscopic depth perception: Roles of the middle temporal area in coarse versus fine disparity discrimination. *Journal of Neuroscience, 26,* 6791–6802.

Uka, T., Tanaka, H., Yoshiyama, K., Kato, M., & Fujita, I. (2000). Disparity selectivity of neurons in monkey inferior temporal cortex. *Journal of Neurophysiology, 84,* 120–132.

Vanduffel, W., Tootell, R. B. H., Schoups, A. A., & Orban, G. A. (2002). The organization of orientation selectivity throughout macaque visual cortex. *Cerebral Cortex, 12,* 647–662.

Vapnik, V. (1995). *The nature of statistical learning theory.* New York, NY: Springer.

Wallach, H., & O'Connell, D. N. (1953). The kinetic depth effect. *Journal of Experimental Psychology, 45,* 205–217.

Watt, S. J., & Bradshaw, M. F. (2002). Binocular information in the control of prehensile movements in multiple-object scenes. *Spatial Vision, 15,* 141–155.

Welchman, A. E., Deubelius, A., Conrad, V., Bülthoff, H. H., & Kourtzi, Z. (2005). 3D shape perception from combined depth cues in human visual cortex. *Nature Neuroscience, 8,* 820–827.

# CHAPTER 20

## Dynamic Cue Combination in Distributional Population Code Networks

*Rama Natarajan and Richard S. Zemel*

### INTRODUCTION

In this chapter, we investigate how hierarchical networks of neural populations might code stable representations of transient stimulus variables along with the uncertainty about them, while allowing consistent semantics of inputs and outputs at every level of the neural hierarchy. One effective paradigm to study this question is the integration of information from multiple sensory sources. Significant behavioral and neurophysiological evidence substantiates the notion that when separate sensory modalities receive correlated inputs about an external stimulus, the information is often combined to produce a coherent, unitary percept of the world (Stein & Meredith, 1993). This ability of neural systems to combine information from multiple sources affords considerable, ecologically relevant advantages. For instance, it has been shown to attenuate the effects of input variability owing to noise, thereby reducing the overall uncertainty in the final estimate of the stimulus variable.

Sensory cue integration and sensorimotor combinations involve many important and challenging statistical issues; for example, the different sources of information are not equally reliable, and their reliability can change with changing stimulus conditions and task demands. Bayesian probability theory has provided a normative framework for predicting how sensory systems might integrate information optimally, to make perceptual inferences about the environment from noisy sensory data. These predictions have been quantitatively tested using psychophysical experiments that examine what computations are performed when reliability of the cues changes over time. Results from widely ranging studies of human cue integration are consistent in that subjects behave in a manner that takes the uncertainty in sensory inputs into account, to form statistically optimal estimates of stimulus variables (see Knill & Pouget, 2004, for a review). Several different computational strategies have been proposed and validated; some examples are linear weighted averaging (Hillis, Watt, Landy, & Banks, 2004; Jacobs, 1999; Knill & Saunders, 2003; van Beers, Sittig, & van der Gon, 1999), extensions thereof (Landy, Maloney, Johnston, & Young, 1995), multiplicative interactions, and fully probabilistic linear and nonlinear Bayesian inference (Knill, 2003).

Regardless of the exact inference strategy, the common theme in all these studies is that sensory uncertainty determines the optimal weighting scheme for combining sensory inputs for perceptual judgments. Similarly, studies also demonstrate that sensory and motor uncertainties determine how sensory signals should be transformed and used to plan actions and guide behavior. An example of a commonly used paradigm involves manipulating continuous visual feedback from the hand to control pointing movements. Subjects are able to compensate for experimentally induced changes in sensory (such as position and velocity) and motor uncertainties and optimally adjust the degree to which they rely on the feedback to make corrections (Körding & Wolpert, 2004; Saunders & Knill, 2003, 2004).

What is less clear is how neural systems might represent information about the various cues, to implement these putative computations in a manner sensitive to the uncertainties about the cues. More generally, because of the noise and ambiguities inherent in sensory inputs, many perceptual tasks are better viewed as statistical-inference problems. One normative hypothesis is that the brain represents and computes with probability distributions over all the different stimuli that are consistent with the inputs, as opposed to unitary estimates of stimulus variables (Zemel, Dayan, & Pouget, 1998).

In this chapter, we consider how a network consisting of several neural populations can represent and combine information from multiple cues in a statistically optimal manner, in order to carry out proper probabilistic inference. We then take this aim a step further, considering time-varying inputs. If the neural system can maintain, at each stage of local computation, full distributions over all possible stimulus values, it can allow considerable flexibility in accommodating changing cue uncertainties. This representational scheme thus pushes the envelope on current psychophysical studies of cue combination, yielding a computational network of neural populations where the responses approximate proper inference even when cues' values and uncertainties vary rapidly.

Influential ideas abound regarding how neural systems might encode (Rao, Olshausen, & Lewicki, 2002; Sanger, 1996) and interpret (decode) probability distributions over stimulus variables (Denève, Latham, & Pouget, 1999; Paradiso, 1988; Seung & Sompolinsky, 1993; Snippe & Koenderink, 1992), and how various computations, including uncertainty-sensitive, Bayesian optimal statistical processing, might be performed through feedforward and recurrent connections between neural populations (Denève, Latham, & Pouget, 2001; Pouget, Zhang, Denève, & Latham, 1998). However, theoretical investigations have for the most part neglected the *temporal* dimension of coding; often, the stimuli are treated as being discrete rather than evolving along full trajectories (Brunel & Nadal, 1998; Van Rullen & Thorpe, 2001). Otherwise it is assumed that encoded stimulus variables do not vary quickly with time, and therefore population spike counts as opposed to actual timing of spikes suffice.

In this chapter we consider how a neural system could properly combine cues even as their reliabilities change dynamically and continuously in time. The rest of the chapter is organized as follows: The next section describes a framework for characterizing how uncertain information may be represented in population codes, and how the representation may be optimized to facilitate optimal decoding. We then motivate and present a coding scheme within this framework that applies to time-varying stimulus variables. Next, we describe a hierarchical network setup that utilizes this coding approach, and we demonstrate an application to a dynamic cue-combination task, a novel adaptation of a sensorimotor task (Körding & Wolpert, 2004). Specifically, we consider how a neural population might recursively integrate dynamic inputs from multiple sensory modalities with learned prior information, to determine appropriate motor commands that control behavior. Then, we present results of simulated experiments with this network. Finally, we discuss implications of this scheme and suggest some future directions.

## APPROXIMATING PROBABILISTIC INFERENCE IN POPULATION-CODE NETWORKS

To illustrate the cue-combination process that we address in this chapter, let us consider a simple target-localization task that involves pointing a finger at a visual target. The computational problem entails extracting a task-relevant physical attribute of the environment from multisensory data. In this case, we compute the amount of displacement $s^c$ of the finger from the current location to the target position. Several useful cues (i.e., functions of the sensory input; see definition in Chapter 5) are available in this context. In our example, we employ a visual cue $s^v$ signaling the visual location of the target, and a proprioceptive cue $s^p$ conveying information about the position of the finger.

We begin by assuming that the basic representations in the network are population codes; that is, information about sensory and motor variables is represented in the joint spiking activity of large populations of neurons (Barlow, 1953; Georgopoulos, Schwartz, & Kettner, 1983). It is impossible to infer the exact location of the target or the finger position from the neural activity due to uncertainty that arises from noise in sensation and the sensorimotor transmission process, as well as potential ambiguities in the stimulus such as low-contrast visual information about target location. Hence, the population codes are treated as encoding whole probability density functions (PDFs) over the underlying variables rather than just a single best estimate. The goal is to provide a rich representation of uncertainty in the aspects of the stimuli that are represented (see Pouget, Dayan, & Zemel, 2003, for a review).

We formulate a neural implementation that respects or aims to closely approximate proper combination of probabilistic information. According to the probabilistic population-coding hypothesis, *explicit* activities $\boldsymbol{\rho} = \{\rho_i\}$ of multiple neurons $i = \{1, 2, 3, \ldots, n\}$ represent a probability distribution $p(s|\boldsymbol{\rho})$ over an *implicit* underlying variable $s$ (such as the position of the target), using some encoding scheme; decoding then describes how the distribution can be recovered from the population activity (Anderson, 1994; Rao et al., 2002; Zemel et al., 1998). One proposal for a neural implementation of cue combination using the distributional coding scheme entailed specifying a simple two-layer feedforward network (Zemel & Dayan, 1997). In the context of the target-localization task we described earlier, the first layer consists of separate populations of visual and proprioceptive neurons that encode probability distributions $p(s^v|\boldsymbol{\rho}^v)$ and $p(s^p|\boldsymbol{\rho}^p)$ over visual and proprioceptive positions, in their neural activities $\boldsymbol{\rho}^v$ and $\boldsymbol{\rho}^p$, respectively. Representing a complete distribution in this manner may be essential for correctly combining information from the different sensory sources, if the statistical relationship between the inputs (visual and proprioceptive) and outputs (displacement $s^c$) is to be preserved.

Cue combination can then be cast as the problem of inferring the distribution over $s^c$ based on the inputs $\boldsymbol{\rho}^v$ and $\boldsymbol{\rho}^p$, that is, $p(s^c|\boldsymbol{\rho}^v, \boldsymbol{\rho}^p)$. Given that the inputs specify probability distributions $p(s^v|\boldsymbol{\rho}^v)$ and $p(s^p|\boldsymbol{\rho}^p)$ according to some encoding scheme, the Bayes-optimal method of performing inference in this approach is specified as follows (Zemel & Dayan, 1997):

$$p(s^c|\boldsymbol{\rho}^v, \boldsymbol{\rho}^p) = \int_{s^v, s^p} p(s^v|\boldsymbol{\rho}^v)p(s^p|\boldsymbol{\rho}^p) \times p(s^c|s^v, s^p)ds^v ds^p \tag{20.1}$$

$$\propto p(s^c) \int_{s^v, s^p} p(s^v|\boldsymbol{\rho}^v)p(s^p|\boldsymbol{\rho}^p) \times p(s^v, s^p|s^c)ds^v ds^p, \tag{20.2}$$

where $p(s^c)$ is the prior distribution over $s^c$. We will assume that the information in the different inputs is independent and that there is a probabilistic generative model that specifies how the distribution $p(s^v, s^p|s^c)$ over possible visual target and proprioceptive finger locations is produced, for any given displacement $s^c$. Eq. 20.2 establishes the ideal observer, or the standard by which inferences about the distribution over $s^c$ should be judged.

Computations in the network are guided by this probabilistic formulation. The feedforward connections determine how $\boldsymbol{\rho}^v$ and $\boldsymbol{\rho}^p$ are combined to produce $\boldsymbol{\rho}^c$, such that $\boldsymbol{\rho}^c$ defines a distribution that approximates Eq. 20.2 as closely as possible. Figure 20.1 illustrates the generative and recognition operations, showing the activities, the distributions that they represent, and the various probabilistic relationships.

This formulation requires specifying a form for the decoder that determines how the distribution is derived from the activities, and then optimizing the network synaptic connections to approximate the ideal observer under the specified encoding and decoding schemes. One possible form of decoding is a kernel density

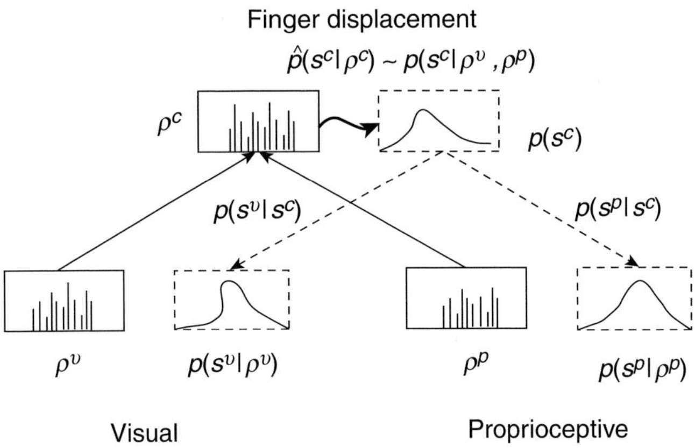


**Figure 20.1** An example of a network formulated to combine population code representations of PDFs. The elements shown in solid lines depict explicit network components, including the population responses ($\boldsymbol{\rho}^v$, $\boldsymbol{\rho}^p$, $\boldsymbol{\rho}^c$). The elements shown in dashed lines are the implicit components, that is, the probabilistic information represented by the explicit network components. The probabilistic combination provides the target for the network population codes and weights; the decoded distribution $\hat{p}(s|\boldsymbol{\rho})$ should match the posterior distribution $\hat{p}(s|\boldsymbol{\rho})$ obtained by Bayesian inference given the input PDFs $p(s^v|\boldsymbol{\rho}^v)$ and $p(s^p|\boldsymbol{\rho}^p)$.

estimate, in which the PDF is a sum of PDFs proposed by each neuron in the population weighted by its activity (Anderson, 1994); a second is a more optimal but complicated maximum-likelihood scheme (Zemel et al., 1998). An alternative decoding approach decodes the PDF as a log-linear combination of the PDFs proposed by each neuron (Hinton, 1999):

$$\hat{p}(s|\boldsymbol{\rho}) \propto \prod_i \hat{p}_i(s|\rho_i)^{\rho_i} = \exp\left(\sum_i \rho_i \log \hat{p}_i(s|\rho_i)\right). \qquad (20.3)$$

We have applied this *product-of-experts* formulation (Huys, Zemel, Natarajan, & Dayan, 2007; Natarajan, Huys, Dayan, & Zemel 2008) and shown that this scheme has the attractive feature of allowing each neuron to be considered independently of the others, while permitting a wide variety of PDFs. Note in particular that this product representation can produce much more peaked distributions than the kernel density estimate, which involves a linear combination of PDFs.

Given this decoder, computation in neural circuitry can be optimized such that applying this simple decoder to the network outputs will approximate the target distribution (Eq. 20.2) as faithfully as possible. An important point is that we are not proposing that neural circuits actually perform decoding at each level. Rather, the motivation for using this simple decoder is to explore whether a coding scheme can be found that will approximate proper inference, when the information about the relevant variable(s) at each level can be easily accessed, as in a log-linear decoding scheme.

This framework, along with this product-of-experts decoder, bears an interesting relationship to other recent proposals, notably the probabilistic population codes of Pouget and colleagues (Ma, Beck, Latham, & Pouget, 2006). Adopting the same decoder, they show that under some limited assumptions about the individual neuron's PDFs ($\hat{p}_i(s|\rho_i)$), several natural computations can be carried out by linear operations on activities in the input populations.

## DYNAMIC PROBABILISTIC POPULATION CODES

### Time-Varying Continuous Inputs

The formulation described earlier readily applies to static cue-integration problems, in which cue weights are assumed to remain constant over time. In this section, we consider a more realistic situation in which the input forms a continuous stream and the underlying variable of interest follows some trajectory. Hence, information from each cue can accrue over time in ways that affect how the different cues are combined dynamically.

To consider continuous, dynamic inputs, we switch the description of the neural activity from rate based to spike trains. We also adopt a different version of the decoder, which ignores correlations in the inputs and treats each spike independently, linearly integrating the information conveyed by them. The log-linear spike decoder (Hinton & Brown, 2000) fits these desiderata, and it can be seen as a simple extension of the product-of-experts decoder described in the previous section to spiking inputs, where the effect of past spikes decays exponentially over time. Here again, the motivation for this decoder is that the information necessary to perform proper probabilistic inference is available in a form that biological neurons might reasonably be expected to access.

***Deriving an Optimal Time-Varying Target Distribution*** Consider a dynamic stimulus variable, say the position of a visual target, that evolves over time forming a *trajectory* defined by $\vec{s}_T = \{s_1, \cdots, s_t, \cdots, s_T\}$, where $s_t$ is the position at time $t$. Thus, $\vec{s}_T$ defines the trajectory through which this object moves in the world. Note that we employ a discrete time representation. A population of neurons $i = \{1, 2, \ldots, N\}$ that responds selectively to the position generates a population spike sequence $\vec{\boldsymbol{\xi}}_T = \{\boldsymbol{\xi}_1, \cdots, \boldsymbol{\xi}_t, \cdots, \boldsymbol{\xi}_T\}$, where $\boldsymbol{\xi}_t$ is a binary spike vector at time $t$, such that $\boldsymbol{\xi}_t^i$ is 1 when neuron $i$ spikes at time $t$.[1]

We assume that the spikes $\vec{\boldsymbol{\xi}}_T$ are generated by an encoding model $P(\vec{\boldsymbol{\xi}}_T|\vec{s}_T)$ that specifies the probability of a particular population spike sequence being evoked by the trajectory $\vec{s}_T$. Since neural spiking is stochastic and not capable of representing the stimulus value exactly, we consider the population response to implicitly define a distribution over likely stimulus trajectories. Then, the posterior distribution $p(s_T|\vec{\boldsymbol{\xi}}_T)$ over stimulus positions can be estimated as a Bayesian inverse of the respective encoding model. Thus, we adopt the filtering goal of estimating the posterior distribution over trajectories implied by the input spikes, rather than the prediction one of making an estimate about the future course of the trajectory.

***Spike-Generation Model*** We adopt a standard (tuning curve plus noise) spike-generation model for the set of all the $J$ spikes $\boldsymbol{\xi}_\varsigma \equiv \{\xi_{t_j}^i\}_{j=1}^J$ at times $0 < \{t_j\}_{j=1}^J \leq T$ evoked by the trajectory $\vec{s}_T$, where $\varsigma$ is a collection of all spike times. Under this model, the population response is governed by neurons whose expected responses are defined by partially overlapping Gaussian tuning functions, and whose stochastic observed responses are modeled as Poisson variables. The spikes are probabilistically related to the stimulus by means of a tuning function defined for each neuron $i$ in the population as follows:

$$f_i(s_{t_j}) = r_{\max} \exp\left(-\frac{(s_{t_j} - \theta_i)^2}{2\sigma^2}\right), \tag{20.4}$$

where $s_{t_j}$ is the value of the stimulus variable at time $t_j$, $\theta_i$ is the preferred stimulus value of neuron $i$, $r_{\max}$ is the maximum input firing rate and $\sigma$ is the tuning width. By this simple Gaussian definition, each neuron fires maximally at its preferred value $\theta_i$ and the activity drops off monotonically according to $\sigma$, as the stimulus $s_{t_j}$ drifts away from $\theta_i$.

The actual observed spikes are generated as inhomogeneous and instantaneous Poisson processes governed by the tuning functions (Barbieri et al., 2004; Brown, Frank, Tang, Quirk, & Wilson, 1998):

$$P(\vec{\boldsymbol{\xi}}_\varsigma|\vec{s}_T) \propto \left(\prod_j f_{i(j)}(s_{t_j})\right) \exp\left(-\sum_i\sum_t f_i(s_t)\right). \tag{20.5}$$

[1] Regarding notation: throughout this chapter we use a boldface variable to denote responses in a population of neurons; we use the arrow notation, e.g., $\vec{s}_T$, to denote a time-series vector, in this case of length $T$.

This spiking model entails some assumptions about the tuning properties and response of the input neurons. In our abstraction, the spikes are conditionally independent events given the stimulus and the current response is independent of past activity. The tuning properties of the input population are constrained such that each neuron has the same maximum firing rate and tuning width. Furthermore, the tuning functions are assumed to span the stimulus state-space evenly and densely such that $\sum_i \sum_t f_i(s_t)$ is approximately a constant. This leads to:

$$P(\vec{\boldsymbol{\xi}}_{\varsigma}|\vec{s}_T) \propto \prod_j f_{i(j)}(s_{t_j}). \tag{20.6}$$

Substituting for the tuning function from Eq. 20.4, the input spike generation model is then:

$$P(\vec{\boldsymbol{\xi}}_{\varsigma}|\vec{s}_T) \propto r_{\max} \times \exp\left(-\frac{\left(\vec{s}_{\varsigma} - \vec{\theta}(T)\right)^T \left(\vec{s}_{\varsigma} - \vec{\theta}(T)\right)}{2\sigma^2}\right), \tag{20.7}$$

where $\vec{s}_{\varsigma}$ is the vector of all the stimulus positions ordered by spike time, and $\vec{\theta}(T)$ is the corresponding vector of preferred stimulus values of the spiking neurons.

***Ideal Observer*** In Huys et al. (2007) we investigated the computational consequences of probabilistically encoding such stimulus trajectories in the spiking activity of populations of neurons. We summarize the basic setup and findings here. We first specify a prior over trajectories. The trajectories are defined over continuous time, and they are assumed to be drawn from a Gaussian Process (GP). This means that for any finite collection of times $\mathfrak{I} = \{t_i\}$, the stimulus values $s_{\mathfrak{I}}$ are drawn from a multivariate Gaussian distribution with mean $\boldsymbol{m}$ and covariance matrix $C$:

$$p(\varphi_{(0,T)}) \sim N(\boldsymbol{m}, C)$$

$$C_{t_i t_j} = c \exp\left(-\alpha \left\| t_i - t_j \right\|^{\zeta}\right), \tag{20.8}$$

where $C$ is the matrix of $C_{t_i t_j}$ at the discretized times. Different values of $\zeta$ determine the different classes of prior distributions over trajectories, and $c$ parameterizes the overall scale of the process. The value of $\alpha$ scales the temporal extent of the interactions in the stimulus.

Under the assumptions described above, the posterior distribution for an observed population spike train can be derived as a Gaussian distribution with a mean $\mu(T)$ that is a weighted sum of the preferred positions of neurons that fired, and a variance $\nu^2(T)$ that depends only on $C$ and the tuning width $\sigma^2$:

$$\mu(T) = \boldsymbol{k}(\vec{\boldsymbol{\xi}}_{\varsigma}, T) \cdot \vec{\theta}(T) \tag{20.9}$$

$$\nu^2(T) = C_{TT} - \boldsymbol{k}(\vec{\boldsymbol{\xi}}_{\varsigma}, T) \cdot C_{\varsigma T}. \tag{20.10}$$

Here $\vec{\theta}(T)$ is the vector of preferred stimulus values of the spiking neurons, ordered by spike time, $\varsigma$ is a collection of all spike times, $C_{TT} = c$ is the static stimulus variance at the observation time, and $C_{\varsigma T}$ is a vector of the cross-covariance between the spike times and observation time $T$. Recall that $C$ depends only on the times of spikes, not on their identities. The posterior variance is similar to a Kalman filter and depends only on when data are observed, not what data. The weight on each spike depends strongly on the time at which the spike occurred:

$$\boldsymbol{k}(\vec{\boldsymbol{\xi}}_{\varsigma}, T) = C_{T\varsigma}(C_{\varsigma\varsigma} + \boldsymbol{I}\sigma^2)^{-1}. \tag{20.11}$$

Here, $C_{\varsigma\varsigma}$ is the covariance matrix of the stimulus at all the spike times. A spike that occurred in the distant past will be given small weight.

Even under such a constrained and analytically tractable formulation of the encoding model (Eq. 20.5), the population spike trains tend to be sparse, so decoding trajectory information as a Bayesian inverse of the encoding model turns out to be ill posed. Prior information about what trajectories are likely plays a critical role. For the simple GP prior, the form of the dynamics is controlled by the various parameters, and particularly by the parameter $\zeta$. If $\zeta = 1$, stimuli undergo Markovian dynamics, and the posterior distribution can be written in a recursive form that depends on only current spikes and a single population vector summarizing information in past spikes. But when $\zeta = 2$, stimulus correlations extend further back in time, producing stimuli with *smooth* autocorrelations. This regime is the most ecologically relevant, as natural trajectories tend to vary smoothly over time. In this case, however, a simple recursive decoding is not possible, as instead decoding couples together the spikes, which means that the entire population spiking history is required to properly interpret a new spike.

Thus, our analyses show that neural correlations induced by naturalistic, smooth stimuli lead to a decoding problem that can only be resolved by access to information that is nonlocal both in time and across neurons. This makes trajectory inference computationally very hard. In a network of neurons, the downstream neural population that obtains these spikes as inputs faces a complicated inference problem, because computational and behavioral constraints do not permit retaining the full spiking history.

### Optimizing a Network to Approximate Time-Varying Target Distributions

We now turn to the network version of the dynamic population-code combination problem, that is, the continuous analog to Figure 20.1. In Natarajan et al. (2008), we considered the distribution produced by the ideal observer in the previous section as the optimal target distribution for the network. The decoder for the population spikes was a spike-based version of the product of experts, in which each spike is considered independently of the others in the spike sequence, and spikes from different neurons can be combined without taking correlations into account. We then formulated a recurrent network, the connection strengths of which can be optimized so that this simple decoder approximates the dynamic target distribution. The details of the recurrent network and the decoding model are provided next.

***Nonlinear Recurrent Network Approximating Optimal Inference*** Let $j = \{1, 2, \ldots, M\}$ be a population of recurrently connected output neurons in a network, receiving inputs $\vec{\boldsymbol{\xi}}_T$ from the population $i = \{1, 2, \ldots, N\}$. We ascribe simple dynamics to the recurrent population, similar to the general spiking-neuron model of Kistler, Gerstner, and van Hemmen (1997). The output population spikes are specified by $\vec{\boldsymbol{\rho}}_T$, where $\rho_t^j = 1$ if neuron $j$ spikes at time $t$. Like the inputs, the output spikes also convey information about $\vec{s}_T$.

The strength of the synaptic connection from an input neuron $i$ to an output neuron $j$ is characterized by the weight $W_{ij}$, and lateral connections between neurons $j$ and $k$ in the output population by $U_{jk}$. This scheme is illustrated in Figure 20.2. In a discrete time representation, the internal state (analogous to the membrane potential) of a neuron $j$ at time $T$ can be characterized by a continuous variable $h_T^j$:

$$h_T^j = \sum_{\tau=0}^{T-1} \sum_{i=1}^{N} \xi_{T-\tau}^i W_{ij} \eta(\tau) + \sum_{\tau=0}^{T-2} \sum_{k=1}^{M} \rho_{T-\tau-1}^k U_{kj} \eta(\tau). \quad (20.12)$$

The term $\eta(\tau)$ specifies the effect of a past spike on the current membrane potential; this typically has a form where temporally distant spikes have diminishing effects compared to more recent ones. Note that the feedforward and lateral weights can be negative. Thus, $h_T^j$ is a signed variable where large negative values make spikes unlikely; large positive values make them likely.

For each neuron $j$ in the population, its response is governed by a stochastic binary spiking rule:

$$P(\rho_T^j = 1) = \sigma(h_T^j). \quad (20.13)$$

The spikes are generated independently among the population. This implies that the probability of any population binary (spike/no-spike) vector $\rho_T$ at time $T$ is:

$$P(\vec{\boldsymbol{\rho}}_T | \vec{\boldsymbol{\xi}}_T) = \prod_j \sigma(h_T^j)^{\rho_T^j} (1 - \sigma(h_T^j))^{(1-\rho_T^j)}, \quad (20.14)$$

where the sigmoid function is defined by $\sigma(h_T^j) = \frac{1}{1+\exp(-h_T^j)}$.

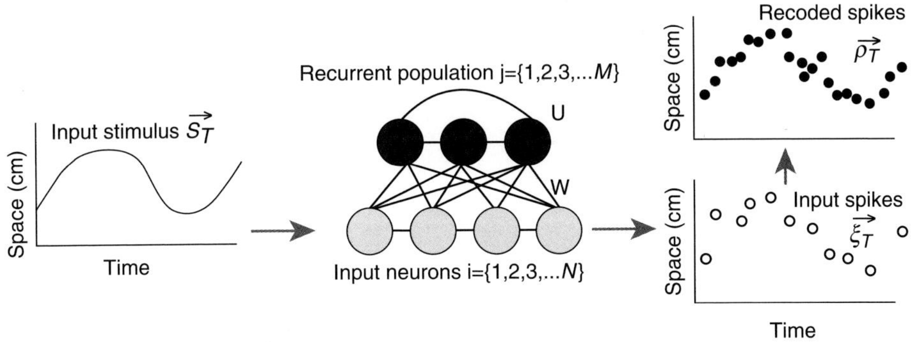


**Figure 20.2** Schematic description of our network. Sensory *input* neurons $i = 1, \ldots, N$ generate population spikes in response to a stimulus trajectory. Downstream *output* population $j = 1, \ldots, M$ receives the input via feedforward synapses **W**; recurrently processes the input using learned lateral synaptic weights **U** to recode the input into a representation that is independently decodeable by downstream neurons. Note the convention for this and subsequent figures: The neurons are arranged based on their preferred stimulus values, and a circle indicates that the neuron at that position spiked at the particular time.

Note that the dynamics can be simplified considerably if the influence of past spikes is defined as:

$$\eta(\tau) = \exp(-\beta\tau), \tag{20.15}$$

where $\beta$ is the *temporal decay constant.* Using an exponentially decaying function to characterize the postsynaptic potential of a neuron allows us to express the dynamics of the output population in a recursive formulation:

$$h_T^j = \sum_i \xi_T^i W_{ij} + \sum_k \rho_{T-1}^k U_{kj} + \eta(1) h_{T-1}^j. \tag{20.16}$$

Then the probability of a population spike vector is a function solely of the membrane potential and population outputs at the previous time step, and the current input spikes:

$$P(\boldsymbol{\rho}_T | \vec{\boldsymbol{\xi}}_T) = P(\boldsymbol{\rho}_T | \boldsymbol{h}_{T-1}; \boldsymbol{\rho}_{T-1}; \boldsymbol{\xi}_T). \tag{20.17}$$

Figure 20.2 illustrates our network formulation.

***An Independent Probabilistic Decoder*** The decoding model specifies the probabilities of various stimulus trajectories based on the spike sequence. Rather than considering the complicated space of possible trajectories given an entire spike train, we focus on an instantaneous version of the problem. In mathematical terms, our aim is to decode at time $T$ a distribution over the stimulus position at that time, $s_T$, given all the spike observations up to that particular time, $\vec{\boldsymbol{\rho}}_T = \{\boldsymbol{\rho}_1, \cdots, \boldsymbol{\rho}_T\}$; that is, we want to infer $\hat{p}(s_T | \vec{\boldsymbol{\rho}}_T)$ to approximate closely the true posterior distribution $p(s_T | \vec{\boldsymbol{\xi}}_T)$. In this scheme, the total effect of the spike-train $E(s, T, \vec{\boldsymbol{\rho}}_T)$ is specified as a linear combination of the individual spikes:

$$E(s, T, \vec{\boldsymbol{\rho}}_T) = \sum_{j=1}^{M} \sum_{\tau=0}^{T-1} \kappa_{\text{std}}(j, s, \tau) \rho_{T-\tau}^j, \tag{20.18}$$

where $\kappa_{\text{std}}(j, s, \tau)$ is the spatiotemporal decoding kernel defined as being uniform and separable; uniform in that the shape of the kernel is the same for the entire population, and at all times, and separable as $\kappa_{\text{std}}(j, s, \tau) = \phi_j(s)\psi(\tau)$, where $\phi_j(s)$ is the spatial component and $\psi(\tau)$ is the temporal component. Then the spatiotemporal contribution of the spikes (Eq. 20.18) can be rewritten as follows:

$$E(s, T, \vec{\boldsymbol{\rho}}_T) = \sum_j \left[ \sum_{\tau=0}^{T-1} \psi(\tau) \rho_{T-\tau}^j \right] \phi_j(s). \tag{20.19}$$

The spatial dimension of the kernel is parameterized as

$$\phi_j(s) = \frac{|s - s_j|^2}{\omega}, \tag{20.20}$$

where $\omega$ is the projective width of the neurons and $s_j$ is the preferred stimulus value of neuron $j$. Thus, $\phi_j(s)$ defines the influence of the output of a particular neuron $j$ in the population $j = \{1 \ldots M\}$, on the spatial interpretation of the underlying variable.

The temporal dimension of the kernel is specified as an exponential decay (analogous to the postsynaptic potential of the neuron, $\eta$ in Eq. 20.16): $\psi(\tau) = \exp(-\gamma\tau)$. The parameter $\gamma$, which we refer to as the *temporal integration constant,* specifies the timescale for synaptic integration in the readout. It effectively controls what effect the spiking of a neuron at one time has on the interpretation at future times. Hence, the kernels are very simple, specified using just three parameters: the preferred stimulus value $s_j$ and spatial projective width $\omega$ for neuron $j$, and the temporal integration constant $\gamma$. The approximating probability distribution over stimulus trajectories $\hat{p}(s_T|\vec{\boldsymbol{\rho}}_T)$ is interpreted from the spiking activity as:

$$\hat{p}(s_T|\vec{\boldsymbol{\rho}}_T) \propto \exp(-E(s, T, \vec{\boldsymbol{\rho}}_T)). \tag{20.21}$$

Eqs. 20.18 and 20.21 define our decoding hypothesis. Under this model, a downstream neuron simply has to add the responses of all the neurons that impinge on it; linear functions of these afferent spikes establish the information available in the population inputs. The information is thus readily accessible: if the convolution of spikes with the spatiotemporal kernels $\kappa_{\text{std}}(j, s, \tau)$ can be considered as defining the postsynaptic potentials of neurons, then information about the relative probabilities of stimulus values can be thought of as being accessed by simply adding (and exponentiating) the neuronal excitatory postsynaptic potential (EPSPs). Figure 20.3 illustrates the decoding method.

This choice of decoder is crucial, especially for ecologically relevant, smoothly varying trajectories. If we allow a complex decoder, for example, the Bayesian decoder $p(s_T|\vec{\boldsymbol{\xi}}_T)$ described earlier, then the network needs access to all the input spikes (Huys et al., 2007). To prevent infinite regress, the decoder applied to the output spikes should access the type of information that biological neurons might reasonably be expected to extract. In our case, this is particularly a decoder that does not require access to all spikes at all times. We chose an independent decoder that integrates the information provided by spikes recursively, which provides a more plausible analog to how real neurons may integrate information.

Independent decoding of the input spikes $\vec{\boldsymbol{\xi}}_T$ is far from optimal, especially for the smooth case. This decoder cannot by itself access the information in the input spikes that is due to the stimulus autocorrelations. Thus, this choice of output decoder shifts the onus of providing the information about the stimulus correlations from the decoder onto the network. In essence, the task of the network is to produce spikes that represent the information contained in the stimulus autocorrelations to make up for the fact that the decoder of its output spikes $\vec{\boldsymbol{\rho}}_T$ will, by itself, neglect any such information in the inputs $\vec{\boldsymbol{\xi}}_T$.

In Natarajan et al. (2008), the overall aim of the network was to form output spikes such that the posterior obtained by decoding these spikes according to Eqs. 20.18 and 20.21 would faithfully approximate optimal decoding of input spikes $p(s_T|\vec{\boldsymbol{\xi}}_T)$. The network encoded spatiotemporal stimulus regularities in the lateral connections of the output population. The network was trained to minimize the KL divergence between the decoded distribution $\hat{p}(s_T|\vec{\boldsymbol{\rho}}_T)$ and the analytically-derived optimal distribution $p(s_T|\vec{\boldsymbol{\xi}}_T)$. Results showed that the network obviated the need to maintain a spiking history by making the temporal prior information explicit in the spiking activity of the population. The recurrent structure thus kept the information contained in the past spikes online. It handled noisy and sparse input appropriately by re-expressing the information contained in the input into a set of spikes that were independently decodeable.

This form of temporal recoding can be considered a natural extension of the line-attractor scheme of Pouget et al. (1998). Both methods

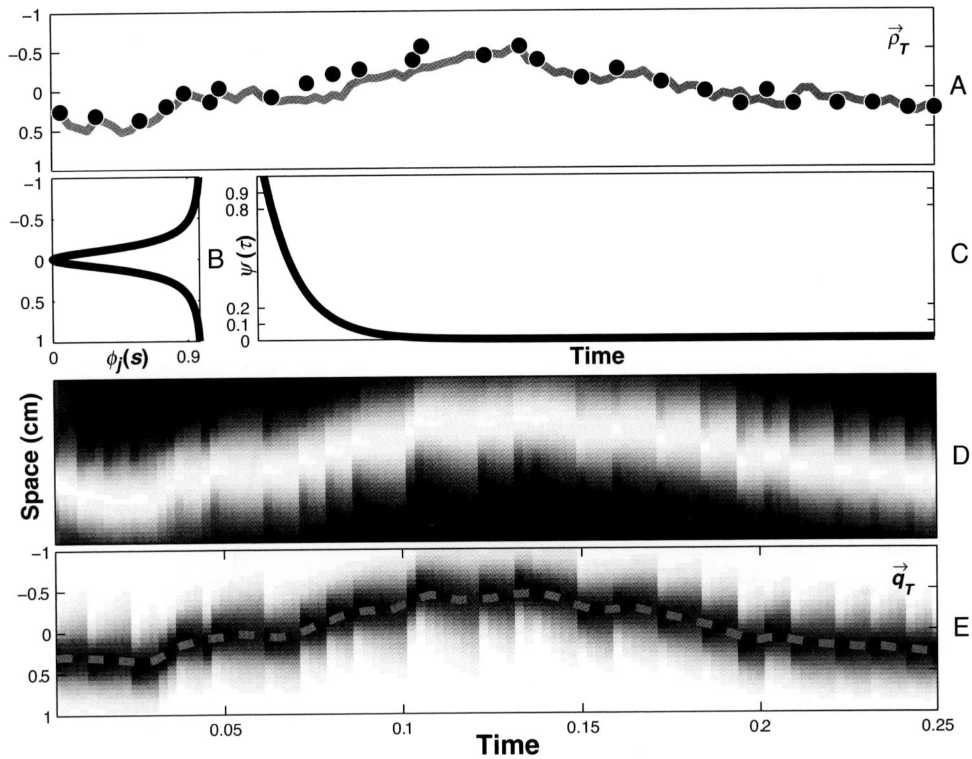


**Figure 20.3** The independent decoding model. (A) Output spikes (solid black circles) of population $j = \{1, 2, \ldots M\}$ convey information about the stimulus trajectory (solid gray line). (B and C) An example of the form of spatial and temporal components of the decoding kernel. (D) Linear contribution of the population spikes through time. (E) Inferred posterior distribution (shaded in gray) over stimulus positions through time; posterior mean is in dashed gray line.

formulate feed-forward and recurrent connections so that a simple decoding of the output can match optimal but complex decoding applied to the inputs. The model presented here extends this approach to spiking networks, and more importantly, to dynamically varying inputs associated with a prior that must be learned.

Our method is also related to some other early proposals where the spiking activity of either a single neuron (Denève, 2005) or a pair of neurons (Gold & Shadlen, 2001) is considered as reporting (logarithmic) probabilistic information about an underlying binary hypothesis. Another approach proposes that a population of neurons directly represents the (logarithmic) probability over the states of a hidden Markov model (Rao, 2004). Like Denève (2005), we consider the transformation of input spikes to output spikes with a fixed assumed decoding scheme so that the dynamics of an underlying process is captured. Our decoding mechanism produces something like the predictive coding apparent in Denève (2005), except that here, a neuron may be silent not only if it itself has recently spiked and thereby conveyed the appropriate information, but also if one of its population neighbors has recently spiked. This is explicitly captured by the recurrent interactions among the population.

## APPLYING THE CODING SCHEME TO DYNAMIC CUE COMBINATION

In this section we consider how a neural system might employ the proposed coding scheme recursively, to dynamically weight and integrate information about a transient stimulus variable from different sensory modalities. Particularly, we evaluate the coding efficacy of our approach when input to the model has the same characteristics as the output representation produced by it; that is, information can be decoded in an (approximately) optimal manner even when the decoder ignores correlations in the inputs and treats each spike independently, linearly integrating the information conveyed by them (Eq. 20.21). We examine whether and how the model can approximate proper inference in a challenging version of a cue-combination task, one in which the inputs and their reliabilities are continuously varying through time, and the information is communicated by spiking neural populations.

The advantage of independent interpretability of spikes is not confined to decoding. Neural computations underlying integration of information from different modalities (e.g., Ernst & Banks, 2002; Hillis, Ernst, Banks, & Landy, 2002) or sensorimotor combination (e.g., Körding & Wolpert, 2004) become straightforward, requiring only an addition in the log domain or multiplication of single-neuron (Chance, Abbott, & Reyes, 2002; Poirazi, Brannon, & Mel, 2003; Salinas & Abbott, 1996) or population (Denève et al., 2001) activity.

In this section, we look beyond decoding as the canonical task; we explore how our dynamic coding scheme can be manipulated easily and integrated efficiently in a hierarchical manner to perform uncertainty-sensitive neural computations through time. Specifically, we consider how we can extend the framework presented earlier (see section on "Approximating Probabilisitic Inference in Population-Code Networks") to handle continuous, dynamic stimulus variables.

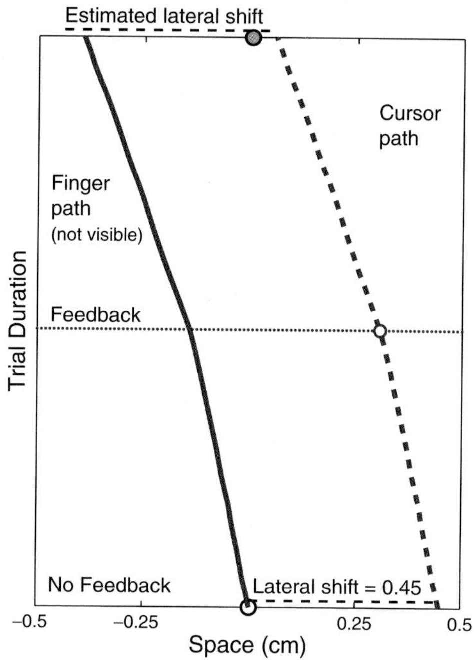


**Figure 20.4** Experimental setup. One-dimensional position of the finger on the screen is represented along the x-axis, and the time course of the trial along the y-axis. The unfilled circle at the bottom of the screen indicates the starting position of the cursor; the green filled circle at the top of screen shows the target position. The task is to reach the target as closely as possible. The invisible finger trajectory is indicated by a solid blue line; the true cursor position by a dashed blue line. On the trial shown here, the cursor is laterally displaced relative to the finger position by 0.45 cm. The midpoint of the trial is indicated by the horizontal black dashed line at the center of the figure; the blue unfilled circle along the cursor path indicates brief visual feedback. Based on this feedback, there is compensatory correction in the finger trajectory from the midpoint onward. Further details of the setup are provided in the text.

## Dynamic Sensorimotor Task

We focus on a version of the sensorimotor integration task where Körding and Wolpert (2004) explored the consequence of manipulating the reliability of visual feedback during reaching. Figure 20.4 illustrates the experimental setup where a starting position and a target position are marked using a white and green circle, respectively, indicated at the bottom and top of a horizontal plane. Subjects were required to reach to the visual target from the starting position, within the virtual-reality environment that blocked the hand from view. A cursor was shown before the start of the movement; it was then hidden except for one point of visual feedback midway through the trial. At the onset of movement, unbeknownst to the subjects, the cursor was laterally displaced relative to the true finger position by an amount drawn randomly from a known prior distribution.

Midway through the movement, brief visual feedback about the cursor position was provided. On each trial, the reliability of the visual feedback was a random draw of positions from a Gaussian distribution, with position indicated using dots. Across trials, the feedback was varied across four conditions, $\sigma_v^0$ (a single precise white dot), $\sigma_v^M$, $\sigma_v^L$ (small translucent dots distributed as a two-dimensional Gaussian with standard deviations of 1 and 2 cm, respectively), and $\sigma_v^\infty$ (no feedback). The task was to land the cursor as close to the target as possible; feedback about the final cursor position was provided only in the high-reliability condition $\sigma_v^0$.

Subjects were trained for about 1000 trials in the task to ensure that they encountered many samples of the lateral shift drawn from the underlying prior distribution. Upon testing, subjects were found to generate compensatory corrections in their finger trajectories in the second half of the movement, in order to offset the imposed lateral displacement of the cursor. The authors assumed a Bayes-optimal strategy and inferred the priors used by subjects based on the measured shifts in final estimates of target position.

On test trials where no visual feedback was given, subjects appeared to learn the prior distribution over offsets: The estimated displacement was equivalent to the mean of the prior distribution. On trials in which feedback was provided, subjects combined prior knowledge of the distribution with sensory (visual) evidence in a manner that was appropriately sensitive to the degree of noise in the visual feedback. The authors accounted for their results within this framework as follows: Adjustments to ongoing motor commands were dependent on both the reliability of sensory inputs and on an estimation of prior probabilities of displacements in a manner consistent with Bayesian computation. Other studies (e.g., Tassinari, Hudson, & Landy, 2006) have employed related experimental paradigms without assuming any strategy, and they have quantitatively demonstrated that human performance does indeed result from a nearly optimal combination of sensory and prior information.

## Dynamic Cue-Combination Network

The objective for our recurrent network model is to compute the distribution over cursor positions on the screen based on information about finger position and visual information about the cursor, each having varying noise levels.

We set up a hierarchical network much like that described earlier (see section, "Approximating Probabilisitic Inference in Population-Code Networks"), where two independent sensory populations (visual and proprioceptive) are connected by means of feedforward weights to a third population of downstream neurons (Fig. 20.5). The first layer re-represents its inputs into a form that is independently decodeable using our log-linear scheme. It is these spikes that serve as inputs to the downstream population, which in turn combines the information with knowledge of the prior distribution over the lateral shifts that is learned in the network

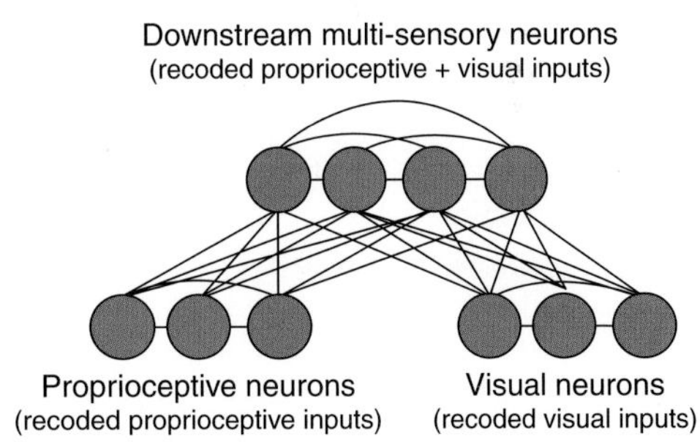


**Figure 20.5** Dynamic combination network. Recurrently connected unisensory populations of proprioceptive and visual neurons recode their inputs into independently decodeable representations that then serve as inputs to a third recurrently connected downstream population that combines them. Feedforward weights connect the two levels of the network. In this recursive scheme, inputs and outputs to the network have consistent semantics; that is, they are independently interpretable using a fixed decoding scheme.

synaptic connections. A posterior distribution is derived from the output spikes of the downstream population using the same decoding scheme. This makes the approach recursive in that the spikes at every level may be interpreted using the same decoding approach. The mean of the posterior distribution provides the final estimate of the cursor position on the screen. In our network model, this mean can be thought of as computing the "motor command" for compensation in the finger position. Details of our simulation, including the setup of each of these elements of recursive computation, are provided next.

***Network Preprocessing: Log-Linear Decodeable Unisensory Inputs*** We create input spikes for our network by applying the recurrent-network approach to Gaussian-Poisson spikes, as described earlier (see section on "Spike-Generation Model"), separately for visual and proprioceptive inputs. Neural populations $i_v = \{1, \cdots, N_v\}$ and $i_p = \{1, \cdots, N_p\}$ are defined such that the preferred stimulus positions of the neurons are evenly distributed in the stimulus space. The neurons are individually tuned to respond across a certain range of the stimulus space. The visual $\vec{\boldsymbol{\xi}}^v$ and proprioceptive inputs $\vec{\boldsymbol{\xi}}^p$ are determined by Gaussian tuning curves with Poisson variability (Eq. 20.4). In the simulations that follow, sparse inputs are generated by assigning a low value to the maximum input firing rate $r_{\max} = 0.144$ Hz and tuning width $\sigma = 0.1$ cm in Eq. 20.4.

Laterally connected visual and proprioceptive neural populations $j_v = \{1, 2, \cdots, M_v\}$ and $j_p = \{1, 2, \cdots, M_p\}$ have preferred stimulus positions distributed evenly across the stimulus space and receive input spikes $\vec{\boldsymbol{\xi}}^v$ and $\vec{\boldsymbol{\xi}}^p$, respectively, in response to the visually observed cursor position and the finger position. The lateral connections of the individual populations are indicated by $\mathbf{U}_v$, $\mathbf{U}_p$; the projective width used in our simulations is $\omega = 0.2$ (Eq. 20.20). Each population individually learns to recode its inputs into representations $\vec{\boldsymbol{\rho}}^v$ and $\vec{\boldsymbol{\rho}}^p$ that are independently decodeable.

For training the preprocessing systems, stimulus trajectories $\vec{s}^p$ and $\vec{s}^v$ are drawn from the Gaussian Process prior distribution (Eq. 20.8). The parameter $\zeta$ of the covariance matrix $C$ determines the smoothness of the trajectories. By changing the value of $\zeta$ we can consider different classes of GP priors, each defining the density over a set of trajectories with similar spatiotemporal dynamics. Since a hallmark of motor behavior is that movements are smooth, relatively straight trajectories (Flash & Hogan, 1985; Morasso, 1981), we choose parameters of the Gaussian Process prior such that the resulting trajectories have smoothly varying dynamics. The particular values used in the simulation are specified in Figure 20.6.

This spike-generation model leads to a simple ideal observer to produce the training signal: the posterior distributions $p(s_T^p|\vec{\boldsymbol{\xi}}_T^p)$ and $p(s_T^v|\vec{\boldsymbol{\xi}}_T^v)$ for an observed population spike train, as described above (see section on "Ideal Observer"). Approximate posterior distributions $\hat{p}(s_T^p|\vec{\boldsymbol{\rho}}_T^p)$ and $\hat{p}(s_T^v|\vec{\boldsymbol{\rho}}_T^v)$ are decoded following Eqs. 20.18 and 20.21. Then each population $j_v = \{1, 2, \cdots, M_v\}$ and $j_p = \{1, 2, \cdots, M_p\}$ individually learns to recode its inputs by minimizing the divergences between the true and approximate posterior distributions over finger and cursor positions: $D_{KL}(p(s_T^p|\vec{\boldsymbol{\xi}}_T^p)||\hat{p}(s_T^p|\vec{\boldsymbol{\rho}}_T^p))$ and $D_{KL}(p(s_T^v|\vec{\boldsymbol{\xi}}_T^v)||\hat{p}(s_T^v|\vec{\boldsymbol{\rho}}_T^v))$, where $D_{KL}(p(s)||\hat{p}(s)) = \sum_s p(s)\log(p(s)/\hat{p}(s))$ is the Kullback-Leibler (KL) divergence, or relative entropy between the true $p(s)$ and model distribution $\hat{p}(s)$.

Note that beyond labeling the two unisensory populations as visual and proprioceptive, we have not detailed how the two modules differ from each other in the information they represent. Typically, in such a sensorimotor context, the proprioceptive neurons are simulated to encode information about finger position in joint-angle space, and the visual neurons would encode information in retinocentric space. However, neural mechanisms underlying sensorimotor transformations have been explored extensively, often formalized as coordinate transformations between body-centric and eye-centric representations (Baraduc, Guigon, & Burnod, 2001; Denève et al., 2001; Pouget et al., 2003). Hence, we assume that the visual and proprioceptive inputs have already been converted into a common frame of reference by

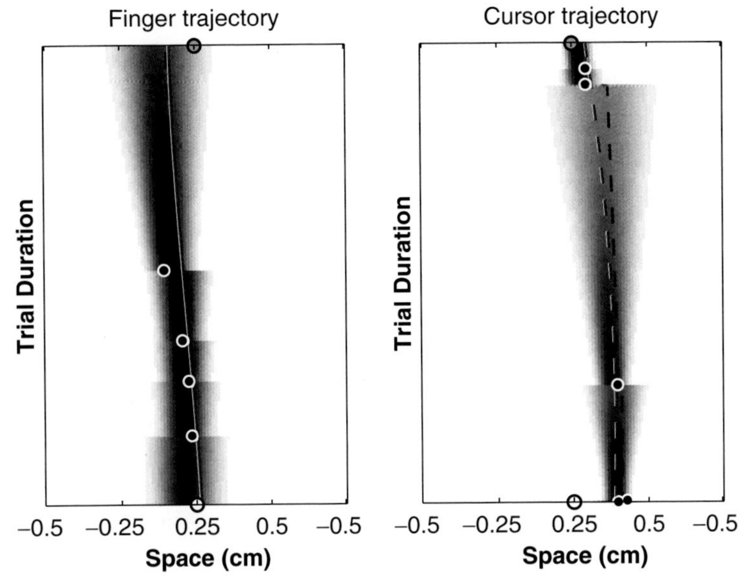


**Figure 20.6** Generating visual and proprioceptive inputs with varying dynamics. The solid red line shows a sample finger trajectory generated from a GP prior with $\zeta = 2, \alpha = 0.05, c = 0.2$. The dashed red line is a sample cursor trajectory; $\zeta = 2, \alpha = 0.15, c = 0.5$. White circles shaded black indicate proprioceptive and visual input spikes in the left and right panels, respectively. The spatiotemporal distributions in grayscale plot the approximate distributions derived from decoding proprioceptive (left) and visual (right) recoded outputs. The dashed white lines show the means of these posterior distributions.

some mechanism (the basis-function approach of Pouget et al. can be readily implemented under our scheme), and we explore differences in the dynamics of the two unisensory networks.

Recall that in our setup, there is a steady stream of proprioceptive inputs from the sensed location of the finger, but visual information is very sparse since it is displayed only as a brief flash as in the original experiment. Therefore, in generating the stimulus trajectories $\vec{s}^p$ and $\vec{s}^v$, we consider slightly different dynamics in specifying the Gaussian-Process prior. Recall (see section on "Ideal Observer") that different values of $\zeta$ determine the different classes of prior distributions over trajectories. We generated the finger trajectories using faster, smoother temporal dynamics by setting $\zeta = 2$ in Eq. 20.8; the cursor trajectories were generated by setting $\zeta = 1$. Accordingly, the proprioceptive and visual inputs in our network reflect the differences in the input dynamics (see the parameter values below Fig. 20.6). Consequently, the learned parameter $\beta$, which specifies the dynamics of the spiking activity (Eqs. 20.15–20.16), is observed to be different for the two submodules. We elaborate on this in the section on "Simulation Results."

***Training the Network*** The recoded visual and proprioceptive inputs are then fed to the next stage of recurrent processing by neurons that combine the information. It is in these feedforward and lateral weights (as well as network dynamics) that we expect the learned prior distribution over lateral shifts to be embedded. Therefore, the trajectories for this second stage of processing are generated such that there is compensation for the imposed lateral shift at the midpoint of each trial. The visual stimulus (cursor $s_t^v$) indicates the position of the finger $s_t^p$ at any time $t$. The cursor $s_t^v$ is shifted laterally from the finger position $s_t^p$ by a value $\delta_{\text{shift}}$ drawn from the known prior distribution $p_{\text{shift}} \propto \mathcal{N}(\mu_{\text{shift}}, \sigma_{\text{shift}})$ that carries information about the probabilistic structure of variations in the task.

Halfway through the trial, at $t = T/2$, the visual stimulus is displayed only for that timestep, with varying degrees of uncertainty for different trials: $\sigma_v^0$ when the exact position of the cursor $s^v_{(t=T/2)}$ is shown with no variability, and $\sigma_v^M$ and $\sigma_v^L$ when the cursor is displayed with medium and large variances. The idea is that based on this visual input, the subsequent finger positions change to compensate for the lateral shift. For this, we estimate the shift in the trial using Bayes rule, given the visual input and the known prior distribution. The posterior distribution over sensed lateral shifts in each trial is computed and the mean of this posterior is selected to be the estimate on that trial; the finger position is compensated by that amount.

The training signal for this stage is the true posterior distribution over cursor positions, derived following Eq. 20.2,

$$P(s_T^c|\vec{\boldsymbol{\rho}}_T^v, \vec{\boldsymbol{\rho}}_T^p) \propto P(\vec{s}_T^c) \int_{\vec{s}_T^v, \vec{s}_T^p} p(s_T^v|\vec{\boldsymbol{\xi}}_T^v) p(s_T^p|\vec{\boldsymbol{\xi}}_T^p) \times P(\vec{s}_T^v, \vec{s}_T^p|\vec{s}_T^c) d\vec{s}_T^v d\vec{s}_T^p. \tag{20.22}$$

Here, the combined stimulus prior $P(\vec{s}_T^v, \vec{s}_T^p|\vec{s}_T^c)$ can be seen as scaling the prior over displacements $P(\vec{s}_T^c)$. The network parameters are optimized to minimize the KL divergence between this distribution and the distribution derived from decoding its outputs $\vec{\boldsymbol{\rho}}^p$ according to Eq. 20.21. The proprioceptive inputs are received at a timescale that fits our general scheme well; the visual inputs are received just as a brief flash. The lateral connections in the top level integrate the inputs and maintain the belief state online.

## SIMULATION RESULTS

In this section, we present results from simulating the network under various experimental conditions. The trained network from the previous section was tested on a set of 500 trials; in the following simulations, we assumed a prior distribution $p_{\text{shift}} \propto \mathcal{N}(\mu_{\text{shift}}, \sigma_{\text{shift}})$, where $\mu_{\text{shift}} = 0.3$ and $\sigma_{\text{shift}} = 0.2$. We first analyze results on a single trial of the experiment followed by results summarized over the 500 test trials.

Figure 20.7 plots the estimated cursor distributions for three different stimulus conditions: $\sigma_v^0, \sigma_v^M$, and $\sigma_v^L$. In each vertical panel, the x-axis represents the stimulus space (i.e., finger/cursor position) and the y-axis represents the time steps in the course of the trial; each trial proceeds from the bottom up. The starting position of the finger movement is indicated by the black circle at the center of stimulus space (0 cm) and the target position by the circle shaded in green at the top of the panel. At the start of a trial, the cursor is shifted laterally by 0.45 cm. The true cursor position is indicated by the dashed line in red ($\sigma_v^0$), blue ($\sigma_v^M$), and white ($\sigma_v^L$). The estimated posterior distribution over cursor positions is plotted in grayscale for each step of the trial.

At the start of the trial the estimated posterior appears to rely heavily on the prior distribution $p_{\text{shift}}(\Delta)$ for all three conditions; the estimated mean is centered around the mean of the Gaussian prior distribution at 0.3 cm. During the first half of the movement, the variance of the posterior distribution is seen to grow with time. The only inputs during this phase are the proprioceptive inputs from the unseen hand and the visual input at $t = 1$; the increasing variance of the posterior distribution indicates increasing unreliability of the finger position estimate.

When visual feedback is presented midway through the trial, the posterior mean shifts toward the cursor position (0.45 cm for the trials presented here) and the posterior variance shrinks. This increased certainty about the position of the cursor reflects augmentation of the sensory inputs with new visual information. From this point on, the posterior distribution appears to rely more on the visual feedback and less on the learned prior information. The variance in general is less during the second half of movement compared to the first. One clear difference between the decoded distributions for the three stimulus conditions is that the posterior variance increases as the visual reliability decreases.

Figure 20.8 plots the estimated mean of the posterior distribution in dashed red, blue, and white lines for each of the conditions discussed earlier. The finger trajectory on the trial is indicated by the solid line. The panels on the

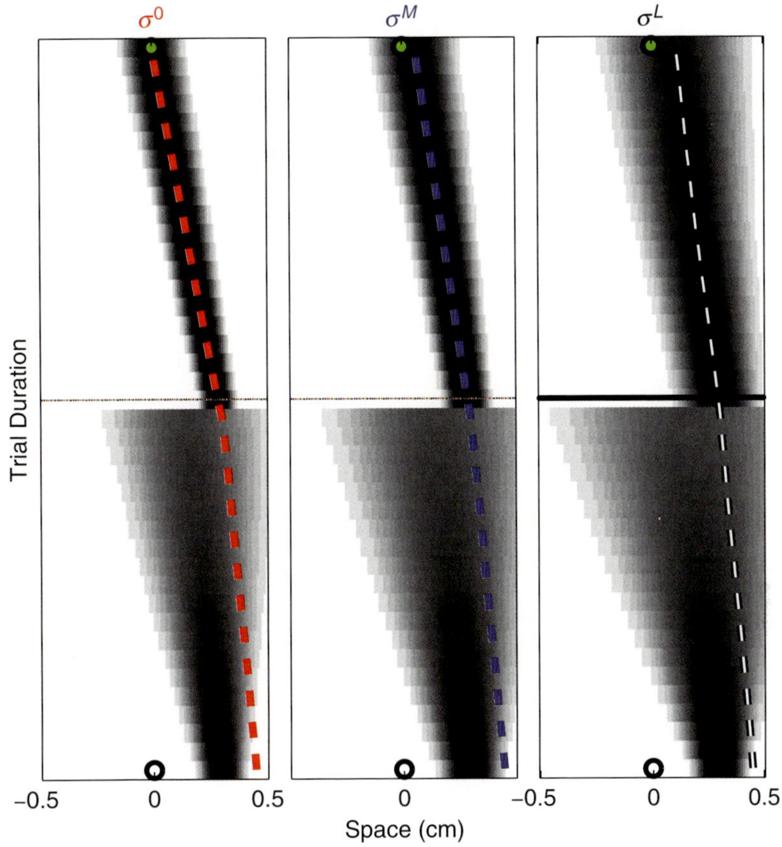


**Figure 20.7** Simulation results. Estimated cursor distributions for three stimulus conditions. True lateral shift of visual cursor on all trials = 0.45 cm. Dashed lines in each panel indicate true cursor position: red, $\sigma_v^0$; blue, $\sigma_v^M$; and white, $\sigma_v^L$. At each time step, the estimated posterior distribution over cursor positions is plotted in grayscale for all three stimulus conditions. At the start of the trial, the estimated posterior mean is centered around 0.3 cm, the mean of the Gaussian prior distribution over lateral shifts. Notice how for all three stimulus conditions, the posterior variance increases during the first half of the movement and shrinks at the midpoint (indicated by the horizontal dashed black line) when visual feedback is provided. At this point, there is also a sudden shift in posterior mean. These results are analyzed in detail in the text.

right of the plot indicate the amount of visual noise for each condition. For the high-reliability condition, $\sigma_v^0$, the final estimate of the target location (i.e., the mean of the estimated posterior at the end of the trial) is right on target. For $\sigma_v^M$ and $\sigma_v^L$, it is shifted away from the target location, toward the true displaced cursor position. The degree of this shift increases with increasing unreliability in visual feedback. These observations show that the sensory inputs were integrated with the learned prior in a manner that was appropriately sensitive to the degree of noise in the visual feedback: As the precision of the visual input decreases, the system relies more on prior knowledge of displacement statistics to adjust finger movement.

To quantify the system behavior, we calculate the average performance of the network over 500 trials. Figure 20.9 summarizes the final deviation of the estimated cursor position from the target, as a function of the true lateral shift on each trial. These values are averaged over the 500 trials for each condition. The results are qualitatively similar to those observed by

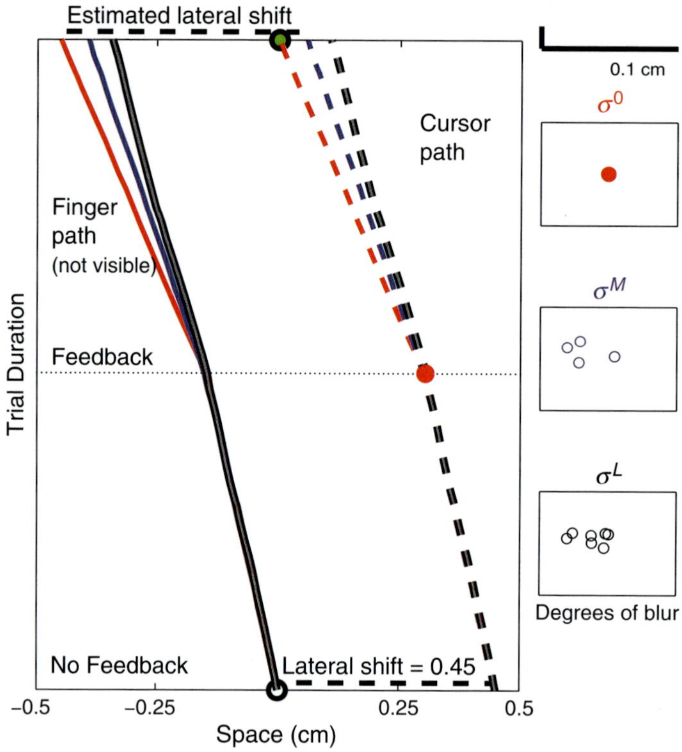


**Figure 20.8** Estimated mean of the posterior distribution. Solid lines, finger trajectory; dashed lines, estimated posterior mean. Illustrations on the right indicate the degree of visual noise for each stimulus condition. For $\sigma_v^0$ (red line), the mean of the estimated posterior at the end of the trial is right on target. For $\sigma_v^M$ and $\sigma_v^L$ (blue and black lines, respectively), it is shifted away from the target location, toward the true displaced cursor position. The degree of this shift increases with increasing unreliability in visual feedback. Results suggest that cue weighting is sensitive to uncertainty in the visual feedback.

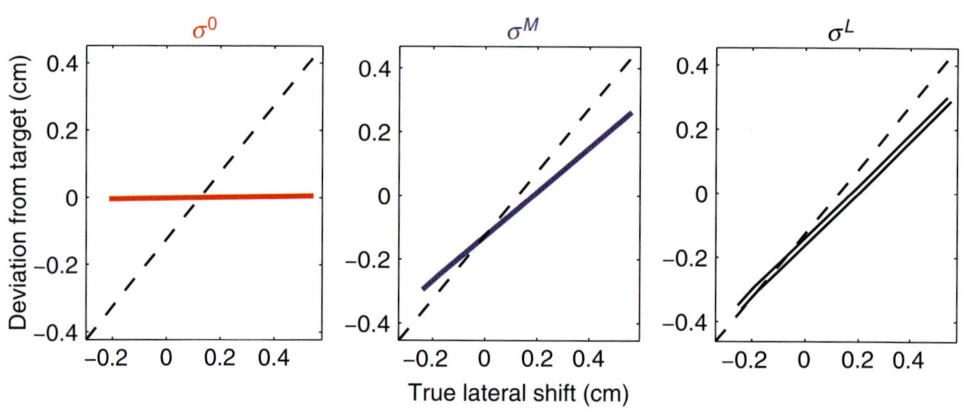


**Figure 20.9** Summary results. Average network performance over 500 trials for each of the three conditions. The x-axis plots the true lateral shifts imposed on different runs of the simulations; the y-axis indicates the final deviation of the cursor from the target. The solid red, blue, and black lines plot the final deviation of the estimated cursor position from the target for the three different stimulus conditions. For $\sigma_v^0$, this plot is almost a horizontal line, indicating that the estimated cursor position lands on average at the true target position. The slope of the blue and black lines increases with visual uncertainty. Results are qualitatively similar to those of Körding and Wolpert (2004).

Körding and Wolpert (2004): The slope of the plotted lines increases with visual uncertainty. For $\sigma_v^0$, the estimated cursor position lands on average at the true target position; with increasing noisiness, the final cursor position is displaced. We conclude from these results that the sensory integration in our dynamic network was appropriately sensitive to the degree of noise in the visual feedback.

## Network Preprocessing: Cue Differentiation

We can gain some insight into how the network achieves this behavior by examining its learned feedforward and lateral weights, temporal decay constant, and the decoding kernels. We first discuss the components of the preprocessing stage. Here, the learned feedforward connectivities for the visual and proprioceptive unisensory networks were qualitatively similar (not shown), displaying a strong local connectivity, with each input neuron having strong excitatory connections to neurons in the recurrent population having the same or very similar stimulus preference and inhibitory connections to their neighboring neurons.

Figure 20.10 plots the learned lateral connection strengths $\mathbf{U}_{\mathrm{v}}$ and $\mathbf{U}_{\mathrm{p}}$ for the recurrently connected visual and proprioceptive neurons. The plot is in the form of a matrix, where the rows $j_v = \{1, 2, \cdots, M\}$ and columns $k_v = \{1, 2, \cdots, M\}$ correspond to the output neurons spatially laid out in the stimulus space. Each cell of the weight matrix $\mathbf{U}$ is shaded according to the strength of the synapse $U_{j_v k_v}$. The connectivities learned by both networks are starkly different. We attribute this to the differences in temporal dynamics of the input stimulus (and therefore the dynamics of the neural inputs) to these networks.

Let us first examine the weights $\mathbf{U}_{\mathrm{p}}$ (Fig. 20.10, left panel). Each neuron is seen to strongly excite its immediate neighbors and also to inhibit the ones further away. The strength of excitation is strongest for neurons tuned to the center of the stimulus space and decreases as the neuron's stimulus preference moves toward the periphery. This is likely a direct consequence of the spatial range of the stimuli the network was trained on. The negative weights allow one neuron's spikes to decrease the membrane potential of another. So the population activity not only indicates where the stimulus is at any given time (by spiking when the stimulus is at the neuron's preferred position) but also actively indicates where the stimulus may not be.

The temporal decay constant adapts to a large value, $\beta = 2.42$ (Eqs. 20.15–20.16). This allows the postsynaptic potential of neurons in the recoding population to decay slowly with time. This means that temporally distant spikes have very slowly diminishing effects on the current population activity. The decay constant reflects the temporal extent of the interactions in the stimulus, specified by $\alpha$ in Eq. 20.8. This same rate of decay is applied to $\gamma$ in the temporal kernel to decode the spikes; it implies that the influence of a spike persists for a while, having a slowly decaying effect on the representation at future times.

Next, we examine the weights $\mathbf{U}_{\mathrm{v}}$ (Fig. 20.10, middle panel). Each neuron has strong positive connections to some (but not its immediate) neighbors, evident in the positive weights. However, the learned temporal decay constant $\beta = 1.85$ is much lower than that of the proprioceptive network.

## Learned Network Components

Next, we analyze the components of the network. The feedforward weights from the visual and proprioceptive ensemble to the recurrently connected multisensory neurons display strong local connectivity. The rightmost panel in Figure 20.10 plots the lateral weights learned during the combination stage, in the same matrix format described earlier. The positive synaptic weight patterns are off diagonal, indicating that at every time step, each neuron is signaling several (again, not immediate) neighboring neurons to fire at subsequent time steps during recurrent processing. The learned temporal decay constant is large again, $\beta = 2.38$.

Since the lateral weights and the decay constant are learned together in an iterative manner with the decoding kernels fixed, they influence each other very closely. Combined with the input spikes to the population, they influence

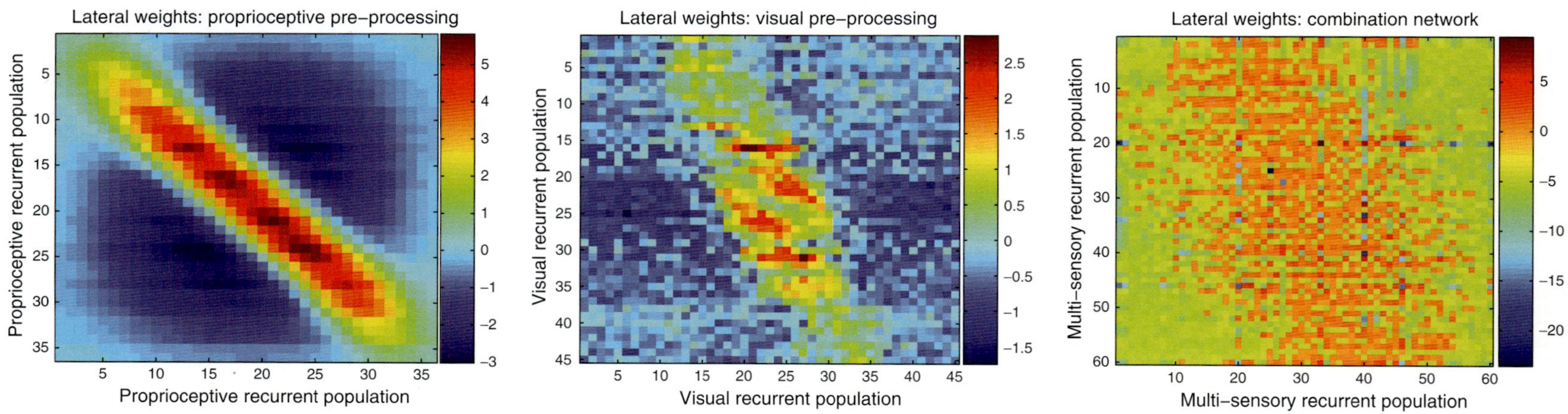


**Figure 20.10** Understanding the lateral synaptic weights. (Left) Learned lateral weights $U_p$, $\beta = 2.42$. (Middle) Lateral weights $U_v$, $\beta = 1.85$. (Right) Lateral connections between the downstream multisensory neurons, $\beta = 2.38$. The connection patterns learned by the three populations are starkly different. These different network dynamics are a reflection of the differences in input stimulus dynamics; additionally, the multisensory neurons also learn to combine their two inputs. The color bars on the right indicate the strength of the lateral connections; warm colors correspond to positive weights and cold colors to negative weights. In the absence of input spikes, recurrent activity contributes to the persistent effect of previously observed spikes.

the membrane potential $\boldsymbol{h}_T$ (Eq. 20.16) of neurons in the recurrently connected population according to how the input population connects to the recurrent population via the feedforward weights. In the absence of input spikes, recurrent activity contributes to the persistent effect of previously observed spikes. This triggers a cascaded pattern of activation among neurons of the recurrent population. This explains the increasing variance with time in the decoded distribution.

## SUMMARY AND DISCUSSION

Our understanding of how the central nervous system might encode and interpret sensory input has significantly progressed in the last decades. Concomitantly, theoretical explorations have provided numerous hypotheses and results on how various ecologically relevant computations might be performed through feedforward and recurrent connections between neural populations (Denève et al., 2001; Pouget et al., 1998). Our study is at the intersection of these two lines of work. We explore the characteristics of neural population codes desirable for uncertainty-sensitive, optimal downstream decoding of the represented information. We focus on time-varying inputs represented by a spiking network and attempt to understand dynamic population codes from a functional perspective, beyond the issue of stimulus representation.

### Summary

In this chapter, we first reviewed our proposal for how uncertainty about time-varying sensory inputs can be represented in population spike times. In our scheme, recoding produces temporally independent spikes, and the decoding kernels convolve them in such a way that information originally encoded in spatiotemporal spike patterns can now be independently decoded to produce a smooth, inferred distribution. Our main contribution here was an extension of the coding scheme to develop a recursive, hierarchical formulation of the system.

The highlights of our proposal are as follows. We first specified a recursive application of our coding scheme; we demonstrated how the recoded information can be manipulated easily and integrated efficiently in two stages to causally reweight and integrate information about the stimulus variable from different modalities. One population encoded dynamic proprioceptive information while another represented visual information; both utilized the recoding scheme to efficiently represent a stimulus variable such as position. Then, a third population received these recoded spikes as inputs, combined them using the same representational scheme, and produced a spike-based representation of the posterior distribution over positions.

Second, in our formulation, the visual and proprioceptive subnetworks receive inputs of varying temporal dynamics. The proprioceptive neurons received inputs corresponding to smoothly varying finger trajectories; the visual neurons received sparser inputs corresponding to a visual stimulus (cursor position on screen) that was only briefly flashed midway through the experimental trial. The main computational advantage of using a fixed independent decoder such as ours is that rather than employing different decoding strategies for different stimulus dynamics, a neural population can recode the input representation into one that can be decoded independently regardless of stimulus dynamics. Our results demonstrated that the visual and proprioceptive subnetworks did in fact learn to reflect the different dynamics underlying their respective inputs. Additionally, our results showed that under this coding scheme, a downstream neural population (recurrently connected multisensory neurons) is able to appropriately compute with inputs from the different sources using the same fixed independent decoder.

The inputs to the visual and proprioceptive neurons were constrained to be sparse. This was meant to simulate those situations where the temporal dynamics of a stimulus are incompatible with (i.e., faster than) neural spiking dynamics. Such input sparsity makes a more challenging case for recoding; if spikes are dense relative to the movement in the stimulus (i.e., the likelihood term in Eq. 20.4 dominates either via very low noise $\sigma$ or high firing rates

$r_{max}$), the contribution of the prior will be small and recoding may not be necessary. On the other hand, if spikes are sparse, the prior will be more important and approximations more costly; recoding will become important due to the need to account for spatiotemporal stimulus dynamics and the desire to decode independently. Our choice of a sparse spiking regime implies that the complexity of the decoding task primarily derives from the smooth dynamics of the finger movements.

Third, our learning rule for the multisensory downstream population was derived by applying the independent decoder to the recoded unisensory inputs. The computational motivation for applying this rule recursively is that at each level of the hierarchy, additional information from other spiking populations is combined, such that the network is effectively consolidating the information in all of its inputs. This implies that the learning objective is to simply preserve the information in the combined inputs. This preservation is itself a form of computation, because it involves combining the distributions implied by the visual and proprioceptive unisensory inputs.

Finally, this model relates to experimental results from Körding and Wolpert (2004) using many simulations with smooth trajectories and varying visual noise levels. We demonstrated that our spiking cue-combination network can account for these data, yielding the same dependence of the final cursor position on the degree of noisiness in the visual feedback. Our implementation possesses some neural plausibility, since it employs a straight-forward nonlinear network requiring access to the type of information that biological neurons might reasonably be expected to extract.

### Related Work

Several sensorimotor-transformation schemes have been proposed that exploit redundancy and broad tuning ubiquitous in the cortex to minimize the deleterious effects of noise (Baraduc et al., 2001; Salinas & Abbott, 1995) or to generate probabilistic population codes to represent Gaussian and more general forms of probability distributions to propagate uncertainty in neural processing (Knill & Pouget, 2004; Pouget et al., 1998; Pouget, Denève, Ducom, & Latham, 1999).

One popular theory is based on a neural architecture that combines basis functions and attractor dynamics. The basis functions are used to recode sensory information into a flexible intermediate representation to facilitate the transformation into a motor command; attractor dynamics are used for optimal statistical inferences. As an example, Denève et al. (2001) proposed a network architecture that uses gain-encoding to combine inputs from two sensory modalities (vision and audition) and perform optimal Bayesian inferences.

This model used basis functions to perform coordinate transformations of the inputs (from retinal to head-centric coordinates) and then decode the maximum-likelihood estimate of the encoded variable (object location) given both inputs. This scheme relaxes noisy population codes into smooth hills of activity over time (stable network states called attractors). As a consequence, the multimodal inputs are integrated with weights proportional to their reliability. Our model presented here can be viewed as extending this approach to spiking networks and, more important, to dynamically varying inputs associated with a prior that must be learned.

Similarly, Salinas and Abbott (1996) demonstrate the use of recurrent architectures in computing the basis functions themselves to produce a useful intermediate representation of visual target location for motor action. Their approach uses recurrently connected populations to produce multiplicative responses as an emergent property of the network, even when individual neurons can only simply sum their synaptic inputs linearly. This scheme is illustrated by modeling the combination of target-retinal-location and gaze-direction inputs in parietal cortex. Such a multiplicative parietal representation has been shown to be very versatile because downstream neurons can readily read out various task-specific linear combinations of inputs. In both these approaches, recurrent connectivity effectively suppresses input noise. Salinas and Abbott (1996) also suggest how their model can select between multiple inputs.

Our proposed decoding scheme also bears an interesting relationship to other recent proposals, notably the probabilistic population codes of Ma and colleagues (2006). Adopting the same decoder, they show that under some limited assumptions about the individual neurons' probability density functions, several natural computations can be carried out by linear operations on activities in the input populations. This means that in these situations, simple neural circuits, namely linear ones, can approximate optimal inference, which makes the optimization of the circuit trivial. The formulation readily applies to static cue-integration problems, in which cue weights are assumed to remain constant over time.

We consider a more realistic situation in which the input forms a continuous stream and the underlying variable of interest follows some trajectory. Hence, information from each cue can accrue over time in ways that affect how the different cues are combined through time. Our framework thus provides a computational characterization of the function of neural populations in a network, combining information from their input populations and performing computations in such a way that simple decoding closely approximates optimal inference.

## Limitations of Our Approach

One limitation in the model is that the learning procedure is driven by supervision. The network assumes access to a global reward signal: knowledge of the optimal posterior based on the available information in the input spikes. The objective of learning in this setup was to assess whether any set of synaptic weights could be found that could perform meaningful computations dynamically, beyond the sole objective of input representation. If the aim extends to making the learning plausible in a biological context, then some feedback about the optimal distribution over stimulus values would be required. While information about the true underlying value can be plausibly derived, it is more challenging to envision how information about the optimal distribution could be obtained.

In our simulation of the Körding and Wolpert (2004) experiment, we are not focusing on how subjects actually learn, but rather how the neural populations can faithfully encode and transmit the information about the stimulus position via multiple cues. So, assuming that the population receptive and projective fields are defined, we only model how the feedforward and recurrent connections, and other network parameters adapt to ensure that the full distributional information is maintained online.

## Predictions

Since we are always in the sparse spike limit in our simulations, the information per spike is of most relevance. If there were dense spiking, the population firing rate (DeCharms & Zador, 2000; Silberberg, Bethge, Markram, Pawelzik, & Tsodyks, 2004; Zhang & Sejnowski, 1999) might carry enough information to overwhelm any prior. The model makes two predictions about dynamically changing uncertainty: *(1)* During the first half of the trial, the variance of the time-varying posterior distribution over cursor positions rapidly increases with time. The variance decreases when visual feedback is received and then increases again much more slowly during the second half of movement. *(2)* The degree of uncertainty is consistent with the degree of noise in visual feedback.

Our model allows further predictions for extended versions of this task. For example, visual feedback could be provided more than once during the trial, and the model would predict the relationship between the estimated displacement and the particular feedback (position and uncertainty) on each trial. Our scheme is general enough to accommodate cases where the prior over cursor displacements is multimodal. Whereas standard dynamic models, such as Kalman filters, are unable to represent and update a multimodal posterior, our model can maintain and generate predictions in this case.

With regard to the population code, our study makes several predictions that may help initiate physiological investigations into representations of dynamic inputs. First, analysis of the visual and proprioceptive network dynamics suggests that the temporal dynamics of spiking reflect the temporal dynamics of the stimuli themselves. Second, lateral connections play a critical role in encoding the temporal prior over stimulus dynamics, so that spikes during periods of limited input can be interpreted as making predictions about the underlying stimulus. In particular, during such periods, we expect to observe the way that the increased uncertainty (i.e., posterior variance) is coded. A future line of work involves examining whether the firing properties of the multisensory neurons in our network resemble those of parietal or motor cortical neurons. Since the firing patterns are by-products of the network dynamics, this investigation may be a useful step toward guiding and constraining our model formulations.

## ACKNOWLEDGMENTS

This work was supported by the National Sciences and Engineering Council of Canada, and the Canadian Institute for Advanced Research. We would like to thank Quentin Huys and Peter Dayan for many useful discussion on the work presented here, and Mike Landy and Julia Trommershäuser for their comments on an earlier draft.

## REFERENCES

Anderson, C. H. (1994). Basic elements of biological computational systems. *International Journal of Modern Physics C, 5*, 135–137.

Baraduc, P., Guigon, E., & Burnod, Y. (2001). Recoding arm position to learn visuomotor transformations. *Cerebral Cortex, 11*, 906–917.

Barbieri, R., Frank, L. M., Nguyen, D. P., Quirk, M. C., Solo, V., Wilson, M. A., & Brown, E. N. (2004). Dynamic analyses of information encoding in neural ensembles. *Neural Computation, 16*, 277–307.

Barlow, H. B. (1953). Summation and inhibition in the frog's retina. *Journal of Physiology, 137*, 69–88.

Brown, E. N., Frank, L. M., Tang, D., Quirk, M. C., & Wilson, M. A. (1998). A statistical paradigm for neural spike train decoding applied to position prediction from ensemble firing patterns of rat hippocampal place cells. *Journal of Neuroscience, 18*, 7411–7425.

Brunel, N., & Nadal, J.-P. (1998). Mutual information, Fisher information, and population coding. *Neural Computation, 10*, 1731–1757.

Chance, F. S., Abbott, L. F., & Reyes, A. D. (2002). Gain modulation from background synaptic input. *Neuron, 35*, 773–782.

DeCharms, C., & Zador, A. (2000). Neural representation and the cortical code. *Annual Review of Neuroscience, 23*, 613–647.

Denève, S. (2005). Bayesian inference in spiking neurons. In L. K. Saul, Y. Weiss, & L. Bottou (Eds.), *Advances in neural information processing systems* (Vol. 17, pp. 353–360). Cambridge, MA: MIT Press.

Denève, S., Latham, P. E., & Pouget, A. (1999). Reading population codes: A neural implementation of ideal observers. *Nature Neuroscience, 2*, 740–745.

Denève, S., Latham, P. E., & Pouget, A. (2001). Efficient computation and cue integration with noisy population codes. *Nature Neuroscience, 4*, 826–831.

Ernst, M. O., & Banks, M. S. (2002). Humans integrate visual and haptic information in a statistically optimal fashion. *Nature, 415*, 429–433.

Flash, T., & Hogan, N. (1985). The coordination of arm movements: An experimentally confirmed mathematical model. *Journal of Neuroscience, 5*, 1688–1703.

Georgopoulos, A. P., Schwartz, A. B., & Kettner, R. E. (1983). Neuronal population coding of movement direction. *Science, 233*, 1416–1419.

Gold, J. I., & Shadlen, M. N. (2001). Neural computations that underlie decisions about sensory stimuli. *Trends in Cognitive Sciences, 5*, 10–16.

Hillis, J. M., Ernst, M. O., Banks, M. S., & Landy, M. S. (2002). Combining sensory information: Mandatory fusion within, but not between, senses. *Science, 298*, 1627–1630.

Hillis, J. M., Watt, S. J., Landy, M. S., & Banks, M. S. (2004). Slant from texture and disparity cues: Optional cue combination. *Journal of Vision, 4*, 967–992.

Hinton, G. E. (1999). Products of experts. In *Ninth International Conference on Artificial Neural Networks, (ICANN 9)* (Vol. 1, pp. 1–6). New York, NY: IEEE.

Hinton, G. E., & Brown, A. D. (2000). Spiking Boltzmann machines. In S. A. Solla, T. K. Leen, & K-R. Müller (Eds.), *Advances in neural information processing systems (NIPS)* (Vol. 12, pp. 122–128). Cambridge, MA: MIT Press.

Huys, Q. J. M., Zemel, R., Natarajan, R., & Dayan, P. (2007). Fast population coding. *Neural Computation, 19*, 404–441.

Jacobs, R. A. (1999). Optimal integration of texture and motion cues to depth. *Vision Research, 39*, 3621–3629.

Kistler, W., Gerstner, W., & van Hemmen, J. L. (1997). Reduction of Hodgkin-Huxley equations to a threshold model. *Neural Computation, 9*, 1069–1100.

Knill, D. C. (2003). Mixture models and the probabilistic structure of depth cues. *Vision Research, 43*, 831–854.

Knill, D. C., & Pouget, A. (2004). The Bayesian brain: The role of uncertainty in neural coding and computation. *Trends in Neurosciences, 27*, 712–719.

Knill, D. C., & Saunders, J. A. (2003). Do humans optimally integrate stereo and texture information for judgments of surface slant? *Vision Research, 43*, 2539–2558.

Körding, K., & Wolpert, D. M. (2004). Bayesian integration in sensorimotor learning. *Nature, 427*, 244–247.

Landy, M. S., Maloney, L. T., Johnston, E. B., & Young, M. J. (1995). Measurement and modeling of depth cue combination: In defense of weak fusion. *Vision Research, 35*, 389–412.

Ma, W. J., Beck, J. M., Latham, P. E., & Pouget, A. (2006). Bayesian inference with probabilistic population codes. *Nature Neuroscience, 9*, 1432–1438.

Morasso, P. (1981). Spatial control of arm movements. *Experimental Brain Research, 42*, 223–227.

Natarajan, R., Huys, Q. J., Dayan, P., & Zemel, R. S. (2008). Encoding and decoding spikes for dynamic stimuli. *Neural Computation, 20*, 2325–2360.

Paradiso, M. A. (1988). A theory for the use of visual orientation information which exploits the columnar structure of striate cortex. *Biological Cybernetics, 58*, 35–49.

Poirazi, P., Brannon, T., & Mel, B. W. (2003). Arithmetic of subthreshold synaptic summation in a model CA1 pyramidal cell. *Neuron, 37*, 977–987.

Pouget, A., Dayan, P., & Zemel, R. S. (2003). Inference and computation with population codes. *Annual Review of Neuroscience, 26*, 318–410.

Pouget, A., Denève, S., Ducom, J.-C., & Latham, P. E. (1999). Narrow vs wide tuning curves: What's best for a population code? *Neural Computation, 11*, 85–90.

Pouget, A., Zhang, K., Denève, S., & Latham, P. E. (1998). Statistically efficient estimation using population codes. *Neural Computation, 10*, 373–401.

Rao, R. P. N. (2004). Bayesian computation in recurrent neural circuits. *Neural Computation, 16*, 1–38.

Rao, R. P. N., Olshausen, B. A., & Lewicki, M. S. (Eds.). (2002). *Probabilistic models of the brain: Perception and neural function.* Cambridge, MA: MIT Press.

Salinas, E., & Abbott, L. F. (1995). Transfer of coded information from sensory to motor networks. *Journal of Neuroscience, 15*, 6461–6474.

Salinas, E., & Abbott, L. F. (1996). A model of multiplicative neural responses in parietal cortex. *Proceedings of the National Academy of Sciences USA, 93*, 11956–11961.

Sanger, T. D. (1996). Probability density estimation for the interpretation of neural population codes. *Journal of Neurophysiology, 76*, 2790–2793.

Saunders, J. A., & Knill, D. C. (2003). Humans use continuous visual feedback from the hand to control fast reaching movements. *Experimental Brain Research, 152*, 341–352.

Saunders, J. A., & Knill, D. C. (2004). Visual feedback control of hand movements. *Journal of Neuroscience, 24*, 3223–3234.

Seung, S. H., & Sompolinsky, H. (1993). Simple models for reading neuronal population codes. *Proceedings of the National Academy of Sciences USA, 90*, 10749–10753.

Silberberg, G., Bethge, M., Markram, H., Pawelzik, K., & Tsodyks, M. (2004). Dynamics of population rate codes in ensembles of neocortical neurons. *Journal of Neurophysiology, 91*, 704–709.

Snippe, H. P., & Koenderink, J. J. (1992). Information in channel-coded systems: Correlated receivers. *Biological Cybernetics, 67*, 183–190.

Stein, B. E., & Meredith, M. A. (Eds.). (1993). *The merging of the senses.* Cambridge, MA: MIT Press.

Tassinari, H., Hudson, T. E., & Landy, M. S. (2006). Combining priors and noisy visual cues in a rapid pointing task. *Journal of Neuroscience, 26,* 10154–10163.

van Beers, R. J., Sittig, A. C., & Denier van der Gon, J. J. (1999). Integration of proprioceptive and visual position-information: An experimentally supported model. *Journal of Neurophysiology, 81,* 1355–1364.

Van Rullen, R., & Thorpe, S. J. (2001). Rate coding versus temporal order coding: What the retinal ganglion cells tell the visual cortex. *Neural Computation, 13,* 1255–1283.

Zemel, R. S., & Dayan, P. (1997). Combining probabilistic population codes. *International Joint Conference on Artificial Intelligence, 15,* 1114–1119. San Mateo, CA: Morgan Kaufmann.

Zemel, R. S., Dayan, P., & Pouget, A. (1998). Probabilistic interpretation of population codes. *Neural Computation, 10,* 403–430.

Zhang, K., & Sejnowski, T. J. (1999). Neuronal tuning: To sharpen or to broaden. *Neural Computation, 11,* 75–84.

# CHAPTER 21

## A Neural Implementation of Optimal Cue Integration

*Wei Ji Ma, Jeff Beck, and Alexandre Pouget*

### INTRODUCTION

This chapter discusses a theoretical framework for how optimal cue integration can be performed by populations of neurons. Cue integration is an interesting behavior from the perspective of neural computation for at least two reasons. First, it is one of the simplest tasks that demonstrate that humans take uncertainty into account when perceiving the world; in other words, the brain keeps track of "error bars" on its estimates. How neurons encode and manipulate uncertainty (or more generally, probability distributions) has traditionally not been a topic of study in systems neuroscience. Therefore, explaining cue integration from a neural point of view can yield new insights into the format in which neurons represent information and the mechanisms by which they process it. The second, related reason is that cue integration is a textbook example of how a large body of psychophysical data can be used to not only constrain but also construct neural models. Many studies in computational neuroscience focus on constructing neural models that are biophysically realistic and reproduce dynamics observed in physiological experiments. Even when behavioral data are used to constrain such models, there are often many parameter settings that satisfy those constraints. Following an alternative approach, we start from a normative theory of behavior (in this case, optimal cue integration) and use theories of neural coding to link behavioral to neural quantities. This results in a theory stating which neural operations *should* be performed if the brain is to execute certain behaviors optimally. In this approach, biophysical realism is important but only a last step, serving merely to make concrete an implementation that has been found in terms of more abstract neural operations.

This chapter is based on a recent paper by the authors (Ma, Beck, Latham, & Pouget, 2006). Here, however, we will attempt a more didactic approach and highlight the broader context of the work. In previous chapters, we have seen that the problem of cue integration can be formulated in terms of the multiplication of probabilities,

$$p\left(s|x_V, x_A\right) \propto p\left(x_V|s\right) p\left(x_A|s\right) \tag{21.1}$$

(see Eq. 1.7), where $s$ is the stimulus, and $x_V$ and $x_A$ are the noisy observations from two cues (for concreteness, we use the subscripts $V$ for visual and $A$ for auditory). Our first goal is to establish how a neural population can encode a probability distribution over the stimulus. After that, we will examine how the multiplication is implemented.

Before delving into specifics, it is important to comment on the use of the word *optimality*, which has different meanings depending on context and author. In this chapter, we discuss optimality in a very specific sense, namely one in which an observer computes the posterior probability distribution over the task variable of interest (as defined later). This is not necessarily the same meaning as that of the term "ideal observer," which commonly indicates an observer who extracts all information that is present in a physical stimulus. In contrast, a Bayes-optimal observer is optimal in the sense that *during a particular computation*, such as cue integration, no information is lost. However, it is possible that input information is lost before the computation, that is, that the probability distributions that enter the computation are broader than the ones that could be extracted from the stimulus.

## NEURAL VARIABILITY

Our first task is to understand how populations of neurons encode a stimulus. Our starting point is a variable $s$ that is of interest to the organism. This can be the slant of a surface, the width of an object, the spatial location of an event, the speed of a moving object, the identity of a spoken syllable, and so forth. We assume that each presentation of a particular value of this stimulus variable (this particular value is also denoted $s$) elicits activity in a large population of neurons. Activity is characterized as the total number of evoked action potentials (spikes). An important feature of this response is that when the same value $s$ is presented repeatedly, this spike count typically varies (Tolhurst, Movshon, & Dean, 1982). This variability has been measured in many areas of cortex. In an attempt to model it, people often assume that it obeys a Poisson distribution. This reflects the absence of temporal correlations between the spikes and implies that the probability of a spike count $r$ in response to a stimulus $s$ is

$$p(r|s) = \frac{e^{-\lambda}\lambda^r}{r!}. \tag{21.2}$$

In this equation, $\lambda$ stands for the mean spike count, which in a Poisson process is identical to the variance of the spike count. Observed variability is not exactly Poisson—we will address this issue later. The mean spike count $\lambda$ depends on two things: the stimulus presented, $s$, and which neuron in the population is considered, $i$. Therefore, it can be written as $\lambda = gf_i(s)$, where $g$ is an overall scaling factor (the gain). As a function of $s$, $f_i(s)$ is called the tuning curve of the $i$'th neuron; it is typically bell shaped or monotonic. If $s$ is a spatial variable, then $f_i(s)$ is a receptive field. An example of a set of tuning curves (for different $i$) is shown in Figure 21.1A.

Since there are multiple neurons in the population, their responses to $s$ have to be considered jointly. A population pattern of activity is a set of spike counts $(r_1, r_2, \ldots, r_N)$, where $N$ is the number of neurons in the population. An example is shown in Figure 21.1B.

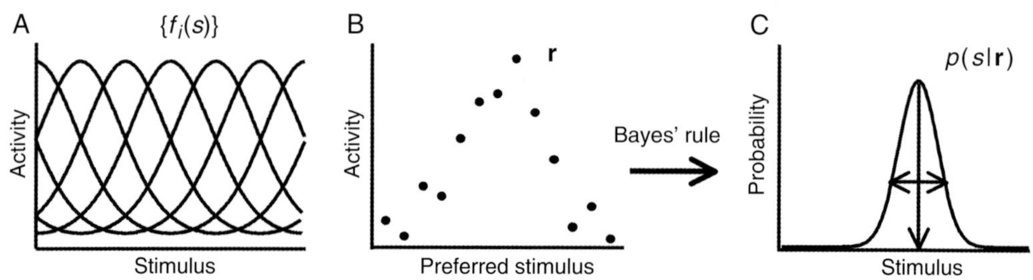


**Figure 21.1** Schematic illustration of probabilistic population coding. (A) Bell-shaped tuning curves of six neurons in a hypothetical population. (In real data, these do not look nearly as smooth and identical.) Notation: $s$ is the stimulus value, $i$ labels the neuron, and $f_i(s)$ is the average activity of the $i$'th neuron in response to $s$. (B) Population pattern of activity elicited by a stimulus (e.g., the orientation of a line segment) on a single trial. Neurons are ordered by their preferred stimuli. (C) Based on this pattern of activity $\mathbf{r}$, Bayes' rule computes the probability distribution $p(s|\mathbf{r})$ over the stimulus (right), providing not only the most likely value of the stimulus (indicated by the arrow) but also its uncertainty (indicated by the double arrow). One can think of the probability distribution in (C) as being *encoded* in the pattern of activity in (B).

The simplest assumption regarding the neurons' joint activity is that all neurons are uncorrelated. In other words, for a given $s$, the responses $r_i$ taken across all possible $i$ are independent of each other. That means that the probability of observing pattern $(r_1, r_2, \ldots, r_N)$ is equal to the product of the probabilities of all individual responses $r_i$ under their respective distributions $p(r_i|s)$:

$$p\left(r_1, r_2 \ldots, r_N|s\right) = p\left(r_1|s\right) \cdot p\left(r_2|s\right) \cdots \times p\left(r_N|s\right). \quad (21.3)$$

From now on, we will use shorthand notation $\mathbf{r}$ for the vector $(r_1, r_2, \ldots, r_N)$, and $\Pi$ for a product. Combining Eqs. 21.2 and 21.3, and $\lambda_i = \langle r_i \rangle = gf_i(s)$, we find for neural population variability:

$$p(\mathbf{r}|s) = \prod_{i=1}^{N} p\left(r_i|s\right) = \prod_{i=1}^{N} \frac{e^{-gf_i(s)}\left(gf_i(s)\right)^{r_i}}{r_i!}. \quad (21.4)$$

If you know $g$ and $f_i(s)$, this equation allows you to calculate for each possible pattern of activity $\mathbf{r}$ (and there are a lot of them) the probability that it will occur when the stimulus was $s$. These probabilities will normally be different for different $s$. Therefore, the activity pattern $\mathbf{r}$ is informative about $s$. The observer's brain does not have knowledge of $s$, and its task is exactly to make a guess about $s$ based on $\mathbf{r}$—in other words, to decode $s$ from $\mathbf{r}$. There are many recipes in the literature to make such a guess, such as winner take all, population vector, and maximum likelihood. Some of these decoding methods are better than others, but they have in common that they all return a single value of $s$ on a single trial.

## PROBABILISTIC POPULATION CODES

For optimal cue integration, it is critical that a population of neurons encodes a *probability distribution* over the stimulus on a single trial, not just a best guess about the stimulus. This is where Bayes' rule comes in. In Eq. 21.4, we fixed $s$ and considered the probabilities of different $\mathbf{r}$. Now, we do the reverse: We fix $\mathbf{r}$ (interpreted as the observed pattern of activity on a single trial) and we consider the probabilities of different $s$. This is the "inverse problem" that the brain has to solve. Bayes' rule explains the latter probability, $p(s|\mathbf{r})$, in terms of the former, $p(\mathbf{r}|s)$:

$$p(s|\mathbf{r}) = \frac{p(\mathbf{r}|s)\, p(s)}{p(\mathbf{r})}. \quad (21.5)$$

This type of coding is called *probabilistic population coding*. The left-hand side is called the posterior distribution, while $p(\mathbf{r}|s)$ is called the likelihood function when considered as a function of $s$. (This is somewhat confusing: Even though $\mathbf{r}$ is the first argument in $p(\mathbf{r}|s)$, one can still regard it as a function of $s$ by fixing $\mathbf{r}$ and considering different possible values of $s$. Some people use a notation like $L_{\mathbf{r}}(s)$ to denote a likelihood over $s$.) In this equation, the distribution $p(s)$ reflects prior knowledge that the observer has about the stimulus, that is, beliefs held about $s$ before any data ($\mathbf{r}$) are observed. In this chapter, we will choose this prior distribution to be uniform (flat); that is, the observer is completely agnostic (if this distribution is not flat, it is still possible to perform optimal cue integration using neural populations, essentially by regarding the prior information as another cue). Moreover, since the left-hand side is a probability distribution over $s$, factors on the right-hand side that do not depend on $s$ are irrelevant except for the fact that they serve as a normalization. Therefore, we will from now on use the formulation

$$p(s|\mathbf{r}) \propto p(\mathbf{r}|s). \quad (21.6)$$

Combining Eqs. 21.4 and 21.6 allows us to write down the posterior distribution for a population pattern of activity drawn from an independent Poisson distribution:

$$p(s|\mathbf{r}) \propto \exp \sum_{i=1}^{N} \left(-gf_i(s) + r_i \log f_i(s)\right), \quad (21.7)$$

where we have absorbed factors independent of $s$ into the proportionality sign.

Note that $p(s|\mathbf{r})$ is not a probability distribution in the classical, frequentist sense of "expected frequencies of possible outcomes of a random variable," since we are considering only a single trial. Based on a single **r**, frequentists would only reconstruct a single value of $s$, the "best guess" we mentioned earlier. Instead, $p(s|\mathbf{r})$ is to be interpreted as the degree of belief in a hypothesized value of the stimulus. Given a single observation **r**, one asks to what extent one believes that stimulus value $s$ caused **r**. It should be emphasized that in this view, Bayesian inference is not characterized by the presence of a nontrivial prior distribution. The framework allows for incorporation of prior beliefs, but the mere fact that we consider $p(s|\mathbf{r})$ a legitimate distribution over $s$ makes our approach Bayesian.

Although Bayes' rule follows directly from the basic properties of probability distributions, its implications in our context are profound. It means that based on a single pattern **r**, one cannot only reconstruct the value of $s$ most likely to have caused **r** (which is what a maximum-likelihood decoder would do) but also the probability that *any* value of $s$ caused **r**. This was first proposed in the 1990s (Földiák, 1993; Sanger, 1996). An example is shown in Figure 21.1C. The width of this probability distribution over $s$ is interpreted as the uncertainty about the stimulus (the terms *certainty*, *reliability*, or *fidelity* are sometimes used for the inverse quantity). Note that this width is in general different from the width of the tuning curve. Even though the probability distribution and the population pattern of activity are related and can both be bell shaped, their relationship is indirect, as indicated by Eq. 21.7.

As a consequence, if the task is to estimate $s$ from **r**, the observer has knowledge of the confidence in the decision without the need of a confidence-estimation mechanism separate from the stimulus representation. However, the merits of this type of coding are not limited to representing the confidence about a decision. Since any neural population that encodes a stimulus variable simultaneously also encodes uncertainty about this variable, this code allows for the easy propagation of uncertainty through all brain areas involved in a perceptual computation. The population activity **r** that encodes a probability distribution over the stimulus will carry uncertainty information with it whenever it is manipulated. This is the main argument we will lay out in the rest of this chapter.

Other schemes have been proposed to encode probability distributions in neural activity. In some, neural activity (either on a single trial or averaged over many trials) is linearly related to probability ("explicit" coding) or to the log of probability. In those schemes, the width of the tuning curve (when bell shaped) is equal to the width of the probability distribution. Probabilistic population coding stands out by being the only scheme that bases beliefs about the stimulus on the observed neural variability. When tuning curves are not bell shaped but monotonic, the difference between probabilistic population codes and "explicit" coding becomes very clear (see Ma, Beck, & Pouget, 2008, for a review).

## CAN ONE "MEASURE" THE POSTERIOR DISTRIBUTION?

Before we consider cue integration using probabilistic population codes, we first address the common question of how the posterior distribution relates to behavior as measured through a psychophysical experiment. It is tempting to identify the posterior distributions with the distribution of stimulus estimates across many trials, but this is a mistake. The posterior distribution, $p(s|\mathbf{r})$, reflects the observer's beliefs about the stimulus on a single trial. When a decision needs to be made, a single value $\mu$ is extracted from the posterior distribution (for example, its mode, mean, or median, depending on the cost function one uses). This value is the model observer's response, $\hat{s} = \mu$. These responses can be collected over many trials, keeping the true stimulus, $s_0$, the same. This creates a response distribution, $p(\hat{s}|s_0)$. There is no reason why $p(\hat{s}|s_0)$ should have the same shape or functional form as $p(s|\mathbf{r})$. The reason that this is nevertheless often believed is because only the Gaussian case is considered. In behavioral modeling, the internal representation of a stimulus is typically taken to be $\mu$, not **r**, and from the outset, a Gaussian distribution $p(\mu|s)$ is assumed. Under uniform priors, this choice makes both $p(s|\mu)$ and $p(\hat{s}|s_0)$ Gaussian with the same variance. Operations performed on $p(s|\mu)$ are then directly mirrored in operations on $p(\hat{s}|s_0)$, just like we will see in this chapter. However, in the presence of nonuniform priors (Stocker & Simoncelli, 2006), or when the posterior is non-Gaussian (Körding et al., 2007), this is no longer true and identifying the posterior with the response distribution leads to wrong predictions. It is important to keep this caveat in mind.

## OPTIMAL CUE INTEGRATION WITH INDEPENDENT POISSON POPULATIONS

Now we can turn to the problem of cue integration. Suppose there are two cues to the same stimulus attribute, which we will call auditory (A) and visual (V) for convenience. Each cue is represented by a neural population of $N$ neurons; we will denote their patterns of activity by $\mathbf{r}_A$ and $\mathbf{r}_V$. We assume that these patterns are both drawn from independent Poisson distributions, and even that they have identical tuning curves $f_i(s)$ (there are a lot of assumptions here, and we will relax all of them eventually). They only differ in their gains: The mean activities of the auditory neurons are equal to $g_A f_i(s)$, whereas the mean activities of the visual neurons are $g_V f_i(s)$. A higher gain implies narrower posteriors and less uncertainty. Choosing different gains for the auditory and the visual cues reflects that they come with different degrees of uncertainty. Moreover, gain can change from trial to trial.

We are now interested in the optimal posterior distribution that is encoded by $\mathbf{r}_A$ and $\mathbf{r}_V$ together, because the psychophysics of cue integration suggests that this distribution is computed in the brain. Using Bayes' rule, the posterior takes the following form:

$$p(s|\mathbf{r}_A,\mathbf{r}_V) \propto p(\mathbf{r}_A,\mathbf{r}_V|s) = p(\mathbf{r}_A|s)\,p(\mathbf{r}_V|s). \tag{21.8}$$

In going from the second to the third expression, we have assumed that the cues are conditionally independent given the stimulus, just as in the behavioral theory. We substitute Eq. 21.4 and absorb all factors independent of $s$ into the proportionality sign. This gives

$$p(s|\mathbf{r}_A,\mathbf{r}_V) \propto \left(\prod_{i=1}^{N} e^{-g_A f_i(s)} f_i(s)^{r_{Ai}}\right) \times \left(\prod_{i=1}^{N} e^{-g_V f_i(s)} f_i(s)^{r_{Vi}}\right). \tag{21.9}$$

This can be rewritten as:

$$p(s|\mathbf{r}_A,\mathbf{r}_V) \propto \exp \sum_{i=1}^{N} \left(-\left(g_A+g_V\right) f_i(s) + \left(r_{Ai}+r_{Vi}\right)\log f_i(s)\right). \tag{21.10}$$

This is the posterior distribution encoded by $\mathbf{r}_A$ and $\mathbf{r}_V$ together. However, $\mathbf{r}_A$ and $\mathbf{r}_V$ are separate populations—what we want instead is a single multisensory population. To implement optimal cue integration neurally means to ask what operation we can perform on $\mathbf{r}_A$ and $\mathbf{r}_V$ such that the resulting multisensory population encodes the optimal posterior distribution, Eq. 21.10. In that way, we would not lose any information about $s$. The right-hand side of Eq. 21.10 suggests the answer: addition. We construct a new population pattern of activity, $\mathbf{r}_{AV}$, by summing the activities of corresponding pairs of neurons in the auditory and visual populations:

$$\mathbf{r}_{AV} = \mathbf{r}_A + \mathbf{r}_V. \tag{21.11}$$

The output population pattern, $\mathbf{r}_{AV}$, will still obey independent Poisson variability across many trials, since the sum of two Poisson processes is again Poisson. The mean activity of the $i$'th neuron in the output population in response to $s$ is $(g_A + g_V)f_i(s)$. Therefore, it encodes a posterior distribution that is given by:

$$p(s|\mathbf{r}_{AV}) \propto \exp \sum_{i=1}^{N} \left(-\left(g_A+g_V\right) f_i(s) + \left(r_{Ai}+r_{Vi}\right)\log f_i(s)\right). \tag{21.12}$$

This distribution is identical to the one in Eq. 21.10. We conclude that adding independent Poisson population patterns of activity implements a multiplication of the probability distributions over the stimulus that are encoded in those patterns. We will now attempt to generalize this framework to other forms of neural variability.

## POISSON-LIKE VARIABILITY

We assumed earlier that neurons fire with Poisson statistics and that their noise is independent. Both assumptions are often not completely satisfied. In cortical neurons, spike count variance is often proportional to, but not equal to, spike count mean. The ratio variance/mean is called the *Fano factor*, and its measured values range from 0.3 to 1.8 (Gur & Snodderly, 2006; Tolhurst et al., 1982). Moreover, neurons are not independent (when conditioned on the stimulus) but exhibit correlations (Averbeck, Latham, & Pouget, 2006). Therefore, a more general treatment is needed. Fortunately, there is a family of distributions that is more general than independent Poisson variability but leaves the mechanism for implementing optimal cue integration intact. This family is the exponential family with linear sufficient statistics, also called Poisson-like variability. It takes the following form:

$$p(\mathbf{r}|s) = \frac{\Phi(\mathbf{r})}{\eta(s)} e^{\mathbf{h}(s)\cdot\mathbf{r}}, \tag{21.13}$$

where $\Phi(\mathbf{r})$ is an arbitrary function of $\mathbf{r}$, $\mathbf{h}(s)$ is a vector-valued function of $s$ that we will specify later, and $\eta(s)$ serves as a normalization (since this is a probability distribution over $\mathbf{r}$). The exponent contains the inner product of $\mathbf{h}(s)$ with the population pattern of activity. To gain some intuition for Eq. 21.13, it helps to see what $\Phi$, $\mathbf{h}$, and $\eta$ are for independent Poisson variability:

$$\Phi(\mathbf{r}) = \frac{1}{\prod_i r_i!}, \quad \eta(s) = e^{g\sum_i f_i(s)},$$

$$h_i(s) = \log f_i(s). \tag{21.14}$$

Thus, $\mathbf{h}$ and $\eta$ both depend on the tuning curve, whereas $\Phi$ contains all factors that only depend on $\mathbf{r}$. In general, when variability is Poisson-like but not necessarily independent Poisson, there is a relationship between $\mathbf{h}(s)$ and the tuning curve. By using the definition, Eq. 21.13, it is possible to show that the derivative of $\mathbf{h}$ satisfies:

$$\mathbf{h}'(s) = \Sigma^{-1}(s)\,\mathbf{f}'(s), \tag{21.15}$$

where $\Sigma^{-1}(s)$ is the inverse of the covariance matrix of the population and $\mathbf{f}(s)$ is the mean activity. For independent neurons, the covariance matrix is a diagonal matrix, with the variances of the neural activities on the diagonal. In the case of independent Poisson variability, it is

$$\Sigma(s) = \begin{pmatrix} f_1(s) & 0 & \cdots & 0 \\ 0 & f_2(s) & \ddots & \vdots \\ \vdots & \ddots & \ddots & 0 \\ 0 & \cdots & 0 & f_N(s) \end{pmatrix}. \tag{21.16}$$

Therefore, Eq. 21.15 implies that $h_i'(s) = \frac{f_i'(s)}{f_i(s)}$, which is, up to a constant, equivalent to the second part of Eq. 21.14. This confirms that independent Poisson variability is indeed a special case of Poisson-like variability.

## DEALING WITH "IRRELEVANT" VARIABLES

When a task involves estimating a stimulus, such as a spatial location of an event, the size of a visual object, or the direction of motion of a moving object, neural activity is often affected by parameters that are not of interest to the observer. For example, the visual object might come with greater or lesser contrast, or the motion might be more or less coherent. Such variables, which affect the difficulty of the task but are irrelevant when estimating the stimulus, are called *nuisance parameters*. Nuisance parameters are extremely common in any real-world perceptual task, for example, in object recognition (Kersten, Mamassian, & Yuille, 2004). The brain is faced with this problem of estimating the stimulus while not knowing the value of the nuisance parameters. In this section, we describe under what conditions Poisson-like variability solves this problem. This section is more technical than the rest of this chapter and can be skipped without affecting the understanding of the overall line of reasoning. The main results of this section are Eqs. 21.21 and 21.22.

We will examine the specific situation in which nuisance parameters affect the gain of the population. For example, if $\mathbf{r}$ is a visual population, then the gain $g$ could be determined by the contrast of the stimulus. In the formulation of the Poisson-like family, Eq. 21.13, we did not include the gain. Yet each of the factors in Eq. 21.13 could in principle depend on it. For example, in Eq. 21.14, the expression for $\eta(s)$ contains the gain. This does not pose a problem if the gain is known, but in general this is not the case. There are two types of solutions to this problem. The first is to use an external mechanism to estimate the gain and substitute its estimated value. However, this requires extra computational resources and it is not an optimal solution. The second solution is the Bayes-optimal one: When a parameter whose value is unknown influences the observations, it is averaged out (also called "integrated out" or "marginalized out"). This is done as follows:

$$p(s|\mathbf{r}) \propto p(\mathbf{r}|s) = \int p(\mathbf{r}|s,g)\,p(g)\,dg, \tag{21.17}$$

where $p(g)$ is some prior distribution over $g$. In writing this integral, we have assumed that $g$ does not depend on $s$. To avoid the complications of marginalizing out gain, we will restrict ourselves to the situation where the $s$ and $g$ dependencies of $p(\mathbf{r}|s,g)$ can be separated, that is, where $p(\mathbf{r}|s,g)$ can be written as the product of a factor that only depends on $s$ and $\mathbf{r}$ and one that only depends on $g$ and $\mathbf{r}$. Looking back at Eq. 21.13, this means that it would take the following form:

$$p(\mathbf{r}|s,g) = \frac{\Phi(\mathbf{r},g)}{\eta(s)}e^{\mathbf{h}(s)\cdot\mathbf{r}}. \tag{21.18}$$

How does this help? If we substitute Eq. 21.18 into the integral of Eq. 21.17, then we find:

$$\begin{aligned} p(s|\mathbf{r}) &\propto \int \frac{\Phi(\mathbf{r},g)}{\eta(s)}e^{\mathbf{h}(s)\cdot\mathbf{r}}p(g)\,dg \\ &= \frac{e^{\mathbf{h}(s)\cdot\mathbf{r}}}{\eta(s)}\int \Phi(\mathbf{r},g)\,p(g)\,dg \\ &\propto \frac{e^{\mathbf{h}(s)\cdot\mathbf{r}}}{\eta(s)}, \end{aligned} \tag{21.19}$$

where we can go from the second to the third line because the integral does not depend on $s$, no matter what $p(g)$ is.

It turns out that another constraint must be satisfied. To derive this constraint, we first compute the derivative of $\eta(s)$ with respect to $s$, keeping in mind that $\eta(s)$ is a normalization factor:

$$\begin{aligned} \frac{d}{ds}\log\eta(s) &= \frac{1}{\eta(s)}\frac{d}{ds}\int \Phi(\mathbf{r},g)\,e^{\mathbf{h}(s)\cdot\mathbf{r}}\,d\mathbf{r} \\ &= \mathbf{h}'(s)\cdot\int \frac{\mathbf{r}\,\Phi(\mathbf{r},g)\,e^{\mathbf{h}(s)\cdot\mathbf{r}}}{\eta(s)}\,d\mathbf{r} \\ &= \mathbf{h}'(s)\cdot\langle\mathbf{r}\rangle = \mathbf{h}'(s)\cdot g\mathbf{f}(s). \end{aligned} \tag{21.20}$$

Now, differentiating both sides with respect to $g$ gives $0 = \mathbf{h}'(s)\cdot\mathbf{f}(s)$. Substituting this back into Eq. 21.20 implies that $d\eta/ds = 0$. Surprisingly, this condition is not very hard to meet. For example, in the independent Poisson case, Eq. 21.14, it seems as though $\eta$ depends both on $s$ and on $g$. However, if tuning curves are translation invariant and many of them span the stimulus space, as in Figure 21.1A, then the sum $\sum_i f_i(s)$ will be nearly independent of $s$. This means that $\eta$ only depends on $g$ and can therefore be absorbed into $\Phi(\mathbf{r},g)$.

To allow Eq. 21.19 to be true, it is also important that $\mathbf{h}(s)$ does not depend on $g$. Both the mean activity and the covariance matrix can depend on the gain g, and in general they will, but the combination $\mathbf{\Sigma}^{-1}(s,g)\mathbf{f}'(s,g)$ (from Eq. 21.15) cannot. Since $\mathbf{f}(s,g) = g\mathbf{f}(s)$, this means that the covariance matrix must be of the form $\mathbf{\Sigma}(s,g) = g\mathbf{\Sigma}(s)$. On the diagonal, this means that the variance scales with the gain, in other words, that the Fano factor is constant but not necessarily equal to 1 (as it is in a Poisson process). Off diagonal, it means that the entries $\langle r_i r_j \rangle - g^2 f_i(s) f_j(s)$ should be proportional to $g$ as well. In conclusion, we find that neural variability must be of the form

$$p(\mathbf{r}|s) = \Phi(\mathbf{r}, g)\, e^{\mathbf{h}(s)\cdot\mathbf{r}}, \tag{21.21}$$

and the posterior distribution over $s$ is simply

$$p(s|\mathbf{r}) \propto e^{\mathbf{h}(s)\cdot\mathbf{r}}. \tag{21.22}$$

In the more general case in which nuisance parameters $\mathbf{c}$ exist that affect the tuning curves and the covariance matrix, but not through a simple gain modulation, then Poisson-like variability requires that $\boldsymbol{\Sigma}^{-1}(s,\mathbf{c})\mathbf{f}'(s,\mathbf{c})$ be independent of $\mathbf{c}$.

Whether cortical variability is approximately Poisson-like is an open question that can in principle be addressed by analyzing population recordings. We just stated that Poisson-like variability requires that the elements of the covariance matrix, including the variance, scale with the gain of the population. This condition seems to be roughly satisfied in cortical neurons (Gur & Snodderly, 2006; Tolhurst et al., 1982), but further study is needed. Furthermore, if variability is Poisson-like, the locally optimal linear decoder (Seriès, Latham, & Pouget, 2004) should extract all available information. This property can be falsified by trying other decoders, such as support vector machines (Bishop, 2006). Moreover, the optimal decoder of Poisson-like activity is completely determined by $\mathbf{h}(s)$ and should therefore be independent of nuisance parameters.

## OPTIMAL CUE INTEGRATION WITH POISSON-LIKE POPULATIONS

We claim that the same addition operation that implements optimal cue integration in the independent Poisson case, $\mathbf{r}_{AV} = \mathbf{r}_A + \mathbf{r}_V$, does the same in the more general Poisson-like case. We verify this by first calculating the distribution of the sum random variable, $\mathbf{r}_{AV}$, for a given stimulus $s$ and input gains $g_V$ and $g_A$. That is done in the same way one would calculate the distribution of the total number rolled with two dice, namely by summing (or integrating) over all possible values of one of the terms in the sum:

$$\begin{aligned} &p(\mathbf{r}_{AV}|s, g_V, g_A) \\ &= \int p(\mathbf{r}_V|s, g_V) \\ &\quad \times p(\mathbf{r}_A = \mathbf{r}_{AV} - \mathbf{r}_V|s, g_A)\, d\mathbf{r}_V \\ &= \int \Phi_V(\mathbf{r}_V, g_V)\, e^{\mathbf{h}(s)\cdot\mathbf{r}_V} \\ &\quad \times \Phi_A(\mathbf{r}_{AV} - \mathbf{r}_V, g_A)\, e^{\mathbf{h}(s)\cdot(\mathbf{r}_{AV} - \mathbf{r}_V)} d\mathbf{r}_V \\ &= \int \Phi_V(\mathbf{r}_V, g_V) \\ &\quad \times \Phi_A(\mathbf{r}_{AV} - \mathbf{r}_V, g_A)\, e^{\mathbf{h}(s)\cdot\mathbf{r}_{AV}} d\mathbf{r}_V \\ &= e^{\mathbf{h}(s)\cdot\mathbf{r}_{AV}} \int \Phi_V(\mathbf{r}_V, g_V) \\ &\quad \times \Phi_A(\mathbf{r}_{AV} - \mathbf{r}_V, g_A)\, d\mathbf{r}_V. \end{aligned} \tag{21.23}$$

Note that in the transition from the second to the third line, it is essential that $\mathbf{h}(s)$ is the same in both populations. As a consequence of Eq. 21.23, the posterior encoded in a multisensory population pattern of activity can be computed in analogy to Eq. 21.22. We find

$$p(s|\mathbf{r}_{AV}) \propto e^{\mathbf{h}(s)\cdot\mathbf{r}_{AV}}. \tag{21.24}$$

When we substitute $\mathbf{r}_{AV} = \mathbf{r}_A + \mathbf{r}_V$ (i.e., giving the random variable $\mathbf{r}_{AV}$ the value $\mathbf{r}_A + \mathbf{r}_V$), it follows that

$$p(s|\mathbf{r}_{AV} = \mathbf{r}_A + \mathbf{r}_V) \propto p(\mathbf{r}_A|s)\, p(\mathbf{r}_V|s), \tag{21.25}$$

where we again assumed that $\mathbf{h}(s)$ is the same function for auditory and visual inputs. Thus, just like for independent Poisson variability, optimal cue integration is achieved in Poisson-like populations by adding input population activities.

Our assumption that $\mathbf{h}(s)$ is the same in both input populations is violated if tuning curves or covariance matrices differ between auditory and visual areas. However, different $\mathbf{h}(s)$ can be dealt with as long as they can be linearly mapped onto a common basis of functions, that is, $\mathbf{h}_A(s) = \mathbf{W}_A\mathbf{H}(s)$ and $\mathbf{h}_V(s) = \mathbf{W}_V\mathbf{H}(s)$, where $\mathbf{W}_A$ and $\mathbf{W}_V$ are stimulus-independent matrices and $\mathbf{H}(s)$ is the common basis. Then, it can be shown that the linear combination

$$\mathbf{r}_{AV} = \mathbf{W}_A^{\mathrm{T}}\mathbf{r}_A + \mathbf{W}_V^{\mathrm{T}}\mathbf{r}_V \tag{21.26}$$

(where the superscript "T" denotes a transpose) implements optimal cue integration (for details, see the Supplement of Ma et al., 2006). This more general operation is depicted in Figure 21.2. Notably, the weights do not depend on neural gain or on uncertainty. Having to adjust the weights every time gain or uncertainty changes would make a neural implementation much more difficult. By using Poisson-like variability, the brain can avoid this problem, since the weights are learned once and for all.

## A PHYSIOLOGICAL PREDICTION

Our most general prediction for physiology is that the activity in a multisensory area involved in optimal cue integration is equal to a linear combination of the activities in the input populations (Eq. 21.26). If one would present only one of both inputs, then only one of the terms in $\mathbf{r}_{AV}$ (either $\mathbf{W}_A^{\mathrm{T}}\mathbf{r}_A$ or $\mathbf{W}_V^{\mathrm{T}}\mathbf{r}_V$) would be nonzero. It follows that the activity evoked in a multisensory area by both cues presented simultaneously is predicted to be approximately equal to the sum of the activities evoked by each individual cue separately. This property is called *additivity*. Recent physiological studies have begun to test this prediction (see Chapter 16). Earlier work had claimed that multisensory interactions are characterized by *superadditivity* of multisensory responses (Stein & Meredith, 1993), that is, that the multisensory activity evoked by both cues is more than the sum of the activities evoked

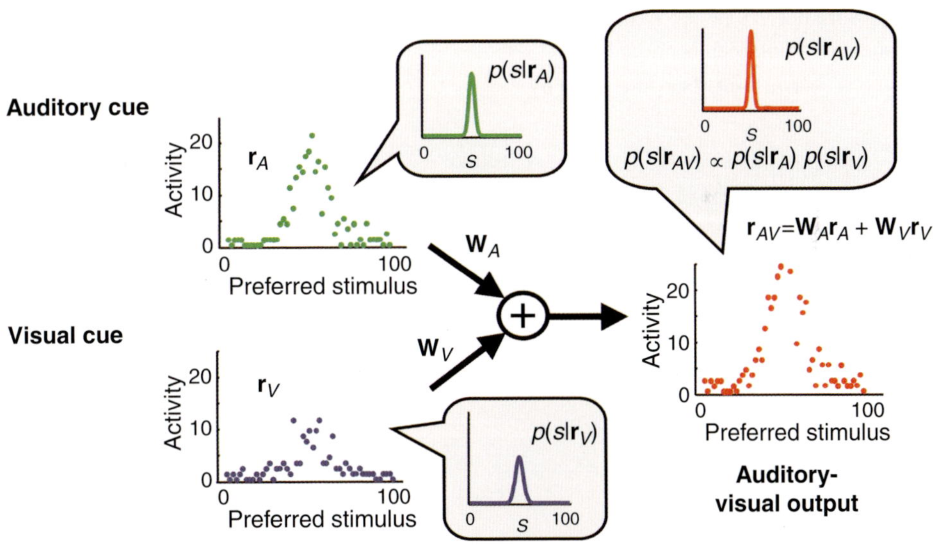


**Figure 21.2** Optimal cue integration with probabilistic population codes. The cues elicit activity in input populations $\mathbf{r}_A$ and $\mathbf{r}_V$, indicated by green and blue dots. The dialogue boxes show the probability distributions over the stimulus encoded in each population on a single trial. A simple linear combination of the population patterns of activity, $\mathbf{r}_{AV} = \mathbf{W}_A\mathbf{r}_A + \mathbf{W}_V\mathbf{r}_V$, guarantees optimal cue integration, if neural variability is Poisson-like. Optimal cue integration means that the probability distribution over the stimulus encoded in the multisensory population is a product of the distributions encoded in the unisensory populations, i.e. $p(s|\mathbf{r}_{AV}) \propto p(s|\mathbf{r}_A)p(s|\mathbf{r}_V)$. The synaptic weight matrices $\mathbf{W}_A$ and $\mathbf{W}_V$ depend on the tuning curves and covariance matrices of the input populations, but they do not have to be adjusted over trials.

by the individual cues. However, this notion has become largely discredited, based on new physiological data (see Ma & Pouget, 2008, for a review).

## RELATING BACK TO BEHAVIOR

We will now examine how the neural operation $\mathbf{r}_{AV} = \mathbf{r}_A + \mathbf{r}_V$ relates to the behavioral equations for multisensory mean and variance that we encountered in Chapter 1. In behavioral modeling of cue integration discussed in this book, it is assumed that the posterior distribution $p(s|\mathbf{r})$ is Gaussian. Therefore, it is exponential with a quadratic function of $s$ in the exponent:

$$p\,(s|\mathbf{r}) \propto e^{-\frac{1}{2}s^2 a(\mathbf{r}) + sb(\mathbf{r})}, \tag{21.27}$$

where $a(\mathbf{r})$ and $b(\mathbf{r})$ are functions of $\mathbf{r}$. Comparing with Eq. 21.22, we see that these functions must be of the form $a(\mathbf{r}) = \mathbf{a}{\cdot}\mathbf{r}$ and $b(\mathbf{r}) = \mathbf{b}{\cdot}\mathbf{r}$, where now $\mathbf{a}$ and $\mathbf{b}$ are constant vectors. From Eq. 21.27, we can find the mean $\mu$ and variance $\sigma^2$ of the Gaussian, since the exponent of a Gaussian is of the form $-\frac{(s-\mu)^2}{2\sigma^2} = -\frac{s^2}{2\sigma^2} + \frac{s\mu}{\sigma^2} +$ constant. They are given by

$$\frac{1}{\sigma^2} = a\,(\mathbf{r}) = \mathbf{a} \cdot \mathbf{r} \tag{21.28}$$

and

$$\frac{\mu}{\sigma^2} = b\,(\mathbf{r}) = \mathbf{b} \cdot \mathbf{r}. \tag{21.29}$$

Since $\mathbf{r}_{AV} = \mathbf{r}_A + \mathbf{r}_V$ for optimal cue integration, applying the inner product with $\mathbf{a}$ gives (from Eq. 21.28):

$$\frac{1}{\sigma_{AV}^2} = \frac{1}{\sigma_A^2} + \frac{1}{\sigma_V^2}, \tag{21.30}$$

which is the *single-trial* version of our well-known equation for optimal combination of variances. For the mean, Eq. 21.29 gives

$$\frac{\mu_{AV}}{\sigma_{AV}^2} = \frac{\mu_A}{\sigma_A^2} + \frac{\mu_V}{\sigma_V^2} \tag{21.31}$$

(the extra assumption here is that the trial-to-trial fluctuations in the inverse variance are small). This is the *single-trial* version of the optimal combination of means. Now, we can look at the effect across many trials. This requires a way to turn $p(s|\mathbf{r})$ into a single estimate of the stimulus, $\hat{s}\,(\mathbf{r})$, on each trial. The optimal estimator is the maximum-likelihood estimator, which chooses the $s$ that makes $p(\mathbf{r}|s)$ maximal. Since we have assumed that the prior is uniform, this is also the estimator that maximizes $p(s|\mathbf{r})$. For a Gaussian $p(s|\mathbf{r})$, this is simply the mean of the Gaussian. We can now calculate the variance of this estimate using the so-called Cramèr-Rao bound, which states that the inverse variance (sampled across many trials) of an optimal estimator is given by the *Fisher information*:

$$\frac{1}{\sigma_{\text{estimator}}^2} = I\,(s) \equiv -\left\langle \frac{\partial^2}{\partial s^2} \log p\,(\mathbf{r}|s) \right\rangle, \tag{21.32}$$

where the average $\langle\cdot\rangle$ is over $\mathbf{r}$ drawn from $p(\mathbf{r}|s)$. Fisher information and the Cramèr-Rao can be applied to any distribution. For Poisson-like variability, there are several ways to express Fisher information:

$$\begin{aligned} I\,(s) &= -\mathbf{h}''\,(s) \cdot g\mathbf{f}\,(s) = g\mathbf{h}'\,(s) \cdot \Sigma\,(s)\,\mathbf{h}'\,(s) \\ &= g\mathbf{f}'\,(s) \cdot \Sigma^{-1}\,(s)\,\mathbf{f}'\,(s). \end{aligned} \tag{21.33}$$

This offers a particularly easy way to check optimality of $\mathbf{r}_{AV} = \mathbf{r}_A + \mathbf{r}_V$. Taking the average on both sides, we find $g_{AV} = g_A + g_V$, and since $I(s)$ is proportional to $g$ according to Eq. 21.33, it follows from Eq. 21.32 the estimate's inverse variances sum:

$$\frac{1}{\sigma_{\text{estimator},AV}^2} = \frac{1}{\sigma_{\text{estimator},A}^2} + \frac{1}{\sigma_{\text{estimator},V}^2}. \tag{21.34}$$

This is the relationship found in behavior. Similarly, for the mean estimate, we have from Eq. 21.29:

$$\langle\hat{s}\rangle = \sigma^2\mathbf{b} \cdot \langle\mathbf{r}\rangle = \sigma_{\text{estimator}}^2\mathbf{b} \cdot g\mathbf{f}\,(s), \tag{21.35}$$

and therefore, $g_{AV} = g_A + g_V$ implies

$$\frac{\langle\hat{s}\rangle_{AV}}{\sigma^2_{\text{estimator},AV}} = \frac{\langle\hat{s}\rangle_{A}}{\sigma^2_{\text{estimator},AV}} + \frac{\langle\hat{s}\rangle_{V}}{\sigma^2_{\text{estimator},AV}}, \tag{21.36}$$

which is the behavioral result for the mean multisensory estimate.

## OPTIMAL CUE INTEGRATION WITH BIOPHYSICAL POPULATIONS

So far, we have used abstract neurons completely characterized by their firing rates and therefore without any dynamics. As a proof of principle, it is important to show that the same scheme can be implemented with a population of biologically more realistic neurons. We did this by tuning the parameters of a network of conductance-based integrate-and-fire neurons such that the network would mimic the linear combination operation (Eq. 21.26). The output of this network satisfied the same equations that describe human observers (Eqs. 21.34 and 21.36). It is not known how to capture, in general, the network behavior of conductance-based integrate-and-fire neurons in equations only involving firing rates, and therefore a direct mapping between this network and the firing-rate neurons cannot be made. However, our approach provides an example of top-down driven neural modeling: The computational model at the behavioral level is used to construct the neural theory at an abstract level, and this in turn is used to guide a more physiologically realistic implementation. The more realistic implementation thus serves as a feasibility check, not as the centerpiece of the computational approach.

## WHAT IS OPTIMAL ABOUT CUE INTEGRATION?

One might wonder whether an optimal perceptual strategy would not lead to separate, veridical percepts of the auditory and the visual stimuli. This is not necessarily the case. Although in cue-integration experiments, small conflicts between the *presented* stimuli are introduced by the researcher, small conflicts between the best *estimates* of the auditory and visual stimuli exist even in the absence of artificial conflict. This is due to the variability in the neural response, which leads to variability in the perceived auditory and visual stimuli ($\mu_A$ and $\mu_V$ in Eq. 21.31). Thus, even when the true auditory and visual stimuli are physically completely in agreement, the brain still has to solve the cue-integration problem. Of course, it is important that in experimental settings, the artificial conflicts are kept sufficiently small and infrequent, so that they can be mistaken for naturally occurring ones. If conflicts are too large or too frequent, subjects may notice that the stimuli have different sources and develop a tendency to separate their percepts. Such perception can still be modeled using Bayesian models (Körding et al., 2007; Sato, Toyoizumi, & Aihara, 2007; also Chapters 1 and 2 in this volume).

## THE BIG PICTURE

In this chapter, we have laid out a theoretical framework for how optimal cue integration can be implemented by neural populations. The main significance of this framework does not merely lie in understanding multisensory perception in a principled manner, but in the fact that it provides a blueprint for finding neural implementations of other forms of Bayes-optimal computation. Evidence for Bayesian optimality of human behavior has been found in many perceptual tasks, including decision making (Beck et al., 2008), visual search (Ma, Navalpakkam, Beck, & Pouget, 2008; Vincent, Baddeley, Troscianko, & Gilchrist, 2009), causal inference (Körding et al., 2007), oddity detection (Hospedales & Vijayakumar, 2009), and multiple-trajectory tracking (Ma & Huang, 2009). Probabilistic population coding provides a roadmap for identifying a neural implementation of each of these computations: First work out the Bayesian model at the behavioral level, then assume that probability distributions in this model are encoded in neural populations with Poisson-like variability, and finally identify the neural operations that

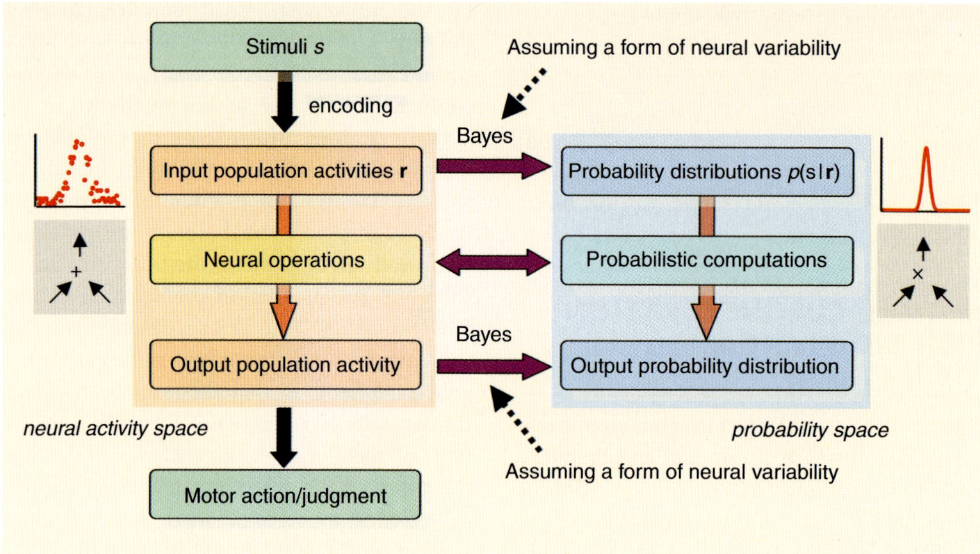


**Figure 21.3** Schematic of perceptual computation using probabilistic population codes. One or multiple stimuli elicit population patterns of activity. Each pattern encodes a probability distribution over the stimulus through Bayes' rule. In perceptual tasks, these probability distributions have to be manipulated in specific ways to achieve optimality (e.g., multiplication in cue integration). The key problem is to establish a "dictionary" between such probabilistic computations (e.g., multiplication) and neural operations on population patterns of activity (e.g., addition), assuming a form of neural variability (e.g., Poisson-like). Using those neural operations, the brain will retain full probabilistic information about the variable(s) of interest at all stages of computation. Eventually, a motor action is generated or a high-level judgment is made. (From Ma, Beck, & Pouget 2008).

map onto the desired operations on probability distributions. This general scheme for neural computation is illustrated in Figure 21.3. We believe that this approach to neural computation provides unprecedented power for relating mental functions to their underlying neural mechanisms.

## REFERENCES

Averbeck, B. B., Latham, P. E., & Pouget, A. (2006). Neural correlations, population coding, and computation. *Nature Reviews Neuroscience, 7*, 358–366.

Beck, J. M., Ma, W. J., Kiani, R., Hanks, T. D., Churchland, A. K., Roitman, J. D., ... Pouget, A. (2008). Bayesian decision-making with probabilistic population codes. *Neuron, 60*, 1142–1145.

Bishop, C. M. (2006). *Pattern recognition and machine learning.* Cambridge, England: Springer.

Földiák, P. (1993). The "ideal homunculus": Statistical inference from neural population responses. In F. Eeckman & J. Bower (Eds.), *Computation and neural systems* (pp. 55–60). Norwell, MA: Kluwer Academic Publishers.

Gur, M., & Snodderly, D. M. (2006). High response reliability of neurons in primary visual cortex (V1) of alert, trained monkeys. *Cerebral Cortex, 16*, 888–895.

Hospedales, T., & Vijayakumar, S. (2009). Multisensory oddity detection as Bayesian inference. *PLoS ONE, 4*(1), e4205.

Kersten, D., Mamassian, P., & Yuille, A. (2004). Object perception as Bayesian inference. *Annual Review of Psychology, 55*, 271–304.

Körding, K. P., Beierholm, U., Ma, W. J., Quartz, S., Tenenbaum, J. B., & Shams, L. (2007). Causal inference in multisensory perception. *PLoS ONE, 2*(9), e943.

Ma, W. J., Beck, J. M., Latham, P. E., & Pouget, A. (2006). Bayesian inference with probabilistic population codes. *Nature Neuroscience, 9*, 1432–1438.

Ma, W. J., Beck, J. M., & Pouget, A. (2008). Spiking networks for Bayesian inference and choice. *Current Opinion in Neurobiology, 18*, 217–222.

Ma, W. J., & Huang, W. (2009). No capacity limit in attentional tracking: Evidence for probabilistic inference under a resource constraint. *Journal of Vision, 9*(11):3, 1–30.

Ma, W. J., Navalpakkam, V., Beck, J. M., & Pouget, A. (2008). *Bayesian theory of visual search.* Program No. 616.1. 2008 Neuroscience Meeting Planner. Washington, DC: Society for Neuroscience. Online.

Ma, W. J., & Pouget, A. (2008). Linking neurons to behavior in multisensory perception: A computational review. *Brain Research 1242*, 4–12.

Sanger, T. (1996). Probability density estimation for the interpretation of neural population codes. *Journal of Neurophysiology, 76*, 2790–2793.

Sato, Y., Toyoizumi, T., & Aihara, K. (2007). Bayesian inference explains perception of unity and ventriloquism aftereffect: Identification of common sources of audiovisual stimuli. *Neural Computation, 19*, 3335–3355.

Seriès, P., Latham, P., & Pouget, A. (2004). Tuning curve sharpening for orientation selectivity: Coding efficiency and the impact of correlations. *Nature Neuroscience, 10*, 1129–1135.

Stein, B. E., & Meredith, M. A. (1993). *The merging of the senses.* Cambridge, MA: MIT Press.

Stocker, A. A., & Simoncelli, E. P. (2006). Noise characteristics and prior expectations in human visual speed perception. *Nature Neuroscience, 9*, 578–585.

Tolhurst, D., Movshon, J., & Dean, A. (1982). The statistical reliability of signals in single neurons in cat and monkey visual cortex. *Vision Research, 23*, 775–785.

Vincent, B. T., Baddeley, R. J., Troscianko, T., & Gilchrist, I. D. (2009). Optimal feature integration in visual search. *Journal of Vision, 9*(5):15, 1–11.

# CHAPTER 22

## Contextual Modulations of Visual Receptive Fields: A Bayesian Perspective

*Sophie Denève and Timm Lochmann*

### INTRODUCTION

We live in an unpredictable and perpetually changing world, with noisy sensory receptors and motor effectors. A wealth of recent experimental and theoretical results (some of them presented in this book) shows that humans and animals optimize their perceptual and motor decisions in the presence of uncertainty (Ernst & Banks, 2002; Gold & Shadlen, 2002; Knill & Pouget, 2004; Körding & Wolpert, 2004; Trommershäuser, Maloney, & Landy, 2008; Yuille & Bülthoff, 1996). In particular, human performance can be well predicted as inferring the best explanation for sensory data, or maximizing the expected outcome of an action, under a given world model and priors (Knill & Richards, 1996; Körding, 2007).

In particular, different chapters in this book describe how cues are combined optimally, that is, how the common cause of several sensory events can be inferred optimally (e.g., recognizing a word from both the image and sound of the human speaker pronouncing it). They also treat another important problem in perceptual inference, which is "explaining away": In the presence of several possible causes of the same sensory inputs, humans are able to decide which one is really responsible for the sensory observations. Thus, in the cocktail-party effect, speech sounds can be properly attributed to multiple speakers using visual and localization cues. These elementary problems of perceptual inference can be expressed and combined in a "normative model" that graphically describes the causal structure of the sensory world or behavioral task.

In this chapter, we suggest that this same Bayesian framework and normative approach is useful to describe information processing at a much more microscopic level, that is, at the level of single neurons or microcircuits of neurons. In other words, probabilistic approaches that have proved useful recently to describe human and animal behaviors can be adapted to understand how the dynamics and biophysical properties of neural systems are related to behavioral performance and the statistics of the natural sensory world. In particular, the interplay between "cue combination" and "explaining away" can explain many puzzling and nonlinear aspects of neural sensory processing.

For example, we showed recently that single neurons can be interpreted as Bayesian integrators. They accumulate synaptic evidence and fire spikes when the probability of their preferred stimulus exceeds a threshold, resulting in integrate-and-fire dynamics (Denève, 2008a, 2008b). These neurons can be seen as performing optimal integration of multiple cues, corresponding to their synaptic inputs, with a common cause, that is, the preferred stimulus.

Here we go one step further and explore the implication of this approach for spatial and temporal visual processing. In particular, we concentrate on the problem of analyzing a dynamic visual scene.

Since similar visual activations can be caused by different visual objects (e.g., overlapping visual features, two-dimensional (2D) projections of different three-dimensional objects) "explaining away," that is, deciding among different possible interpretations of the visual input, is absolutely crucial. If "cue integration" can be performed by single neurons with feedforward connections, explaining away requires competition and collective dynamics to "segment" the scene and interpret ambiguous inputs.

To formalize the implications of this "normative approach" for visual processing, we describe each visual neuron as a predictor rather than a filter of its input. Thus, neurons are defined by their "causal field," that is, how their preferred stimulus is expected to affect (cause) the sensory input. This contrasts with the more traditional interpretation of sensory neurons in terms of their receptive fields, that is, as filters that are applied to the sensory input. We apply this approach to early stages of visual processing, and we consider what it implies for the spike trains of visual neurons, the spatiotemporal dynamics of their receptive fields, and the contextual interactions with stimuli outside of their receptive fields.

While the concept of the visual receptive field (RF) has been seminal in our understanding of visual neural processing (DeAngelis, Ohzawa, & Freeman, 1995; Hubel & Wiesel, 1962; Jones & Palmer, 1987), receptive fields from retinal ganglion cells to primary and secondary visual cortices are not invariant but depend drastically on the context in which they are recorded. For example, stimuli in the surround of the classical receptive field (cRF) of a visual neuron, which would elicit no response when presented alone, can nevertheless strongly modulate the cell's response to stimuli inside the cRF (Alitto & Usrey, 2008; Jones, Grieve, Wang, & Sillito, 2001; Naito, Sadakane, Okamoto, & Sato, 2007; Polat, Mizobe, Pettet, Kasamatsu, & Norcia, 1998; Sillito, Grieve, Jones, Cudeiro, & Davis, 1995; Solomon, Lee, & Sun, 2006; Walker, Ohzawa, & Freeman, 2000; Wielaard & Sajda, 2006). These nonlinear, nonclassical receptive-field (ncRF) properties can drastically change the neuron's behavior, for example, its preferred orientation (Sillito et al., 1995). Moreover, the extent and influence of the cRFs and ncRFs vary as a function of time, luminance, contrast, and light adaptation. For example, receptive fields of retinal ganglion cells and V1 neurons sharpen and their preferred spatial frequency increases for longer stimulus duration and higher contrasts (Bair & Movshon, 2004; Chander & Chichilnisky, 2001; Duong & Freeman, 2007; Sceniak, Ringach, Hawken, & Shapley, 1999). Similarly, dark adaptation can drastically change the size of the receptive fields of ganglion cells (Korth, Ilschner, & Sembritzki, 1987). These observations hint at a coarse-to-fine continuum for the coding properties of visual neurons as more information becomes available: At low contrast, for short presentations or for fast stimuli, visual neurons integrate information from a wider range of channels, decreasing detection threshold at the cost of lower precision. At high contrast, for slower stimuli and for longer stimulus presentations, the central receptive field decreases in size and the inhibitory surround strengthens as neurons achieve higher precision.

We provide a normative theory of these effects based on a model of optimal Bayesian spatiotemporal visual processing. We assume that layers of visual spiking neurons integrate their noisy input in order to detect objects appearing and disappearing in a dynamic visual scene. The predicted receptive fields are not invariant but vary strongly with the context in which they are recorded. In particular, receptive fields vary dynamically as a function of time and contrast, and they can be strongly reshaped as a function of the stimuli shown outside their receptive fields, that is, in the surround. In addition, this simple model accounts for a wide range of visual response properties, such as the statistics and correlation of visual spike trains or the transient nature of visual responses. All these effects are due to the interplay between feedforward integration (cue combination) from input pixels and the lateral competition (explaining away) that modulates the gain of this input.

The performance of this network depends crucially on divisive inhibition among neurons with similar selectivity: Neurons that can successfully predict the sensory input shunt the input to neurons coding for alternative but less probable objects. Thus, this model proposes a new form of inhibitory interaction among sensory neurons based on input-selective divisive inhibition. Divisive inhibition has been widely reported in visual cortices (Carandini, Heeger, & Movshon, 1997; Simoncelli & Heeger, 1998b) but is usually interpreted as a rather nonselective form of gain modulation (Heeger, 1993; Simoncelli & Heeger, 1998a; Webb, Tinsley, Barraclough, Parker, & Derrington, 2003). According to our theory, the role of divisive inhibition is crucial in shaping the selectivity of visual neurons.

## STRUCTURE OF THE MODEL NETWORK

The perceptual interpretation of a sensory scene implies inferring the external events $X$, for example, the objects composing a visual scene like different people and cars appearing and disappearing on a busy crossroads, responsible for the sensory input $S$. A generative model represents a set of assumptions about the underlying causes of this sensory input; that is, it predicts the noisy sensory responses caused by these underlying events, $P(S|X)$.

Next we describe a simple generative model for the input received by a sensory layer. We propose that the role of sensory processing is to compute the posterior probability P(X|S), for example, to infer from the input $S$ which objects $X$ are currently present. In other words, the sensory system inverts the generative model using Bayes' rule: $P(X|S) = \dfrac{P(S|X)P(X)}{\sum_{X'} P(S|X')P(X')}$.

As a first approximation, we consider that "natural" movies are composed of visual objects appearing and disappearing at random times. These objects increase or decrease the instantaneous firing rates (i.e., the probability of emitting a spike) of visual input neurons, called sensory receptors. The task of the visual system is to infer online which objects are currently present in the scene by integrating the noisy input spike trains of these receptors.

The assumptions about the origin of the visual input and their corresponding implementation in a neural structure are represented in Figure 22.1A. This causal model represents assumptions about the likelihood of the sensory input $\mathbf{s}_t$ given the composition $\mathbf{x}_t$ of the visual scene, $P(\mathbf{s}_t|\mathbf{x}_t)$, and the probability of changes in the scene $P(\mathbf{x}_{t+1}|\mathbf{x}_t)$. In the "real" world, objects (circular nodes) appear and disappear randomly (loopy arrows). The probability of appearance and disappearance of an object defines how often it appears and how long it typically stays in the visual scene. These objects in turn cause changes in the firing rates of sensory receptors (triangularly shaped neurons).

The task of "object-detector" neurons (star shaped) is to respond selectively to one object and thus to infer the composition of the visual scene. To do so, object detectors integrate the activity of the sensory receptors and compete among themselves.

The "causal model" (above the dashed line in Fig. 22.1A) describes how events in the outside world predict the visual input. In contrast, the neural network (below the dashed line) represents a biophysical system whose goal is to infer the underlying causes of the sensory input, that is, which objects compose the scene. In other words, the neural structure implements Bayes' rule and computes $P(\mathbf{x}_t|\mathbf{s}_{0\to t})$, where $\mathbf{s}_{0\to t}$ is the activity of receptor units up to time $t$. This neural network is a "mirror image" of the (implicit) causal model: Feedforward connections from receptors to detectors (see Fig. 22.1A) integrate inputs from the causal fields, that is, from the subset of receptor neurons whose activity is influenced by this particular object. This performs optimal cue combination, where each cue is the input received from a receptor. In addition, however, feedforward inputs are modulated by the activity of other detector neurons through lateral "shunting" connections (dotted lateral connections in Fig. 22.1A).

Note that the role of "sensory receptors" and "object detectors" could be played alternatively by different neuron types. Thus, retinal ganglion

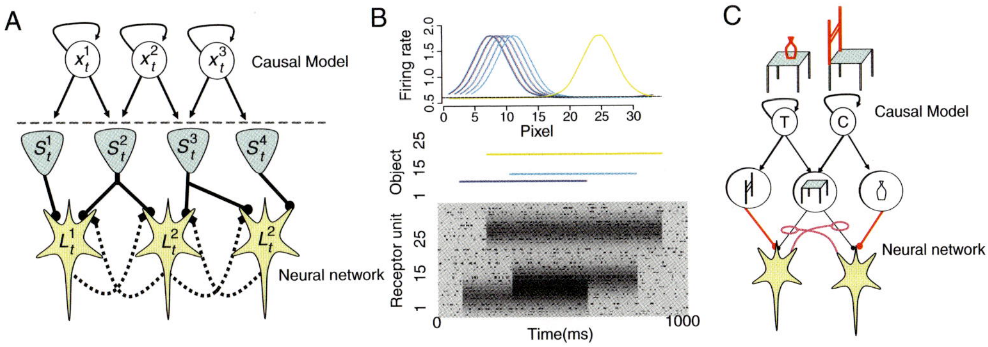


**Figure 22.1** Causal model for dynamic visual processing. (A) Schematic representation of the causal "implicit" model (above the dashed line) and the neural network inferring the composition of the dynamic visual scene (below the dashed line). (B) Causal model used for visual inputs: objects are "blobs" of luminance increase. Top panel: baseline (dashed line) and object-triggered (plain lines) firing rates. Objects are color coded according to their position. Bottom panel: example visual input (activity of visual receptors) caused by presentation of three objects (middle panel). Levels of shading represent the firing rate of the receptor units, while black dots are the input spikes sampled from these rates. (C) Toy model illustrating the need for competition among detector units for their input. See text for details.

cells could correspond to sensory receptors and LGN neurons to object detectors. Alternatively, LGN neurons could play the role of sensory receptors and V1 cells the role of object detectors. This two-layer network describes neural processing in two successive levels in the hierarchical and compositional structure of the visual world: From pixels to elementary features, from elementary features to complex features, from complex features to object. Notably, this model is self-consistent and generalizes to multiple processing stages: Output spikes from the detector neurons can be used in turn as input spikes by the next neural layer (see Mathematical Appendix and Denève, 2008a, 2008b).

To generate predictions for visual responses, we used an idealized generative model for the visual input as described later. This model is compatible with the high level of local spatial correlations in natural images, and, at the same time, it is simple enough to allow straightforward interpretation of the predicted visual responses.

The generative model assumes overlapping Gaussian-shaped "blobs" as causal fields (Fig. 22.1B). A visual object corresponds to a local, spatially correlated increase in luminance, resulting in an increase in receptor-unit firing rates. Receptor units fire spikes according to a Poisson process, resulting in a highly variable response. This variability captures the strong noise observed in the responses of visual neurons and/or the "photon noise" inherent in light stimulation. The shape of the causal fields captures the spatial extent of correlations in natural movies. Moreover, since each object has "slow" temporal dynamics as parameterized by its probability of appearance and disappearance, the model also captures temporal correlations in natural movies. Since objects appear and disappear randomly and independently of other objects, inference based on this generative model results in a decorrelation of the visual inputs in space and time. Redundancy reduction applied to natural images has been shown to account for the center-surround RF structures found in retinal ganglion and LGN cells (Atick & Redlich, 1992; Srinivasan, Laughlin, & Dubs, 1982).

## NEURAL NETWORK DYNAMICS

Detecting visual objects is difficult for three reasons: The presence of *sensory noise* (the trial-to-trial fluctuations in spike trains from receptor neurons), *unpredictable changes* in the visual scene (random appearance and disappearance of objects, as represented by the loopy arrows in Fig. 22.1A), and *ambiguities* (different objects can activate the same set of receptors, as represented by several arrows pointing to the same receptor in Fig. 22.1A). As a result, it will not be possible to decide with absolute confidence the composition of the scene. Instead, detector neurons compute the *probability* that their object is present given the past visual inputs. As shown in the Mathematical Appendix, this can be approximated by the following network dynamics. Object detectors are leaky integrate-and-fire neurons whose membrane potentials evolve as

$$\tau_i \frac{\partial V_i}{dt} = -(V_i - V^o) + I_i(t)$$
$$V_i \geq 0 \rightarrow V_i = -g, \qquad (22.1)$$

where $V^o$ is the rest potential and $\tau_i$ the time constant of integration for the neuron detecting object $i$. Whenever the membrane potential crosses zero, an output spike is fired and the membrane potential is reset to $-g$. The membrane potential of this model neuron can be interpreted as signaling the difference between the evidence accumulated so far for the presence of the object (based on the past inputs from receptors) and the evidence expressed so far by the output spike train (i.e., the past response of the detector). A new output spike represents a "prediction error" that updates the probability of presence of the object compared to what could be predicted from previous output spikes. After a spike, this prediction is removed from the input (hence the reset), resulting in a predictive encoder. As a result, the output spike train tracks efficiently the probability of presence of the object and can easily be read out.

The probability $p_i$ that object $i$ is present at time $t$ can be decoded by integrating the output spike train $O_i(t)$ from detector neuron $i$, as follows:

$$\tau_o \frac{\partial p_i}{dt} = -(p_i - p_o) + g\frac{p_i(1-p_i)}{1+gp_i}O_i(t). \qquad (22.2)$$

All parameters with the exception of the reset potential $g$ are constrained by the parameters of the generative model (see Mathematical Appendix).

The synaptic input is provided by feedforward connections from the sensory receptors, which are gain modulated by the activity of other detector neurons. Thus, the synaptic input to detector neuron $i$ is given by:

$$I_i(t) = \tau_i \sum_j \frac{w_{ij}}{1 + \sum_{k \neq i} w_{kj}\, p_k(t)} s_j(t), \qquad (22.3)$$

where $w_{ij}$ is the weight of the feedforward synaptic connection from receptor neuron $j$ to detector neuron $i$, and $s_j(t)$ describes the input spike train from receptor $j$. The input from receptor neuron $j$ to detector neuron $i$ is thus gain modulated by its prediction from other detector neurons, as provided by the term $\sum_{k \neq i} w_{kj}\, p_k(t)$. This divisive inhibition could be implemented by lateral connections within the layer of detector neurons or feedback modulation of inputs from receptor neurons.

Why input-selective divisive inhibition? Past models performed redundancy reduction either through center-surround "decorrelating" receptive fields (Atick & Redlich, 1992), lateral subtractive inhibition (Srinivasan et al., 1982), or by divisive normalization (Schwartz & Simoncelli, 2001). Our model requires a much more selective form of interaction, since each individual synaptic input can be selectively shunted by the prediction of this synapse's firing rate from other detectors. Why should competition between object detectors take this form?

We provide here an intuitive explanation based on a toy example. Mathematical derivations are provided in the Mathematical Appendix. Consider two neurons selective for similar objects, a "chair" and a "table" (Fig. 22.1C). "Chairs" and "tables" predict the presence of low-level features, some of them specific, many of them shared by the two objects. The corresponding receptors have overlapping "causal fields," and consequently share a large portion of their connections. If these two receptors did not compete, this would often result in a coactivation of the two neurons, such that the "chair" neuron would report a chair if it sees a table, or vice versa.

If one object predicts some of the features present in the scene, these same features should not be taken into account as much by other objects. This effect is called "explaining away." Thus, when the chair neuron is activated, it should prevent the table neuron from responding to the feature that they have in common (e.g., four legs). However, it should not affect features that are specific to tables (e.g., a bottle). Gain modulating the input sent to each object detector by its prediction from other objects allows the output layer to respond appropriately when only a table, only a chair, or both a table and a chair are present, depending on what is required to account for the visual scene. They could not do so if object detectors competed directly and nonselectively (e.g., by subtractive inhibition).

As a result of explaining away, detector units are most strongly activated by features that are most important for discrimination, that is, salient features that are not shared by other objects in the scene (in red). These relevant features will vary with time and the composition of the scene, resulting in a dynamic reshaping of receptive fields as different part of receptive fields are differentially shunted by the context.

In our "blob" model, shared features correspond simply to pixels in the overlap between blobs. Each detector needs to compete with surrounding detectors for these shared inputs.

## NETWORK PERFORMANCE AND DIVISIVE INHIBITION

The network described earlier performs approximate inference. Computing the posterior object probabilities exactly would require computing the probability of all $2^N$ possible combinations of objects, which is clearly intractable. Our proposed neural mechanism computes instead $N$ marginal probabilities, one per object. We found, however, that this approximation performs strikingly well.

In contrast, a purely feedforward network (with no lateral divisive inhibition) cannot efficiently solve ambiguities and thus fails at discriminating between similar objects. In Figure 22.2, we illustrate the importance of divisive inhibition by comparing the network estimates with (Fig. 22.2A) and without (Fig. 22.2B) divisive inhibition.

The failure of the feedforward network is due to the overlap between causal fields for different objects, that is, that several objects can potentially predict the same receptor-neuron activities. This is translated into a strong degree of shared inputs among different detector neurons. If detector neurons sharing most of their inputs did not compete, their output would also be strongly correlated and redundant (Fig. 22.2B, middle panel). Lateral divisive inhibition gain modulates and reassigns the feedforward input among competing detectors. In effect, most feedforward connections that a neuron receives at any time are strongly inhibited by other detectors. The only inputs that have an impact are from "diagnostic" input features (i.e., receptors) that are unambiguous, that is, that support this neuron's preferred object and not other objects in the scene. The process ensures that neurons sharing most of their feedforward connections respond nevertheless selectively to their preferred object (the network estimates in Fig. 22.2A, middle panel, efficiently track the objects truly present in the visual scene, shown in Fig. 22.1B) and respond independently from other neurons in the detector layer.

## PREDICTIONS FOR VISUAL RESPONSES

To illustrate the predicted effects on visual receptive fields, we characterized the response properties of the detectors by studying their responses to visual stimuli.

### Transient Visual Responses

Detector neurons exhibit a transient response to the presentation of a visual stimulus followed by a decay, as illustrated in the bottom panels of Figure 22.2. This apparent temporal adaptation of visual responses is reminiscent of transient and sustained responses reported in ganglion cells (Enroth-Cugell & Robson, 1966; Victor, 1987). However, while transients are often interpreted as the result of local activity-dependent adaptation such as receptor bleaching

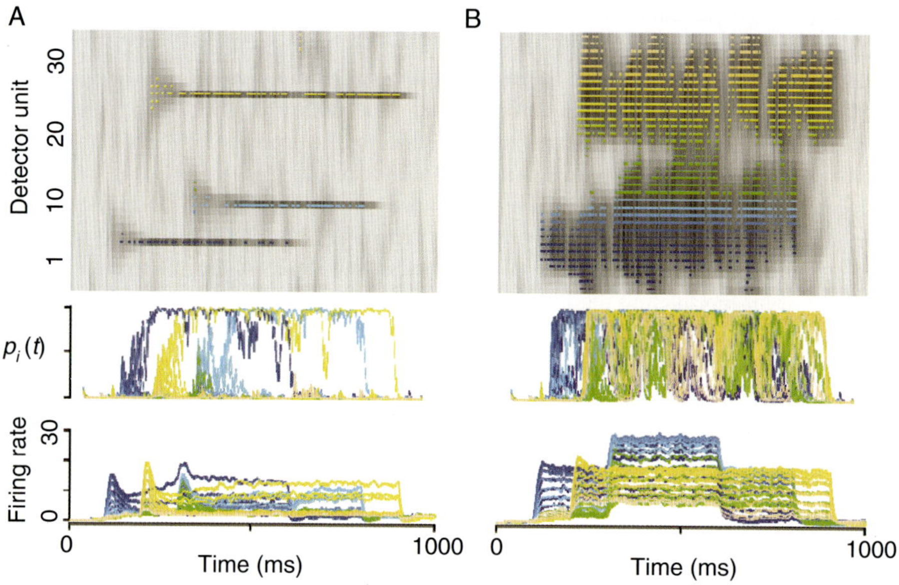


**Figure 22.2** Response of the model network to the input in Figure 22.1B. (A) Response of the intact network with divisive inhibition. (B) Response of the network with divisive inhibition removed. Top panel: Response of the detector neurons as a function of time and the position of their causal field (same color code as in Fig. 22.1B). Levels of gray indicate average firing rate over 1000 repetitions of the same object sequence (as in Fig. 22.1B). Colored dots correspond to output spikes in an example trial. Middle panel: Probability of object presence as a function of time, decoded from the output spike trains in the top panel. Bottom panel: Instantaneous firing rates of the detector units over 1000 repetitions of the same object sequence (as in Fig. 22.1B).

or adaptation, in our case it is a nonlocal network effect entirely due to the dynamic competition among detector neurons.

More precisely, the transient is due to the interplay between a quasi-instantaneous response to feedforward inputs (Eq. 22.1) and a more delayed, slowly building divisive inhibition (Eq. 22.3). The strength and speed of the decay in firing rates varies with the stimulus. Decays are stronger for stimuli in the periphery of the RF. For example, in Figure 22.2A, bottom panel, notice that the poststimulus time histograms of detectors that have a causal field similar to the "optimal" detector (as represented by their similar colors) decay after an initial transient response, while the optimal detector (the one coding for the object that was actually present) keeps a high sustained firing rate. These result in the sparsening of neural responses over time and dynamic changes (sharpening) in the receptive fields described next.

### Variability and Decorrelation of Output Spike Trains

The output spike trains in response to repeated presentations of the same visual stimuli are irregular, asynchronous, and variable from trial to trial (see output spike trains in Fig. 22.2A, top panel). Since detector neurons are deterministic, this variability is entirely due to random fluctuations in the noisy inputs from receptor neurons. The inter-spike-interval (ISI) distributions are close to exponential and the variance of the spike counts scales with the mean (Fig. 22.3A). In a previous study, we showed that this is expected from integrate-and-fire neurons performing Bayesian integration of their noisy synaptic inputs (Denève, 2008a). The variability of output spike trains is a consequence of the noisy input and the integrate-and-fire dynamics of single units.

In addition, divisive inhibition between detector neurons in the network results in

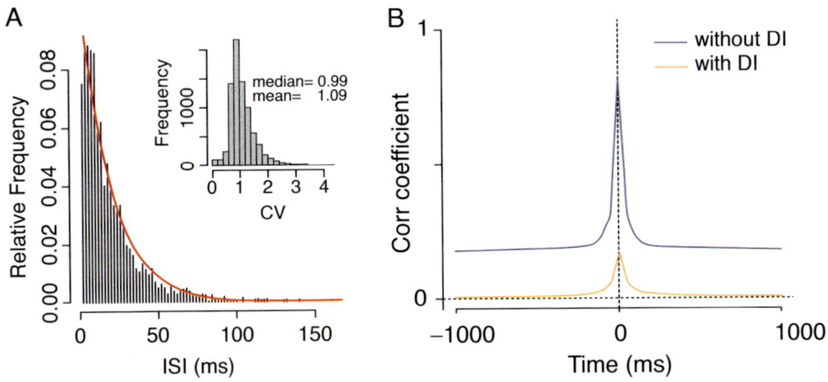


**Figure 22.3** Firing statistics of model visual neurons. (A) Interspike interval distribution in response to repeated presentation of the preferred stimulus. Red line: predicted exponential for a Poisson process. Inset: Distribution of measured coefficient of variation (CV). (B) Cross-correlation between two neighboring detectors when the network is driven by its natural input (i.e., receptor responses generated from the causal model in Fig. 22.1B). These plots represent the probability of observing a spike in unit $k$ conditioned on a spike at time 0 in unit $k + 1$. Orange line: intact network. Blue line: network without divisive inhibition (DI).

a drastic reduction of pairwise correlations between detector neurons due to shared inputs, as illustrated in Figure 22.3B. Indeed, since detector neurons share their input from sensory receptors, the output spikes are highly correlated in the absence of divisive competition (see Fig. 22.2B, middle panels). Input-selective divisive inhibition, however, decorrelates the spiking neural responses. By integrating from multiple input streams but also by competing for their inputs, visual neurons detect the independent events underlying their temporally and spatially correlated sensory inputs. The level of shared inputs is likely to be higher in our schematic model than it is in the visual cortex. However, noise correlations due to shared inputs have a substantial impact on the information transmitted by visual neurons (Bair, Zohary, & Newsome, 2001; Kohn & Smith, 2005; Latham, Denève, & Pouget, 2003; Schneidman, Berry, Segev, & Bialek, 2006; Zohary, Shadlen, & Newsome, 1994).

### Structure of the Receptive Fields (Blob Model)

We mapped the receptive fields of the detector neurons by using methods analogous to those used to map receptive fields experimentally. We manipulated the contrast of the visual stimulus by increasing the firing rate changes of receptor neurons when a pixel is intensified at the corresponding location. Increasing contrast results in a higher signal-to-noise ratio (SNR) in the input. “Dense-noise” mapping of receptive fields was performed by presenting a quick succession of random “pictures” corresponding to randomly intensifying half of the pixels, that is, increasing the firing rate of half of the receptor neurons. The spike-triggered average, that is, the average image present at different delays before each spike, provides a dynamic picture of the neuron’s receptive field (Fig. 22.4A). Another commonly used method maps receptive fields by measuring responses to expanding stimuli, that is, by intensifying all the pixels in a circular patch centered on the receptive field and measuring neural response as a function of patch radius (Fig. 22.4B). The radius at which the response saturates provides an estimate of the size of the central receptive field. We simulated both of these methods, and results are shown in Figures 22.4A and 22.4B.

Receptive fields have a center-surround interaction, as illustrated by the negative lobes on both sides of the central receptive field in Figure 22.4A and the decay of responses to

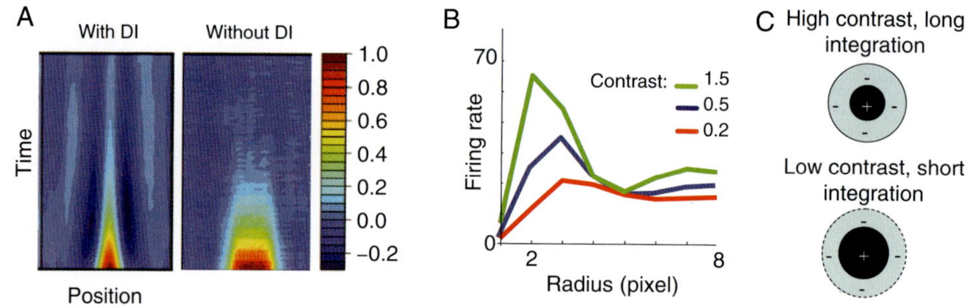


**Figure 22.4** Spatiotemporal dynamics of receptive fields. (A) Spike-triggered average of a model detector neuron as a function of position and time preceding the spike. Left panel: intact network; right panel: network without divisive inhibition. (B) Response of a model detector as a function of the radius of stimulation, starting from the center of its causal field. Optimal stimulus size corresponds to the size of the "receptive field" center. Red: low contrast (C = 0.2); blue: average contrast (C = 0.5); green: high contrast (C = 1.5). (C) Schema representing the changes in receptive-field structure as a function of contrast and integration time.

larger stimuli in Figure 22.4B. This "inhibitory surround" is not implemented by feedforward connections (all excitatory) from the receptor layers. Rather, it is due to divisive lateral competition: Intensifying pixels in the periphery tends to favor competing detector neurons (with overlapping causal fields), resulting in a reduction of the response of the recorded neuron. As in other models (Atick & Redlich, 1992; Srinivasan et al., 1982; Tokutake & Freed, 2008) this "center-surround" interaction reflects the redundancy reduction performed by the detector layer.

We found, however, that the predicted spatial receptive fields are not fixed but depend on contrast and time since stimulus onset. The size of the receptive field center diminishes and the strength of the inhibitory surround increases for longer delays between the stimulus and the response (Fig. 22.4A) and at higher contrast (Fig. 22.4B). These effects are due to input-selective divisive inhibition. Without divisive inhibition the receptive fields would be much larger and their shapes would not vary with contrast and time (Fig. 22.4A, right panel).

Figure 22.4C illustrates the overall effect of input-selective divisive inhibition. The receptive fields switch from performing integration (coarse and mainly excitatory receptive field) to performing discrimination (fine receptive field with inhibitory surround) as more information becomes available (i.e., when contrast is higher or inputs are integrated for a longer period).

### Change in Selectivity Due to Surround Interactions

The consequence of input-selective divisive inhibition goes beyond global changes in the shape of receptive fields. The presence of competition between detector neurons can selectively reshape to which part of its "causal field" a neuron responds. We illustrate this effect once again with a toy example (Fig. 22.5A) before considering what it implies for visual receptive fields (Fig. 22.5B).

Consider the receptive field of a "chair-detector neuron" in two different contexts: in the presence of a table (top panel) or in the presence of a ladder (bottom panel). Both tables and ladders share a different set of features with the chair. In the presence of a table the "chair" neuron should rely on the feature corresponding to the back of the chair, which distinguishes chairs from tables. On the other hand, in the presence of a ladder, the "chair neuron" should respond to the seat of the chair, which distinguishes chairs from ladders. As a consequence, the chair neuron will appear to be selective to different features in the presence of different objects in the surround, even if its

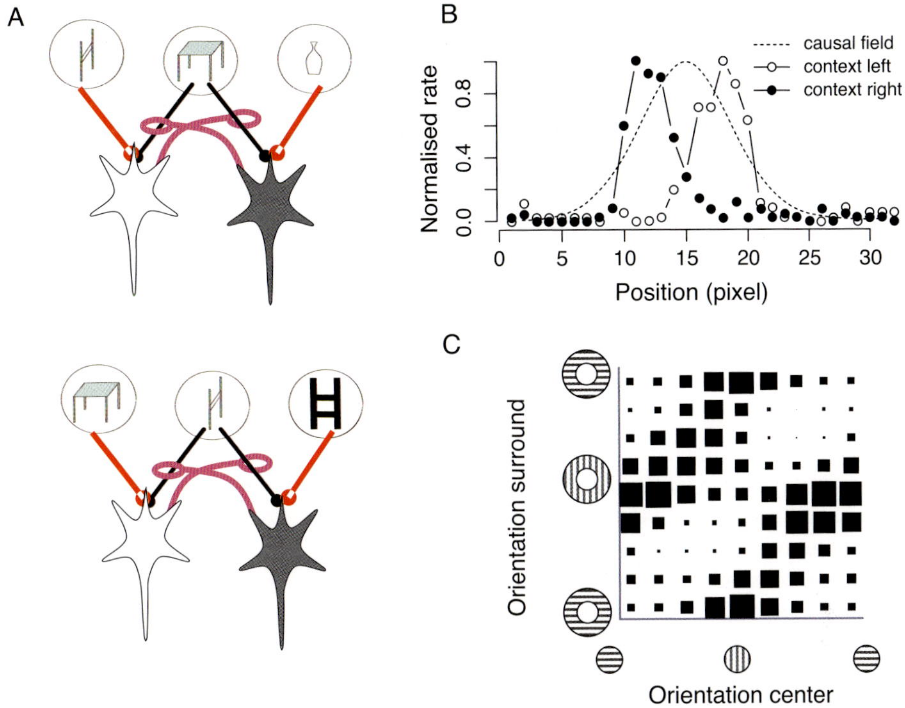


**Figure 22.5** Selective reshaping of the receptive field by context. (A) Toy model illustrating how competing objects in the scene can shape the receptive field of a visual neuron, favoring integration of the most discriminative cues (see text for details). (B) Receptive field (spike-triggered average) of a detector neuron when the right or left neighboring unit's probability is clamped to 1. The receptive field is repelled away from the competing object. (C) Illustration of one of the consequences of selective divisive inhibition. Neurons respond to salient features that are not predicted by the context. This figure plots the response (size of the black square) of a detector unit as a function of the orientation in the central receptive field and the surround (see text for details).

causal field (i.e., the set of features predicted by a chair) is invariant.

In the case of "blob-like" causal fields, the receptive fields will in effect be repelled by competing stimuli. For example, in Figure 22.5B, we plot the receptive field (i.e., the spike-triggered average) of neuron $k$ when the probabilities of the competing detector neurons to the left or right are clamped to 1, that is, we set $p_{k-1} = 1$ or $p_{k+1} = 1$. This could be the case, for example, if a blob of luminance corresponding to the preferred objects of these competitors were shown for a long period of time (adaptation period), and the receptive field of neuron $k$ was mapped immediately afterward. Because probabilities are updated by slow integration of the input, the probability of the competitor is still high in the period immediately following the disappearance of the adapting stimulus. Divisive inhibition prevents nearby detectors from responding to inputs within the causal field of the adapted detector, resulting in a repulsion of the receptive field away from the adapting stimulus. This also biases the interpretation of the sensory input after adaptation, since detectors away from the adapted detector are favored by this competition. Thus, this model explains the repulsive effects of adaptation in both neural tuning and perception, as best documented for orientation and motion direction (Carandini, Movshon, & Ferster, 1998; Dragoi, Sharma, & Sur, 2000; Felsen, Touryan, & Dan, 2005; Schwartz, Hsu, & Dayan, 2007; Wiese & Wenderoth, 2007).

More generally, we predict that visual cells will respond most strongly to the most salient stimuli, that is, stimuli that are not explained by what is shown in the surround. In Figure 22.5C, we illustrate one of the consequences of this competition. Here, we consider a model neuron (e.g., a complex V1 cell) selective both for the position and orientation of a visual stimulus. When stimuli of different orientations are shown in the periphery of the (spatial) receptive field, tuning to the center orientation shifts away from the surround orientation. The response is maximally suppressed when the surround is co-oriented with the center. This dependency of surround suppression on what is shown in the center has been reported in V1 (Cavanaugh, Bair, & Movshon, 2002; Sillito et al., 1995).

According to our model, divisive gain modulation, transient visual responses, the coarse-to-fine changes in receptive fields as a function of time and contrast, stimulus adaptation, and saliency effects might all have the same origin: the competition between visual detectors for their input. This in turn is necessary to resolve ambiguities between similar visual objects, and to set the tradeoff between integration (for detecting noisy stimuli) and discrimination (for differentiating between similar objects).

## CONCLUSION

We have proposed a normative neural model of visual processing under the assumption that visual spiking neurons optimally detect the presence of independent objects in dynamic visual scenes. Rather than by their receptive fields, these neurons are better described by their causal field, that is, by what they predict for the sensory input. As a result, visual layers can discover the set of objects that probably explains the input from the previous layer, solving two problems at once: integrating the sensory input optimally to detect visual objects efficiently, that is, performing optimal combination of visual cues, and resolving ambiguities between similar objects, that is, performing explaining away. This model provides a fresh view of sensory processing at the level of spiking neurons and small circuits as a form of redundancy reduction in time and space.

Despite the fact that it is derived from principles of Bayesian inference, the predicted responses of model visual neurons share many characteristics with those observed in biological neurons in the retina, LGN, and visual cortex. These units can be described as integrate-and-fire neurons with balanced excitatory and inhibitory inputs (Shadlen & Newsome, 1994). They generate asynchronous, weakly correlated, Poisson-like output spike trains (Vogels, Spileers, & Orban, 1989). They respond to the presentation of visual stimuli with a strongly transient response. Their response properties are shaped by lateral divisive inhibition (Carandini et al., 1997). Their receptive fields have center-surround structure (Bradley & Andersen, 1998; Bullier & Norton, 1979; Hartline, 1938). They respond best to the most salient stimuli, that is, stimuli not predicted by their surround (Nothdurft, Gallant, & Van Essen, 1999). And their response properties can be reshaped by surround stimuli and by stimuli presented previously. In most cases, contextual stimuli create a repulsion effect: The preferred stimulus (e.g., the preferred orientation) shifts away from surround stimuli or stimuli presented previously.

These contextual effects depend on the capacity to discriminate between similar objects. If the SNR in the input is low, either because the stimulus is brief, noisy, or at low contrast, these fine distinctions cannot be made. To use the available information optimally, detector neurons should integrate inputs from a larger set of features for a longer time after stimulus presentation, resulting in larger receptive fields with weak or no inhibitory surround. Peripheral parts of the receptive field can switch from being excitatory at low SNR to being suppressive at high SNR, and surround and adaptive stimuli can switch from being repulsive to being attractive. This coarse-to-fine gradient is automatically implemented by the divisive, selective inhibition predicted by Bayesian inference, without changing the parameters of the model. This explains a large number of contextual effects in early visual processing, such as changes of the receptive field with contrast (Sceniak et al., 1999; Sceniak, Hawken, & Shapley, 2002), time (Malone, Kumar, & Ringach, 2007; Ringach, Hawken, & Shapley, 1997; Shapley, Hawken, & Ringach, 2003), surround stimuli (Alitto & Usrey, 2008; Jones et al., 2001; Naito et al., 2007; Polat et al., 1998; Sillito et al., 1995; Solomon et al., 2006; Walker et al., 2000; Wielaard & Sajda, 2006), and previous stimuli as in adaptation to orientation or direction of motion (Dragoi et al., 2000; Felsen et al., 2005; Schwartz et al., 2007; Wiese & Wenderoth, 2007). Our model proposes both a functional role and a possible mechanism to account for these phenomena.

This model contrasts with previous approaches that aimed at describing visual responses with simplified models of linear processing followed by nonlinear transfer functions (Heeger, Simoncelli, & Movshon, 1996; Pillow, Paninski, Uzzell, Simoncelli, & Chichilnisky, 2005) or using the known anatomy of thalamico-cortical, lateral, and feedback cortico-cortical connections (Schwabe, Obermayer, Angelucci, & Bressloff, 2006). Interestingly, however, these models also incorporated divisive inhibition and a fine balance between excitation and inhibition.

Our approach is closely related to "information-maximization" approaches such as redundancy reduction (Srinivasan et al., 1982), independent-component analysis (Bell & Sejnowski, 1997), sparse coding (Olshausen & Field, 1996), or slow feature analysis (Wiskott & Sejnowski, 2002). It also aims at finding independent causes for the visual input. Our approach differs from these previous models by incorporating both spatial and temporal statistics and by assuming that the visual system is mainly interested in the *composition* of the visual scene. Rather than *estimating* the coefficients of a linear superposition of features, our model neurons report the *probability* of presence of each object. As a result, a visual layer does not necessarily commit to a single interpretation of the dynamic visual scene. Unresolved ambiguities can be transmitted to the next layer and resolved later in the hierarchy of visual processing.

Furthermore, while we proposed a specific implementation with spiking neurons, contextual effects are predicted by generic inference principles. They do not depend on the neural code for probability, or whether individual objects are represented by single neurons or populations. A similar statement can be made for the model implementation in cortical circuits. Thus, we labeled the connections from the receptors to the detectors as "feedforward" and the divisive inhibition as "lateral." However, the anatomical implementation of such a system might be more intricate. For example, in primary visual cortex, pooling from the causal field could be implemented not only by feedforward connections from LGN to V1 but also by lateral connections within V1 and feedback connections from V2, yielding significant spatial summation at low contrast. Similarly, input-selective divisive inhibition is more likely the result of processing in cortical columns and/or inhibitory feedback from the detector to the receptor layer than direct lateral inhibition exerted on each synapse.

Another prediction of the model that has not been explored here is that dynamic properties of neurons and synaptic strengths should be matched to the spatial and temporal statistics of the visual input. For example, the time constant of synaptic integration and resting potential should be matched to the temporal statistics of the stimulus, with slower stimuli corresponding to a longer time constant. We have previously derived learning rules for these parameters based on a slow integration of synaptic inputs (Denève, 2008b; Mongillo & Denève, 2008).

## MATHEMATICAL APPENDIX

### Mathematical Derivation

The presence or absence of visual objects in the scene at time $t$ is formalized by a set of binary variables $x_j^t$, equal to 1 when object $j$ is present and zero otherwise. These objects appear and disappear randomly, appearing with rate $r_{on}^j$ (e.g., $r_{on}^j = 0.1$ means that on average the object appears once every 10 seconds) and disappearing with rate $r_{off}^j$. We suppose that the effect of objects combine linearly at the receptor layer, that is, the instantaneous firing rate of receptor

$i$ is defined as $q_i + \sum_j dq_j^i x_j^t$, where $dq_j^i$ is the increase in firing rate of pixel $i$ predicted by the presence of unit $j$ and $q_i$ is the background firing rate.

We have shown previously that in the absence of overlap between the causal fields, that is, when no competition is required between objects, the log ratio $L_j(t) = \log\left(\frac{p(x_j^t = 1|s_{0\to t})}{p(x_j^t = 0|s_{0\to t})}\right)$ for object $j$ can be computed dynamically as follows:

$$\frac{\partial L_j}{dt} = r_{on}^j(1+\exp(-L_j)) - r_{off}^j(1+\exp(L_j)) + \sum_j w_{ij}s_j^t - \theta_j, \qquad (22.4)$$

where $\theta_j$ is a constant and the synaptic weights are given by $w_{ij} = \log\left(\frac{q_i + dq_j^i}{q_i}\right)$ (Denève, 2008a).

This equation describes synaptic integration. We derived a firing mechanism that insured that the model is self-consistent and output spikes represent the probability of presence of the object accurately. This is done by comparing each $L_j(t)$ with "threshold" variables $G_j(t)$. This threshold computes the probability of the object given the output spike train, that is, $G_j(t) = \log\left(\frac{p(x_j^t = 1|O_{o\to t})}{p(x_j^t = 0|O_{o\to t})}\right)$ where $O_{o\to t}$ corresponds to the *output* spike train up to time $t$. If the integrated input $L_j(t)$, representing what is known about the object given past inputs, exceeds the integrated output $G_j(t)$, representing the information conveyed by the output spikes, a new spike is fired. As a result, the output spike train tracks the probability of the presence of the stimulus and can be decoded using Eq. 22.2, where $p_j(t) = \frac{\exp(G_j(t))}{1+\exp(G_j(t))}$. The output weight $w_o$ and the baseline probability $p_o$ are learned in an unsupervised way from the output spike train (Denève, 2008b; Mongillo & Denève, 2008).

We have shown (Denève, 2008b) that the dynamics of this neuron can be approximated by linearizing the equations, resulting in integrate-and-fire neurons with membrane potentials $V_j(t) = L_j(t) - G_j(t)$. In its simplest expression, this leads to Eq. 22.1 with $\tau_j = r_{on}^j + r_{off}^j$ and the input given by $I_j(t) = \sum_i w_{ij} S_j^t$.

This, however, does not take into account possible ambiguities in the input, that is, the fact that the same changes in firing rates can be explained by other objects. To solve this, we use a "mean-field approximation" of the impact of neighboring objects on the firing rate of receptor neuron $i$; that is, we add to the baseline firing rate $q_i$ and the "object-triggered firing rate" $q_i + dq_j^i$ the firing rate predicted by other objects in the scene, $\sum_{k\neq j} dq_k^i p_k(t)$. As a result, the input to the model neuron becomes:

$$I_i(t) = \sum_j \log\left(\frac{q_i + dq_j^i + \sum_{k\neq j} dq_k^i p_k(t)}{q_i + \sum_{k\neq j} dq_k^i p_k(t)}\right) s_j^t. \qquad (22.5)$$

If, in addition, $q_i \gg dq_j^i$, we can simplify this expression to Eq. 22.3.

## Parameters Used in Simulations

In all simulations, we used a circularly symmetric "retina," where the position of each pixel is defined by circular variable $\theta_i$. We used 30 input pixels, corresponding to 33 receptor neurons, spaced by $\frac{2\pi}{32}$. We used 35 detector neurons, also on a circularly symmetric grid at positions spaced by $\frac{2\pi}{35}$.

The causal fields were defined as follows. The baseline firing rate was $q_i = 10$ Hz, and the stimulus-triggered increases in firing rate were overlapping circular Gaussians, $dq_j^i = 5\exp(3(\cos(\theta_i - \theta_j) - 2))$ Hz. For all neurons we used transition rates $r_{on} = 0.1$ Hz and $r_{off} = 2$ Hz.

To generate visual stimuli, we intensified "pixels" by increasing the firing rates of the corresponding receptors from $q_i$ to $q_i(1 + C)$, where C is the contrast. The inputs spike trains $s_j^t$ were obtained by randomly sampling spikes from the corresponding firing rates. In the figure, "low contrast" corresponds to C = 0.2 and "high contrast" to C = 2. To map receptive fields with dense noise, we randomly intensified half of the pixels every 30 ms. Spike-triggered averages were obtained by averaging this binary image at various delays before a spike.

To map the receptive fields with expanding stimuli, we increased the firing rate of the central pixel (radius 1) for 500 ms and measured the firing rate in response to 1000 presentations of this stimulus. For stimuli of radius 2, we increased the firing rate of the central pixel and the pixel on either side. For radius 3, we intensified the central pixel and two pixels on either side, and so on.

Finally, for Figure 22.5C, we used a 2D circularly symmetric "retina," one axis representing orientation and the other spatial position. Intensifying one pixel in this model corresponds to a specific orientation shown at a specific location, for 500 ms. Causal fields were 2D circular Gaussians $dq_j^i = 5\exp(3(\cos(\theta_j^{ori} - \theta_i^{ori}) + \cos(\theta_j^{pos} - \theta_i^{pos}) - 2)$ Hz. The central receptive field (along the position axis) is mapped by using expanding stimuli at high contrast ($C = 2$) at the preferred orientation. We present an orientation in the center by intensifying pixels in this central receptive field at the corresponding orientation. We present an orientation in the surround by intensifying pixels for all other positions at the corresponding orientation.

## REFERENCES


Alitto, H. J., & Usrey, W. M. (2008). Origin and dynamics of extraclassical suppression in the lateral geniculate nucleus of the macaque monkey. *Neuron, 57*, 135–146.

Atick, J. J., & Redlich, A. N. (1992). What does the retina know about natural scenes? *Neural Computation, 4*, 196–210.

Bair, W., & Movshon, J. A. (2004). Adaptive temporal integration of motion in direction-selective neurons in macaque visual cortex. *Journal of Neuroscience, 24*, 7305–7323.

Bair, W., Zohary, E., & Newsome, W. T. (2001). Correlated firing in macaque visual area MT: Time scales and relationship to behavior. *Journal of Neuroscience, 21*, 1676–1697.

Bell, A. J., & Sejnowski, T. J. (1997). The "independent components" of natural scenes are edge filters. *Vision Research, 37*, 3327–3338.

Bradley, D. C., & Andersen, R. A. (1998). Center-surround antagonism based on disparity in primate area MT. *Journal of Neuroscience, 18*, 7552–7565.

Bullier, J., & Norton, T. T. (1979). Comparison of receptive-field properties of X and Y ganglion cells with X and Y lateral geniculate cells in the cat. *Journal of Neurophysiology, 42*, 274–291.

Carandini, M., Heeger, D. J., & Movshon, J. A. (1997). Linearity and normalization in simple cells of the macaque primary visual cortex. *Journal of Neuroscience, 17*, 8621–8644.

Carandini, M., Movshon, J. A., & Ferster, D. (1998). Pattern adaptation and cross-orientation interactions in the primary visual cortex. *Neuropharmacology, 37*, 501–511.

Cavanaugh, J. R., Bair, W., & Movshon, J. A. (2002). Selectivity and spatial distribution of signals from the receptive field surround in macaque V1 neurons. *Journal of Neurophysiology, 88*, 2547–2556.

Chander, D., & Chichilnisky, E. J. (2001). Adaptation to temporal contrast in primate and salamander retina. *Journal of Neuroscience, 21*, 9904–9916.

DeAngelis, G. C., Ohzawa, I., & Freeman, R. D. (1995). Receptive-field dynamics in the central visual pathways. *Trends in Neurosciences, 18*, 451–458.

Denève, S. (2008a). Bayesian spiking neurons I: Inference. *Neural Computation, 20*, 91–117.

Denève, S. (2008b). Bayesian spiking neurons II: Learning. *Neural Computation, 20*, 118–145.

Dragoi, V., Sharma, J., & Sur, M. (2000). Adaptation-induced plasticity of orientation tuning in adult visual cortex. *Neuron, 28*, 287–298.

Duong, T., & Freeman, R. D. (2007). Spatial frequency-specific contrast adaptation originates in the primary visual cortex. *Journal of Neurophysiology, 98*, 187–195.

Enroth-Cugell, C., & Robson, J. G. (1966). The contrast sensitivity of retinal ganglion cells of the cat. *Journal of Physiology, 187*, 517–552.

Ernst, M. O., & Banks, M. S. (2002). Humans integrate visual and haptic information in a statistically optimal fashion. *Nature, 415*, 429–433.

Felsen, G., Touryan, J., & Dan, Y. (2005). Contextual modulation of orientation tuning contributes to efficient processing of natural stimuli. *Network, 16*, 139–149.

Gold, J. I., & Shadlen, M. N. (2002). Banburismus and the brain: Decoding the relationship between sensory stimuli, decisions, and reward. *Neuron, 36,* 299–308.

Hartline, H. K. (1938). The response of single optic nerve fibers of the vertebrate eye to illumination of the retina. *American Journal of Physiology, 121,* 400–415.

Heeger, D. J. (1993). Modeling simple-cell direction selectivity with normalized, half-squared, linear operators. *Journal of Neurophysiology, 70,* 1885–1898.

Heeger, D. J., Simoncelli, E. P., & Movshon, J. A. (1996). Computational models of cortical visual processing. *Proceedings of the National Academy of Sciences USA, 93,* 623–627.

Hubel, D. H., & Wiesel, T. N. (1962). Receptive fields, binocular interaction and functional architecture in the cat's visual cortex. *Journal of Physiology, 160,* 106–154.

Jones, H. E., Grieve, K. L., Wang, W., & Sillito, A. M. (2001). Surround suppression in primate V1. *Journal of Neurophysiology, 86,* 2011–2028.

Jones, J. P., & Palmer, L. A. (1987). The two-dimensional spatial structure of simple receptive fields in cat striate cortex. *Journal of Neurophysiology, 58,* 1187–1211.

Knill, D. C., & Pouget, A. (2004). The Bayesian brain: The role of uncertainty in neural coding and computation. *Trends in Neuroscience, 27*(12), 712–719.

Knill, D. C., & Richards, W. (Eds.). (1996). *Perception as Bayesian inference.* Cambridge, MA: Cambridge University Press.

Kohn, A., & Smith, M. A. (2005). Stimulus dependence of neuronal correlation in primary visual cortex of the macaque. *The Journal of Neuroscience, 25,* 3661–3673.

Körding, K. P. (2007). Decision theory: What "should" the nervous system do? *Science, 318,* 606–610.

Körding, K. P., & Wolpert, D. M. (2004). Bayesian integration in sensorimotor learning. *Nature, 427,* 244–247.

Korth, M., Ilschner, S., & Sembritzki, O. (1987). Retinal receptive fields under different adaptation levels studied with pattern-evoked ERG. *Graefes Archive for Clinical and Experimental Ophthalmology, 225,* 63–69.

Latham, P. E., Denève, S., & Pouget, A. (2003). Optimal computation with attractor networks. *Journal of Physiology Paris, 97,* 683–694.

Malone, B. J., Kumar, V. R., & Ringach, D. L. (2007). Dynamics of receptive field size in primary visual cortex. *Journal of Neurophysiology, 97,* 407–414.

Mongillo, G., & Denève, S. (2008). Online learning with hidden markov models. *Neural Computation, 20,* 1706–1716.

Naito, T., Sadakane, O., Okamoto, M., & Sato, H. (2007). Orientation tuning of surround suppression in lateral geniculate nucleus and primary visual cortex of cat. *Neuroscience, 149,* 962–975.

Nothdurft, H. C., Gallant, J. L., & Van Essen, D. C. (1999). Response modulation by texture surround in primate area V1: Correlates of "popout" under anesthesia. *Visual Neuroscience, 16,* 15–34.

Olshausen, B. A., & Field, D. J. (1996). Emergence of simple-cell receptive field properties by learning a sparse code for natural images. *Nature, 381,* 607–609.

Pillow, J. W., Paninski, L., Uzzell, V. J., Simoncelli, E. P., & Chichilnisky, E. J. (2005). Prediction and decoding of retinal ganglion cell responses with a probabilistic spiking model. *Journal of Neuroscience, 25,* 11003–11013.

Polat, U., Mizobe, K., Pettet, M. W., Kasamatsu, T., & Norcia, A. M. (1998). Collinear stimuli regulate visual responses depending on cell's contrast threshold. *Nature, 391,* 580–584.

Ringach, D. L., Hawken, M. J., & Shapley, R. (1997). Dynamics of orientation tuning in macaque primary visual cortex. *Nature, 387,* 281–284.

Sceniak, M. P., Hawken, M. J., & Shapley, R. (2002). Contrast-dependent changes in spatial frequency tuning of macaque V1 neurons: Effects of a changing receptive field size. *Journal of Neurophysiology, 88,* 1363–1373.

Sceniak, M. P., Ringach, D. L., Hawken, M. J., & Shapley, R. (1999). Contrast's effect on spatial summation by macaque V1 neurons. *Nature Neuroscience, 2,* 733–739.

Schneidman, E., Berry, M. J., Segev, R., & Bialek, W. (2006). Weak pairwise correlations imply strongly correlated network states in a neural population. *Nature, 440,* 1007–1012.

Schwabe, L., Obermayer, K., Angelucci, A., & Bressloff, P. C. (2006). The role of feedback in shaping the extra-classical receptive field of cortical neurons: A recurrent network model. *Journal of Neuroscience, 26,* 9117–9129.

Schwartz, O., Hsu, A., & Dayan, P. (2007). Space and time in visual context. *Nature Reviews Neuroscience, 8*, 522–535.

Schwartz, O., & Simoncelli, E. P. (2001). Natural signal statistics and sensory gain control. *Nature Neuroscience, 4*, 819–825.

Shadlen, M. N., & Newsome, W. T. (1994). Noise, neural codes and cortical organization. *Current Opinion in Neurobiology, 4*, 569–579.

Shapley, R., Hawken, M. J., & Ringach, D. L. (2003). Dynamics of orientation selectivity in the primary visual cortex and the importance of cortical inhibition. *Neuron, 38*, 689–699.

Sillito, A. M., Grieve, K. L., Jones, H. E., Cudeiro, J., & Davis, J. (1995). Visual cortical mechanisms detecting focal orientation discontinuities. *Nature, 378*, 492–496.

Simoncelli, E. P., & Heeger, D. J. (1998a). A model of neuronal responses in visual area MT. *Vision Research, 38*, 743–761.

Simoncelli, E. P., & Heeger, D. J. (1998b). A model of neuronal responses in visual area MT. *Vision Research, 38*, 743–761.

Solomon, S. G., Lee, B. B., & Sun, H. (2006). Suppressive surrounds and contrast gain in magnocellular-pathway retinal ganglion cells of macaque. *Journal of Neuroscience, 26*, 8715–8726.

Srinivasan, M. V., Laughlin, S. B., & Dubs, A. (1982). Predictive coding: A fresh view of inhibition in the retina. *Proceedings of the Royal Society of London B: Biological Sciences, 216*, 427–459.

Tokutake, Y., & Freed, M. A. (2008). Retinal ganglion cells—spatial organization of the receptive field reduces temporal redundancy. *European Journal of Neuroscience, 28*, 914–923.

Trommershäuser, J., Maloney, L. T., & Landy, M. S. (2008). Decision making, movement planning and statistical decision theory. *Trends in Cognitive Sciences, 12*, 291–297.

Victor, J. D. (1987). The dynamics of the cat retinal X cell centre. *Journal of Physiology, 386*, 219–246.

Vogels, R., Spileers, W., & Orban, G. A. (1989). The response variability of striate cortical neurons in the behaving monkey. *Experimental Brain Research, 77*, 432–436.

Walker, G. A., Ohzawa, I., & Freeman, R. D. (2000). Suppression outside the classical cortical receptive field. *Visual Neuroscience, 17*, 369–379.

Webb, B. S., Tinsley, C. J., Barraclough, N. E., Parker, A., & Derrington, A. M. (2003). Gain control from beyond the classical receptive field in primate primary visual cortex. *Visual Neuroscience, 20*, 221–230.

Wielaard, J., & Sajda, P. (2006). Extraclassical receptive field phenomena and short-range connectivity in V1. *Cerebral Cortex, 16*, 1531–1545.

Wiese, M., & Wenderoth, P. (2007). The different mechanisms of the motion direction illusion and aftereffect. *Vision Research, 47*, 1963–1967.

Wiskott, L., & Sejnowski, T. J. (2002). Slow feature analysis: Unsupervised learning of invariances. *Neural Computation, 14*, 715–770.

Yuille, A. L., & Bülthoff, H. H. (1996). Bayesian decision theory and psychophysics. In D. C. Knill & W. Richards (Eds.), *Perception as Bayesian inference* (pp. 123–161). New York, NY: Cambridge University Press.

Zohary, E., Shadlen, M. N., Newsome, W. T. (1994). Correlated neuronal discharge rate and its implication for psychophysical performance. *Nature, 370*, 140–143.

# INDEX

Note: The page numbers followed by "*f*" and "*t*" refer to figures and tables, respectively.